DATE DUE

JAN 26 1996			
FEB 16 1996			
AUG 0 7 1997			

Demco, Inc. 38-293

R.J.G. Rycroft T. Menné P. J. Frosch (Eds.)

Textbook
of Contact Dermatitis

Second, Revised and Enlarged Edition

With 210 Illustrations, 95 in Colour, and 122 Tables

Springer-Verlag

Berlin Heidelberg New York
London Paris Tokyo
Hong Kong Barcelona
Budapest

Dr. Richard J.G. Rycroft
St. John's Institute of Dermatology,
St. Thomas's Hospital,
London SE1 7EH, UK

Prof. Dr. med. Torkil Menné
Department of Dermatology,
Gentofte Hospital,
University of Copenhagen,
Niels Andersens Vej 65,
2900 Hellerup, Denmark

Prof. Dr. med. Peter J. Frosch
Hautklinik der Städtischen Kliniken
Dortmund, Abteilung Dermatologie,
Universität Witten/Herdecke,
Beurhausstraße 40,
44123 Dortmund, Germany

2nd Edition
ISBN 3-540-57943-5 Springer-Verlag Berlin Heidelberg New York
ISBN 0-387-57943-5 Springer-Verlag New York Berlin Heidelberg

1st edition
ISBN 3-540-54562-X Springer-Verlag Berlin Heidelberg New York
ISBN 0-387-54562-X Springer-Verlag New York Berlin Heidelberg

Library of Congress Cataloging-in-Publication Data. Textbook of contact dermatitis/R.J.G. Rycroft, T. Menné, P.J. Frosch. – 2nd. rev. and enlarged ed. p. cm. Includes bibliographical references and index. ISBN 3-540-57943-5. – ISBN 0-387-57943-5 1. Contact dermatitis. I. Rycroft, R.J.G. (Richard J.G.) II. Menné, Torkil. III. Frosch, Peter J. RL244.T49 1995 616.5'1-dc20 94–34409

Typesetting: Macmillan India Ltd., Bangalore-25
SPIN: 10132859   23/3130/SPS – 5 4 3 2 1 0 – Printed on acid-free paper

We honour the memory of Claude Benezra,
our coeditor for the first edition of this textbook,
who was killed in a tragic accident in January 1992.

Foreword to the Second Edition

The growth of contact dermatitis as a subspecialty of dermatology has been impressive in the past couple of decades. Each new textbook that is published reflects the considerable increase in information coming from many parts of the world. An important advance was made 3 years ago with the appearance of this new comprehensive textbook, brought to fruition from the contributions of nearly all the workers active in this field throughout Europe.

In the Foreword to the previous edition, Dr. Etain Cronin described the greatest pitfalls of patch testing as the lack of knowledge in selecting the correct allergen and the difficulty encountered in interpreting the results. It is works such as this that bring together the knowledge of the past, in such a way that the reader/investigator can have readily available the information necessary to study the patients, patch test them, and interpret the results with accuracy and precision. Millions of patients worldwide experience contact dermatitis each year; not nearly enough of them are studied in detail to determine the precise cause of their affliction. In almost no other branch of medicine is it possible to pinpoint a specific, often removable, cause of a recurring, disabling disease. With the assistance of the information that is so prolifically available in this text, physicians will be able to bring help to many of these patients.

The 22 chapters of this volume cover every aspect of contact dermatitis, even including the addresses of physicians worldwide who work in this field. This work brings together dermatologists from many different countries and is an excellent example of what can be accomplished by the cooperation of those from a variety of nationalities and languages; truly a "European union" of contact dermatology!

The editors, including the late Dr. Claude Benezra, worked with devotion and care in the creation of this fine book. Dr. Rycroft, especially, deserves congratulations for bringing everyone together and organizing this textbook, which will surely remain a model of its kind for many years.

ROBERT M. ADAMS, M.D.
Department of Dermatology
Stanford University Medical Center
Stanford, CA 94035, USA

Foreword to the First Edition

Ideally every patient with eczema should be patch tested and the importance of this investigation is now universally accepted. The simplicity of the technique belies its many pitfalls, the greatest being to lack the knowledge required to select the correct allergens and to interpret the results. The introduction, nearly 20 years ago, of the journal *Contact Dermatitis* greatly stimulated the reporting of the clinical side of contact dermatitis but a vast amount of laboratory work has also been published in other journals on the mechanisms and theory of these reactions. The literature on the subject is now quite vast and a comprehensive book on the clinical and research aspects of contact dermatitis has been sorely needed. This textbook was carefully planned to gather together what is known of the subject into a cohesive whole and it has succeeded admirably. It consists of 22 chapters written by 41 contributors, each selected for their special study of particular subjects. Every feature of contact dermatitis has been covered, beginning with its history and even concluding with the names and addresses of those worldwide who have a specific interest in the subject. The text is illustrated and well laid out; it has been broken up into clearly demarcated sections making it easy to read and its information readily accessible. One's own writing concentrates the mind but editing the texts of authors from so many different countries was a task of considerable proportions. The editors are greatly to be congratulated, particularly Dr Rycroft who has worked tirelessly to mould this multi-authored book into an integrated whole. This Textbook of Contact Dermatitis is an impressive achievement; it will instruct and help all who read it and stimulate many to take a greater interest in this fascinating subject.

ETAIN CRONIN
St. John's Institute of Dermatology
St. Thomas's Hospital
London SE1 7EH, UK

Contents

5 Individual Predisposition to Contact Dermatitis
(TORKIL MENNÉ and JOHN D. WILKINSON)

6 Epidemiology
(PIETER-JAN COENRAADS and JET SMIT)

7 Clinical Features
(NIELS K. VEIEN)

8 Hand Eczema
(ETAIN CRONIN)

9   Noneczematous Contact Reactions
(CHEE LEOK GOH)

10   Diagnostic Tests

10.1   Patch Testing
(JAN E. WAHLBERG)

12   Contact Dermatitis in Children
(CARLO LUIGI MENEGHINI)

13   Allergens from the Standard Series
(KLAUS E. ANDERSEN, DESMOND BURROWS
and IAN R. WHITE)

14   Allergens Related to Specific Exposures

14.1   Cosmetics and Skin Care Products
(ANTON C. DE GROOT and IAN R. WHITE)

14.2   Topical Drugs
(GIANNI ANGELINI)

14.3   Clothing
(JEAN FOUSSEREAU)

17 Principles of Prevention and Protection in Contact Dermatitis
(JEAN-MARIE LACHAPELLE)

18 Predictive Assays: Animal and Man, and In Vitro and In Vivo
(ESTHER PATRICK and HOWARD I. MAIBACH)

19 International Legal Aspects of Contact Dermatitis
(PETER J. FROSCH and RICHARD J. G. RYCROFT)

List of Contributors

KLAUS E. ANDERSEN
  Algade 33, 4000 Roskilde, Denmark
  Dermatology Department I, Odense Hospital, 5000 Odense C,
  Denmark

GIANNI ANGELINI
  2nd Department of Dermatology, University of Bari, 70100 Bari, Italy

DONYA BAGHERI
  CCS Associates, 1285 Hamilton Drive, Palo Alto, Ca, USA

CLAUDE BENEZRA[†]
  Laboratoire de Dermatochimie, Université Louis Pasteur, Clinique
  Dermatologique, 1 Place de l'Hôpital, 67091 Strasbourg Cedex, France

BERT BJÖRKNER
  Department of Occupational Dermatology, General Hospital,
  214 01 Malmö, Sweden

B. MARY E. VON BLOMBERG
  Department of Pathology, Free University Hospital,
  de Boelelaan 1117, 1081 HV Amsterdam, The Netherlands

DESMOND BURROWS
  Dermatology Department, Royal Victoria Hospital, Grosvenor Road,
  Belfast BT12 6BA, UK

JOSÉ G. CAMARASA
  Department of Dermatology, Hospital de N. S. del Mar,
  Paseo Maritimo S/n, 08003 Barcelona, Spain

PIETER-JAN COENRAADS
  Occupational and Environmental Dermatology Unit, State University,
  Academic Hospital, P.O. Box 30001, 9700 RB Groningen,
  The Netherlands

ETAIN CRONIN
   Contact Dermatitis Clinic, St. John's Dermatology Centre,
   St. Thomas's Hospital, London SE1 7EH, UK

M. DOOMS
   Contact Dermatitis Unit, University Hospital, Kapucijnenvoer 33,
   3000 Leuven, Belgium

AN DOOMS-GOOSSENS
   Contact Dermatitis Unit, University Hospital, Kapucijnenvoer 33,
   3000 Leuven, Belgium

J. DRIEGHE
   Contact Dermatitis Unit, University Hospital, Kapucijnenvoer 33,
   3000 Leuven, Belgium

GEORGES DUCOMBS
   Clinique Dermatologique, Hôpital Saint André, Université de
   Bordeaux, Rue Jean Burguet 1, 33075 Bordeaux, France

JEAN FOUSSEREAU
   Clinique Dermatologique, Université Louis-Pasteur,
   1 Place de l'Hôpital, 67091 Strasbourg Cedex, France

ROSSANA FRAGINALS[†]
   Laboratoire de Dermatochimie, Université Louis Pasteur,
   Clinique Dermatologique, 1 Place de l'Hôpital,
   67091 Strasbourg Cedex, France

PETER J. FROSCH
   Hautklinik, Städtische Kliniken Dortmund,
   Beurhausstraße 40, 44123 Dortmund, Germany

CHEE LEOK GOH
   Contact and Occupational Dermatoses Clinic, National Skin Centre,
   1 Mandalay Road, Singapore 1130, Republic of Singapore

ANTON C. DE GROOT
   Department of Dermatology, Carolus Hospital, P.O. Box 1101,
   5200 BD's-Hertogenbosch, The Netherlands

MATTI HANNUKSELA
   Department of Dermatology, University of Oulu, Kajaanintie 50,
   90220 Oulu, Finland

JEAN-MARIE LACHAPELLE
  Unit of Occupational and Environmental Dermatology,
  Catholic University of Louvain, 30 Clos Chapelle-aux-Champs,
  UCL 3033, 1200 Brussels, Belgium

ARTO LAHTI
  Department of Dermatology, University of Oulu, 90220 Oulu, Finland

JEAN-PIERRE LEPOITTEVIN
  Laboratoire de Dermatochimie, Université Louis Pasteur, Clinique
  Dermatologique, 1 Place de l'Hôpital, 67091 Strasbourg Cedex, France

HOWARD I. MAIBACH
  Department of Dermatology, University of California, School of
  Medicine, Box 0989, Surge 110, San Francisco, CA 94143-0989, USA

CLIFFORD MCMILLAN
  Dermatology Department, City Hospital, Belfast, UK

CARLO LUIGI MENEGHINI
  Department of Dermatology, Post-Graduate Medical School,
  University of Bari, Via Abate Gimma 99, 70100 Bari, Italy

TORKIL MENNÉ
  Department of Dermatology, Gentofte Hospital, University of
  Copenhagen, Niels Andersens Vej 65, 2900 Hellerup, Denmark

HIDEO NAKAYAMA
  Department of Dermatology, Saiseikai Central Hospital, 1-4-17 Mita,
  Minato-ku, Tokyo 108, Japan

ESTHER PATRICK
  Department of Dermatology, University of California, School of
  Medicine, San Francisco, CA 94143-0989, USA

PATRICIA PODMORE
  Department of Dermatology, Altnagelvin Hospital, Waterside,
  Londonderry BT47 1SB, UK

RICHARD J.G. RYCROFT
  Contact Dermatitis Clinic, St. John's Institute of Dermatology,
  St. Thomas's Hospital, London SE1 7EH, UK

RIK J. SCHEPER
Department of Pathology, Free University Hospital, de Boelelaan 1117, 1081 HV Amsterdam, The Netherlands

RICHARD J. SCHMIDT
Welsh School of Pharmacy, UWCC, PO Box 13, Cardiff CF1 3XF, UK

HANS J. SCHUBERT
Klinik und Poliklinik für Hautkrankheiten der Medizinischen Akademie, Postfach 434, Erfurt, Germany

JØRGEN SERUP
Department of Dermatology, Bispebjerg Hospital, University of Copenhagen, Copenhagen, Denmark

CAROLINE C. SIGMAN
CCS Associates, 1285 Hamilton Drive, Palo Alto, Ca, USA

JET SMIT
TNO-Institute of Preventive Health Care, Leiden, The Netherlands

NIELS K. VEIEN
Dermatology Clinic, Vesterbro 99, 9000 Aalborg, Denmark

JAN E. WAHLBERG
Karolinska Sjukhuset, Box 60500, 104 01 Stockholm, Sweden

LEON M. WALL
Sir Charles Gairdner Hospital, 5th Floor, G Block, Nedlands, Western Australia 6009, Australia

IAN R. WHITE
Contact Dermatitis Clinic, St. John's Institute of Dermatology, St. Thomas's Hospital, London SE1 7EH, UK

JOHN D. WILKINSON
Department of Dermatology, Amersham General Hospital, Amersham, Bucks, HP7 0JD, UK

Chapter 1
Historical Aspects

Historical Aspects

JEAN-MARIE LACHAPELLE

Contents

1.1 Introduction

Contact dermatitis, an inflammatory skin reaction to direct contact with noxious agents in our environment, was most probably recognized as an entity even in ancient times, since it must have accompanied mankind throughout its history. Early recorded reports include Pliny the Younger, who in the first century AD noticed that some individuals experienced severe itching when cutting pine trees (quoted in [1]). A review of the ancient literature could provide dozens of similar, mostly anecdotal examples and some are cited in modern textbooks, monographs and papers [2–4].

It is interesting to note that the presence of idiosyncrasy was suspected in some cases of contact dermatitis reported in the 19th century, many decades before the discovery of allergy by von Pirquet. For instance, in 1829, Dakin [5], describing *Rhus* dermatitis, observed that some people suffered from the disease, whereas others did not. He therefore posed the question: 'Can it be possible that some peculiar structure of the cuticule or rete mucosum constitutes the idiosyncrasy?'

The modern history of contact dermatitis cannot be separated from the history of patch testing, which is the only tool that we have to unmask the causative chemical culprits. In the rest of this introductory chapter, I will therefore review briefly the history of this important technique.

1.2 Historical Aspects of Patch Testing

Historical aspects of patch testing have been reviewed by Foussereau [6] and Lachapelle [7]. A selection of important steps forward has been made for this short survey.

1.2.1 The Pre-Jadassohn Period

During the 17th, 18th and 19th centuries [6], some researchers occasionally reproduced contact dermatitis by applying the responsible agent (chemical, plant, etc.) to intact skin. Most of the observations are anecdotal, but some deserve special attention.

In 1847, Städeler [8] described a method devised to reproduce on human skin the lesions provoked by *Anacardium occidentale* (Städeler's blotting paper strip technique), which can be summarized as follows: 'Balsam is applied to the lower part of the thorax on an area measuring about 1 cm². Then a piece of blotting paper previously dipped in the balsam is applied to the same site. 15 min later, the subject experiences a burning sensation which increases very rapidly and culminates about half an hour after. The skin under the blotting paper turns whitish and is surrounded by a red halo. As the burning sensation decreases, the blotting paper is kept in place for 3 h'. This observation is important because it was the first time that any test was actually designed and described in full detail [6].

Another description of a patch test technique was given by the French entomologist Jean Henri Fabre (1823–1915), who lived in Sérignan-du-Comtat, a village in Provence. This work was contemporaneous with Jadassohn's experiments, but it is described here because it was not designed primarily for dermatological diagnosis [9]. Fabre reported in 1897 (in the 6th volume of the impressive encyclopedia *Souvenirs entomologiques,* translated into more than 20 languages) that he had studied the effect of processionary caterpillars on his own skin. A square of blotting paper, a novel kind of plaster, was covered by a rubber sheet and held in place with a bandage. The paper used was a piece of blotting paper folded four times, so as to form a square with one-inch sides, which had previously been dipped into an extract of caterpillar hair. The impregnated paper was applied to the volar aspect of the forearm. The next day, 24 h later, the plaster was removed. A red mark, slightly swollen and very clearly outlined, occupied the square which had been covered by the 'poisoned' paper.

In these and further experiments, he dissected various anatomical parts of the insects in order to isolate noxious ones that provoked burning or itching. Rostenberg and Solomon [10] have emphasized the importance to dermatology of Fabre's methodology, so often used in the past decades by dermato-allergologists. For instance, many similar attempts have been made during the 20th century to isolate noxious agents (contact allergens and irritants), not only from different parts of plants, woods and animals, but also from various other naturally occurring substances and industrial products encountered in our modern environment.

1.2.2 Josef Jadassohn, the Father of Patch Testing in Dermatology

Among the various scientists who undoubtedly used patch testing to repeat experimentally their clinical observations, one name is traditionally quoted as the true pioneer in the field: Josef Jadassohn [11] (Fig. 1).

By applying chemicals (on pieces of blotting paper) to the skin, Jadassohn [12, 13] was able to reproduce the clinical picture of contact dermatitis from iodoform or mercury salts in patients suffering from skin intolerance to those substances. He suspected the specific significance of such tests ('specific intolerance') at a time when the term 'allergy' had not yet been created and defined. As pointed out by Foussereau [6], Jadassohn most probably applied and expanded – in a practical way – observations and interpretations previously made by Neisser in 1884 [14]. The tests were performed at the University of Breslau, a city that – in those days – was part of Germany (now Wroclaw in Poland). The room where Jadassohn most probably carried out his first patch tests has not been altered since his time, but its function has changed since it has now been transformed into a tiny museum devoted to dermatology. A survey of Jadassohn's life and work has been made by Sulzberger [15, 16].

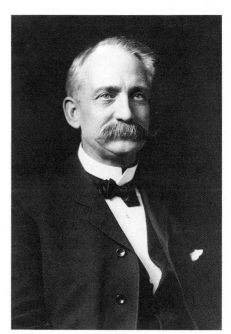

Fig. 1. Josef Jadassohn (1863–1936) (with the kind permission of the Institut für Geschichte der Medizin der Universität Wien)

Summing up the different sources of information available, we can reasonably conclude that Jadassohn first presented the results of the patch test technique at the meeting of Graz (Austria) in 1895; these results were published in 1896 [12]. Therefore, 1995 will be celebrated as the centenary of patch testing.

1.2.3 Other Important Steps Forward

It is difficult, in retrospect, to assess the importance of the patch test technique to the diagnosis of contact dermatitis between 1895 and the 1960s. Some points are neverthless clear:
- The technique was used extensively in some European clinics, and ignored in others.
- No consensus existed concerning the material, the concentration of each allergen, the time of reading, the reading score, etc.
- Differential diagnosis between irritant and allergic contact dermatitis was very often unclear.

It is no exaggeration to say that patch testers were acting like skilled craftsmen [17]; though – step by step – they provided new information on contact dermatitis.

When covering this transitional period, we should recall the names of some outstanding dermatologists who directly contributed to our present knowledge and to the dissemination of the patch test technique throughout the world. Bruno Bloch is very often quoted as one of the pioneers in the field, continuing and expanding Jadassohn's clinical and experimental work [18]. Marion Sulzberger, who spent a long time at Jadassohn's clinic, introduced the patch test technique to the United States; he is considered to be the father of contact dermatology in that country [19]. At the same time, in Paris, Tzanck and Sidi [20] were also very active in diagnosing and treating patients suffering from contact dermatitis. Surprisingly enough, they worked in a 'vacuum', surrounded by the general (almost proverbial) indifference of most French dermatologists of that time.

We may consider that patch testing first blossomed in the Scandinavian countries in the late 1930s. In 1938, a list of the most common allergens used routinely in the patch test clinic was proposed by Poul Bonneve and published in his justly famous textbook of environmental dermatology [21]. This list (Table 1) can be considered as the prototype of the standard series of patch tests. It was built on the experience gained at the Finsen Institute in Copenhagen regarding the occurrence of positive reactions to various chemicals among patch-tested patients. It is remarkable that the list was used in Copenhagen without any change from 1938 until 1955, which allowed Marcussen to publish in 1962 [22] a most impressive epidemiological survey concerning time fluctuations in the relative occurrence of contact allergies. Seven of the 21 allergens listed by Bonnevie are still present in the standard series of patch tests used currently.

Table 1. The standard series of patch tests proposed by Poul Bonnevie (1939) [21]

Allergen	Concentration (%)	Vehicle
Turpentine	50	Olive oil
Colophony	10	Olive oil
Balsam of Peru	25	Lanolin
Salicylic acid	5	Lanolin
Formaldehyde	4	Water
Mercuric chloride	0.1	Water
Potassium dichromate	0.5	Water
Silver nitrate	2	Water
Nickel sulphate	5	Water
Resorcinol	5	Water
Primula obconica	as is	
Sodium perborate	10	Water
Brown soap	as is	
Coal tar	pure	
Wood tars	pure	
Quinine chlorhydrate	1	Water
Iodine	0.5	Ethanol
Pyrogallol	5	Petrolatum
Phenylenediamine	2	Petrolatum
Aminophenol	2	Petrolatum
Adhesive plaster	as is	

The idea of developing a standard series of allergens was also developed extensively by Bruno Bloch in Zurich [23]. The substances with which standard tests were made were the following: formaldehyde (1%–5%), mercury (1% sublimate or ointment of white precipitate of mercury), turpentine, napthalene (1%), tincture of arnica, primula (piece of the leaf), adhesive plaster, iodoform (powder), and quinine hydrochloride (1%).

1.2.4 The Founding of Groups

A Scandinavian Committee for Standardization of Routine Patch Testing was formed in 1962. In 1967 this committee was enlarged, resulting in the formation of the International Contact Dermatitis Research Group (ICDRG). The founder members of the ICDRG were H.J. Bandmann, C.D. Calnan, E. Cronin, S. Fregert, N. Hjorth, B. Magnusson, H.I. Maibach, K.E. Malten, C. Meneghini, V. Pirilä and D.S. Wilkinson. The major task for its members was to standardize at an international level the patch testing procedure, for example the vehicles used for allergens, the concentration of each allergen, and so on.

Niels Hjorth (1919–1990) in Copenhagen was the vigorous chairman of the ICDRG for more than 20 years. He organized the first international symposium on contact dermatitis at Gentofte, Denmark, in October 1974; this symposium was followed by many others, which led to an increasing interest in contact dermatitis throughout the world and, consequently, to the establishment of numerous national contact dermatitis groups (see Chap. 21). Hjorth's contribution to promoting our knowledge of contact dermatitis was enormous; it is true to say that he ushered in a new era of environmental dermatology. All contributors to this textbook are greatly indebted to him: he showed us the way forward.

1.3 References

1. Castagne D (1976) Dermatoses professionnelles provoquées par les bois tropicaux. Thesis, Bordeaux
2. Avenberg KM (1980) Footnotes on allergy. Pharmacia, Uppsala
3. Mitchell J, Rook AJ (1979) Botanical dermatology. Greengrass, Vancouver
4. Rostenberg A (1955) An anecdotal biographical history of poison ivy. Arch Dermatol 72: 438–445
5. Dakin R (1829) Remarks on a cutaneous affection produced by certain poisonous vegetables. Am J Med Sci 4: 98–100
6. Foussereau J (1984) History of epicutaneous testing: the blotting-paper and other methods. Contact Dermatitis, 11: 219–223
7. Lachapelle JM (1986) Le test épicutané: aperçu historique. Servinfo. Gist-Brocades, Brussels
8. Städeler J (1847) Über die eigenthümlichen Bestandtheile der Anacardium Früchte. Ann Chemie Pharmacie 63: 117–165
9. Fabre JH (1897) Souvenirs entomologiques, vol 6. Delagrave, Paris, pp 378–401
10. Rostenberg A, Solomon LM (1968) Jean Henri Fabre and the patch-test. Arch Dermatol 98: 188–190
11. Lachapelle JM (1989) Contact Dermatitis 1988: historical reflections and current problems in patch testing. In: Frosch PJ, Dooms-Goossens A, Lachapelle JM, Rycroft RJ, Scheper RJ (eds) Current topics in contact dermatitis Springer, Berlin Heidelberg New York, pp 50–56
12. Jadassohn J (1896) Zur Kenntnis der Arzneiexantheme. Arch Dermatol Forsch 34: 103
13. Jadassohn J (1896) Zur Kenntnis der medicamentösen Dermatosen. Verhandlungen der Deutschen Dermatologischen Gesellschaft, V Congress, Wien (1895). Braumüller, Vienna, pp 103–129
14. Neisser A (1884) Ueber Jodoform-Exantheme. Dtsch Med Wochenschr 30: 467
15. Sulzberger MD (1936) Josef Jadassohn (1863–1936). Arch Dermatol 33: 1063
16. Sulzberger MD (1986) In: Skin and allergy news. From there to here. My many lives. Institute for Dermatologic Communication and Education
17. Sézary A (1936) Méthodes d'exploration biologique de la peau. Les tests cutanés en dermatologie. Encycl Méd Chir 12010: 1–8
18. Bloch B (1911) Experimentelle Studien über das Wesen der Jodoformidiosynkrasie. Exp Pathol Ther 9: 509–538
19. Sulzberger MB (1940) Dermatologic allergy. Thomas, Baltimore
20. Tzanck A, Sidi E (1952) Dermites allergiques. Statistiques des dermatoses allergiques étudiées au laboratoire des tests de l'Hôpital Saint-Louis durant les années 1949, 1950 et 1951. Sem Hôp Paris 81: 3267–3269
21. Bonnevie P (1939) Aetiologie und Pathogenese der Ekzemkrankheiten. Klinische Studien über die Ursachen der Ekzeme unter besonderer Berücksichtigung des Diagnostischen Wertes der Ekzemproben. Busch, Copenhagen and Barth, Leipzig
22. Marcussen PV (1962) Variations in the incidence of contact hypersensitivities. Trans St Johns Hosp Dermatol Soc 48: 40–48
23. Bloch B (1929) The rôle of idiosyncrasy and allergy in dermatology. Arch Dermatol Syphilis 19: 175–197

Chapter 2
Basic Features

2.1 Cellular Mechanisms in Allergic Contact Dermatitis

RIK J. SCHEPER and B. MARY E. VON BLOMBERG

Contents

2.1.1 Delayed Hypersensitivity and Allergic Contact Dermatitis

2.1.1.1 Cell-Mediated Immunity

In the last two decades, our understanding of the basic mechanisms underlying induction, expression and regulation of allergic contact dermatitis (ACD) has rapidly increased. Highlights in this period include the discovery of T-cell lymphoid tissue domains related to cell-mediated immunity, the discovery of the thymus as the cradle for these T lymphocytes, and how such T cells may bear specificity to just one or few allergens out of the vast number of allergens known. Progress has also resulted from the development of reagents (monoclonal antibodies) that allow better identification of various inflammatory cells and the bioindustrial production of large amounts of peptide-mediators like interferon-γ and interleukin-2 (IL-2), which allow in-depth analysis of skin inflammatory processes such as those taking place in ACD.

Although, in ACD, humoral antibody-mediated reactions can be a factor, ACD depends primarily on the activation of specifically sensitized T cells [1, 2]. Evolutionarily, cell-mediated immunity has fully developed in vertebrates, for their benefit, by facilitating effective eradication of microorganisms and toxins. Elicitation of ACD by nontoxic doses of small molecular allergens indicates that the T-cell repertoire is often slightly broader than one might wish. ACD thus represents an untoward side effect of a well-functioning immune system.

Subtle differences can be noted in macroscopic appearance, time course and histopathology of allergic contact reactions in various vertebrates, including rodents and man. Nevertheless, essentially all basic features are shared. As both mouse and guinea pig models have strongly contributed to our present knowledge of ACD, in this chapter data from animal studies have been taken together with results obtained from studies on T-cell-mediated reactions in man. ACD can be regarded as a prototype of delayed hypersensitivity, as classified by Turk [3] and Gell and Coombs (type IV hypersensitivity [4]).

2.1.1.2 Development of Allergic Contact Dermatitis

It is convenient to distinguish between afferent and efferent limbs in the development of ACD [3, 5, 6] (Fig. 2.1.1). The afferent limb includes the events following a first contact with the allergen and is complete when the individual is sensitized and capable of giving a positive elicitation reaction. The efferent limb is activated during the elicitation (challenge) phase. The entire process of the afferent limb requires from at least 3 days to several weeks, whereas full development of the elicitation phase only requires 1–2 days. The main afferent (1–4) and efferent (5) events are:

1. *Binding of allergen to skin components.* Allergen penetrating the skin readily associates with class II molecules. These molecules, coded in humans by HLA-D-region genes, are abundantly present in the epidermis on dendritic cells, the Langerhans cells (LCs). This association may be due to a covalent bond, as in the case of poison oak/ivy allergens, or to a coordination bond, as with nickel cations. Allergen-carrying LCs travel via the afferent lymphatics to the regional lymph nodes, where they settle in the T-cell (paracortical) areas.

2. *Recognition of allergen-modified LCs by specific T cells.* In the paracortical areas, conditions are optimal for allergen-carrying LCs to encounter T cells that specifically recognize the allergen – class II molecule complexes. Notably, in nonsensitized individuals the frequency of T cells with corresponding specificities is far below 1 per 1000. The dendritic

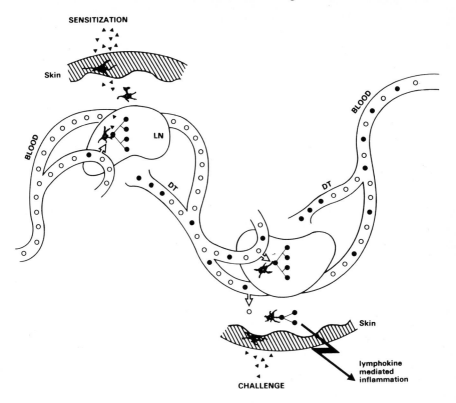

Fig. 2.1.1. Pathogenesis of allergic contact dermatitis: sensitization (*top left*) and challenge (*bottom right*). Allergen-bearing Langerhans cells (✶) travel to the draining lymph nodes (*LN*), where they present the allergen (▲) to specific T lymphocytes (●; T lymphocytes with irrelevant specificities, ○). Their progeny reaches the blood through the thoracic duct (*DT*). Subsequent challenge of the skin with allergen results in a local lymphokine-mediated inflammation and further increases the frequency of allergen-specific cells in the circulation

morphology of the LC strongly facilitates multiple cell contacts, ultimately leading to binding and activation of sufficient numbers of allergen-specific T cells.

3. *Proliferation of specific T cells in draining lymph nodes.* Supported by interleukin-1, (IL-1), a mediator released by the allergen-presenting cells, activated T cells start producing several other mediators called lymphokines, including IL-2. A partly autocrine cascade follows in which the density of IL-2 receptors on activated T cells increases transiently, leading to full reception of the IL-2 signal, and resulting in vigorous blast formation and proliferation within a few days.

4. *Propagation (dissemination) of specific T-cell progeny over the body.* The expanded progeny (effector cells) is subsequently released into the circulation and may enter the peripheral tissues including the skin.

5. *Efferent action.* The efferent limb of the cellular immune response is based on the increased frequency of T cells with a given specificity throughout the body of a sensitized individual, as well as on the enhanced capacity of effector cells to enter peripheral tissues. At sites of primary allergenic skin contact, too few specific T cells are available locally to allow for macroscopically detectable skin reactivity. When a sensitized individual is challenged, a local inflammatory reaction follows. Allergen-presenting cells and specific T cells meet locally, leading to cytokine production within the skin. The release of these mediators, many of which have a proinflammatory action, causes the arrival of more T cells, thus further amplifying local mediator release. This leads to a gradually developing eczematous reaction which reaches a maximum after 18–48 h. Cytokines that play a major role in the development of ACD are those with stimulatory effects on other lymphocytes (MIP-1β, IL-2, interferon-γ), on mononuclear phagocytes (chemotactic factor, migration inhibition factor, interferon-γ), and on mast cells and vasculature (skin reactive factor, interferon-γ).

2.1.1.3 Allergen-Presenting Cells

2.1.1.3.1 Langerhans Cells

In healthy skin, the epidermal dendritic Langerhans cell (LC), bearing high numbers of class II molecules on its cell membrane, is the primary allergen-presenting cell (APC). LCs stem from the bone marrow, but their continuous presence in the epidermis is at least partly maintained by local LC proliferation [7–9]. In mice the sensitization rate was found to be determined by the density of LCs at the site of allergen application. Moreover, absence or functional inactivation of LCs, e.g. by UV treatment, was associated with tolerance induction [10, 11] (see Sect. 2.1.2).

Fortunately, in several ways the risk of full-blown skin inflammation at the first encounter with an allergen has been kept low. This is important in view of the extreme amplification power of the lymphokine cascade, as illustrated by experimental studies in which measurably oedema could be triggered by only one specific T cell [12]. Besides rigid activation requirements and limited entry of naive (unprimed) T cells into the skin (see Sect. 2.1.4.), the necessity for LCs to mature further before full presenting power is obtained also appears important [13–15]. Such maturation may occur when LCs travel from the skin and settle within the paracortical areas of the lymph nodes, or farther away within the periarteriolar lymph sheaths in the spleen. So-called dendritic cells isolated from these organs display rapid and efficient allergen-presentation towards naive T cells. Similar stimulatory capacity with LCs freshly isolated from skin blister roofs was observed only after 1–2 days of preculturing. Notably, even without delay, LCs are excellent in stimulating primed memory T cells with contact allergens [2, 6, 15–17].

2.1.1.3.2 Allergen Presentation

Most contact allergens are small chemically reactive molecules. Upon penetration through the epidermis they readily bind to LC surface-exposed MHC class II molecules, besides binding to a plethora of other skin constituents. The ability to associate with MHC class II molecules, or with peptides present in the grooves of these molecules, is a prerequisite for contact sensitization. Whereas most allergens bind spontaneously, some need enzyme- or photo-induced activation before they bind. MHC class II modification may also result from allergen binding to nearby cell-surface molecules or even free proteins. Allergen-binding proteins, however, require degradation by allergen-presenting cells, or nearby macrophages, to small fragments, before being presented at the cell membrane. Close association with class II molecules, essential for T-cell triggering, is facilitated by peptide-binding sites present on class II molecules [18, 19].

It should be recalled that effective presentation of contact allergens to T lymphocytes depends not just simply on MHC class II molecule expression by LCs, but also on their capacity to create and maintain close cell contacts with T lymphocytes (clustering). To this end, the intricate structure of paracortical areas in the lymph nodes and the characteristic membrane ruffling of LCs and dendritic cells provide optimal conditions for T-cell triggering. Intimate cellular contacts are further facilitated by sets of specialized interaction molecules. All together, these sets of interaction molecules resemble a delicate zipper which has to be drawn together for turning on T cells.

2.1.1.4 Lymphocytes

2.1.1.4.1 Naive and Effector/Memory T Cells

The nature of the cells that mediate contact sensitivity has intrigued dermatologists and immunologists for decades. The earliest relevant information was obtained in experimental studies by transferring immune cells to naive recipients. In both guinea pigs and mice, contact hypersensitivity could be transferred with thymus-derived T, and not with B, lymphocytes [5]. Then monoclonals became available, discriminating between primarily lymphokine-producing ($CD4^+$, 'helper') and cytotoxic ($CD8^+$, 'cytotoxic/suppressor') T lymphocytes. Although cytotoxic T cells can mediate distinct skin damage in ACD, the helper subset is held to be primarily responsible for mediating delayed hypersensitivity and ACD [2, 6, 20, 21].

Within the helper T-cell population different subsets can now be distinguished. The ability to mount delayed-type hypersensitivity reactions resides in the 'Th1' subset, able to produce IL-2, IFN_γ and $TNF\beta$ [22, 23]. The 'Th2' subset produces IL-4, IL-5 and IL-10, and may account for both the persistent production of antibodies (notably IgE) and eosinophilia observed in helminthic infections and immediate type I hypersensitivity reactions. Both subsets produce IL-3, $TNF\alpha$, and granulocyte-macrophage colony-stimulating

Table 2.1.1. Some characteristics of CD4$^+$ naive and effector/memory T cells

	Naive Relative expression	Effector/memory of surface molecules
CD2 (LFA-3 receptor)[a]	+	++
CD3 (TCR-assoc. mol: T3)	+	+
CD11a (LFA-1)	+	++
CD29 (VLA β-chain)	+	++
CD45RA (LCA)	+++	+
CD45RO (truncated LCA)	+	++++
CD58 (LFA-3)	+	+++
	Relative functional capacity	
Interleukin-2 production	+++ (late)	+++ (early)
Interferon-γ production	+	+++
Allergen-driven proliferation in vitro	+	+++
Mitogen-driven proliferation in vitro	++++	++

[a] Cluster designation (CD) number (recognized membrane component) [30, 31, 79]

factor (GM-CSF). Th2 cytokines such as IL-4 shift T-cell differentiation away from the production of Th1 cytokines, whereas the Th1 cytokine IFN$_\gamma$ is very potent in preventing the development of Th2 cells [24–26]. Bacteria, viruses and most contact allergens may preferentially induce Th1 responses through stimulation of interleukin-12 (IL-12) production by macrophages or other cells. IL-12 stimulates IFN$_\gamma$ production by T cells. Allergenic contacts and infections along the mucosal surfaces rather induce the differentiation of Th2 cells [24, 27, 28]. Here, IL-4 production by cells of the mast cell/basophil lineages, in the absence of local IFN$_\gamma$ release, determines T-cell differentiation. Development of antigen-specific Th2 cells along mucosal surfaces bears the advantage that responsiveness focuses on rapid antibody (IgE/IgA) mediated effector mechanisms, preventing microorganisms from entering the body, in the absence of potentially damaging tissue inflammatory reactions. In line with these recent insights, nickel-specific CD4$^+$ effector T cell clones were found to exhibit the Th1 cytokine profile, whereas human atopical allergen-specific CD4$^+$ T cell clones released typical Th2 cytokines [29]. Thus, CD4$^+$ Th1 type T effector cells may be considered as central in causing allergic contact dermatitis.

Recently, a qualitative distinction between (difficult to stimulate, afferently acting) naive and (easy to stimulate, efferently acting) effector/memory cells was also confirmed. A high molecular weight isoform of the leucocyte common antigen (CD45RA) characterizes naive T cells, whereas only a truncated form of the molecule is expressed on effector/memory T cells (CD45RO) (Table 2.1.1). Importantly, T cells with the naive phenotype show excellent proliferative capacity and good (albeit slow-onset) IL-2 production. On the other hand, effector/memory (T cells not only show additional interferon-γ production, but also full-scale IL-2 production as early as 24 h after simulation [30, 31]. These results strongly suggest that the major effector cells in ACD belong to the latter subset. These cells indeed dominate in the skin [31]. In contrast to naive cells, which really need LCs/dendritic cells for allergen-presentation, effector/memory lymphocytes can also be stimulated by other cell types presenting allergen-modified class II-molecules, e.g. monocytes, endothelial cells and B cells [32–34]. Clearly, effector/memory cells display higher numbers of 'cellular adhesion modecules' (CAMs), allowing for more promiscuous cellular interactions.

2.1.1.4.2 Cellular Adhesion Molecules

Presentation of allergen by MHC class II molecules alone does not provide sufficient binding strength. Additional sets of CAMs facilitate the strongest binding and full activation of T cells (Fig. 2.1.2). Four of these sets deserve mention here. First, the CD4 ('helper') molecule bears affinity to a constant region of the class II molecule, providing additional binding stability in T cell/APC interactions. Secondly, LFA-1 (leukocyte function associated antigen, a 180/95-kDa two-chain cell surface molecule) is abundantly present on T cells, and one of its counter-structures (ICAM-1) is present on LC. For CD2 (a T-cell antigen formerly used for its binding to sheep red blood cells) the counter-structure is a 25- to 29-kDa molecule (LFA-3), anchored in the plasma membrane of most nucleated cells. CD2/LFA-3 interaction may provide an activational signal synergizing with the T cell-receptor/class II allergen mediated signal [35, 36]. Also CD28-B7 receptor-ligand binding provides costimulatory signals. CD28 is expressed at high levels on all

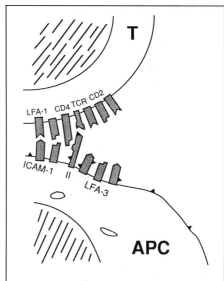

Fig. 2.1.2. The cellular adhesion molecule zipper connecting an allergen-presenting cell (*APC*) and a specific CD4+ T cell (▲, allergen). The T-cell receptor (*TCR*) recognizes a modified MHC class II molecule, thereby allowing receptor-associated CD3 chains (not depicted) to transduce a signal for cellular activation. Additional binding and signals result from CD4/class II, CD2/LFA-3 and LFA-1/ICAM-1 interactions

Th cells, and B7 on dendritic cells and, after activation, on B cells and monocytes [37].

Importantly, triggering of sensitized (effector/memory) T cells in ACD is facilitated by enhanced expression of various CAMs. Moreover, expression of the counterstructures on several (epi)dermal cells is upregulated by T-cell lymphokines, notably interferon-γ. This further promotes development of ACD, as eventually T cells may also be triggered by allergen bound to various skin cells [38–41].

On the other hand, priming of T cells may lead to the loss of L-selectin and other CAMs which facilitate interactions with high endothelial venules in peripheral lymph nodes [42, 43]. Apparently, after sensitization T cells are less capable of recirculating through the lymphoid organs, but gain in ability to migrate into the peripheral tissues, including the skin. Indeed, interactions with endothelia within inflamed skin are facilitated by the enhanced expression of CAMs like the cutaneous lymphocyte associated antigen CLA [43, 44]. Moreover, the recent progeny of allergen-activated T cells shows a strongly increased random migratory capacity [45–47].

2.1.1.4.3 T-Cell Specificity:
Cross-reactions and Concomitant Sensitization

Allergen-specific T cells display strong specificity for both the MHC class II molecules involved and for the allergen: if, for example, nickel-specific T cells are cultured in vitro with nickel (bivalent cations) presented by cells with incompatible MHC class II molecules, they do not react, even if all the other CAMs and counter-structures fit nicely. On the other hand, if the same cells are cultured with fully compatible APCs, but with the physicochemically very similar metal allergen cobalt, they do not react either [21, 48]. Such in vitro studies confirm the notion that simultaneously occurring allergies often derive from concomitant sensitization rather than from immunological cross-reactivity. Multiple sensitization may readily occur as allergens frequently go together (like nickel and cobalt in alloys, or drugs and preservatives in medicaments). Moreover, ongoing allergic reactions have strong immunopotentiating power (e.g. from local IL-2 and interferon-γ release) and, thus, the risk of developing new allergies at these sites is high [49].

Still, molecular mimicry may occur. The T-cell receptor (TCR) recognizes rather small molecular moieties, e.g. peptides with at least 7–8 amino acids. Thus, it can be envisaged that to some degree binding of truly different allergens to APCs may generate similar class II epitopes, thus triggering T cells unable to discriminate between these allergens. Evidence supporting this view was obtained in the above-mentioned studies: nickel-specific T-cell clones were, depending on the MHC class II type of the original donor, either truly nickel specific, or equally stimulated by copper or palladium cations (R. J. Scheper, unpubl. work).

Interestingly, both these metals immediately surround nickel in the periodic table. Thus, it may well be that development of nickel allergy in some patients inevitably also leads to palladium or copper allergy. Actually, the latter allergies have, to our knowledge, never been reported to occur in the absence of nickel allergy [50]. It can be concluded that skin testing alone does not reveal to what extent positive reactions to different allergens are based on the same T-cell clone(s), rather than on separate coexisting clones. Nevertheless, clinical consequences for patient and treatment are similar, whether allergies to different compounds stem from separate, overlapping or identical sets of T-cell clones.

2.1.1.4.4 T-Cell and Allergen Retention in the Skin, Flare-up Reactions

From the basic mechanisms of ACD it can be inferred that allergen-specific flare-up reactions depend either on local allergen or T-cell retention at distinct skin sites. The former type of flare-up reactions can readily be observed in man when, from about 1 week after primary sensitization, sufficient effector T cells have entered the circulation to react with residual allergen at the sensitization site [51]. Another example is the inadvertent flare-up reaction that may be observed at a site of patch testing with a compound providing two different allergenic moieties: previously induced allergic reactivity and, thus, positive reactivity to one (e.g. penicillin) may potentiate primary sensitization to the other (e.g. formaldehyde), which may then cause a flare-up 1 week after skin testing. Local allergen retention is usually of short duration only. In experimental guinea pig studies using dinitrochlorobenzene (DNCB), chromium and penicillin allergens, we never found local allergen retention in the skin to mediate flare-up reactions for periods exceeding 2 weeks (R. J. Scheper, unpubl. work).

In contrast, allergen-specific T cells may persist for much longer in the skin (up to several months) (Fig. 2.1.3). Thus, locally increased allergen-specific hyperreactivity, detectable through either accelerated 'retest' reactivity (after repeated allergenic contacts at the same skin site) or flare-up reactivity (after repeated allergen entry from the circulation, e.g. derived from food), may be observed for several months at former skin reaction sites [52, 53]. Interestingly, histological examination of such previous skin reaction sites shows that only few T cells remain present for such periods. Still, the remarkable flare-up reactivity at such sites can be understood by considering that only very few specific T cells are required for macroscopic reactivity. Moreover, a high frequency of the residual T cells may bear specificity to the allergen: allergic skin reactions tend selectively to recruit allergen-specific T cells from the circulation, whereas subsequent allergen-driven proliferation and retention of those cells further increase the local frequency of allergen-specific cells [45, 54].

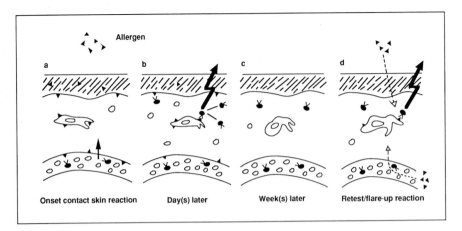

Fig. 2.1.3a–d. T-cell-mediated flare-up reactivity in allergic contact dermatitis. T lymphocytes with irrelevant specificities (O), but in particular specific T lymphocytes (⚫), enter a challenged skin site (*a, b*). Lymphokine release and proliferation ensues. A small residual infiltrate, with a relatively high frequency of allergen-specific T cells, persists (*c*) and may give rise to accelerated (specific cells already presente) local reactivity upon renewed allergenic contacts, either via the skin (retest reactivity) or the circulation (flare-up reactivity) (*d*)

2.1.2 Regulatory Mechanisms in Allergic Contact Dermatitis

2.1.2.1 Tolerance Induction, Suppressor Cells

Uncontrolled development and expression of T-cell-mediated immune function would be detrimental to the host. During evolution, several mechanisms developed to prevent lymph node 'explosion' or excessive skin ulceration upon persisting antigen exposure. Epicutaneous allergenic contacts not only induce T effector cells, but also lymphocytes that curtail further T effector cell proliferation (afferently acting suppressor cells) or decrease the intensity of skin reactions upon subsequent allergen contacts (efferently acting suppressor cells). Sensitization, therefore, seems to be the resultant of a delicate balance between effector and suppressor mechanisms. Upon preferential stimulation of suppressor cells, a strong and stable allergen-specific unresponsiveness may develop, known as immunological tolerance (Table 2.1.2). This phenomenon can be demonstrated by administering allergen intravenously or orally to nonsensitized, immunologically naive individuals [5, 55–57]. The cell type critical in determining whether exposure to an allergen leads to hypersensitivity or tolerance is the LC. By oral or intravenous administration, appropriate allergen presentation by LCs is prevented. In support of this view, tolerance may be induced by applying allergens on skin sites where LCs have been functionally damaged, e.g. by UV irradiation, or are naturally absent (e.g. in the tail skin of mice; [58, 59]).

Table 2.1.2. Effects of various routes of allergen administration on the clinical outcome

Allergen route	Nonsensitized individual		Hypersensitive individual	
	Sensitization	Tolerance	ACD	Flare-up/ Desensitization
Skin	++	−	++	(+)
Intravenous, oral	−	++	−	++

Clinical outcome may, depending on the immune status (nonsensitized vs hypersensitive), vary from sensitization or tolerance induction to allergic skin reactions, flare-ups and/or desensitization.
In this table, effects of different doses of allergen and frequencies of allergenic contacts have been omitted. Generally, higher doses and frequencies favour involvement of suppressor cell-mediated (tolerance) and flare-up or desensitization phenomena, also with the skin route.
The tolerogenic routes may include skin deficient in, or depleted of, functionally active Langerhans cells.

The concept of suppressor cells controlling ACD is based on two main facts. First, allergen-specific tolerance can be transferred from tolerant to normal (naive) animals by lymphoid cells. Secondly, contact sensitization can be enhanced, and tolerance reversed, by treatment with certain cytostatic drugs, including cyclophosphamide [5, 60]. In mice, guinea pigs and man (precursors of) suppressor cells have been demonstrated to be particularly sensitive to cytostatic drugs, thus allowing for exaggerated effector cell development. Interferons have also been shown to inhibit the suppressor action in mice and to stimulate effector cell function [61]. Still, suppressor cells are not a well-defined subpopulation of cells, and several different mechanisms of action have been proposed recently. These may involve a subset of allergen-specific T cells shedding truncated T-cell receptor moieties which can block allergen presentation [62], and Th2 cells releasing cytokines which interfere with effector T-cell functions (IL-4[63]; IL-10[64]).

Both clinical and experimental findings make clear that full and persistent tolerance can only be induced prior to any sensitizing allergen contacts. Experimentally, even subsensitizing doses of nickel applied to the skin prevented subsequent tolerance induction by feeding the metal allergen [65]. This may have contributed to incomplete tolerance induction in earlier clinical studies when feeding with poison ivy/oak-derived allergens [66]. Apparently, the progeny of naive allergen-specific cells, once 'on the stage,' has escaped susceptibility to suppressor cell action. This explains why, to our knowledge, permanent reversal of existing ACD has never been achieved clinically. Nevertheless, effector cells still seem to be susceptible to (transient) downregulation of allergen reactivity, as observed in desensitization procedures [5, 66].

2.1.2.2 Skin Hyporeactivity, Desensitization

For dermatologists, methods by which patients might be desensitized of an existing ACD would be a welcome addition to the available therapies, and investigators have made a wide variety of attempts. A limited and transient degree of hyposensitization was obtained by Chase [67] when feeding DNCB-contact-sensitized guinea pigs with the allergen, whereas, for achieving persistent chromium-unresponsiveness in presensitized animals, Polak and Turk [68] needed a harsh protocol involving up to lethal doses of the allergen. Unfortunately, results from clinical studies on hyposensitization in ACD were in line with these experimental data. Therapeutic protocols involving ingestion of poison ivy allergen or penicillin were of only transient benefit to the patients [66, 69]. The mechanism underlying specific desensitization in ACD depends primarily on direct interference of allergen with effector T-cell function, by blocking or downregulating T-cell receptors [70]. No suppressor cell mechanisms are involved, as the onset of desensitization does not require time. Moreover, T cells can be 'desensitized' in vitro in the absence of putative suppressor cells [71]. Interestingly, the latter study also pointed towards class II-bearing non-LCs (here, keratinocytes) as being most effective in rendering allergen-specific effector cells refractory to further effector function. A major problem with desensitization in vivo may lie in the rapid replacement of peripherally inactivated effector cells from the relatively protected lymphoid organs [70].

Upon repeated administration of allergens to sensitized individuals, suppressor cells may, however, still be triggered and contribute to desensitization. It was found that local desensitization by repeatedly applying allergen at the same skin site resulted not from local skin hardening or LC inactivation, as local reactivity to a nonrelated allergen at the site was unimpaired [72]. The role of suppressor cells in such local desensitization was further supported by the persistence of a cellular infiltrate at the site. Upon discontinuation of allergen exposure, local unresponsiveness rapidly dispersed (within 1 week). Collectively, these data illustrate the problems encountered in attempting to eradicate established effector cell function.

2.1.3 Preventive Allergen Screening

From the foregoing it can be concluded that the safest option for reducing the incidence of ACD is to prevent it from its very roots by eliminating potential allergens wherever possible. For each known allergen this may require special measures, including legislative action. For example, frequencies of nickel allergy might be reduced by avoiding industrial and consumer use of nickel-containing alloys from which the allergen is released too readily [73]. This view has also provided the incentive for developing screening procedures for potential allergenicity of newly produced substances, including new drugs, cosmetics and preservatives. The guinea pig model, which has proved so useful in studying mechanisms of ACD, also allows for the prospective testing of materials that are possible contact allergens in man. An assumption of such studies is that materials that sensitize man are indeed sensitizers of guinea pigs, and conversely. Indeed, it turns out that, generally, sensitizers rank in parallel in man and guinea pig, so that materials that are strong or weak contact sensitizers in man are similarly strong or weak contact sensitizers in the guinea pig, and conversely [74–76].

Although few guinea pigs are sufficient to identify a strong sensitizer, weak sensitizers would require unacceptably large numbers of animals, if simply applied to the skin. To increase screening power, several immunopotentiation techniques have been elaborated in order to achieve maximum sensitization (see Sect. 18.3).

These techniques include repeated skin applications under occlusion and series of intradermal injections with or without adjuvants, usually Freund's complete adjuvant (FCA). This is a mineral oil containing heat-killed tubercle bacilli. Through the use of FCA, weak contact allergens that might otherwise be missed have become accessible to prospective testing. Similar procedures, including additional UV treatments, are employed in testing compounds for photoallergenicity [77]. Cautiousness remains warranted, however, as potentially very weak allergens may still escape detection and present clinical problems when applied in a potentially very sensitizing way, notably involving repeated skin contacts. This was recently demonstrated by the development of clonidine allergies in patients transdermally treated with this antihypertensive drug [78].

Further improvements in sensitization and evaluation techniques in mouse ACD models have made this species, too, very attractive for prospective allergenicity testing (see Sect. 18.3.10). As well as for economical reasons, the availability of many genetically well-defined strains and appropriate immunological reagents would favour more extended use of this species in ACD studies. A rapid screening technique for contact sensitizers was recently developed, based on early assessment of draining lymph node proliferative activity upon administration of compounds onto the ears (Kimber assay [79, 80]). The results from these tests all contribute to the decisions which have to be made concerning the health and safety of any population which might be exposed to a given material.

2.1.4 Summary and Conclusions

Extensive research has recently led to the unravelling of the basic immunological mechanisms of ACD. Major cell types and mediators involved can be identified. How T cells specifically recognize distinct allergens, and how these and other inflammatory cells interact to generate inflammation, has begun to be understood. This rapid advance sharply contrasts with the slow progress in unravelling the regulatory mechanisms in cell-mediated immunity, including ACD. Putative suppressor cell actions are still heavily disputed. The poor understanding of regulatory mechanisms in ACD hampers further therapeutic progress. So far, no methods of permanent desensitization have been devised.

Nevertheless, recently defined cellular interaction molecules and mediators provide promising targets for antiinflammatory drugs, some of which have already entered clinical trials. Clearly, drugs found to be effective in preventing severe T-cell-mediated conditions, e.g. rejection of a vital organ graft, should be very safe before their use in ACD would seem appropriate. To date, prudence favours any measure to prevent ACD, be it through legal action to outlaw the use of certain materials or through avoiding personal contact with these materials. In the meantime, for difficult-to-avoid allergens, further studies on the potential value of tolerogenic treatment prior to possible sensitization seem warranted.

2.1.5 References

1. Boerrigter GH, Bril H, Scheper RJ (1988) Hapten-specific antibodies in allergic contact dermatitis in the guinea pig. Int Arch Allergy Appl Immunol 85: 385–391
2. Bergstresser PR (1989) Sensitization and elicitation of inflammation in contact dermatitis. In: Norris DA (ed) Immune mechanisms in cutaneous disease. Dekker, New York, pp 219–246
3. Turk JL (1975) Delayed hypersensitivity, 2nd edn. North-Holland, Amsterdam
4. Gell PDH, Coombs RRA, Lachman R (1975) Clinical aspects of immunology, 3rd edn. Blackwell, London
5. Polak L (1980) Immunological aspects of contact sensitivity. An experimental study. Monogr Allergy 15: 4–60
6. Von Blomberg BME, Bruynzeel DP, Scheper RJ (1991) Advances in mechanisms of allergic contact dermatitis: in vitro and in vitro. In: Marzulli FN, Maibach HI (eds) Dermatotoxicology, 4th edn. Hemisphere, Washington, pp 255–362
7. Stingl G, Katz SI, Clement L et al. (1978) Immunological functions of Ia-bearing epidermal Langerhans cells. J Immunol 121: 2005–2013
8. Czernielewski JM, Demarchez M (1987) Further evidence for the self-reproducing capacity of Langerhans cells in human skin. J Invest Dermatol 88: 17–20
9. Breathnach SM (1988) The Langerhans cell. Centenary review. Br J Dermatol 119: 463–469
10. Toews G, Bergstresser P, Streilein J et al. (1980) Epidermal Langerhans cell density determines whether contact hypersensitivity or unresponsiveness follows skin painting with DNCB. J Immunol 124: 445–453
11. Halliday GM, Muller HK (1986) Induction of tolerance via skin depleted of Langerhans cells by a chemical carcinogen. Cell Immunol 99: 220–227
12. Marchal G, Seman M, Milon M et al. (1982) Local adoptive transfer of skin delayed type hypersensitivity initiated by a single T Lymphocyte. J Immunol 129: 954–958
13. Schuler G, Steinman RM (1985) Murine epidermal Langerhans cells mature into potent immuno-stimulatory dendritic cells in vitro. J Exp Med 161: 526–546
14. Shimada S, Caughman SW, Sharrow SO et al. (1987) Enhanced antigen-presenting capacity of cultured Langerhans cells is associated with markedly increased expressior of Ia antigen. J Immunol 139: 2551–2555
15. Inaba K, Steinman RM (1986) Accessory cell-T lymphocyte interactions. Antigen-dependent and -independent clustering. J Exp Med 163: 247–261
16. Braathen LR, Thorsby E (1983) Human epidermal Langerhans cells are more potent than blood monocytes in inducing some antigen-specific T cell-responses. Br J Dermatol 108: 139–146

17. Res P, Kapsenberg ML, Bos JD et al. (1987) The crucial role of human dendritic antigen-presenting cell subsets in nickel-specific T cell proliferation. J Invest Dermatol 88: 550–554

18. Cresswell P (1987) Antigen recognition by T lymphocytes. Immunol Today 8: 67–69

19. Claverie JM, Prochnicka-Chalufour A, Bougueleret L (1989) Implications of a Fab-like structure for the T cell receptor. Immunol Today 10: 10–14

20. Shimada S, Katz SI (1985) TNP-specific Lyt-2^+ cytolytic T cell clones preferentially respond to TNP-conjugated epidermal cells. J Immunol 135: 1558–1563

21. Sinigaglia F, Scheidegger D, Garotta G et al. (1985) Isolation and characterization of Ni-specific T cell clones from patients with Ni-contact dermatitis. J Immunol 135: 3929–3932

22. Mosmann TR, Coffmann RL (1989) Thl and Th2 cells: different patterns of lymphokine secretion lead to different functional properties. Annu Rev Immunol 7: 145–173

23. Cher DJ, Mossmann TR (1987) Two types of murine helper T cell clone. Delayed type hypersensitivity is mediated by Th1 clones. J Immunol 138: 3688–3694

24. Romagnani S (⊠) Induction of Th1 and Th2 responses: a key role for the 'natural' immune response? Immunol Today 13(10): 379–381

25. Bloom BR, Salgame P, Diamons B (1992) Revisiting and revising suppressor T cells. Immunol Today 13(4): 131–136

26. Hsieh CS, Macatonia SE, Tripp CS, Wolf S, O'Garra A, Murphy KM (1993) Development of Thl CD4+ T cells through IL-12 produced by listeria-induced macrophages. Science 260: 547–549

27. Lehner T, Bergmeier LA, Panagiotidi C, Tao L, Brookes R, Klavinskis LS, Walker P, Ward RG, Hussain L, Gearing AJH, Adams SE (1992) induction of mucosal and systemic immunity to a recombinant simian immunodeficiency viral protein. Science 258: 1365–1369

28. Scott P (1993) IL-12: initiation cytokine for cell-mediated immunity. Science 260: 496–497

29. Kapsenberg ML, Bos JD, Wierenga EA (1992) cells in allergic responses to haptens and proteins. Springer Semin Immunopathol 13: 303–314

30. Sanders ME, Makgoba MW, Shaw S (1988) Human naive and memory T cells: reinterpretation of helper-inducer and suppressor-inducer subsets. Immunol Today 9: 195–198

31. Dohlsten M, Hedlund G, Sjogren H et al. (1988) Two subsets of human CD4+ T helper cells differing in kinetics and capacities to produce interleukin 2 and interferon-gamma can be defined by the Leu 18 and UCHL1 monoclonal antibodies. Eur J Immunol 18: 1173–1178

32. Bos JD, Zonneveld I, Das PK et al. (1987) The skin immune system (SIS): distribution and immunophenotype of lymphocyte subpopulations in normal human skin. J Invest Dermatol 88: 569–573

33. Yon Blomberg BME, van der Burg CKH, Pos O et al. (1987) In vitro studies in nickel allergy: diagnostic value of a dual parameter analyis. J Invest Dermatol 88: 362–368

34. Hirschberg H, Braathen LR, Thorsby E (1982) Antigen presentation by vascular endothelial cells and epidermal Langerhans cells: the role of HLA-DR. Immunol Rev 65: 57–77

35. Breitmeyer JB (1987) Lymphocyte activation. How T cells communicate. Nature 329: 760–761

36. Bierer BE, Burakoff SJ (1988) T cell adhesion molecules. FASEB J 2: 2584–2590

37. Jenkins MK, Johnson JG (1993) Molecules involved in T-cell costimulation. Curr Opin Immunol 5: 361–367

38. Issekutz TB, Stoltz JM, von der Meide P (1988) Lymphocyte recruitment in delayed hypersensitivity; the role of interferon-gamma. J Immunol 140: 2989–2993

39. Messadi DV, Pober JS, Fiers W et al. (1987) Induction of an activation antigen on postcapillary venular endothelium in human skin organ culture. J Immunol 139: 1557–1562
40. Haskard DO, Cavender D, Fleck RM et al. (1987) Human dermal microvascular endothelial cells behave like umbilical vein endothelial cells in T cell adhesion studies. J Invest Dermatol 88: 340–344
41. Dustin ML, Rothlein R, Bhan AK et al. (1986) Induction by IL-1 and interferon-gamma:tissue distribution, biochemistry, and function of a natural adherence molucule (ICAM-1). J Immunol 137: 245–254
42. Hamann A, Jablonski-Westrich D, Scholz KW et al. (1988) Regulation of lymphocyte homing. I. Alterations in homing receptor expression and organ-specific high endothelial venule binding of lymphocytes upon activation. J Immunol 140: 737–741
43. Mackay CR (1993) Homing of naive, memory and effector lymphocytes. Curr Opin Immunol 5: 423–427
44. Picker LJ, Kishimoto TK, Smith CW et al. (1991) ELAM-1 is an adhesion molecule for skin-homing T cells. Nature 349: 796–779
45. Scheper RJ, von Blomberg BME (1989) Allergic contact dermatitis: T cell receptors and migration. In: Frosch PJ, Dooms-Goossens A, Lachapelle JM, Rycroft RJG, Scheper RJ (eds) Current topics in contact dermatitis. Springer, Berlin Heidelberg New York, pp 12–17
46. Pals ST, Horst E, Scheper RJ et al. (1989) Mechanisms of human lymphocyte migration and their role in the pathogenesis of disease. Immunol Rev 108: 111–133
47. Duijvesteijn A, Hamann A (1989) Mechanisms and regulation of lymphocyte migration. Immunol Today 10: 23–28
48. Silvennoinen-Kassinen S, Jakkula H, Karvonen J (1986) Helper T cells carry the specificity of nickel sensitivity reaction in vitro in humans. J Invest Dermatol 86: 18–20
49. Scheper RJ, von Blomberg BME, Velzen D et al. (1976) Effects of contact sensitization and delayed hyper-sensitivity reactions on immune responses to non-related antigens. Modulation of immune responses. Int Arch Allergy Appl Immunol 50: 243–255
50. Camarasa JG, Serra-Baldrich E, Lluch M et al. (1989) Recent unexplained patch test reactions to palladium. Contact Dermatitis 20: 388–399
51. Skog E (1966) Spontaneous flare-up reactions induced by different amounts of 1,3-dinitro-4-chlorobenzene. Acta Derm Venereol (Stockh) 46: 386–395
52. Scheper RJ, von Blomberg BME, Boerrigter GH et al. (1983) Induction of local memory in the skin. Role of local T cell retention. Clin Exp Immunol 51: 141–151
53. Yamashita N, Natsuaki M, Sagami S (1989) Flare-up reaction on murine contact hypersensitivity. I. Description of an experimental model: rechallenge system. Immunology 67: 365–369
54. Scheper RJ, van Dinther-Janssen ACHM, Polak L (1985) Specific accumulation of hapten-reactive T cells in contact sensitivity reaction sites. J Immunol 134: 1333–1336
55. Miller SD, Sy M-S, Claman HN (1977) The induction of hapten-specific T cell tolerance using hapten-modified lymphoid membranes. II. Relative roles of suppressor T cells and clone inhibition in the tolerant state. Eur J Immunol 7: 165–170
56. Mowat A (1987) The regulation of immune responses to dietary protein antigens. Immunol Today 8: 93–98
57. van Hoogstraten IMW, Andersen JE, von Blomberg BME et al. (1989) Preliminary results of a multicenter study on the incidence of nickel allergy in relationship to previous oral and cutaneous contacts. In: Frosch PJ, Dooms-Goosens A, Lachapelle JM, Rycroft RJG, Scheper RJ (eds) Current topics in contact dermatitis. Springer, Berlin Heidelberg New York, pp 178–184
58. Semma M, Sagami S (1981) Induction of suppressor T cells to DNFB contact sensitivity by application of sensitizer through Langerhans cell-deficient skin. Arch Dermatol Res 271: 361–364

59. Elmets CA, Bergstresser PR, Tigelaar RE et al. (1983) Analysis of the mechanism of unresponsiveness produced by haptens painted on skin exposed to ultraviolet radiation. J Exp Med 158: 781–794
60. Zembala M, Asherson GL (1973) Depression of T cell phenomenon of contact sensitivity by T cells from unresponsive mice. Nature 244: 227–228
61. Knop J. Stremmer R, Neumann C, De Maeyer D, Macher E (1982) interferon inhibits the suppressor T cell response of delayed-type hypersensitivity. Nature 296: 775–776
62. Kuchroo VK, Byrne MC, Atsumi Y, Greenfeld E, Connol JB, Whitters MJ, O'Hara RM, Collins M, Dorf ME (1991) T cell receptor alpha chain plays a critical role in antigen-specific suppressor cell function. Proc Natl Acad Sci USA 8700–8704
63. Gautam SC, Chikkala NF, Hamilton TA (1992) Anti-inflammatory action of IL-4. Negative regulation of contact sensitivity to trinitrochlorobenzene. J Immunol 148: 1411–1415
64. Fiorentino DF, Zlotnik A, Mosmann TR, Howard M, O'Garra A (1991) IL-10 inhibits cytokine production by activated macrophages. J Immunol 147: 3815–3822
65. van Hoogstraten IMW, von Blomberg BME, Boden D, Kraal G, Scheper RJ (1994) Non-sensitizing epicutaneous skin tests prevent subsequent induction of immune tolerance. J Invest Dermatol 102: 80–83
66. Epstein WL (1987) The poison ivy picker of Pennypack Park: the continuing saga of poison ivy. J Invest Dermatol 88: 7–9
67. Chase MW (1946) Inhibition of experimental drug allergy by prior feeding of the sensitizing agent. Proc Soc Exp Biol Med 61: 257–259
68. Polak L, Turk JL (1968) Studies on the effect of systemic administration of sensitizers in guinea pigs with contact sensitivity to inorganic metal compounds. I. The induction of immunological unresponsiveness in already sensitized animals. Clin Exp Immunol 3: 245–251
69. Wendel GD, Stark BJ, Jamison RB et al. (1985) Penicillin allergy and desensitization in serious infections during pergnancy. N Engl J Med 312: 1229–1232
70. Polak L, Rinck C (1978) Mechanism of desensitization in DNCB-contact sensitive guinea pigs. J Invest Dermatol 70: 98–104
71. Gaspari AA, Jenkins MK, Katz SI (1988) Class II MCH-bearing keratinocytes induce antigen-specific unresponsiveness in hapten-specific TH1 clones. J Immunol 141: 2216–2220
72. Boerrigter GH, Scheper RJ (1987) Local and systemic desensitization induced by repeated epicutaneous hapten application. J Invest Dermatol 88: 3–7
73. Menné T, Brandrup F, Thestrup-Pedersen K et al. (1987) Patch test reactivity to nickel alloys. Contact Dermatitis 16: 255–259
74. Magnusson B, Kligman AM (1977) Usefulness of guinea pig tests for detection of contact sensitizers. In: Marzulli FN, Maibach HI (eds) Dermatotoxicology and pharmacology. Wiley, London, pp 551–560
75. Klecak G (1983) Identification of contact allergens: predictive tests in animals. In: Marzuli FN, Maibach HI (eds) Dermatotoxicology. McGraw-Hill, New York, pp 193–237
76. Maguire HC (1985) Estimation of the allergenicity of prospective human contact sensitizers in the guinea pig. In: Maibach HI, Lowe N (eds) Models in dermatology, vol 2. Karger, Basel, pp 234–239
77. Maurer T (1983) Contact and photocontact allergens: a manual of predictive test methods. Dekker, New York
78. Maibach H (1985) Clonidine: irritant and allergic contact dermatitis assays. Contact dermatitis 12: 192–195
79. Kimber I, Mitchell JA, Griffin AC (1986) Development of a murine local lymph node assay for the determination of sensitizing potential. Food Chem Toxicol 24: 585–586
80. Kimber I (1988) Immunotoxicology and allergy: old problems and new approaches. Toxic in Vitro 2: 309–311
81. Knapp W, Rieber P, Dorken B et al. (1989) Towards a better definition of human leucocyte surface molecules. Immunol Today 10: 253–258

2.2 Cutaneous Irritation

PETER J. FROSCH

Contents

2.2.1 Definition

Irritant contact dermatitis may be defined as a nonimmunological inflammatory reaction of the skin to an external agent. The acute type comprises two forms, the *irritant reaction* and acute irritant contact dermatitis, and usually has only a single cause. In contrast, the chronic form is a multifactorial disease in most cases. Toxic chemicals (*irritants*) are the major cause, but mechanical, thermal and climatic effects are important contributory cofactors. The clinical spectrum of irritant contact dermatitis is much wider than that of allergic contact dermatitis and ranges from slight scaling of the stratum corneum, through redness, wealing, and deep caustic burns, to an eczematous condition indistinguishable from allergic contact dermatitis. Acute forms of irritant contact dermatitis may be painful and may be associated with sensations such as burning, stinging or itching. Individual susceptibility to irritants is extremely variable.

2.2.2 Clinical Pictures

The morphology of cutaneous irritation varies widely and depends on the type and intensity of the irritant(s). Based on clinical criteria we may distinguish the following types:
1. chemical burns,
2. irritant reactions,
3. acute irritant contact dermatitis and
4. chronic irritant contact dermatitis (cumulative insult dermatitis).

Folliculitis, acneiform eruptions, miliaria, pigmentary alterations, alopecia, contact urticaria and granulomatous reactions may result from irritancy to chemicals (Table 2.2.1), but in the following only the first four types, clinically the most important, will be discussed in detail.

Table 2.2.1. Clinical effects of chemical irritants (adapted from [1])

Ulcerations
Strong acids (chromic, hydrofluoric, nitric, hydrochloric, sulphuric)
Strong alkalis (especially calcium oxide, calcium hydroxide, sodium
hydroxide, sodium metasilicate, sodium silicate, potassium cyanide, trisodium phosphate)
Salts (arsenic trioxide, dichromates)
Solvents (acrylonitrile, carbon disulphide)
Gases (ethylene oxide, acrylonitrile)
Folliculitis and acneiform lesions
Arsenic trioxide
Fibreglass
Oils and greases
Tar
Asphalt
Chlorinated naphthalenes
Polyhalogenated biphenyls
Miliaria
Occlusive clothing and dressing
Adhesive tape
Aluminium chloride

Table 2.2.1. (Continued)

Hyperpigmentation	
Any irritant (especially phototoxic agents such as psoralens, tar, asphalt)	
Metals (inorganic arsenic, silver, gold, bismuth, mercury)	
Hypopigmentation	*Urticaria*
p-tert-Amylphenol	Chemicals (dimethylsulphoxide)
p-tert-Butylphenol	Cosmetics (sorbic acid)
Hydroquinone	Animals
Monobenzyl ether of hydroquinone	Foods
p-tert-Catechol	Plants
3-Hydroxyanisole	Textiles
1-tert-Butyl-3, 4-catechol	Woods
Alopecia	*Granulomas*
Borax	Silica
Chloroprene dimers	Beryllium
	Talc

2.2.2.1 Chemical Burns

Highly alkaline or acid materials can cause severe tissue damage even after short skin contact. Painful erythema develops at exposed sites, usually within minutes, and is followed by vesiculation and formation of necrotic eschars (Figs. 2.2.1–2.2.5). Occasionally, intense wealing can be observed in the erythematous phase due to toxic degranulation of mast cells. The shape of lesions is bizarre and 'artificial' in most cases and does not follow the usual pattern of known dermatoses. This is an important hallmark in differentiating accidental and self-inflicted lesions from genuine skin disease (Fig. 2.2.6)

Strong acids and alkalis are the major causes of chemical burns. The halogenated acids are particularly dangerous because they may lead to deep continuous tissue destruction even after short skin contact (Fig. 2.2.1). Holes in protective gloves may result in serious injuries with scar formation. Caustic chemicals are also often trapped by clothing and footwear, resulting in deep ulceration down to the subcutaneous tissue, whereas other, open, areas are less severely affected because of the possibility of rapid removal (Figs. 2.2.2 and 2.2.3).

It is important to realize that a number of other chemicals, including dust and solids, may also cause severe necrotic lesions after prolonged skin contact, particularly under occlusion (cement, amine hardeners, etc.).

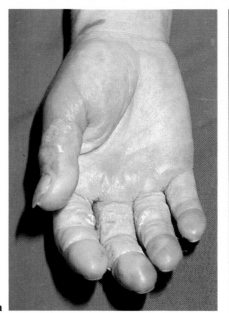
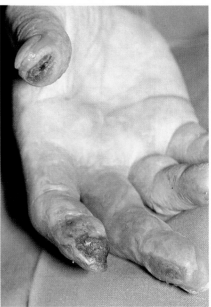

a

b

Fig. 2.2.1a, b. Severe chemical burn caused by bromoacetic acid. **a** Immediate effect. **b** After 21 days there are still erythema, edema and deep necrotic lesions

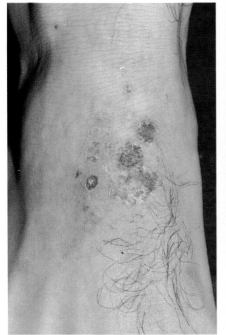

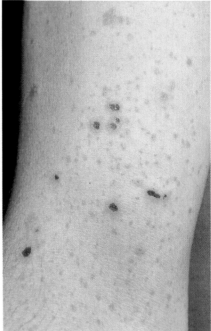

Fig. 2.2.2. Sharply demarcated ulcerative lesions on the dorsum of a chemistry student's foot caused by sodium hydroxide

Fig. 2.2.3. Multiple follicular papules and necrotic lesions on the arm of a factory worker caused by sodium hydroxide being trapped in the clothes after explosion of a container

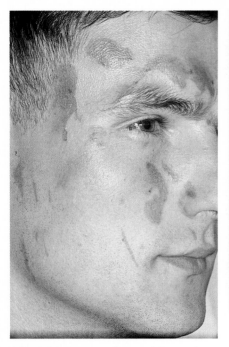

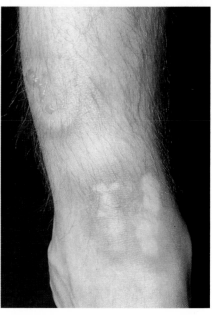

Fig. 2.2.4. Brown-yellow staining and superficial epidermal damage induced by splashes of nitric acid. Note the streaky pattern

Fig. 2.2.5. Erythema and blistering on the lower leg caused by undiluted isothiazolinone (Kathon WT) trapped in the rubber boot of a machinist who wanted to add the biocide to cutting oil

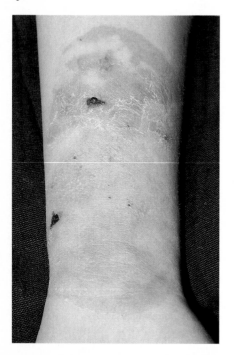

Fig. 2.2.6. Artificial dermatitis with erythema, scaling and crusting in a psychotic patient caused by rubbing in a harsh floor cleanser. Typical of an artefact is the sharp demarcation

2.2.2.2 Irritant Reactions

Irritants may produce cutaneous reactions which do not meet the clinical definition of a 'dermatitis'. In English-speaking countries the term 'dermatitis' is held to be synonymous with 'eczema' by most authors, though this can be disputed. The diagnosis 'acute irritant reaction' is thus increasingly used if the clinical picture is monomorphic rather than polymorphic and characterized by one or more of the following signs: scaling (including the initial stage of 'dryness'), redness (starting with faint follicular spots, up to dusky red areas with haemorrhages), vesicles (blisters), pustules, and erosions (follicular and planar). Severe cutaneous damage reaching down to dermal structures should be termed a 'chemical burn' (German, *Verätzung*; French, *cautérisation*). In practice, of course, some overlap will exist which provides general information based on literature reports of both clinical and experimental studies (see also Sect. 8.3.2 for a discussion of irritant reactions).

Chemicals which can cause irritant reactions are listed in Table 2.2.2, and typical clinical effects are shown in Figs. 2.2.7 and 2.2.8. The substances are mainly 'mild irritants', i.e. ones that do not cause a severe skin reaction on short contact (<1 h). The resulting skin lesion may vary with the type of exposure, body region and individual susceptibility (Fig. 2.2.9).

Table 2.2.2. Common irritants which are important causes of occupational dermatitis (adapted from [14, 28, 91])

Water
and its additives (salts and oxides of calcium, magnesium, and iron)

Skin cleansers
Soaps, detergents, 'waterless cleansers' and additives (sand, silica)

Industrial cleaning agents
Detergents, surface-active agents, sulphonated oils, wetting agents, emulsifiers, enzymes

Alkalis
Soap, soda, ammonia, potassium and sodium hydroxides, cement, lime, sodium silicate, trisodium phosphate, and various amines

Acids
Severe irritancy (caustic): sulphuric, hydrochloric, nitric, chromic, and hydrofluoric acids
Moderate irritancy: Acetic, oxalic, and salicylic acids

Oils
Cutting oils with various additives (water, emulsifiers, antioxidants, anticorrosive agents, preservatives, dyes and perfumes)
Lubricating and spindle oils

Table 2.2.2. (Continued)

Organic solvents
White spirit, benzene, toluene, trichloroethylene, perchloroethylene, methylene chloride, chlorobenzene
Methanol, ethanol, isopropanol, propylene glycol
Ethyl acetate, acetone, methyl ethyl ketone, ethylene glycol monomethyl ether, nitroethane, turpentine, carbon disulphide
Thinners (mixtures of alcohols, ketones, and toluene)

Oxidizing agents
Hydrogen peroxide, benzoyl peroxide, cyclohexanone peroxide, sodium hypochlorite

Reducing agents
Phenols, hydrazines, aldehydes, thioglycolates

Plants
Citrus peel and juice, flower bulbs, garlic, onion, pineapple, pelargonium, iris, cucumbers, buttercups, asparagus, mustard, barley, chicory, corn
Various plants of the spurge family (Euphorbiaceae), Brassicaceae family (Cruciferae) and Ranunculaceae family (for further details see [25])

Animal products
Pancreatic enzymes, body secretions

Miscellaneous irritants
Alkyl tin compounds and penta-, tetra-, and trichlorophenols (wood preservatives)
Methylchloroisothiazolinone and methylisothiazolinone (irritant at high concentrations during production or misuse)
Components of plastic processing (formaldehyde, phenol, cresol, styrene, diisocyanates, acrylic monomers, diallyl phthalate, aliphatic and aromatic amines, epichlorohydrin)
Metal polishes
Fertilizers
Rust-preventing products
Paint removers (alkyl bromide)
Acrolein, crotonaldehyde, ethylene oxide, mercuric salts, zinc chloride, bromide, chlorine

---

2.2.2.3 Acute Irritant Contact Dermatitis

The clinical appearance of acute irritant contact dermatitis is very variable and it may even be indistinguishable from the allergic type. There are numerous reports in the literature of even experienced dermatologists being misled into an initial assumption of allergic contact dermatitis which later, after a careful work-up, turned out to be 'only irritation'.

Most instructive is the report by Malten et al. [69] on hexanediol diacrylate. The UV-cured paint used in a door factory contained hexanediol diacrylate, which caused an epidemic of papular and burning, rather than itching, dermatitis among the workers. Retrospectively, it is clear that the irritant contact dermatitis did not show the typical polymorphic picture of

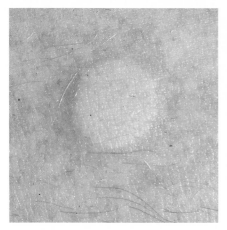

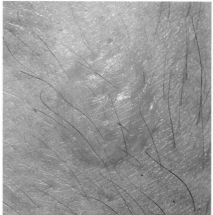

Fig. 2.2.7. Marked wealing induced by undiluted dimethylsulphoxide (DMSO) applied in a cup for 5 min

Fig. 2.2.8. Superficial blister after the application of 0.1% cantharidin in acetone for 24 h

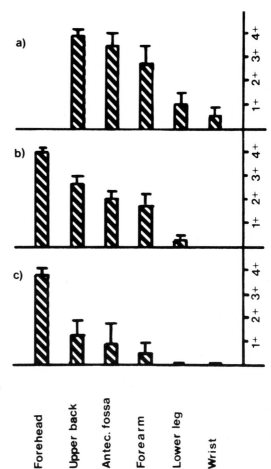

Fig. 2.2.9a–c. Regional variation in cutaneous reactivity to the irritant dimethylsulphoxide (DMSO). The wealing response is most intense in the facial region and least on the palms of the hands. **a** 100% DMSO, **b** 95% DMSO, **c** 90% DMSO (*antec.*, antecubital)

contact allergy, with synchronous presence of macules, papules and vesicles. These lesions developed one after another over the course of a few days (metachronic polymorphism). Malten et al. used the term 'delayed irritation' for this type of cutaneous irritancy.

Delayed irritation may be more common than generally thought so far. Further substances causing it include benzalkonium chloride, dithranol and tretinoin. Irritant patch test reactions to benzalkonium chloride may be papular and increase in intensity with time [11,13]. On the normal skin surrounding psoriatic plaques, dithranol causes redness and edema, which may become very severe on the legs due to venous stasis. Irritation due to tretinoin develops after a few days and is characterized by mild to fiery redness, followed by large flakes of stratum corneum. The dermatitis is burning rather than itching. The skin becomes sensitive to touch and to water.

Acute irritant contact dermatitis includes other well-known entities such as irritation from adhesive tapes, diaper dermatitis, perianal dermatitis and airborne irritant contact dermatitis due to dusts and vapours (Table 2.2.3, Fig. 2.2.10). Dooms-Goossens et al. [20] have compiled a long list of airborne irritants that caused a dermatitis which initially was often thought to be allergic (Table 2.2.4). Cosmetics are not infrequently the cause of mild irritant contact dermatitis on the face, particularly the eyelids, where contact allergy has to be excluded by appropriate patch testing.

The active ingredients of topical medicaments (tretinoin, benzoyl peroxide, dithranol) as well as vehicle constituents (propylene glycol, emulsifiers) may mimic allergic contact dermatitis.

Table 2.2.3. Dermatoses where irritants play a major role in the pathogenesis

Hand eczema
Cosmetic dermatitis
Eyelid eczema
Reactions to therapeutics
Tape irritation
Diaper dermatitis
Perianal and stoma dermatitis
Asteatotic eczema
'Status eczematicus'
Juvenile plantar dermatosis
Photoirritation
Plant dermatitis
Reactions to wool and textiles
Contact urticaria
Subjective irritation ('stinging')
Airborne irritant contact dermatitis

Depending on individual susceptibility and intensity of exposure to the irritant(s) the dermatitis may be more acute or more chronic.

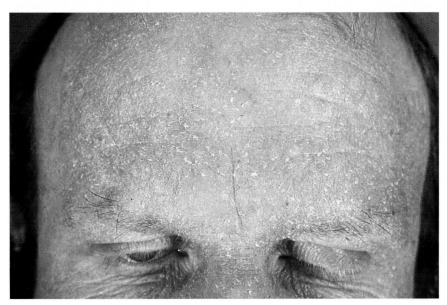

Fig. 2.2.10. Airborne irritant contact dermatitis with slight erythema and scaling caused by irritating stone dust (lime and chalk)

Table 2.2.4. Causes of airborne irritant contact dermatitis (from [20])

Acids and alkalis
Aluminium
Ammonia
Anhydrous calcium sulphate
Arsenic
Bromacetoxy-2-butene
Calcium silicate
Cement
Diallylglycol carbonate monomer
Dichlorvos
Domestic products (e.g. cleaning products)
Epoxy resins
Formaldehyde
Fibreglass
Hexanediol diacrylate
Industrial solvents
Metallic oxide powders (slag)
Paper, carbonless copy paper
Phenol vapours
Phenol formaldehyde resins
Quinine dust
Sawdust from toxic woods
Sewage sludge
Silver
Sodium sesquicarbonate (trona)
Urea-formaldehyde insulating foam, dust from
Wool dust (in atopic individuals)

Table 2.2.5. Materials causing irritant reactions on human skin

Irritant	Cutaneous reaction
Detergents (anionic), soaps	Dryness, erythema, scaling, fissuring, (rarely vesicles)
Benzalkonium chloride (and other cationic detergents)	Erythema, pustules (rarely delayed reactions) with papules
Dimethylsulphoxide	Erythema, wealing (strong)
Methyl nicotinate	Erythema, wealing (weak)
Capsaicin	Erythema, vesiculation
Sodium hydroxide	Erythema, erosions (follicular initially)
Lactic acid	Erythema
Croton oil	Erythema, pustules, purulent bullae
Kerosene	As croton oil
Cantharidin	Erythema, bullae
Metal salts (mercury chloride, cobalt chloride, nickel sulphate, potassium dichromate)	Erythema, follicular papules, pustules
Formic acid	Erythema, superficial blistering (removal of stratum corneum)
Xylene	Dryness, erythema
Toluene	Dryness, erythema, purpura

The reaction's intensity depends on numerous exogenous and endogenous factors. Under experimental conditions a full range of lesions may be produced with the same irritant by varying its dose. In this table, the most typical skin changes are given as observed frequently after more or less 'normal' exposure. Most irritants can produce severe bullous reactions if applied under occlusion at high concentration for 24 h. For further details, see [11, 29, 49, 99, 100, 109].

Various irritants have been tested under experimental conditions and it has been shown that a wide range of lesions can be produced by varying the dose and mode of exposure (Table 2.2.5).

2.2.2.4 Chronic Irritant Contact Dermatitis

Other terms synonymous with chronic irritant contact dermatitis include 'cumulative insult dermatitis', 'traumiterative dermatitis' and 'wear and tear dermatitis' (German, *Abnutzungsdermatose, chronisch degeneratives Ekzem*). Although never clearly defined, this diagnosis applies to an eczematous condition which persists for a considerable time period (minimum 6 weeks) and for which careful diagnostic investigation has failed to demonstrate an allergic cause. Taking a detailed history usually reveals the dermatitis to be caused by repetitive contact with water, detergents, organic solvents, irritating food or other known mild or moderate irritants.

The prime localization is on the hands ('housewives' eczema'). In a fully developed case, redness, infiltration and scaling with fissuring is seen all

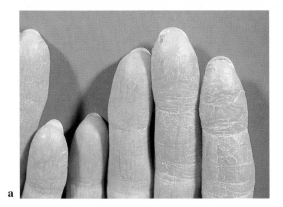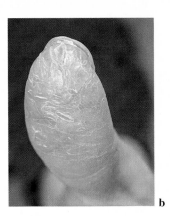

a   b

Fig. 2.2.11a, b. Chronic irritant contact dermatitis (cumulative insult dermatitis) **a** House-wives' eczema due to wet work and a number of irritants. **b** Close-up view of the thumb

over the hands (Fig. 2.2.11). The dermatitis includes the fingers, initially starting in the webs, but spreading later to the sides and backs of the hands and finally including the palmar aspect. The volar aspect of the wrist is usually unaffected, in contrast to allergic hand eczema. Occasionally, there is a nummular pattern on the backs of the hands. If there is extensive occupational contact with moderate irritants (organic solvents, detergents), the dermatitis may be limited to those fingers with most exposure. Friction is a further contributing factor and plays an important part in determining the localization of the dermatitis [44, 72, 73].

The hallmark of chronic irritant contact dermatitis may be the absence of vesicles and the predominance of dryness and chapping, and a number of studies on hand eczema have confirmed that vesiculation is less frequent in the irritant type than in allergic and atopic types [5, 6, 55, 71]. However, the diagnosis is often complicated by so-called hybrids, where there is a combination of irritancy and contact allergy, or of irritancy and atopy, or even all three [71, 86]. For further information see Chap. 8.

Dermatitis due to metalworking fluids is irritant in most cases and shows a variable morphological pattern. Some workers exhibit only dryness and scaling of the hands, whereas others develop an itchy nummular type of dermatitis spreading to the forearms and sometimes other exposed body regions. The correct diagnosis can often only be made after careful patch testing and reexposure to the work environment.

In atopic hand eczema, irritant factors often play a major role in the pathogenesis. It is sometimes a matter of definition whether these cases are diagnosed primarily as atopic or irritant contact dermatitis.

High-risk occupations for chronic irritant contact dermatitis are listed in Table 2.2.6, and the major irritants in various occupations are summarized in Table 2.2.7.

Table 2.2.6. High-risk occupations for chronic irritant (cumulative insult) contact dermatitis

Baker
Butcher
Canner
Caterer
Cleaner
Cook
Construction worker
Dental assistant or technician
Fisherman
Hairdresser
Horticulture and nursery gardening
Masseur
Metal worker
Motor mechanic
Nurse (hospitals and nursing homes for elderly)
Printer

Table 2.2.7. List of irritants in various occupations (based on [1, 14, 16, 28])

Agricultural workers	Pesticides, artificial fertilizers, disinfectants and cleansers for milking utensils, petrol, diesel oil, plants, animal secretions
Artists	Solvents used for cleansing and degreasing, soaps and detergents, paint removers
Bakers and pastry makers	Soaps and detergents, oven cleaners, fruit juices, acetic, ascorbic and lactic acids, spices, enzymes
Bartenders	Wet work, soaps and detergents, fruit juices, alcohol
Bathing attendants	Wet work, soaps and detergents, free or combined chlorine/bromine
Bookbinders	Glue, solvents
Building workers	Cement, chalk, hydrochloric and hydrofluoric acids, wood preservatives, glues
Butchers	Soaps and detergents, wet work, spices, meat, entrails
Canning and food industry workers	Soaps and detergents, wet work, brine, syrup, vegetables and vegetable juices, fruit and fruit juices, fish, meat, crustaceans
Carpenters, cabinet makers	French polish, solvents, glues, cleansers, wood preservatives
Chemical and pharmaceutical industry workers	Soaps and detergents, wet work, solvents, numerous other irritants that are specific for each work-place
Cleaners	Wet work, detergents, solvents
Coal and other miners	Oil, grease, cement, powdered limestone
Cooks, catering industry	Soaps and detergents, wet work, vegetable and fruit juices, spices, fish, meat, crustaceans, dressing, vinegar
Dentists and dental technicians	Soaps and detergents, wet work, soldering fluxes, adhesives, acrylic monomers, solvents

Table 2.2.7. (Continued)

Dyers	Solvents, oxidizing and reducing agents, hypochlorite, hair removers
Electricians, electronics industry	Soldering flux, metal cleaners, epoxy resin hardeners
Fishermen	Wet work, oils, petrol, fish, crustaceans, entrails
Floor layers	Detergents, solvents, cement, adhesives
Florists, gardeners, plant growers	Manure, fertilizers, pesticides, irritating plants and plant parts
Foundry workers	Cleansers, oils, phenol-formaldehyde, other resins
Hairdressers and barbers	Soap, wet work, shampoos, permanent wave liquids, bleaching agents
Histology technicians	Solvents, formaldehyde
Hospital workers	Soaps and detergents, wet work, hand creams, disinfectants, quaternary ammonium compounds
Housework	Soap and detergents, wet work, cleaners, polishes, food
Jewellers	Acids and alkalis for metal cleaning, polishes, soldering fluxes, rust removers, adhesives
Laundry workers	Detergents, wet work, bleaches, solvents, stain removers
Masons	Cement, chalk, acids
Mechanics	Detergents, hand cleansers, degreasers, lubricants, oils, cooling system fluids, battery acid, soldering flux
Metalworkers	Hand cleansers cutting and drilling oils solvents
Office workers	Ammonia from photocopy paper, carbonless copy paper
Painters	Solvents, emulsion paints, paint removers, organic tin compounds, hand cleansers
Photographers	Alkalis, acids, solvents, oxidizing and reducing agents
Plastics industry workers	Solvents, acids, oxidizing agents, styrene, diisocyanates, acrylic monomers, phenols, formaldehyde, diallyl phthalate, ingredients in epoxy resin systems
Plating industry workers	Acids, alkalis, solvents, detergents
Plumbers	Wet work, hand cleansers, oils, soldering flux
Printers	Solvents, hand cleansers, acrylates in radiation-curing printing lacquers and inks
Radio and television repairers	Organic solvents, metal cleansers, soldering fluxes
Roofers	Tar, pitch, asphalt, solvents, hand cleansers
Rubber workers	Talc, zinc stearate, solvents
Shoemakers	Solvents, polishes
Shop assistants	Detergents, vegetables, fruit, fish, meat
Tanners	Wet work, acids, alkalis, oxidizing and reducing agents, solvents, proteolytic enzymes
Textile workers	Solvents, bleaching agents, detergents
Veterinarians	Soaps and detergents, hypochlorite, cresol, entrails, animal secretions
Welders	Oils, metal cleansers, degreasing agents
Wood workers	Detergents, solvents, oils, wood preservatives

2.2.3 Epidemiology

Hard data on the incidence of irritant contact dermatitis are still very limited. In many studies on contact dermatitis no clear distinction is made between irritant and allergic types. The source population is also often either ill-defined or highly selected (patients attending a contact dermatitis clinic, for example), and cases of slight cutaneous irritation where medical attention is not sought are therefore missed. Four studies are, however, worth mentioning.

In a large multicentre prospective study on reactions caused by cosmetics, Eiermann et al. [22] found irritancy to account for 16% of 487 cases of contact dermatitis due to cosmetics. Over a time period of 40 months approximately 179800 patients were seen by 11 dermatologists and 8093 patients were tested for contact dermatitis. 487 cases (6%) were caused by cosmetics, the majority of them (407) being due to a contact allergy. The authors pointed out that during the course of the study irritation was more frequently diagnosed once the physicians had been mentally 'sensitized' to this type of reaction.

In Heidelberg, Germany, a retrospective study of 190 cases of hand dermatitis revealed the following distribution of diagnoses: atopic dermatitis 40%, chronic irritant contact dermatitis 27%, allergic contact dermatitis 23%, and various other diseases 10% [55]. The 50 patients with chronic irritant hand dermatitis (without clinical or laboratory signs of atopy) came from the typical high-risk occupations: housework, nursing, hairdressing and cleaning.

Bäurle and coworkers [5, 6] studied 683 patients with hand eczema in Erlangen, Germany. They considered 24.2% to suffer from chronic irritant contact dermatitis, 15.8% from allergic contact dermatitis and 38.5% from atopic hand dermatitis.

Meding [71] made an extensive study of hand eczema in Gothenburg, an industrial city in southern Sweden. After a questionnaire was sent out to 20000 inhabitants the point prevalence of hand eczema was determined to be 5.4% (1-year period prevalence 11%). Females outnumbered males by 2:1. The distribution of the three main diagnoses in her panel of 1585 patients who were investigated further was: 35% irritant contact dermatitis, 22% atopic hand dermatitis and 19% allergic contact dermatitis. The author pointed out that, due to careful clinical examination, a considerable number of mild cases of irritant contact dermatitis were recognized, hence the relatively high figure for irritant contact dermatitis. In this study the most harmful exposures turned out to be to 'unspecified chemicals', water, detergents, dust and dry dirt. For irritant contact dermatitis of the hand, a significantly higher period prevalence was found in people doing service work (15.4%; even higher in hairdressers), medical and nursing work and administrative work (11.8%). The lowest prevalence was found in female computer operators (3.2%).

Based on the clinical criteria used by dermatologists, slight chronic irritant contact dermatitis of the hands may affect nearly 100% of exposed persons in certain occupations such as food processing, fishing, hairdressing, construction, or veterinary medicine. In the metal industry at least 50% of dermatoses due to cutting oils are of the irritant type (see Sect. 11.16.1). Most workers do not seek medical attention because the effect is not serious and is accepted as 'normal' in that occupation.

2.2.4 Pathogenesis

A number of factors have now been identified as being involved in the pathogenesis of irritant contact dermatitis, particularly of the chronic cumulative type [25, 27, 42, 52, 62, 68, 85]. These can be divided into exogenous and endogenous factors (Table 2.2.8).

2.2.4.1 Exogenous Factors

Table 2.2.8 lists the numerous exogenous factors influencing the irritant response. These include the type of chemical, the mode of exposure, and the body site, but the most important are the inherent toxicity of the chemical for human skin and its penetration.

Agner et al. [3] have recently studied the penetration of sodium lauryl sulphate (SLS) into human skin using an in vitro model. Different formulations of SLS applied to the skin for 24 h (aqueous solution and gels) were studied, but irrespective of the vehicle used permeation of SLS into the recipient phase was poor. Results were compared to in vivo patch testing in 12 subjects. Approximately 70% of SLS applied in aqueous solution was released from the patch test system. Release from gels was poorer. Good agreement was found between the in vivo results and the in vitro model. No correlation was found between the amount of SLS left in the filter disc and the strength of the clinical reaction in vivo.

Apart from strong acids and alkalis, it is not possible to predict the irritant potential of a chemical on the basis of its molecular structure as, to a certain extent, can be done for contact allergens (Chap. 4). The pH is not strictly

Table 2.2.8. Exogenous and endogenous factors influencing the irritant response of human skin

Exogenous factors	Endogenous factors
Type of irritant (chemical structure, pH)	Individual susceptibility to irritant(s)
Amount of irritant penetrating (solubility, vehicle, concentration, method and time of application)	Primary hyperirritable ('sensitive') skin
Body site	Atopy (particularly atopic dermatitis)
Body temperature	Inability to develop hardening
Mechanical factors (pressure, friction, abrasion)	Secondary hyperirritability (status eczematicus)
Climatic conditions (temperature, humidity, wind)	Racial factors
	Age
	Sensitivity to UV light

correlated with irritancy, as studies with detergents, alkaline soaps and α-hydroxy acids have shown [32, 34, 97, 98].

The intensity of the resulting irritation depends greatly on the body region. The face and the postauricular and genital regions are particularly sensitive skin areas, a major reason being a reduced barrier and the abundance of 'holes' in the skin (sweat ducts and hair follicles) [26]. Figure 2.2.9 shows the large regional variation in reactivity to the solvent dimethylsulphoxide (DMSO), which causes toxic degranulation of mast cells [37]. Cua, et al. [17] studied the reactivity to SLS in ten body regions; the thigh had the highest sensitivity and the palm the lowest.

Important but frequently unrecognized cofactors of irritant reactions are mechanical, thermal and climatic influences. Rough sheets have produced facial dermatitis in babies, and rough table tops and paper have aggravated hand dermatitis in post office workers [18, 62, 73]. One detergent caused an epidemic in hospital kitchen workers, mainly because it was used at too high a temperature [88]. Cold windy climates produce drying of the skin due to the reduced capacity of the stratum corneum to retain water at lower temperatures. The condition is aggravated by frequent bathing or showering and the use of soaps and detergent bars. An eczema-like picture is seen in elderly persons. Atopic dermatitis is frequently aggravated by these climatic influences [53].

2.2.4.2 Endogenous Factors

Relevant endogenous factors include atopy and skin sensitivity. A number of studies from Scandinavia, such as those by Nilsson et al. [75], Rystedt [92] and Lammintausta and Kalimo [59], have confirmed the supposition of experienced clinicians that previous or current atopic dermatitis is a risk factor for the development of hand eczema in occupations involving wet work. Further confirmation came recently from a large study of 1600 hand eczema patients in Erlangen, Germany [5, 6]. It is important to point out that, on the basis of these studies, persons with a history of hay fever and/or bronchial asthma do not show a markedly increased risk of developing hand eczema in comparison to nonatopic controls. However, in Meding's study [71] there was a statistically significant but weak correlation between hand eczema and atopic mucosal symptoms.

Persons with atopic dermatitis in childhood often have dry skin for the rest of their lives. Histologically, dry skin shows some similarities to subclinical eczema. Clinically, overt irritation may therefore be precipitated more easily by a number of irritant factors.

2.2.4.3 Sensitive (Hyperirritable) Skin

Individuals with sensitive, hyperirritable skin do exist. This may be due to a genetic predisposition, independent of atopy. Racial differences in cutaneous irritability have been well documented [29, 37, 101, 102]. Blacks in general have less irritable skin than whites of northern (Celtic) extraction. In two recent studies this view has been challenged. Using noninvasive techniques such as TEWL measurements a higher susceptibility to SLS has been found in blacks compared to whites [9]. Similarly a greater sensitivity to SLS was reported in hispanic skin than in white skin [10]. It has been shown that subjects with light skin complexions (types 1 and 2) not only have high UVB sensitivity but also skin that is hyperirritable to chemicals in general [36]. Hyperirritable skin can also develop secondarily during the course of hand or leg eczema. Status eczematicus and 'angry back syndrome' fall into this category.

The cause of hyperirritable skin is still unknown. There is good evidence so far that a thin and/or permeable stratum corneum plays a key role. Based on Fick's law for penetration, the thickness of the stratum corneum influences the flux of the penetrating chemical. Weigand et al. [102] have shown that the stratum corneum of blacks has more cell layers on average than that of whites. This group also found that the buoyant density of black stratum corneum was higher, which may indicate a more compact barrier. Marks' group was able to demonstrate a relationship between the minimal irritancy dose for dithranol and the mean corneocyte surface area: the smaller the corneocyte area, the lower the irritancy threshold [45]. They also found a positive correlation between the minimal blistering time with ammonium hydroxide and the skin surface contour. This was also true for other irritants.

Regional variations in irritability are related to differences in keratinization and to the density of transepidermal shunts allowing penetration (sweat ducts, hair follicles). The intercellular lipids of the stratum corneum play an important part in the barrier function of the skin, as has been shown by a number of investigators [21, 23, 24, 63, 103]. Based on recent reports, it seems that the ceramides and glycosylceramides may be the key elements in storage of water in the stratum corneum. In animals fed a diet free of essential fatty acids, administering linoleic acid either topically or systemically has been shown to improve the stratum corneum barrier [19]. There is also some clinical evidence that this may have an effect in humans [83], but initial therapeutic trials with linoleic acid or ceramide-containing medicaments in atopic eczema and dry skin have not been very encouraging [7].

Individuals with hyperirritable skin are also more reactive when tested on scarified or stripped skin, i.e. after removal of the stratum corneum, the major rate limiting factor for penetration [108]. This is also the basis for the assumption that these individuals may release more inflammatory mediators or may be more reactive to them in comparison to normal or hyporeactive skin.

Recently, using noninvasive bioengineering methods, it has been possible to demonstrate that female skin is more reactive to the anionic detergent SLS in the premenstrual phase than in the remaining menstrual cycle [3]. In general, however, females do not seem to have more sensitive skin than males [11, 29, 60]. Rather, it is assumed that females are exposed more frequently to potential irritants than males (household products, cosmetics) and are therefore more prone to develop irritant contact dermatitis, of both acute and chronic types.

Cutaneous irritability is influenced by age. In one study, susceptibility to detergents was found to increase with age, whereas the pustulogenic effect of croton oil decreased [15]. The same group found no difference with the irritants thymoquinone and croton aldehyde. In another study with SLS the old age group showed significantly less reactivity than young adults [17]. This was quantified by visual scoring and measurements of TEWL. TEWL in the elderly is usually lower than in the young, which might be related to a better stratum corneum barrier against water [105]. There is now increasing evidence that for several compounds the percutaneous penetration in the old age group is less than in the young one [87, 89]. The phenomenon of 'hardening' has been little studied, despite its common occurrence in many occupations. The skin becomes slightly erythematous and hyperkeratotic from daily contact with a mild irritant, and high concentrations of the irritant can then be tolerated. If the hardening stimulus stops, the skin shows desquamation and reactivity returns to its previous level. Hardening can be induced by SLS. It seems to be an irritant-specific phenomenon because the reactivity to other irritants may even be increased [70].

2.2.5 Diagnostic Tests

The diagnostic tests used to quantify a patient's susceptibility to irritants are (see [33, 29, 36]):
- Alkali resistance (sodium hydroxide)
- Ammonium hydroxide
- Dimethylsulphoxide
- Threshold response to various irritants (sodium lauryl sulphate, benzalkonium chloride, kerosene, croton oil, anthralin)
- Lactic acid stinging
- Minimal erythema dose of UVB light
- Measurement of baseline TEWL

None is really so simple and reliable that it can be used clinically on a large scale, and the diagnostic value of the older tests such as Burckhardt's alkali resistance test has been overestimated, particularly in regard to their capacity to distinguish between allergic and irritant eczema. The diagnostic methods listed, however, are very useful in determining threshold responses to various irritants. Subjects with increased reactivity to one or more irritants can be identified and various influences such as the effect of repeated UVB exposure, the cumulative effects of mild irritants, or the protective effects of 'barrier' creams can be quantified. Using these techniques, Frosch [29] demonstrated that in a normal population with healthy skin the proportion of subjects with hyperirritable skin was 14%; 25% were regarded as 'hypoirritable' and 61% as 'normal'. The distinction between the three groups was made by use of cluster analysis, a statistical method which can compare and validate a number of criteria in one subject. Although some individuals seem to have hyperirritable skin *per se*, one finds that the correlation between some irritants is rather weak if a large number of irritants of very different chemical structure are used. In one study, we found a good correlation between the responses to sodium hydroxide, ammonium hydroxide and water-soluble irritants, but a very weak and nonsignificant one between SLS and lipid-soluble irritants such as croton oil and kerosene [36]. As early as 1968, Björnberg showed that one may not necessarily be able to predict the reactivity to one irritant on the basis of reactivity to another irritant [11].

The measurement of the baseline TEWL may be a useful indicator of reactivity to irritants. After 3 weeks treatment with SLS, TEWL showed significant linear correlation with pretreatment TEWL values [107]. This supported an earlier study [81]. However, when a single 24-h occlusive SLS application was employed, no correlation was found [104].

2.2.6 Action of Irritants

Irritants may affect the skin in various ways. Table 2.2.9 lists some targets of major irritants. Detergents have a very broad spectrum of attack. At low doses they primarily affect the horny layer and produce drying and scaling, while at higher doses they dissolve membranes of cells and lysosomes [50]. If applied repeatedly at low doses, signs of chronic inflammation develop, with acanthosis, increased DNA synthesis and changes in cellular metabolism [82, 84]. It has been shown that SLS, and anionic detergent, and Hyamine 3500, a cationic detergent, are chemokinetic as well as chemotactic for polymorphonuclear leucocytes [31]. The motility of these cells is activated at low, nontoxic concentrations and they show a directional response towards the detergents at higher but still nontoxic doses. Marked individual differences were noted in this study, neutrophils from some donors barely reacting to the detergents and others showing a very strong response.

Organic solvents such as methanol or chloroform attack the blood vessels directly by causing hyperaemia [96]. Some irritants such as croton oil stimulate the migratory activity of polymorphonuclear leucocytes [43]. The phorbol esters have been shown to be potent chemotactic attractants [46,

Table 2.2.9. Cellular targets of various irritants (from [29, 82])

Horny layer	Detergents, NaOH, DMSO
Cellular membranes	Detergents
DNA synthesis	Detergents, tretinoin
Epidermal metabolism	Detergents, tributyltin
Blood vessels	Organic solvents
Leucocytes	Croton oil, xylene, detergents
Mast cells	DMSO

77]. Dimethylsulphoxide (DMSO) is a very effective degranulator of mast cells [37]. Imokawa's group and others [47, 84] have shown that detergents cause scaling of the skin by destroying the lysosomal enzymes in the uppermost horny layer. Keratohyaline granules release acid phosphatase. Kunkel [56] recently developed a new assay using superficial stratum corneum biopsies to evaluate the damage to corneocytes both morphologically and by measuring the acid phosphatase. The visible damage caused by detergents depends on the concentration and on the time of incubation. With SLS 2.5% for 24 h, marked destruction of corneocytes was evident in most subjects. Alkylbenzene sulphonate and alkylether sulphate are also active in this assay. Marked individual differences in resistance to a group of detergents was found. Patients with atopic dermatitis reacted significantly more to SLS than subjects with normal skin. The measurement of acid phosphatase using a fluorescent technique based on umbellipherol phosphate may have a potential for distinguishing between chemicals with high, moderate, and low capacities for damaging human stratum corneum.

2.2.7 Inflammatory Mediators

The histological appearance in contact dermatitis is of a mononuclear inflammation consisting of lymphocytes and some monocytes. This arises through selective mechanisms including expression of adherence molecules on endothelial. cells and gradients of mediators responsible for the specific attraction of the mononuclear cells.

Several mediators have been studied in contact dermatitis. Histamine is present, but not in increased amounts. Mast cell activation has been studied in allergic patch tests by estimating tryptase release into suction blister fluid 6 and 24 h after allergen application, but the level was within normal limits [19]. Further studies are needed, however, especially for irritant reactions and contact urticarial disorders.

Prostaglandins can be detected in suction blister fluid 48 h after injection of relevant antigens, but the amount is the same as after injection of physiological saline. Injection of an irritant, 0.05% benzethonium chloride, induced significant increases of prostaglandin I_2, thromboxane B_2, and prostaglandin $F_2\alpha$ [93].

The importance of leukotrienes for contact dermatitis is controversial. Some of the effects of leukotriene B_4, such as chemotaxis of neutrophils, are not prominent features of contact dermatitis, and leukotriene B_4 has been found in low levels in some, but not all, positive patch tests [8].

However, leukotriene B_4 can attract certain lymphocytes, it can augment interleukin-1, interferon-γ and prostaglandin release from monocytes, and it can, by stimulating CD8$^+$ T cells, also induce suppression of these factors. Thus, it may be important for both augmentation and inhibition of contact reactions.

Other mediators like lactoferrin, myeloperoxidase, lysozyme and eosinophil cationic protein have also been studied in allergic reactions using a skin window technique. This technique, however, produces an accumulation of neutrophils and not lymphocytes. It seems that nickel exposure in nickel-allergic patients leads to a slighly increased level of the mediators mentioned above [67].

Recent interest has concentrated on cytokines. The term 'cytokine' is used to refer to a heterogeneous group of short-range, cell-derived peptides which can be released from a variety of nucleated cells and influence the function, growth or differentiation of other cells. The induction and release of cytokines is regulated in a cascade reaction, i.e. certain signals induce production of certain cytokines, which then induce other cytokines. These signals include bacterial products like lipopolysaccharide or serine proteases from *Staphylococcus aureus*, mitogens and UV light, as well as antigen stimulation.

It is highly likely that skin irritation also induces cytokine expression. They are found in many inflammatory disorders and so are probably not of primary aetiological importance, but the strength of an inflammatory response may be significantly influenced by cytokines. It is possible that the quantitative regulation, i.e. transcription of DNA and the release of cytokines, determines whether an inflammatory response is started or not, because apart from their immunostimulating activity, cytokines also induce expression of adherence molecules enabling cells to enter the area [48].

Interferon-γ induces the expression of class I and II antigens and ICAM-1 (intercellular adhesion molecule 1), which is responsible for the adhesion between endothelial cells, keratinocytes and T lymphocytes [74]. Addition of as little as 0.04 U/ml of affinity-purified human interleukin-1 to human umbilical endothelial cells increases the binding of both human B and T lymphocytes by a factor of approximately 2, and this is due to the enhanced expression of adherence molecules and is a first step in lymphocyte migration.

Recent studies have shown that interleukin-1 is increased three-fold in epidermis overlying a positive allergic patch test [64], but not an irritant skin reaction [65]. Time-course studies have revealed that the increase in interleukin-1 is seen as early as 6 h after application of allergen at a time when the clinical reaction is not present [54]. Epidermal homogenate contains an activity which specifically attracts T lymphocytes of the CD4$^+$ subset [66, 110].

This activity is not present in normal nontested skin from healthy persons, but it is increased in both positive patch tests to allergen and to 3% SLS [65]. It can also be detected in nontested healthy skin of patients with an ongoing eczematous reaction (excited skin). The nature of this activity remains to be determined, but preliminary results have shown that it can partly be inhibited using anti-interleukin-8 antibodies (Zachariae et al., unpublished). Other possible mediators should also be considered, however. The fact that the activity is obtained using suction blister homogenate makes it likely, although not proven, that it stems from epidermal cells.

Nickel-positive patients and patients tested with SLS showed expression of interleukin-6, but not of tumour necrosis factor-α (TNF-α), in both allergic and irritant patch tests [78]. Recently, interesting findings were reported using a microsurgery technique for the draining superficial lymph vessel. After induction of an irritant contact dermatitis with SLS a large increase in Langerhans' cells was observed [12a]. In parallel with the clinical symptoms of the dermatitis the levels of the cytokine IL-6 and TNF-α increased 8- to 10-fold, whereas for IL-1β, IL-2, IL-2 receptors and GM-CSF there was a delayed, 2- to 3-fold increase [45a]. Irritant contact dermatitis still needs extensive studies in order to obtain more firm knowledge about the pathophysiological mechanisms involved. The development of new techniques, especially in situ hybridization, will together with time-course studies hopefully lead to a better insight into the important mechanisms, and thereby open ways for new treatment modalities.

Maibach's group [80] has performed a number of elegant experiments in animals using various inhibitors of inflammatory mediators such as antihistamines (cimetidine, mepyramine maleate), 5-hydroxytryptamine antagonists (methysergide maleate), inhibitors of prostaglandin synthesis (indomethacin) and kinins (aprotinin), complement-depleting agents (cobra venom factor) and neutropenia-inducing agents (mechlorethamine). They showed that these had very different effects on the responses to three irritants, ethyl phenylpropiolate, croton oil and methyl salicylate. Recently, the same group demonstrated using this model that there are important species-specific differences. It can be assumed that in humans such differences might account for the marked racial and interindividual variations.

2.2.8 Quantification of the Irritant Response

A very worthwile approach in studying cutaneous toxicity is the use of noninvasive methods to quantify the irritant response. Many groups are now using evaporimeters to measure transepidermal water loss (TEWL) [81, 97], and the Periflux laser flowmeter can quantify blood flow using the Doppler principle [12, 76, 99, 100]. Both techniques are quite sensitive and measurements can be made in minutes without damaging the skin or requiring a biopsy.

Limitations of these instruments have been demonstrated, however: very high rates of TEWL, as well as very intense hyperaemia due to venous stasis, may be evaluated inaccurately by these instruments. Despite this, they are very useful in attempts to measure objectively the degree of skin damage, and have been successfully used to measure the toxic effects of surfactants and organic solvents. Recently, the atrophogenicity of corticosteroids and the protective function of barrier creams have also been assessed [30, 49].

The combined measurement of TEWL and blood flow seems to allow allergic and irritant reactions to be differentiated. When weak or doubtful allergic reactions were compared with clinically similar irritant reactions we found that in most irritant reactions there was a relatively large increase in TEWL with little or no change in blood flow. By contrast, in weak allergic reactions there was no change in TEWL but a relatively large increase in blood flow [94].

Lammintausta et al. [61] have shown that subjects with increased susceptibility to stinging have more vulnerable skin. After applying various irritants they found a greater increase in blood flow and TEWL in 'stingers' than in 'nonstingers'. These differences in cutaneous reactivity were not detected on clinical examination. This supports the view that the measurement of skin functions is worthwhile and should be promoted in future studies.

Studying the dose-response relationship for SLS in humans, Agner and Serup [2] found measurement of TEWL to be the method best suited overall for quantification of patch test results, whereas colorimetry was found to be the least sensitive of the methods tested. Wilhelm et al. [106] quantified the cutaneous response to 6 concentrations of SLS using visual scores, skin color reflectance, TEWL and laser Doppler flow (LDF) measurements. All noninvasive techniques were more sensitive than the human eye in detecting irritation to the lowest concentration of SLS (0.125%). TEWL showed the highest discriminating power and the best correlation with visual scores. Change in total color (ΔE^*) correlated better than redness (Δa^*) to the SLS dose applied and to visual score, whereas Δa^* correlated better with TEWL and with LDF than ΔE^*.

Ultrasound A-mode scanning was found to be a promising method for quantification of the inflammatory response, being consistently more sensitive than measurement of skin colour. Wahlberg has successfully used the laser Doppler flow technique in assessing the irritant response to organic solvents [100], and van der Valk and coworkers [97, 98] have used evaporimetry in a series of studies quantifying the irritant potential of various detergents. Pinnagoda et al. [81] have described a repetitive exposure test for 3 weeks on human forearm skin using SLS. Baseline TEWL before exposure to the irritant correlated with the resulting cumulative irritancy caused by the detergent. The authors concluded that baseline TEWL may be a valuable predictor of cutaneous irritability. Further studies are needed to confirm this idea (see also Sect. 10.7).

2.2.9 Therapy and Prevention

In the acute stage of irritant contact dermatitis topical corticosteroids are indicated. If there is deep tissue destruction or signs of bacterial infection, systemic corticosteroids and antimicrobial agents should be administered.

In all cases of chronic irritant contact dermatitis a systematic approach on a wide front must be undertaken. Potential irritants in the work and home environments must be identified and, whenever possible, eliminated (replacement by other less irritant substances, reduction of exposure, use of protective gloves, etc.). Skin cleansing should be as mild as possible (liquid detergents based on alkylether sulphates or sulphosuccinate esters, avoiding organic solvents and hard brushes or other abrasives), and regular application of bland emollients to counteract desiccation should be encouraged [53]. The use of barrier creams is still controversial (see Sect. 17.3.2) Few well-controlled clinical studies have been conducted (for review [38]). In a model called the *repetitive irritation test*

(RIT), designed for guinea pigs as well as for human volunteers, Frosch and coworkers [35, 39–41] were able to demonstrate large differences in efficacy among commercial products. While some were quite effective in suppressing the irritation of SLS, sodium hydroxide and lactic acid, others were not or even aggravated the irritation. Long-term administration of potent corticosteroids is dangerous because of the risk of atrophy and further impairment of the stratum corneum [30].

If all measures fail, the diagnosis of an irritant contact dermatitis must be reevaluated: atopy may be the dominant cause or contact allergy (e.g. to preservatives or fragrances in hand creams) may be preventing recovery. As chronic irritant contact dermatitis is commonly a multifactorial disease, psychological factors and lack of compliance by the patient must also be kept in mind.

2.2.10 Subjective Reactions to Irritants ('Stinging')

While the subjective hallmark of allergic cutaneous reactions is an often unbearable pruritus, many irritants cause painful sensations described as burning, stinging or smarting. We may distinguish two types of reactions regarding the time course: 1. immediate-type stinging, and 2. delayed-type stinging.

2.2.10.1 Immediate-Type Stinging

A few chemicals cause painful sensations within seconds of contact with normal intact skin. Best known is a mixture of chloroform and methanol (1:1). Depending on the body region and, to some extent, on individual susceptibility, a sharp pain develops within a few seconds or a few minutes of exposure. This phenomenon has been used for assessment of the cutaneous barrier, which mainly resides in the stratum corneum [29, 51]. On the volar forearm of healthy white subjects, discomfort is experienced after an average exposure time of 47 s (range 13–102 s). The irritant mixture is applied in abundant quantity in a small plastic cup (8 mm diameter). Regional differences in sensitivity can be easily documented (mastoid region – upper back – forearm – palmar region; in order of decreasing sensitivity). Once they have started, subjective reactions to chloroform: methanol increase in intensity within seconds to such an extent that the irritant must be removed in order to avoid torturing the subject. The pain abates quickly, with some individual differences. In most cases only faint erythema is visible for a short duration. Rarely, superficial necrosis of the epidermis is seen in 'tough' subjects who endure the pain for a longer exposure of several minutes.

Undiluted ethanol (95%) causes a short-lasting sharp stinging sensation in most individuals in sensitive skin regions (face, neck, genital area). If the skin has slight abrasions, e.g. due to shaving, this phenomenon is experienced by everybody. The immediate type of stinging can also be observed with strong caustic chemicals, primarily acids in irritant concentrations. Typical of these agents is that severe cutaneous damage is nearly always associated with the subjective reaction. The latter is the warning signal of imminent somatic destruction if exposure is continued.

2.2.10.2 Delayed-Type Stinging

When a sunscreen containing amyldimethyl-p-aminobenzoic acid (ADP, Padimate) was marketed on a wide scale in Florida, many users experienced disagreeable stinging or burning after application. The discomfort usually occurred 1 or 2 min after application and intensified over the next 5–10 min. Attempts to remove the sunscreen by washing brought no relief. The pain slowly abated over the next half hour. Objective signs of irritation did not develop. The condition was primarily experienced on the face after sweating and contact with salt water [79].

This is a typical example of the phenomenon of delayed-type stinging, which can be induced by a number of substances. Frosch and Kligman [32] were the first to study this systematically on human skin. The key observation was that this type of discomfort is not experienced by everybody but only by certain 'stingers'. A panel of subjects can be screened for stingers by the application of 5% aqueous lactic acid to the nasolabial fold after induction of profuse sweating in a sauna. Stinging is scored on an intensity scale of 0–3 (severe) at 10 s, 2.5 min, 5 min and 8 min. A subject is regarded a stinger if he or she complains of severe (3+) discomfort between 2.5 and 8 min.

In the *stinging assay* the material to be evaluated is applied to the cheek of preselected sensitive subjects after intensive sweating has been induced. The stinging score of a material is the mean score of three readings taken at 2.5, 5.0 and 8.0 min. Substances with average scores falling between 0.4 and 1.0 are arbitrarily regarded as having 'slight' stinging potential, the range 1.1–2.0 signifies 'moderate' stinging, and the range 2.1–3.0 indicates 'severe' stinging. The immediate and, in most cases, transient type of stinging is identified by questioning the subject 10 s after application of the material. Thus, the subjective tolerance of a cosmetic or topical drug can be evaluated under exaggerated test conditions on subjects with increased sensitivity.

Although a very subjective and seemingly unreliable method, this stinging assay has stood the test of time and proven valuable in screening various agents for subjective discomfort. The existence of the stinging phenomenon was, however, frequently disputed because signs of objective irritation are missing and there is no method of validation. In Table 2.2.11 are listed several substances with which this phenomenon has been observed for years. Among them are the sunscreens ADP and 2-ethoxyethyl-p-methoxycinnamate, the insect repellent N, N-diethyltoluamide, the solvent propylene glycol (undiluted), and dermatological therapeutics such as phenol, salicylic acid, aluminium chloride, benzoyl peroxide and crude coal tar. The intensity of stinging depends on the concentration of the agent and its vehicle. For further details the reader is referred to the original publication and to a recent update [32, 95].

Based on extensive experience with this test, Soschin and Kligman [95] found the classification of a substance to be more reliable if the cumulative score in a 12-member panel is used:

<10   insignificant stinging potential in normal use

11–24   modest stinging potential, creating a problem for persons with sensitive skin

>25   definite stinging potential, certain to be troublesome

These authors confirmed that stingers have a higher susceptibility to a number of diverse chemical irritants and have a history of 'sensitive' skin due to reactions to toiletries and cosmetics. Stingers also usually suffer from generalized dry skin in winter time, and persons with a past history of atopic dermatitis of the face usually sting severely.

The eye area is the most sensitive portion of the entire face. Certain eye-shadows may pass the stinging test on the nasolabial fold but produce subjective discomfort upon regular use. Therefore, eye cosmetics should be tested in this region to assure optimal compatibility.

2.2.10.3 Pathogenesis of Stinging and Influencing Factors

The pathogenesis of the stinging phenomenon is still uncertain, although it clearly involves excitation of sensory nerve endings. These being more abundant around hair follicles may explain why the stinging threshold is lowest on the face, particularly on the cheek and nasolabial fold. Sweating and increase in body temperature might further enhance penetration of the sting-inducing agent.

Initially it was thought that stingers were primarily females with a fair complexion and very sensitive (hyperirritable) skin. Further experience on larger panels of subjects failed to confirm this in regard to the fair complexion: dark-skinned individuals can be stingers, too. However, a recent study by Lammintausta et al. provided evidence that hyperirritability is associated with the stinging phenomenon [61]. The repeated application of the anionic detergent SLS to the skin of the upper back damaged the stratum corneum barrier in stingers more than in nonstingers. This was quantified by visual scoring and measurements of TEWL. Furthermore, in the facial region of stingers lactic acid produced an increase in blood flow recognized by the laser Doppler technique but not with the naked eye. Subjects who did not experience stinging with lactic acid showed less or no change in blood flow.

Blacks develop stinging less frequently than whites. This is Frosch and Kligman's experience as well as that of Weigand and Mershon [101] when evaluating the tear gas o-chlorobenzylidene malononitrile.

Table 2.2.10. Agents causing subjective reactions of the skin in the form of stinging or burning (from [32])

	Concen-tration	Vehicle
Immediate-type stinging		
Chloroform	50%	ethanol
Methanol	100%	
Ethanol (primarily on abraded skin)	100%	
Strong acids		
Hydrochloric acid	1%	water
Trichloracetic acid	5%	water
Weak acids		
Ascorbic, acetic, citric and sorbic acids	5%	water
Retinoic acid	0.05%	ethanol
Delayed-type stinging		
Slight stinging		
Benzene	1%	ethanol
Phenol	1%	ethanol
Salicylic acid	5%	ethanol
Resorcinol	5%	water
Phosphoric acid	1%	water
Aluminium chloride	30%	water
Zirconium hydroxychloride	30%	water
Moderate stinging		
Sodium carbonate	15%	water
Trisodium phosphate	5%	water
Propylene glycol	100%	
Propylene carbonate	100%	
Propylene glycol diacetate	100%	
Dimethylacetamide	100%	
Dimethylformamide	100%	
Dimethylsulphoxide	100%	
Diethyltoluamide (Deet)	50%	ethanol
Dimethyl phthalate	50%	ethanol
2-Ethyl-1,3-hexanediol (Rutgers 612)	50%	ethanol
Benzoyl peroxide	5%	greasefree washable lotion base
Severe stinging		
Crude coal tar	5%	dimethylformamide
Lactic acid	5%	water
Phosphoric acid	3,3%	water
Hydrochloric acid	1.2%	water
Sodium hydroxide	1.3%	water
Amyldimethyl-*p*-aminobenzoic acid (Escalol 506)	5%	ethanol
2-Ethoxyethyl-*p*-methoxy-cinnamate (Giv-Tan FR)	2%	ethanol

The *immediate type of stinging* develops after short exposure (seconds or minutes) and abates quickly after removal of the irritant. The *delayed type of stinging* builds up over a certain time period, does not disappear quickly after removal of the causative agent, and is experienced only by predisposed individuals ('stingers').

A set of experiments has elucidated further factors influencing delayed-type stinging [32]. They can be summarized as follows:
- Stinging is markedly reduced after inhibition of sweating.
- Prior damage to the skin increases stinging (sunburn, tape stripping, chemical irritation by detergents).
- The intensity of stinging is dose-dependent with regard to concentration and frequency of application.
- The vehicle plays an important role (solutions in ethanol or propylene glycol are more effective than fatty ointments).
- There are marked regional differences: the intensity of stinging decreases in the order nasolabial fold > cheek > chin > retroauricular region > forehead; scalp, back and arm are virtually unreactive in respect of stinging.

The correlation of stinging with irritancy is inconsistent. With the α-hydroxy acids a positive correlation was found (pyruvic > glycolic > tartaric > lactic acid) [32]. pH did not account for the differences in either stinging or irritancy. Laden [58] also found that acids of the same pH could have quite different stinging capacities. The esters of p-aminobenzoic acid are examples of divergent action with regard to irritancy and stinging. A stinging ester such as ADP was found to be nonirritating on scarified skin, while an irritating one (glyceryl-p-aminobenzoic acid) was nonstinging.

Strong irritants (undiluted kerosene, benzalkonium chloride) may cause severe blistering reactions if applied under occlusion for 24 h, and yet they do not induce delayed- or immediate-type stinging.

In summary, our knowledge about the stinging phenomenon is still very limited. It undoubtedly exists and causes considerable discomfort in affected persons. They may as a result discontinue the use of a cosmetic or a medicament prescribed by a dermatologist.

Acknowledgement The section on inflammatory mediators (Sect. 2.2.7) was prepared with the help of Professor K. Thestrup-Pedersen, Aarhus. Dr. K.-P. Wilhelm, Lübeck, provided helpful comments for the revision of this chapter for the second edition.

The photographs of this chapter and of others provided by the author (P.J.F.) are mainly from the collection of the Department of Dermatology, University of Heidelberg (Head: Prof. Dr. D. Petzoldt). The skillful technical assistance of S. Preussmann and S. Kaute is gratefully acknowledged.

2.2.11 References

1. Adams R (1990) Occupational skin diseases, 2nd edn. Saunders, Philadelphia
2. Agner T, Serup J (1990) Sodium lauryl sulphate for irritant patch testing – a dose-response study using bioengineering methods for determination of skin irritation. J Invest Dermatol 95: 543–547
3. Agner T, Fullerton A, Broby-Johnson U, Batsberg W (1990) Irritant patch testing: penetration of sodium lauryl sulphate into human skin. Skin Pharmacol 3: 213–217

4. Agner T, Damm P, Skouby SO (1991) Menstrual cycle an skin reactivity. J Am Acad Dermatol 24: 566–570
5. Bäurle G (1986) Handekzeme. Studie zum Einfluß von konstitutionellen und Umweltfaktoren auf die Genese. Schattauer, Stuttgart
6. Bäurle G, Hornstein OP, Diepgen TL (1985) Professionelle Handekzeme und Atopie. Dermatosen 33: 161–165
7. Bamford JTM, Gibson RW, Renier CM (1985) Atopic eczema unresponsive to evening primrose oil (linoleic and gammalinolenic acids). J Am Acad Dermatol 13: 959–965
8. Barr RM, Brain SC, Camp RD, Cilliers J, Greawes MW, Mallet AI, Misch K (1984) Levels of arachidonic acid and its metabolites in the skin in human allergic and irritant contact dermatitis. Br J Dermatol, 111: 23–28
9. Berardesca E, Maibach HI (1988) Racial differences in sodium lauryl sulphate induced cutaneous irritation: black and white. Contact Dermatitis 18: 65–70
10. Berardesca E, Maibach HI (1988) Sodium-lauryl-sulphate-induced cutaneous irritation: comparison of white and hispanic subjects. Contact Dermatitis 19: 136–140
11. Björnberg A (1968) Skin reactions to primary irritants in patients with hand eczema. Isacsons, Göteborg
12. Blanken R, van der Valk PGM, Nater JP (1986) Laser-Doppler flowmetry in the investigation of irritant compounds on human skin. Dermatosen 34: 5–9
12a. Brand CU, Hunziker T, Limat A, Braathen LR (1993) Large increase of Langerhans cells in human skin lymph derived from irritant contact dermatitis. Br J Dermatol 128: 184–188
13. Bruynzeel DP, van Ketel WG, Scheper RJ, von Blomberg-van der Feier BME (1982) Delayed time course of irritation by sodium lauryl sulfate: observations on threshold reactions. Contact Dermatitis 8: 236–239
14. Bruze M, Emmett EA (1990) Occupational exposures to irritants. In: Jackson EM, Goldner R (eds) Irritant contact dermatitis. Dekker, New York, pp 81–106
15. Coenraads PJ, Bleumink E, Nater JP (1975) Susceptibility to primary irritants. Age dependance and relation of contact allergic reactions. Contact Dermatitis 1: 177–181
16. Cronin E (1980) Contact dermatitis. Churchill Livingston, Edinburgh
17. Cua AB, Wilhelm KP, Maibach HI (1990) Cutaneous sodium lauryl sulfate irritation potential: age and regional variability. Br J Dermatol 123: 607–613
18. Dahlquist I, Fregert S (1979) Skin irritation in newborns. Contact Dermatitis 5: 336–337
19. Deleuran B, Kristensen M, Larsen CG, Matsson P, Enander I, Andersson AS, Thestrup-Pedersen K (1991) Increased tryptase levels in suction blister fluid from patients with urticaria. Br J Dermatol 125: 14–17
20. Dooms-Goossens AE, Debusschere KM, Gevers DM et al. (1986) Contact dermatitis caused by airborne agents. J Am Acad Dermatol 15: 1–10
21. Downing DT, Stewart ME, Wertz PW, Colton SW, Abraham W, Strauss JS (1987) Skin lipids: an update. J Invest Dermatol 88: 2s–62
22. Eiermann HJ, Larsen W, Maibach HI, Taylor JS (1982) Prospective study of cosmetic reactions: 1977–1980. J Am Acad Dermatol 6: 909–917
23. Elias PM (1985) The essential fatty acid deficient rodent: evidence for a direct role for intercellular lipid in barrier function. Maibach HI, Lowe N (eds) Models in dermatology, vol 1. Karger, Basel, pp 272–285
24. Elias PM, Brown BE, Zoboh VA (1980) The permeability barrier in essential fatty acid deficiency: evidence for a direct role for linoleic acid in barrier function. J Invest Dermatol 74: 230–233
25. Epstein WL (1990) House and garden plants. In: Jackson EM, Goldner R (eds) Irritant contact dermatitis. Dekker, New York, pp 127–165
26. Feldman RJ, Maibach HI (1967) Regional variations in percutaneous absorption of 14 C cortisol in man. J Invest Dermatol 48: 181–185

27. Fleming MG, Bergfeld WF (1990) The etiology of irritant contact dermatitis. In: Jackson EM, Goldner R (eds) Irritant contact dermatitis. Dekker, New York, pp 41–66
28. Fregert S (1981) Manual of contact dermatitis, 2nd edn. Munksgaard, Copenhagen
29. Frosch P (1985) Hautirritation und empfindliche Haut. Grosse, Berlin
30. Frosch PJ (1985) Human models for quantification of corticosteroid adverse effects. In: Maibach HI, Lowe NJ (eds) Models in dermatology, vol 2. Karger, Basel, pp 5–15
31. Frosch PJ, Czarnetzki BM (1987) Surfactants cause in vitro chemotaxis and chemokinesis of human neutrophils. J Invest Dermatol 88: 52s–55s
32. Frosch PJ, Kligman AM (1977) A method for appraising the stinging capacity of topically applied substances. J Soc Cosmet Chem 28: 197–209
33. Frosch PJ, Kligman AM (1977) Rapid blister formation in human skin with ammonium hydroxide. Br J Dermatol 96: 461–473
34. Frosch PJ, Kligman AM (1979) The soap chamber test: a new method for assessing the irritancy of soaps. J Am Acad Dermatol 1: 35–41
35. Frosch PJ, Kurte A (1994) Efficacy of skin barrier creams. IV. The repetitive irritation test (RIT) with a set of four standard irritants. Contact Dermatitis 31: 161–168
36. Frosch PJ, Wissing C (1982) Cutaneous sensitivity to ultraviolet light and chemical irritants. Arch Dermatol Res 272: 269–278
37. Frosch PJ, Duncan S, Kligman AM (1980) Cutaneous biometrics I: the DMSO test. Br J Dermatol 102: 263–274
38. Frosch PJ, Kurte A, Pilz B (1993) Biophysical techniques for the evaluation of skin protective creams. In: Frosch PJ, Kligman AM (eds) Noninvasive methods for the quantification of skin functions. Springer, Berlin Heidelberg New York, pp 214–222
39. Frosch PJ, Schulze-Dirks A, Hoffmann M, Axthelm I, Kurte A (1993) Efficacy of skin barrier creams. I. The repititive irritation test (RIT) in the guinea pig. Contact Dermatitis 28: 94–100
40. Frosch PJ, Schulze-Dirks A, Hoffmann M, Axthelm I (1993) Efficacy of skin barrier creams. II. Ineffectiveness of a popular "skin protector" against various irritants in the repetitive irritation test in the guinea pig. Contact Dermatitis 29: 74–77
41. Frosch PJ, Kurte A, Pilz B (1993) Efficacy of skin barrier creams. III. The repetitive irritation test (RIT) in humans. Contact Dermatitis 29: 113–118
42. Gehse M, Kändler-Stürmer P, Gloor M (1987) Über die Bedeutung der Irritabilität der Haut für die Entstehung des berufsbedingten allergischen Kontaktekzems. Dermatol Monatsschr 173: 400–404
43. Goldstein IM, Hoffstein ST, Weissmann G (1975) Mechanism of lysosomal enzyme release from human polymorphonuclear leukocytes. J Cell Biol 66: 647–652
44. Gollhausen R, Kligman AM (1985) Effects of pressure on contact dermatitis. Am J Ind Med 8: 323–328
45. Hamami I, Marks R (1988) Structural determinants of the response of the skin to chemical irritants. Contact Dermatitis 18: 71–75
46. Hurley JV, Ham KN, Ryan GB (1967) Acute inflammation: a topographical and electron-microscope study of increased vascular permeability in bacterial and chemical pleurisy in the rat. J Pathol Bacteriol 93: 621–635
47. Imokawa G, Mishima Y (1981) Cumulative effect of surfactants on cutaneous horny layers. Contact Dermatitis 7: 65–71
48. Issekutz TB (1990) Effects of six different cytokines on lymphocyte adherence to microvascular endothelium and in vivo lymphocyte migration in the rat. J Immunol 144: 2140–2146
49. Jackson EM, Goldner R (eds) (1990) Irritant contact dermatitis. Dekker, New York
50. Kästner W, Frosch PJ (1981) Hautirritationen verschiedener anionaktiver Tenside im Duhring-Kammer-Test am Menschen im Vergleich zu tierexperimentellen Modellen. Fette Seifen Anstrichmittel 83: 33–46

51. Klaschka F (1979) Arbeitsphysiologie der Hornschicht in Grundzügen. In: Marchionini A (ed) Jadassohns Handbuch der Haut- und Geschlechtskrankheiten. Ergänzungswerk, vol 1, part 4A. Springer, Berlin Heidelberg New York, pp 153–261

52. Kligman AM (1978) Cutaneous toxicity: an overview from the underside. Curr Probl Dermatol 7: 1–25

53. Kligman AM, Lavker RM, Grove GL, Studemayer T (1982) Some aspects of dry skin and its treatment. In: Kligman AM, Leyden JJ (eds) Safety and efficiency of topical drugs and cosmetics. Grune and Stratton, New York, pp 221–238

54. Kristensen M, Larsen CG, Zachariae COC, Thestrup-Pedersen K (1989) ETAF/IL-1 and epidermal lymphocyte chemotactic factor (ELCF) are expressed early in human epidermis during the development of allergic patch test reactions (Abstr.) J Invest Dermatol 93: 302

55. Kühner-Piplack B (1987) Klinik und Differentialdiagnose des Handekzems. Eine retrospektive Studie am Krankengut der Universitäts-Hautklinik Heidelberg 1982–1985. Thesis, Ruprecht-Karls-University, Heidelberg

56. Kunkel B (1989) Korneozytendestruktion und Freisetzung von saurer Phosphatase durch Irritantien. Thesis, Ruprecht-Karls-University, Heidelberg

57. Lachapelle JM, Mahmoud G, Vanherle R (1984) Anhydrite dermatitis in coal miners. Contact Dermatitis 11: 188–189

58. Laden K (1973) Studies on irritancy and stinging potential. J Soc Cosmet Chem 24: 385–393

59. Lammintausta K, Kalimo K (1981) Atopy and hand dermatitis in hospital wet work. Contact Dermatitis 7: 301–308

60. Lammintausta K, Maibach HI, (1987) Irritant reactivity in males and females. Contact Dermatitis 17: 276–280

61. Lammintausta K, Maibach HI, Wilson D (1988) Mechanisms of subjective (sensory) irritation. Dermatosen 36: 45–49

62. Landman G, Farmer ER, Hood AF (1990) The pathophysiology of irritant contact dermatitis. In: Jackson EM, Goldner R (eds) Irritant contact dermatitis. Dekker, New York, pp 67–77

63. Landmann L (1985) Permeabilitätsbarriere der Epidermis. Grosse, Berlin (Grossc Scripta 9)

64. Larsen CG, Ternowitz T, Larsen FG, Thestrup-Pedersen K (1988) Epidermis and lymphocyte interactions during an allergic patch test reaction. Increased activity of ETAF/IL-1, epidermal derived lymphocyte chemotactic factor and mixed skin lymphocyte reactivity in persons with type IV allergy. J Invest Dermatol 90: 230

65. Larsen CG, Ternowitz T, Larsen FG, and Thestrup-Pedersen K (1989) ETAF/interleukin-1 and epidermal lymphocyte chemotactic factor in epidermis overlying an irritant patch test. Contact Dermatitis 20: 335–40

66. Larsen CG, Anderson AO, Apelle E, Oppenheim JJ, Matsushima K (1989) The neutrophil-activating protein (NAP-1) is also chemotactic for T lymphocytes. Science 243: 1464–1466

67. Lerche A, Bisgaard H, Christensen JD, Venge P, Dahl R, Søndergaard J (1988) Lactoferrin, myeloperoxidase, lysozxyme and eosinophil cationic protein in exudate in delayed type hypersensitivity. Allergy 43: 139–145

68. Malten KE (1981) Thoughts on irritant contact dermatitis. Contact Dermatitis 7: 238–247

69. Malten KE, den Arend J, Wiggers RE (1979) Delayed irritation: hexanediol diacrylate and butanediol diacrylate. Contact Dermatitis 1: 112–116

70. McOsker DE, Beck LW (1967) Characteristics of accomodated (hardened) skin. J Invest Dermatol 48: 372–383

71. Meding B (1990) Epidemiology of hand eczema in an industrial city. Acta Derm Venerol (Stockh) Suppl 153

72. Menné T (1983) Frictional dermatitis in post-office workers. Contact Dermatitis 9: 172–173
73. Menné T, Hjorth N (1985) Frictional contact dermatitis. Am J Ind Med 8: 401–402
74. Nickoloff BJ (1988) The role of gamma interferon in cutaneous trafficking of lymphocytes with emphasis on molecular and cellular adhesion events. Arch Dermatol 124: 1835–1843
75. Nilsson E, Mikaelsson B, Andersson S (1985) Atopy, occupation and domestic work as risk factors for hand eczema in hospital workers. Contact Dermatitis 13: 216–223
76. Nilsson GE, Otto U, Wahlberg JE (1982) Assessment of skin irritancy in man by laser Doppler flowmetry. Contact Dermatitis 8: 401–406
77. O'Flaherty JT et al. (1980) Phorbol myristate acetate: in vivo effects upon neutrophils, platelets and lungs. Am J Pathol 101: 79–92
78. Oxholm AM, Oxholm P, Avnstorp C, Bendtzen K (1991) Keratinocyte-expression of interleukin-6 but not of tumour necrosis factor-alpha is increased in the allergic and the irritant patch test reaction. Acta Derm Venereol (Stockh) 71: 93–98
79. Parrish JA, Pathak MA, Fitzpatrick TB (1975) Facial irritation due to sunscreen products, (Letter to the editor). Arch Dermatol 111: 525
80. Patrick E, Burkhalter A, Maibach HI (1987) Recent investigations of mechanisms of chemically induced skin irritation in laboratory mice. J Invest Dermatol 88: 24s–31s
81. Pinnagoda J, Tupker RA, Coenraads PJ, Nater JP (1989) Prediction of susceptibility to an irritant response by transepidermal water loss. Contact Dermatitis 20: 341–346
82. Prottey C (1978) The molecular basis of skin irritation. In: Breuer MM (ed) Cosmetic science, vol 1. Academic, London, pp 275–349
83. Prottey C, Hartop PJ, Press M (1975) Correction of the cutaneous manifestations of essential fatty acid deficiency in man by application of sunflower seed oil to the skin. J Invest Dermatol 64: 228–234
84. Prottey C, Oliver D, Coxon AC (1984) Prediction and measurement of sufactant action upon human skin under realistic conditions. Int J Cosmet Sci 6: 263–273
85. Rietschel RL (1989) Persistent maleic acid irritant dermatitis in the guinea pig. In: Frosch PJ, Dooms-Goossens A, Lachapelle JM, Rycroft RJG, Scheper RJ (eds) Current topics in contact dermatitis. Springer Berlin Heidelberg New York, pp 429–434
86. Rietschel RL (1990) Diagnosing irritant contact dermatitis. In: Jackson EM, Goldner R (eds) Irritant contact dermatitis. Dekker, New York, pp 167–171
87. Roskos KV, Maibach HI, Guy RH (1989) The effect of aging on percutaneous absorption in man. J Pharmacokinet Biopharm 17: 617–630
88. Rothenberg HW, Menné T, Sjolin KE (1977) Temperature dependent primary irritant dermatitis from lemon perfume. Contact Dermatitis 3: 37–48
89. Rougier A, Lotte C, Corcuff P, Maibach HI (1988) Relationship between skin permeability and corneocyte size according to anatomic site, age, and sex in man. J Soc Cosmet Chem 39: 15–26
90. Rycroft RJG (1986) Occupational dermatoses. In: Rook A, Wilkinson DS, Ebling FJG, Champion RH, Burton JL (eds) Textbook of dermatology, 4th edn. Blackwell, Oxford, pp 569–586
91. Rycroft RJG, Wilkinson JD (1992) The principal irritants and sensitizers. In: Rook A, Wilkinson DS, Ebling FJG, Champion RH, Burton JL (eds) Textbook of dermatology. 5th edn. Blackwell, Oxford, pp 717–754
92. Rystedt I (1985) Atopic background in patients with occupational hand eczema. Contact Dermatitis 12: 247–254
93. Salo H, Oikarinen A, Viinikka L, Ylikorkala O (1985) Prostaglandins in blister fluid after contact with an irritant and contact allergens. Arch Dermatol Res 277: 326–327
94. Simons C (1988) Die Differenzierung von toxischen und allergischen Hautreaktionen durch kombinierte Messung von Hautdurchblutung und transepidermalem Wasserverlust. Thesis, Ruprecht-Karls-University, Heidelberg

95. Soschin D, Kligman AM (1982) Adverse subjective reactions. In: Kligman AM, Leyden JJ (eds) Safety and efficacy of topical drugs and cosmetics. Grune and Stratton, New York, pp 377–388

96. Steele RH, Wilhelm DL (1970) The inflammatory reaction in chemical injury. III. Leukocytosis and other histological changes induced by superficial injury. Br J Exp Pathol 51: 265–279

97. Van der Valk PGM, Crijns MC, Nater JP, Bleumink E (1984) Skin irritancy of commercially available soap and detergent bars as measured by water vapour loss. Dermatosen 32: 87–90

98. Van der Valk PGM, Nater JP, Bleumink E (1984) Skin irritancy of surfactants as assessed by water vapor loss measurements. J Invest Dermatol 82: 291–293

99. Wahlberg JE (1984) Skin irritancy from alkaline solutions assessed by laser Doppler flowmetry. Contact Dermatitis 10: 111

100. Wahlberg JE (1989) Assessment of erythema: a comparison between the naked eye and laser Doppler flowmetry. In: Frosch PJ, Dooms-Goossens A, Lachapelle JM, Rycroft RJG, Scheper RJ (eds) Current topics in contact dermatitis. Springer, Berlin Heidelberg New York, pp 549–553

101. Weigand DA, Mershon MM (1970) The cutaneious irritant reaction to agent o-chlorobenzylidene malononitrile (CS). II. Quantitation and racial influence in human subjects. Edgewood Arsenal Technique No. 4332

102. Weigand DA, Haygood C, Gaylor JR (1974) Cell layers and density of negro and caucasian stratum corneum. J Invest Dermatol 62: 563–568

103. Wertz PW, Miethke MC, Long SA, Strauss JS, Downing DT (1985) The composition of the ceramides from human stratum corneum and from comedones. J Invest Dermatol 84: 410–412

104. Wilhelm KP, Maibach HI (1990) Susceptibility to SLS-induced irritant dermatitis: relation to skin pH, TEWL, sebum concentration, and stratum corneum turnover time. J Am Acad Dermatol 23: 122–124

105. Wilhelm KP, Maibach HI (1993) The effect of aging on the barrier function of human skin evaluated by in vivo transepidermal water loss measurement. In: Frosch PJ, Kligman AM (eds) Noninvasive methods for the quantification of skin functions. Springer, Berlin, Heidelberg New York, pp 181–189

106. Wilhelm KP, Surber C, Maibach HI (1989) Quantification of sodium lauryl sulfate irritant dermatitis in man: comparison of four techniques: skin color reflectance, transepidermal water loss, laser Doppler flow measurement and visual scores. Arch Dermatol Res 281: 293–295

107. Wilhelm KP, Saunders JC, Maibach HI (1990) Increased stratum corneum turnover induced by subclinical irritant dermatitis. Br J Dermatol 122: 793–798

108. Willers P (1984) Die Bedeutung der Hornschicht für die Irritabilität der Haut. Thesis, Westf.-Wilhelms University, Münster

109. Willis CM, Stephens CJM, Wilkinson JD (1988) Experimentally-induced irritant contact dermatitis. Contact Dermatitis 18: 20–24

110. Zachariae COC, Ternowitz T, Larsen CG, Nielsen V, Thestrup-Pedersen K (1988) Epidermal lymphocyte chemotactic factor specifically attracts OKT4 positive lymphocytes. Arch Dermatol Res 280: 354–357

2.3 Immediate Contact Reactions

ARTO LAHTI

Contents

2.3.1 Introduction

Immediate contact reactions of the skin have attracted increasing interest in clinical work and research over the past 10 years. They comprise a heterogeneous group of inflammatory reactions which include not only weals and flares but also transient erythematous and eczematous reactions.

2.3.1.1 Symptoms

Immediate contact reactions appear on normal or eczematous skin within minutes to an hour after agents capable of producing this type of contact reaction have been in contact with the skin, and they disappear within 1 day, usually within a few hours. Symptoms can be classified according to morphology and severity: itching, tingling or burning accompanied by erythema are the weakest type of immediate contact reaction, but are often seen from cosmetics [1] and from fruits and vegetables. A local weal and flare is the prototype reaction of contact urticaria. Generalized urticaria after local contact is a rare phenomenon, but can occur with strong allergens. Microvesicles frequently appear on the fingers in protein contact dermatitis. Apart from the skin, symptoms may also appear in other organs in cases of very strong hypersensitivity, the phenomenon known as contact urticaria

Table 2.3.1. Terminology of immediate contact reactions

Term	Remarks
Immediate contact reaction	Includes urticarial, eczematous and other immediate reactions
Contact urticaria	Allergic and nonallergic contact urticaria reactions
Protein contact dermatitis	Allergic or nonallergic eczematous immediate reactions caused by proteins or proteinaceous material
Atopic contact dermatitis	Immediate urticarial or eczematous IgE-mediated immediate contact reaction
Contact urticaria syndrome	Includes both local and systemic immediate reactions precipitated by contact urticaria agents

syndrome. In some cases, immediate contact reactions can be demonstrated only on slightly or previously affected skin, and can be part of the mechanism responsible for maintenance of chronic eczemas [2–4].

There has been much confusion in the use of such terms as 'contact urticaria', 'immediate contact reaction', 'atopic contact dermatitis', and 'protein contact dermatitis' (Table 2.3.1). Immediate contact reactions include both urticarial and other reactions, whereas protein contact dermatitis refers to allergic or nonallergic dermatitis caused by proteins or proteinaceous materials. Atopic contact dermatitis is an immediate (immunoglobulin (Ig) E-mediated) type of allergic contact reaction in atopic people [2].

2.3.1.2 Aetiology

Depending on the mechanisms underlying contact reactions, they are divided into two main types, namely immunological (IgE-mediated) and nonimmunological immediate contact reactions [5]. However, there are substances causing immediate contact reactions where it is not known whether the mechanism is immunological or not.

Tables 2.3.2–2.3.4 show lists of agents that have been reported to cause immediate contact reactions. They include chemicals in medications, industrial contactants, and components of cosmetic products, foods and drinks, as

Table 2.3.2. Agents which have caused local reactions and anaphylactic symptoms in skin tests

Aminophenazone	Egg
Ampicillin	Epoxy resin
Balsam of Peru	Mechlorethamine
Bacitracin	Neomycin
Chloramphenicol	Penicillin
Diethyltoluamide	Streptomycin

well as many chemically undefined environmental agents. The pathogenic classification (nonimmunological versus immunological) is also given but in many instances it is arbitrary, because the mechanisms of various types of contact reactions are unclear or because a pathogenic evaluation has not been performed.

The increasing awareness of immediate contact reactions will result in the list of aetiologic agents expanding, and more thorough understanding of pathophysiological mechanisms will lead to a better and more rational classification of these reactions than is possible at present.

2.3.2 IgE-Mediated Contact Reactions

Immunological contact urticaria and other immunological immediate contact reactions are immediate allergic reactions occurring in people who have previously become sensitized to the causative agent. In many cases of immunological contact reaction, the respiratory and gastrointestinal tracts have obviously been the routes of sensitization. However, natural latex and some foods can sensitize people through the skin.

On skin challenge, the molecules of a contact reactant penetrate through the epidermis and react with specific IgE molecules attached to mast cell membranes. The cutaneous symptoms, erythema and oedema, are elicited by vasoactive substances, mainly histamine released from the mast cells. The role of histamine is crucial, but other mediators of inflammation, e.g. prostaglandins, leukotrienes and kinins, may also influence the degree of response. However, little is known regarding the dynamics of their interplay in clinical situations.

It has not only been shown that mast cells and circulating basophils have Fc receptors for IgE molecules, but also that eosinophils [6], peripheral B and T lymphocytes [7], platelets [8], monocytes [9] and alveolar macrophages [10] can bind IgE. These findings make the issue of immediate immunological contact reactions more complicated than was previously believed.

It has recently been reported that patients with atopic dermatitis, but not other atopics or normal controls, have IgE on their epidermal Langerhans cells [11–13]. This finding may provide an explanation for the high frequency of positive patch test reactions to inhalant allergens such as house dust mite, birch and grass pollen and animal dander in these patients [14–18]. The most important function of epidermal Langerhans cells is antigen presentation in the delayed-type contact allergic reaction, but it can be hypothesized that protein allergens (inhalant, food, etc.) for type I immediate contact reactions bind to specific IgE molecules present on epidermal Langerhans cells, which become apposed to mononuclear cells [19] and induce a delayed-type hypersensitivity reaction that results in eczematous skin lesions (Fig. 2.3.1). This may be the mechanism whereby repeated immediate contact reactions lead to more persistent eczematous skin lesions.

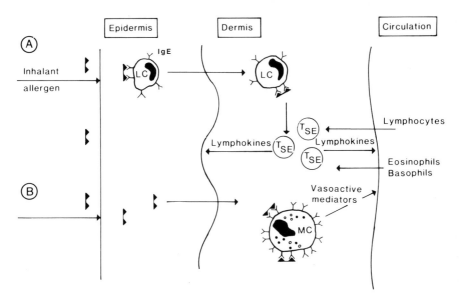

Fig. 2.3.1. Mechanisms by which protein allergens (pollen, mite, food, etc.) may produce delayed-type eczematous reactions (*A*) and immediate-type contact reactions (*B*) in patients with atopic dermatitis. *LC*, Langerhans cell; *MC*, mononuclear cell; T_{SE}, sensitized T lymphocyte (Modified from [11])

Contact urticaria from rubber latex is a typical example of an immediate immunological contact reaction and is more common than was previously thought [20–22]. There have been cases where anaphylactic symptoms and generalized urticaria have occurred after contact with surgical [23, 24] and household rubber gloves [25]. These reactions have been shown to be immediate-type allergic and IgE mediated [25–27]. The allergens are among the proteins that constitute 1%–2% of natural latex. Allergy to latex can be established by skin prick tests or by a latex radioallergosorbent test (RAST), a commercial version of which is available (Pharmacia, Sweden) [28].

Veterinary surgeons can contract contact urticaria of the hands after contact with cows' amniotic fluid, but they do not acquire reactions to cows' dander in clinical provocation tests or in skin prick tests with extracts of cows' epithelium. RAST investigations have shown that antibodies to cows' amniotic fluid and serum, but not to epithelia, can be found in the sera of veterinary surgeons. An interesting finding was that the allergen causing contact urticaria in these cases is a compound of amniotic fluid and serum but not of the epithelium of cows [29].

Foodstuffs are the most common causes of immediate allergic contact reactions (Table 2.3.3). The orolaryngeal area is a site where immediate reactions are frequently provoked by food allergens, most frequently among atopic individuals. Of 230 patients allergic to birch pollen, 152 (66%) had a history of itching, tingling or oedema of the lips and tongue and hoarseness

Table 2.3.3. Agents producing immunological immediate contact reactions

Animal products
  Amniotic fluid
  Blood
  Brucella abortus
  Cercariae
  Cheyletus malaccensis
  Chironomidae, *Chironomus thummi thummi*
  Cockroaches
  Dander
  Dermestes maculatus Degeer
  Gelatine
  Gut
  Hair
  Listrophorus gibbus
  Liver
  Locust
  Mealworm, *Tenibrio molitor*
  Placenta
  Saliva
  Serum
  Silk
  Spider mite, *Tetranychus urticae*
  Wool

Food
  Dairy
    Cheese
    Egg
    Milk
  Fruits
    Apple
    Apricot
    Banana
    Kiwi-fruit
    Mango
    Orange
    Peach
    Plum
  Grains
    Buckwheat
    Maize
    Malt
    Wheat
    Wheat bran
  Honey
  Nuts
    Peanut butter
    Sesame seeds
    Sunflower seeds
  Meats
  Beef

    Chicken
    Lamb
    Liver
    Turkey
  Seafood
    Fish
    Prawns
    Shrimp
  Vegetables
    Beans
    Cabbage
    Carrot
    Celery
    Chives
    Cucumber
    Endive
    Lettuce
    Onion
    Parsley
    Parsnip
    Potato
    Swede (Rutabaga)
    Tomato
    Soybean

Fragrances and flavourings
  Balsam of Peru
  Menthol
  Vanillin

Medicaments
  Acetylsalicylic acid
  Antibiotics
    Ampicillin
    Bacitracin
    Cephalosporins
    Chloramphenicol
    Gentamicin
    Iodochlorhydroxyquin
    Neomycin
    Nifuroxime
    Penicillin
    Rifamycin
    Streptomycin
    Virginiamycin
  Benzocaine
  Benzoyl peroxide
  Clobetasol-17-propionate
  Dinitrochlorobenzene
  Etophenamate
  Mechlorethamine
  Phenothiazines
    Chlorpromazine
    Levomepromazine
    Promethazine

Table 2.3.3. (Continued)

Meats	Pyrazolones
Beef	Aminophenazone
	Methamizole
	Propylphenazone
Metals	Tocopherol
Copper	p-Hydroxybenzoic acid
Nickel	Parabens
Platinum	Phenylmercuric propionate
Rhodium	o-Phenylphenate
Plant products	Polysorbates
Algae	Sodium hypochlorite
Birch	Sorbitan monolaurate
Camomile	Tropicamide
Castor bean	*Miscellaneous*
Chrysanthemum	Acetyl acetone
Cinchona	Acrylic monomer
Colophony	Alcohols (amyl, butyl, ethyl, isopropyl)
Corn starch	Aliphatic polyamide
Cotoneaster	Ammonia
Emetin	Ammonium persulphate
Fennel	Aminothiazole
Garlic	Benzophenone
Grevillea juniperina	Butylated hydroxytoluene
Hakea suaveolens	Carbonless copy paper
Hawthorn, *Crataegus monogyna*	Cu(II)-acetyl acetonate
Henna	Denatonium benzoate
Latex rubber	Diethyltoluamide
Lichens	Epoxy resin
Lily	Formaldehyde resin
Lime	Lanolin alcohols
Mahogany	Lindane
Mustard	Methyl ethyl ketone
Papain	Monoamylamine
Perfumes	Naphtha
Pickles	Naphthylacetic acid
Rose	Nylon
Rouge	Oleylamide
Spices	Para-phenylenediamine
Strawberry	Patent blue dye
Teak	Perlon
Tobacco	Phosphorus sesquisulphide
Tulip	Plastic
Winged bean	Polypropylene
Preservatives and disinfectants	Polyethylene glycol
Benzoic acid	Potassium ferricyanide
Benzyl alcohol	Seminal fluid
Chlorhexidine	Sodium silicate
Chloramine	Sodium sulphide
Chlorocresol	Sulphur dioxide
1,3-diiodo-2-hydroxypropane	Terpinyl acetate
Formaldehyde	Textile finish
Gentian violet	Vinyl pyridine
Hexanetriol	Zinc diethyldithiocarbamate

or irritation of the throat when eating such raw fruits and vegetables as apple, potato, carrot, and tomato [30]. Plum, peach, cherry, kiwi-fruit, celery and parsnip can also elicit immediate contact reactions in people allergic to birch pollen. Positive results on scratch chamber tests with suspected raw fruits and vegetables were noted in 36% of 230 patients. Apple, carrot, parsnip and potato elicited reactions more often than swede (rutabaga), tomato, onion, celery and parsley. The clinical relevance of the skin test results with apple, potato and carrot was 80%–90% per cent. Only 7 of 158 (4%) atopic patients who were not allergic to birch pollen had positive skin test reactions to any of the fruits and vegetables.

RAST and RAST inhibition studies have confirmed the real cross-allergy between birch pollen and fruits and vegetables. All immunological determinants in apple, carrot and celery tuber appeared to be present in birch pollen, too, although the converse was not true [31, 32].

2.3.2.1 Protein Contact Dermatitis

The term 'protein contact dermatitis' was introduced by Hjorth and Roed-Petersen in 1976 [33] for people with hand eczema demonstrating immediate symptoms when the skin was exposed to certain food proteins. Most of these individuals handled food products for a prolonged period as one of the main parts of their job before the symptoms appeared. Itching, erythema, urticarial swelling or small vesicles appear on the fingers or the dorsa of hands within 30 min of contact with, for example, fish or shellfish. Baker's dermatitis is another example of immediate contact reaction and is usually caused by wheat flour. Protein contact dermatitis may appear without previous urticarial rashes but may also be a result of repeatedly occurring contact urticaria [34]. It is probable that both immunological and nonimmunological (irritant) types of protein contact reactions exist. Eczematous reactions are indistinguishable from irritant or allergic contact dermatitis, and careful study of the patient's history and the performance of skin tests are the only ways to ensure a correct diagnosis.

2.3.3 Nonimmunological Immediate Contact Reactions

Nonimmunological immediate contact reactions, which occur without previous sensitization in most exposed individuals, are the most common type of immediate contact reaction. The reaction remains localized and does not spread to become generalized urticaria, nor does it cause systemic symptoms. Typically, the strength of the reaction varies from erythema to an urticarial response, depending on the concentration, the skin area exposed, the mode of exposure and the substance itself [35].

Table 2.3.4. Agents producing immediate nonimmunological contact reactions

Animals	Iodine
Arthropods	Methyl salicylate
Caterpillars	Methylene green
Corals	Myrrh
Jellyfish	Nicotinic acid esters
Moths	Resorcinol
Sea anemones	Tar extracts
Foods	Tincture of benzoin
Cayenne pepper	Witch hazel
Fish	*Metals*
Mustard	Cobalt
Thyme	*Plants*
Fragrances and flavourings	Nettles
Balsam of Peru	Seaweed
Benzaldehyde	*Preservatives and disinfectants*
Cassis (cinnamon oil)	Benzoic acid
Cinnamic acid	Chlorocresol
Cinnamic aldehyde	Formaldehyde
Medicaments	Sodium benzoate
Alcohols	Sorbic acid
Benzocaine	*Miscellaneous*
Camphor	Butyric acid
Cantharides	Diethyl fumarate
Capsaicin	Histamine
Chloroform	Pine oil
Dimethyl sulphoxide	Pyridine carboxaldehyde
Friar's balsam	Sulphur
	Turpentine

The most potent and best studied substances producing nonimmunological immediate contact reactions (Table 2.3.4) are benzoic acid, sorbic acid, cinnamic acid, cinnamic aldehyde and nicotinic acid esters. Under optimal conditions more than half of all individuals react with local erythema and oedema to these substances within 45 min of application if the concentration is high enough. Benzoic acid, sorbic acid and sodium benzoate, which are used as preservatives in cosmetics and other topical preparations, are capable of producing immediate contact reactions at concentrations of 0.1%–0.2% [35, 36].

Cinnamic aldehyde at a concentration of 0.01% may elicit erythema with a burning or stinging feeling in the skin. Some mouthwashes and chewing gums contain cinnamic aldehyde at concentrations high enough to produce a pleasant tingling or 'lively' sensation in the mouth and enhance the sale of the product. Higher concentrations produce lip swelling or contact urticaria in normal skin.

The face, the back, and the extensor aspects of the upper extremities react more readily than other parts of the body, the soles and palms being the least sensitive areas [35, 37]. Scratching does not enhance reactivity, neither does the use of occlusion, at least not where reactions to benzoic acid are concerned.

The mechanism of nonimmunological immediate contact reactions has not been established, but possible mechanisms are a direct influence upon dermal vessel walls or a non-antibody-mediated release of histamine, prostaglandins, leukotrienes, substance P or other inflammatory mediators [5]. No specific antibodies against the causative agent can be found in the serum.

It was previously assumed that substances eliciting nonimmunological immediate contact reactions also result in nonspecific histamine release from the mast cells. However, the antihistamines hydroxyzine and terfenadine did not inhibit reactions to benzoic acid, cinnamic acid, cinnamic aldehyde, methyl nicotinate or dimethyl sulphoxide, though they did inhibit reactions to histamine on prick testing [35, 38]. These results suggest that histamine is not the main mediator in immediate contact reactions to these model substances.

Effect of Nonsteroidal Antiinflammatory Drugs (NSAIDs)

Nonimmunological contact reactions to benzoic acid, cinnamic acid, cinnamic aldehyde, methyl nicotinate and diethyl fumarate can be inhibited by oral acetylsalicylic acid and indomethacin [39, 40] and by topical application of diclofenac or naproxen gels [41]. The duration of inhibition by acetylsalicylic acid can be as long as 4 days [42]. The mechanism by which NSAIDs inhibit contact reactions in human skin has not been defined yet, but it may be ascribed to their common pharmacological action, i.e. inhibition of prostaglandin bioformation.

Role of Sensory Nerves

Capsaicin (*trans*-8-methyl-*N*-vanillyl-6-nonenamide), the most abundant of the pungent principles of the red pepper (*Capsicum*), is known to induce vasodilatation and protein extravasation by specific release of bioactive peptides, for example substance P, from axons of unmyelinated C-fibres of sensory nerves. Pretreatment with capsaicin inhibits erythema reactions in histamine skin tests [43]. However, pretreatment with capsaicin inhibited neither erythema nor edema elicited by benzoic acid or methyl nicotinate [44]. This result suggests that pathways sensitive to capsaicin are not substantially involved.

It was also shown that topical anaesthesia (lidocaine plus prilocaine) can inhibit erythema and oedema reactions to histamine, and also to benzoic acid and methyl nicotinate, but it is not known whether the inhibitory effect is due to the influence on the sensory nerves of the skin only, or if the anaesthetic affects other cell types or regulatory mechanisms of immediate-type skin inflammation [44].

Effect of Ultraviolet Irradiation

Immediate contact reactions to benzoic acid and methyl nicotinate can also be inhibited by exposure ultraviolet B and A light, an effect that lasts for at least 2 weeks [45]. An interesting observation was the fact that UV irradiation had systemic effects: it also inhibited reactions on nonirradiated skin sites [46]. The mechanism of UV inhibition is not known, but it does not seem to be due to thickening of the stratum corneum [46].

2.3.3.1 An Animal Model

Animal skin test methods for determining immediate contact reactions are needed to screen putative agents and to study the mechanisms, but they have not been available. Guinea pig body skin reacts with rapidly appearing erythema to cinnamic aldehyde, methyl nicotinate and dimethyl sulphoxide, but not to benzoic acid, sorbic acid or cinnamic acid. Any of these substances applied to the guinea pig earlobe causes erythema and oedema to appear. Quantification of oedema by measuring changes in the ear thickness with a micrometer is an accurate, reproducible and rapid method [47].

Analogous reactions can be elicited in the earlobes of other laboratory animals. Cinnamic aldehyde and dimethyl sulphoxide produce ear swelling in rat and mouse but benzoic acid, sorbic acid, cinnamic acid, diethyl fumarate and methyl nicotinate produce no response. This suggests that either several mechanisms are involved in immediate contact reactions from different substances or there are differences in the activation of mediators of inflammation between guinea pig, rat and mouse [48, 49].

The swelling response in the guinea pig earlobe is dependent on the concentration of the eliciting substance. The maximal response is a roughly 100% increase in ear thickness, which appears within 50 min of application. Biopsies taken from the guinea pig earlobe 40 min after application of test substances show marked dermal oedema and intra- and perivascular infiltrates of heterophilic granulocytes, which appear to be characteristic of nonimmunological contact urticaria in the guinea pig ear [47, 50].

A decrease in reactivity to contact urticants is noticed after reapplication of the test substances to the guinea pig ear on the following day [51]. The tachyphylaxis is not specific to the substance which produces it, and the reactivity to other agents decreases as well. The length of the refractory period varies with the compound used: it is 4 days for methyl nicotinate, 8 days for diethyl fumarate and cinnamic aldehyde, and up to 16 days for benzoic acid, cinnamic acid and dimethyl sulphoxide.

The reaction of guinea pig earlobe to nonimmunological contact urticants seems to be similar to that of human skin. The similarities include the morphology, the time course of maximal response, the concentrations of the eliciting substances, the tachyphylaxis phenomenon [35], and the lack of an inhibitory effect of antihistamines on contact reactions [38, 50].

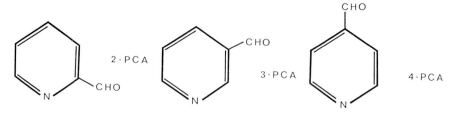

Fig. 2.3.2. Three isomers of pyridine carboxaldehyde (PCA)

2.3.3.2 Specificity

Pyridine carboxaldehyde (PCA) is one of the many substances able to produce nonimmunological immediate contact reactions [52]. It has three isomers, 2-, 3- and 4-PCA, according to the position of the aldehyde group on the pyridine ring (Fig. 2.3.2). In studies of the capacity of these isomers to produce immediate contact reactions, it was found that 3-PCA was the strongest and 2-PCA the weakest contact reactant, in both the human skin and guinea pig ear swelling test [53]. Only a slight change in the molecular structure of a chemical can thus greatly alter its capacity to produce nonimmunological immediate contact reactions.

2.3.4 References

1. Emmons WW, Marks JG (1985) Immediate and delayed reactions to cosmetic ingredients. Contact Dermatitis 13: 258–265
2. Hannuksela M (1980) Atopic contact dermatitis. Contact Dermatitis 6: 30
3. Maibach HI (1976) Immediate hypersensitivity in hand dermatitis: role of food contact dermatitis. Arch Dermatol 112: 1289–1291
4. Veien NK, Hattel T, Justesen O, Nørholm A (1987) Dietary restrictions in the treatment of adult patients with eczema. Contact Dermatitis 17: 223–228
5. Lahti A, Maibach HI (1987) Immediate contact reactions: Contact urticaria syndrome. Semin Dermatol 6: 313–320
6. Capron M, Capron A, Dessaint J, Johansson S, Prin L (1981) Fc-receptors for IgE on human and rat eosinophils. J Immunol 126: 2087–2092
7. Yodoi J, Iskizaka K (1979) Lymphocytes bearing Fc-receptors for IgE. 1. Presence of human and rat lymphocytes with Fc-receptors. J Immunol 122: 2577–2583
8. Joseph M, Auriault C, Capron A, Vorng H, Viens P (1983) A new function for platelets: IgE-dependent killing of schistosomes. Nature 303: 810–812
9. Melewicz F, Spiegelberg H (1980) Fc-receptors for IgE on a subpopulation of human peripheral blood monocytes. J Immunol 125: 1026–1031
10. Joseph M, Tonnel A, Capron A, Voisin C (1980) Enzyme release and super oxide anion production by human alveolar macrophages stimulated with immunoglobulin E. Clin Exp Immunol 40: 416–422
11. Bruynzeel-Koomen C (1986) IgE on Langerhans cells: new insights into the pathogenesis of atopic dermatitis. Dermatologica 172: 181–183
12. Bruynzeel-Koomen C, van Wichen DF, Toonstra J, Berrens L, Bruynzeel PLB (1986) The presence of IgE molecules on epidermal Langerhans cells in patients with atopic dermatitis. Arch Dermatol Res 278: 199–205

13. Barker JNWN, Alegre VA, MacDonald DM (1988) Surface-bound immunoglobulin E on antigenpresenting cells in cutaneous tissue of atopic dermatitis. J Invest Dermatol 90: 117–121

14. Reitamo S, Visa K, Kähönen K, Käyhkö K, Stubb S, Salo OP (1986) Eczematous reactions in atopic patients caused by epicutaneous testing with inhalant allergens. Br J Dermatol 114: 303–309

15. Mitchell EB, Crow J, Williams G, Platts-Mills TAE (1986) Increase in skin mast cells following chronic house dust mite exposure. Br J Dermatol 114: 65–73

16. Leung DY, Schneeberger EE, Siraganian RP, Geha RS, Bhan AK (1987) The presence of IgE on macrophages and dendritic cells infiltrating into the skin lesion of atopic dermatitis. Clin Immunol Immunopathol 42: 328–337

17. Adinoff AD, Tellez P, Clark RA (1988) Atopic dermatitis and aeroallergen contact sensitivity. J Allergy Clin Immunol 81: 736–742

18. Tigalonowa M, Braathen LR, Lea Th (1988) IgE on Langerhans cells in the skin of patients with atopic dermatitis and birch allergy. Allergy 43: 464–468

19. Najem N, Hull D (1989) Langerhans cells in delayed skin reactions to inhalant allergens in atopic dermatitis-an electron microscopic study. Clin Exp Dermatol 14: 218–222

20. Wrangsjö K, Mellström G, Axelsson G (1986) Discomfort from rubber gloves indicating contact urticaria. Contact Dermatitis 15: 79–84

21. Turjanmaa K (1987) Incidence of immediate allergy to latex gloves in hospital personnel. Contact Dermatitis 17: 270–275

22. Turjanmaa K, Reunala T (1988) Contact urticaria from rubber gloves. Dermatol Clin 6: 47–51

23. Carrillo T, Cuevas M, Muñoz T, Hinojosa M, Moneo I (1986) Contact urticaria and rhinitis from latex surgical gloves. Contact Dermatitis 15: 69–72

24. Turjanmaa K, Reunala T, Tuimala R, Kärkkäinen T (1988) Allergy to latex gloves: unusual complication during delivery. Br J Dermatol 297: 1029

25. Seifert HU, Wahl R, Vocks E, Borelli S, Maasch HJ (1987) Immunoglogulin E-vermittelte Kontakturtikaria bzw. Asthma bronchiale durch Latex-enthaltende Haushaltsgummihandschuhe. Dermatosen 35: 137–139

26. Frosch PJ, Wahl R, Bahmer FA, Maasch HJ (1986) Contact urticaria to rubber gloves is IgE-mediated. Contact Dermatitis 14: 241–245

27. Turjanmaa K, Reunala T (1989) Condoms as a source of latex allergen and cause of contact urticaria. Contact Dermatitis 20: 360–364

28. Turjanmaa K, Reunala T, Räsänen L (1988) Comparison of diagnostic methods in latex surgical glove contact urticaria. Contact Dermatitis 19: 241–247

29. Kalveram K-J, Kästner H, Frock G (1986) Detection of specific IgE antibodies in veterinarians suffering from contact urticaria. Z Hautkr 61: 75–81

30. Hannuksela M, Lahti A (1977) Immediate reactions to fruits and vegetables. Contact Dermatitis 3: 79–84

31. Halmepuro L, Løvenstein H (1985) Immunological investigation of possible structural similarities between pollen antigens and antigens in apple, carrot and celery tuber. Allergy 40: 264–272

32. Halmepuro L, Vuontela K, Kalimo K, Björksten F (1984) Cross-reactivity of IgE antibodies with allergens in birch pollen, fruits and vegetables. Int Arch Allergy Appl Immunol 74: 235–240

33. Hjorth N, Roed-Petersen J (1976) Occupational protein contact dermatitis in foodhandlers. Contact Dermatitis 2: 28–42

34. Hannuksela M (1986) Contact urticaria from foods. In: Roe D (ed) Nutrition and the skin. (Contemporary issues in clinical nutrition.) Liss, New York, pp 153–162

35. Lahti A (1980) Non-immunologic contact urticaria. Acta Derm Venereol (Stockh) 60 [Suppl 91]: 1–49

36. Soschin D, Leyden JJ (1986) Sorbic acid-induced erythema and edema. J Am Acad Dermatol 14: 234–241
37. Gollhausen R, Kligman AM (1985) Human assay for identifying substances which induce non-allergic contact urticaria: the NICU-test. Contact Dermatitis 13: 98–106
38. Lahti A (1987) Terfenadine (H_1-antagonist) does not inhibit non-immunologic contact urticaria. Contact Dermatitis 16: 220–223
39. Lahti A, Oikarinen A, Ylikorkala O, Viinikka L (1983) Prostaglandins in contact urticaria induced by benzoic acid. Acta Derm Venerol (Stockholm) 63: 425–427
40. Lahti A, Väänänen A, Kokkonen E-L, Hannuksela M (1987) Acetylsalicylic acid inhibits non-immunologic contact urticaria. Contact Dermatitis 16: 133–135
41. Johansson J, Lahti A (1988) Topical non-steroidal anti-inflammatory drugs inhibit non-immunologic immediate contact reactions. Contact Dermatitis 19: 161–165
42. Kujala T, Lahti A (1989) Duration of inhibition of non-immunologic immediate contact reactions by acetylsalicylic acid. Contact Dermatitis 21: 60–61
43. Bernstein JE, Swift RM, Keyoumars S, Lorincz AL (1981) Inhibition of axon reflex vasodilation by topically applied capsaicin. J Invest Dermatol 76: 394–395
44. Larmi E, Lahti A, Hannuksela M (1989) Effects of capsaicin and topical anesthesia on nonimmunologic immediate contact reactions to benzoic acid and methyl nicotinate. In: Frosch PJ, Dooms-Goossens A, Lachapelle J-M, Rycroft RJG, Scheper RJ (eds) Current topics in contact dermatitis. Springer, Berlin Heidelberg New York, pp 441–447
45. Larmi E, Lahti A, Hannuksela M (1988) Ultraviolet light inhibits nonimmunologic immediate contact reactions to benzoic acid. Arch Dermatol Res 280: 420–423
46. Larmi E (1989) Systemic effect of ultraviolet irradiation on nonimmunologic immediate contact reactions to benzoic acid and methyl nicotinate. Acta Derm Venereol (Stockh) 69: 296–301
47. Lahti A, Maibach HI (1984) An animal model for nonimmunologic contact urticaria. Toxicol Appl Pharmacol 76: 219–224
48. Lahti A, Maibach HI (1985) Contact urticaria from diethyl fumarate. Contact Dermatitis 12: 139–140
49. Lahti A, Maibach HI (1985) Species specificity of nonimmunologic contact urticaria: guinea pig, rat and mouse. J Am Acad Dermatol 13: 66–69
50. Lahti A, McDonald DM, Tammi R, Maibach HI (1986) Pharmacological studies on nonimmunologic contact urticaria in guinea pig. Arch Dermatol Res 279: 44–49
51. Lahti A, Maibach HI (1985) Long refractory period after one application of nonimmunologic contact urticaria agents to the guinea pig ear. J Am Acad Dermatol 13: 585–589
52. Archer CB, Cronin E (1986) Contact urticaria induced by pyridine carboxaldehyde. Contact Dermatitis 15: 308–309
53. Hannuksela A, Lahti A, Hannuksela M (1989) Nonimmunologic immediate contact reactions to three isomers of pyridine carboxaldehyde. In: Frosch PJ, Dooms-Goossens A, Lachapelle J-M, Rycroft RJG, Scheper RJ (eds) Current topics in contact dermatitis. Springer, Berlin Heidelberg New York, pp 448–452

2.4 Phototoxic and Photoallergic Reactions

IAN R. WHITE

Contents

2.4.1 Introduction

Phototoxic and photoallergic reactions may be induced by the topical application of a compound followed by irradiation – phototoxic and photoallergic contact reactions. Alternatively, reactions may be induced after the systemic absorption of a compound followed by irradiation. Most of these latter reactions are probably phototoxic in nature, there being scanty evidence for photoallergy.

This section should be read in conjunction with the section in Chap. 10 on photopatch testing (10.5).

2.4.2 Mechanisms [1]

2.4.2.1 Introduction to Chemistry

A molecule which is able to absorb light is called a *chromophore*. A chromophore will generally absorb UV-light but some may absorb longer wavelengths of light in the visible spectrum. When light energy (a photon) is absorbed there is energy transfer, which promotes the electron status of the molecule to an excited singlet state. Such an excited molecule is short-lived and several things may happen to it.

The excited molecule may return to its ground state with the emission of light (*fluorescence*) or cross to a triplet state, which then returns to the ground state with *phosphorescence*. Alternatively, either state may return to the ground state with release of heat or transfer of energy to another molecule, or the excited molecule may undergo a photochemical reaction, resulting in a chemical alteration to the molecule. These reactions may result in one of several changes occurring, including *cis-trans* isomerization, cycloaddition, rearrangement, fragmentation, and ionization.

2.4.2.2 Mechanisms of Phototoxicity

The term phototoxicity, as used in the context of contact photosensitivity, should be reserved for all those reactions which do not have an immuno-logical basis. Substances causing phototoxicity may reach their target sites either by topical application or systemic absorption. There are several possible mechanisms for phototoxic responses to be caused from the alteration of a chromophore by the absorption of a photon, and these mechanisms have been divided into two main groups: direct and indirect.

1. Direct
   a) Direct interaction of a chromophore in its excited state with a target site. This process necessitates close association between the chromophore and the target site, e.g. furocoumarins.
   b) The formation of stable phototoxic products, e.g. chlorpromazine
2. Indirect (often referred to as photodynamic mechanisms)
   c) Type I reactions. In these reactions there is reduction of an excited chromophore, in its triplet state, by electron transfer, producing free radicals. These free radicals are reactive and may produce damage. The chromophore is chemically changed.
   d) Type II reactions. Here, the excited chromophore transfers energy to oxygen, causing the generation of singlet oxygen ($^1O_2$). Singlet oxygen is a powerful oxidizing agent and is responsible for damage. The chromophore is not chemically altered in reactions of this type.

It is probable that the majority of substances which cause phototoxicity act through a photodynamic mechanism and they may produce damage in more than one way.

2.4.2.2.1 Examples

The following are examples illustrating the mechanisms of phototoxicity:

Furocoumarins (Psoralens). Furocoumarins (Fig. 2.4.1) form complexes between adjacent base pairs on the DNA within the nucleus of a cell, by a mechanism which is now reasonably well understood and is an example of direct interaction.

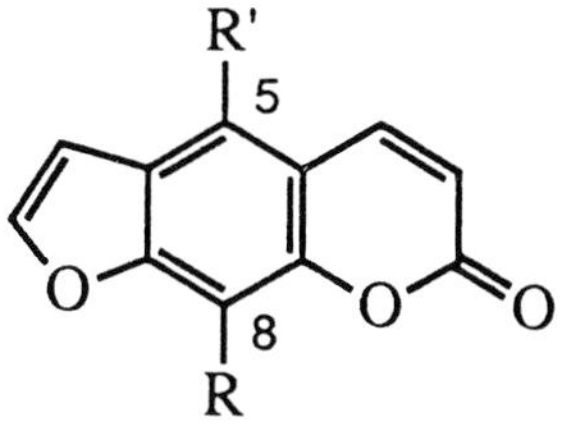

5 - Methoxypsoralen
$R' = CH_3O$, $R = H$

8 - Methoxypsoralen
$R' = H$, $R = OCH_3$

Isopentenyloxypsoralen
$R' = H$, $R = (CH_3)_2 C = CHCH_2O$

Xanthotoxol
$R' = H$, $R = OH$

Fig. 2.4.1. Chemical structures of furocoumarins (psoralens)

With UVA irradiation, a covalent bond is formed between the furocoumarin and a pyrimidine base (thymine rather than cytosine) on a strand of the DNA double helix. This process is an example of cycloaddition and it yields a monoadduct with a furocoumarin molecule linked to one DNA strand. If there is now further absorption of UVA, a similar reaction can take place with a pyrimidine base on the opposite strand of DNA, a process of bifunctional cycloaddition which results in interstrand cross-linking [2].

The mechanism of erythema production from furocoumarin phototoxicity is not fully clear. There is a correlation between the ability of a psoralen to cross-link strands of DNA with the production of an erythematous response [3]. 4,6,4'-Trimethylangelicin, which forms monoadducts only, is far less phototoxic than 8-methoxypsoralen, which engages in bifunctional cycloaddition [4]. However, the erythema from furocoumarin photoxicity may also be related to membrane damage caused by the production of singlet oxygen, a type II photodynamic process [5].

Phenothiazines. Phenothiazines (Fig. 2.4.2) are phototoxic when given systemically but may also produce photoallergic reactions on topical application. The phototoxicity of chlorpromazine is related to the

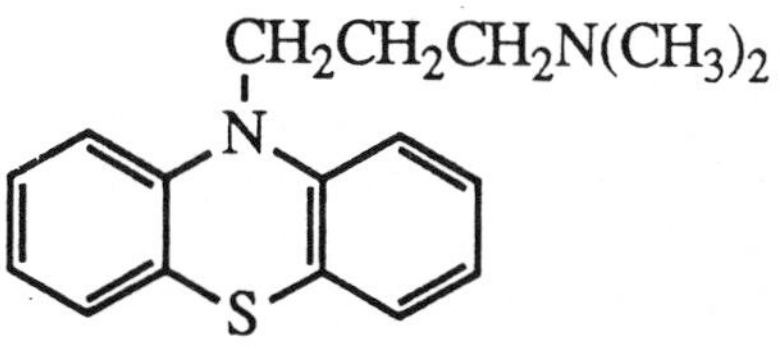

$$CH_2CH_2CH_2N(CH_3)_2$$

Fig. 2.4.2. Chemical structure of chlorpromazine

photodechlorination of several of its metabolic products. Some of these derivatives are able to produce cleavage of DNA and form covalent bond adducts with the DNA [6]. Additionally, by a photodynamic type I mechanism, chlorpromazine can induce cell membrane damage, resulting in photohaemolysis. In promethazine photoxicity there is production of superoxide and free radicals [7].

Dyes. On absorption of light, often in the visible spectrum but also UVA, dyes such as acridine orange cause oxidation by type II photodynamic mechanisms. There is production of singlet oxygen and this is able to diffuse through the cytoplasm of the cell [8]. Because of this diffusion, the site of generation of the singlet oxygen may be different from the site of oxidative damage, that is, the target site.

The more important consequences of oxidation by singlet oxygen are the loss of certain amino acids in proteins (histidine, methionine, tryptophan, tyrosine, cysteine), oxidation of guanine in strands of DNA, and the production of hydroperoxides from unsaturated lipids. As a consequence of these changes, cell membrane damage is a particular sequel.

Nonsteroidal Antiinflammatory Drugs. Nonsteroidal antiinflammatory drugs become decarboxylated and produce photoproducts which generate both singlet oxygen and free radicals. The latter may be incorporated into DNA or biological membranes [9, 10].

Amiodarone. After exposure to UV, amiodarone loses iodine (deiodination) and there is aryl radical formation. This aryl radical is able to take hydrogen from chemical donors such as linoleic acid. A dienyl radical is formed, which can then produce a peroxy radical causing lipid peroxidation. This reaction may be the reason for the deposition of lipofuschin in the skin associated with amiodarone phototoxicity [11].

The minimal erythema dose (MED) for amiodarone-induced phototoxicity is reduced over the range 335–460 nm but normal over 305–330 nm. However, in vitro, the absorption spectrum is in the UVB rather than in the UVA region [12].

2.4.2.3 Mechanisms of Photoallergy

The histology and morphology of a photoallergic contact reaction are similar to those of an ordinary allergic contact reaction and, on immunohistological examination, lymphocytes of the CD4$^+$ type are present in the infiltrate [13].

Many compounds which can cause photoallergy are halogenated aromatic hydrocarbons [14]. In vitro photochemical experiments have shown that irradiation of some substances which are potential photoallergens results in the formation of free radicals. Examples of these compounds include halogenated salicylanilides (Fig. 2.4.3), chlorpromazine and buclosamide. The free radicals are formed by the UV homolysis of a photo-labile carbon-halogen bond. Bithionol, in the presence of oxygen, forms hydroxyl and aryl radicals [15].

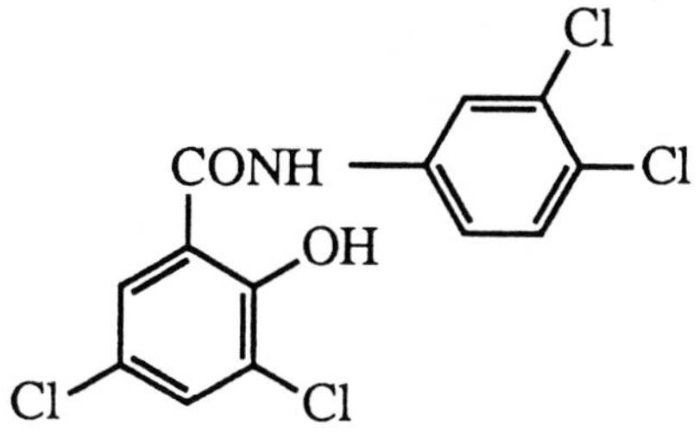

3,3',4,5'-Tetrachlorosalicylanilide; Irgasan BS 200

Fig. 2.4.3. Chemical structure of 3,3',4,5'-Tetrachlorosalicylanilide; Irgasan BS 200

Free aryl radicals are highly reactive compounds which can take hydrogen from suitable donors. Additionally, they may react with other free radicals to form complexes linked by covalent bonds. These may be allergens. Tetrachlorosalicylanilide undergoes photochemical dechlorination with UV irradiation. Free radicals are formed and hydrogen is taken from cysteine. In the presence of human serum albumin, the radicals form photoadducts with the protein, and this may be the antigen [14].

Another mechanism for the formation of photoallergens is that, after the absorption of light, the molecule becomes chemically altered to form a stable compound which is a hapten. After covalent binding to a carrier protein an antigen is formed [14]. Further, after absorption of light, there may be photochemical alteration of a protein hapten complex, which may then be antigenic. Subsequent exposure to UV light may result in the formation of the same or similar photoproducts from endogenous substances. There is evidence for the alteration of carrier proteins in vitro to tetrachlorosalicylanilide [16]. Such a mechanism may explain the phenomenon of persistent light reactivity.

In mice there has been clear demonstration that contact photosensitivity to tetrachlorosalicylanilide is due to a cell-mediated immune response [17] and Langerhans cells are required for the induction of this contact photosensitivity [18]. Such photosensitivity can be transferred into another mouse with lymph-node-derived T cells from the sensitized mouse. Similarly, there is passive transfer of photosensitivity to tetrachlorosalicylanilide in guinea pigs by giving peritoneal exudate cells, rich in T cells, from a sensitized donor to a recipient. Similarly, with systemic photoallergy, the intraperitoneal injection of chlorpromazine or sulphanilamide in mice, with UV irradiation to the skin, causes photosensitivity which can be transferred with lymph node cells [19].

The absorption spectrum of musk ambrette is in the UVB range, but the action spectrum of photoallergic contact reactions in the guinea pig is greater than 320 nm in vivo [20]. It has been pointed out that discrepancies between in vitro absorption spectra and in vivo action spectra may yield closer agreement when consideration of the normal underlying photochemical responses which occur in the skin are considered [21].

2.4.3 Clinical Features of Photosensitivity

2.4.3.1 General Features

A photodermatitis affects the light-exposed areas, although there may be some spread of the reaction in photoallergic reactions. The reaction often occurs in a well-demarcated area with a cut-off at the clothing lines, such as the V of the neck and beyond the sleeves. Sometimes, the reaction may be unilateral. A unilateral reaction may result from assymetric topical application of a photosensitizer, or from greater UV exposure on one side of the body, as may occur when driving a car for instance.

There may be overall similarities between a photodermatitis and an airborne allergic contact dermatitis [22]. In general, however, a photodermatitis tends to spare the shaded areas of exposed skin such as the eyelids and retroauricular and submental areas which are often affected in an allergic contact dermatitis from an airborne allergen [23]. However, this generalization is not always true in every case.

A patchy dermatitis on the face is a presenting feature of a type of photosensitivity to the photoallergen musk ambrette [24], caused by patting an aftershave containing the photoallergen onto the skin. Phototoxic contact reactions to furocoumarins in plants produce a streaky linear reaction.

2.4.3.2 Phototoxic Reactions

Phototoxic reactions appear as an exaggerated sunburn reaction, with erythema which may settle leaving pigmentation. In severe cases, bullae may develop on the erythematous base. The absorption spectra of compounds causing phototoxicity approximate the action spectra of the compounds. These spectra are usually in the range 280–430 nm, although some dyes, e.g. eosin, sensitize with visible light.

2.4.3.2.1 Phytophototoxic Contact Dermatitis

Phytophototoxic contact dermatitis is caused by topical contact with furocoumarins (psoralens) in plants, followed by light exposure. The compounds are lipid soluble and penetrate the epidermis readily, and this may be enhanced by an increased humidity. The absorption spectrum is in the UVA range. Many common plants contain these furocoumarins and examples are listed in Table 2.4.1. After appropriate contact with the plants and light, an acute streaky red eruption develops at the site of contact. The eruption may become bullous and then settles leaving hyperpigmentation. The term dermatitis bullosa striata pratensis has been used to describe the condition.

Table 2.4.1. Plants containing furocoumarins (from [32])

Sources	Family	Common names
Coronilla glauca	Leguminosae	
Psorolea corylifolia	Leguminosae	
Ficus carica	Moraceae	fig
Aegle marmelos	Rutaceae	
Citrus acida	Rutaceae	Seville orange
Citrus aurantifolia	Rutaceae	sweet lime
Citrus bergamia	Rutaceae	bergamot orange
Citrus limonum	Rutaceae	lemon
Dictammus albus	Rutaceae	gas plant
Fagara schinifolia	Rutaceae	
Fagara zanthoxyloides	Rutaceae	
Luvanga scandens	Rutaceae	
Ruta chalepensis	Rutaceae	
Ruta graveolens	Rutaceae	rue
Ruta montana	Rutaceae	
Skimmia laureola	Rutaceae	
Zanthoxylum flavum	Rutaceae	
Ammi majus	Umbelliferae	
Ammi visnaga	Umbelliferae	
Angelica archangelica	Umbelliferae	angelica
Angelica glabra	Umbelliferae	
Angelica keiski	Umbelliferae	
Angelica silvestris	Umbelliferae	
Apium graveolens	Umbelliferae	celery
Bupleurum falcatum	Umbelliferae	
Daucus carota	Umbelliferae	carrot
Heracleum sp.	Umbelliferae	
Levisticum sp.	Umbelliferae	
Ligusticum acutifolium	Umbelliferae	
Ligusticum acutilobum	Umbelliferae	
Pastinaca sativa	Umbelliferae	parsnip
Petroselium sativum	Umbelliferae	
Pimpinella magna	Umbelliferae	
Piminella saxifraga	Umbelliferae	
Prangos sp.	Umbelliferae	
Seseli indicum	Umbelliferae	

2.4.3.2.2 Berloque Dermatitis

Berloque dermatitis was caused by the inclusion of oil of bergamot in some perfumes. The active ingredient, bergapten or 5-methoxypsoralen, caused erythema, leading to hyperpigmentation where the perfume had been placed. The name berloque refers to the drop-like shape of the patches. The erythema could be minimal or marked. The reaction occurred on the sides of the neck or the arms where the perfume had been applied. The hyperpigmentation lasted for months.

2.4.3.2.3 Tar 'Smarts'

Workers exposed to coal tar, or derivatives such as creosote, may develop tar 'smarts'. The reaction consists of burning and smarting of the exposed skin and this is often associated with erythema which leads to hyperpigmentation. The phenomenon occurs in the summer months and is related to the degree of UVA exposure. The reactions may be caused by volatile fumes as well as by direct contact.

2.4.3.2.4 Photoonycholysis

Photoonycholysis has been caused by a number of drugs which induce photo-toxicity. These include tetracyclines, psoralens and benoxaprofen.

2.4.3.3 Photoallergic Contact Dermatitis

Some photoallergens are also contact allergens and may also have both photo-toxic and photoallergic potential. Photoallergy is more common in males due to their greater exposure to potential photoallergens.

A photoallergic contact reaction is clinically similar to a simple allergic contact dermatitis. A spectrum of reactions varying from an erythema alone to a bullous eruption may occur. However, an erythema will most commonly be associated with a phototoxic reaction rather than a photoallergic one. If the dermatitis becomes chronic, lichenification occurs. Although the sun-exposed areas are primarily involved, there may be spread onto unexposed areas and the eruption may become widespread, although the main sites of involvement remain the light-exposed areas.

As a rule, removal from contact with the photoallergen, and from related compounds if cross-reactions occur, will cause resolution of the photocontact dermatitis. In a few cases, however, persistent light reactivity remains.

Clinically, it may be difficult to differentiate between phototoxic and photoallergic contact reactions. Table 2.4.2 lists features which may help in the differentiation. The presence of a sunburn-type erythema alone probably indicates a toxic reaction, which may be confirmed on histological examination. Many case reports allocating the type of photosensitivity reaction to a particular compound often do so on insecure grounds. The majority of systemic photosensitivity reactions are toxic in nature. Substances causing them are listed in Table 2.4.3, and those causing phototoxic contact reactions are in Table 2.4.4. Table 2.4.5 lists photocontact allergens.

2.4.4 Differential Diagnosis

The differential diagnosis of a photocontact dermatitis includes contact dermatitis on the exposed skin, as may occur with toiletries and sunscreens,

Table 2.4.2. Comparison between phototoxic and photoallergic reactions (adapted from [33])

	Phototoxic	Photoallergic
Incidence on exposed skin	high	low
Reaction after single contact?	yes	no
Localization	limited to exposed area	may be spread
Flare-up reactions?	no	possible
Cross-reactions?	no	possible
Appearance	sunburn reaction	eczematous
Action spectrum	absorption spectrum	longer than absorption spectrum
Eliciting concentration	high	low
Eliciting light dose	high	low

Table 2.4.3. Systemic phototoxic substances [34,35]

Amiodarone
Anticancer agents, e.g. dacarbazine, fluoracil, vinblastine
Griseofulvin
Furocoumarins (psoralens)
Nalidixic acid
Nonsteroidal antiinflammatory drugs, e.g. piroxicam, benoxaprofen, azapropazone, tiaprofenic acid
Phenothiazines, e.g. chlorpromazine, phenothiazine
Porphyrins
Quinine, quinidine
Quinoline antimalarials, chloroquine, hydroxychloroquine
Retinoids, e.g. etretinate
Sulphonamides, e.g. sulphamethoxazole
Sulphonylureas
Tetracyclines, e.g. tetracycline, oxytetracycline, doxycycline, chlortetracycline, demethylchlortetracycline
Thiazide diuretics, e.g. chlorothiazide, hydrochlorothiazide, cyclopenthiazide
Tricyclic antidepressents, e.g. protriptyline, clomipramine, dothiepin, imipramine, maprotiline

airborne allergens such as Compositae and phosphorus sesquisulphide, chronic actinic dermatits, and eczematous polymorphic light eruption. Additionally, conditions such as rosacea, seborrhoeic eczema and lupus erythematosus may be photoaggravated.

2.4.5 Investigations

The diagnosis of an allergic photocontact dermatitis is made by patch and photopatch testing. Testing is not ordinarily indicated when a phototoxic

Table 2.4.4. Topical phototoxic substances

Balsam of Peru
Buclosamide
Cadmium sulphide
Chlorpromazine
Coal tar and derivatives, e.g. anthracene, acridine, phenanthrene, pyrene
Dyes, e.g. eosin, acridine orange, acriflavin
Essential oils, e.g. bergamot, cedar, citron, lavender, lime, neroli, petitgrain, sandalwood
2-Ethoxyethyl-p-methoxycinnamate
Fenticlor
Furocoumarins
Halogenated salicylanilides
Isoamyl-$p - N, N'$-dimethylaminobenzoate

Table 2.4.5. Topical photoallergens [35]

Halogenated antimicrobials
bis(2-hydroxy-5-chlorophenyl) sulphide (fenticlor)
5-Bromo-4'-chlorosalicylanilide (multifungin)
Buclosamide (chlorosalicylamide, jadit)
Chlorhexidine
Chloro-2-phenylphenol
4,5-Dibromosalicylanilide (DBS)
Hexachlorophene
Tetrachlorosalicylanilide (TCSA)
2,2'-Thiobis(4,6-dichlorophenol) (bithionol)
Tribromosalicylanilide (TBS)
Trichlorocarbanilide (TCC)
Triclosan

Fragrance ingredients
Cinnamic aldehyde
Oak moss
Methyl coumarin
Musk ambrette
Musk xylol

Sunscreens
Benzophenone-3 (Oxybenzone)
Benzophenone-10 (Mexenone)
Butylmethoxydibenzoylmethane (Parsol 1789)
Digalloyl trioleate
Dimethoxane
2-Ethoxyethyl-p-methoxycinnamate (Cinoxate)
Glyceryl-p-aminobenzoate
4-Isopropyldibenzoylmethane (Eusolex 8020)
3-(4-methylbenzylidene)-camphor (Eusolex 6300)
Octyldimethyl-PABA (Escalol 507)
Octylmethoxycinnamate (Parsol MCX)
PABA (p-aminobenzoic acid)
2-Phenylbenzimidazole sulphate

Table 2.4.5. (Continued)

Colours
Brilliant lake red R (DC-R31)
Erythrocine-AL (FDC-R3)
Lithol red-CA (DC-R11)
Permanent orange (DC-017)
p-Phenylenediamine
Toluidine red (DC-R35)

Others
Benzocaine
Benzydamine
Chlormercaptodicarboximide
Chlorpromazine
Chlorprothixene
Coal tar derivatives
Dibenzthione
Dibucaine
Diphenhydramine
Furocoumarins
Nonsteroidal antiinflammatory drugs, e.g. ketoprofen, tiaprofenic acid, ibuproxam [36]
Promethazine
Quinine sulphate
Stilbenes
Sulphanilamide
Thiourea, dimethylthiourea [37]
Zinc pyrithione

---

contact reaction, such as a phytophotocontact dermatitis, is evident. These reactions are difficult to reproduce and the diagnosis comes from the history and examination alone. Monochromator testing is used to evaluate systemic photosensitivity reactions. Systemic photochallenge, giving 2–3 times the normal dose of a suspected photoactive agent with irradiation of the skin before and at intervals after ingestion, has been advocated [25].

2.4.6 Chronic Actinic Dermatitis

The term chronic actinic dermatitis is now being used to include the conditions of persistent light reactivity, photosensitive eczema, photosensitivity dermatitis and actinic reticuloid [26]. It presents as a persistent eruption with an eczematous character, predominantly affecting the exposed skin but sometimes spreading to covered areas. An erythroderma may sometimes be seen. On monochromator testing, there is a reduction in the MED to UVB on covered skin. The MED may also be reduced to longer wavelengths of light. The histological appearances are those of a chronic eczema and lymphomalike changes may be seen. There are immunohistochemical changes of an allergic contact dermatitis [27].

In photoallergic contact dermatitis there is transient light sensitivity to UVA (normally). When this progresses to persistent light reactivity, the spectrum of sensitivity shifts to UVB, and this is useful in differentiating between the two [28].

As discussed above, in photoallergic reactions there is, after UVA exposure, covalent binding of a hapten to an endogenous protein. If chronic actinic dermatitis follows, there may be an antigenic product formed by the UVB irradiation of a modified endogenous carrier protein alone. There is theoretical support for such a mechanism [29], whereby tetrachlorosalicylanilide causes oxidation of histidine with modification of albumin into a weak allergen. Further irradiation with UVB, in the absence of the initial photosensitizer, may produce sufficient of the oxidized antigenic protein to elicit a cell-mediated immune response at all skin sites [26]. Some cases of polymorphic light eruption may have a similar aetiology [30]. Chronic actinic dermatitis may develop after sensitization to contact allergens such as sesquiterpene lactones [31] and without any identifiable exogenous factor.

2.4.7 References

1. Kornhauser A, Wamer W, Giles A (1987) Light-induced dermal toxicity: effects on the cellular and molecular level. In: Marzulli FN, Maibach HI (eds) Dermatotoxicology, 3rd edn. Hemisphere, Washington, pp 377–412
2. Hearst JE, Isaacs ST, Kanne D, Rapoport H, Straub K (1984) The reaction of the psoralens with deoxyribonucleic acid. Q Rev Biophys 17: 1–44
3. Vedaldi D, Dall'Acqua F, Gennaro A, Rodighiero G (1983) Photosensitized effects of furocoumarins: the possible role of singlet oxygen. Z Naturforsch 38c: 866–869
4. Takashima A, Yamamoto K, Mizuno N (1989) Photobiological activities of a newly synthesized 4,6,4'-trimethylangelicin on human skin. Photomed Photobiol 11: 155–162
5. Kochevar IE (1987) Mechanisms of drug photosensitization. Photochem Photobiol 45: 891–895
6. Kochevar I (1981) Phototoxicity mechanisms: chlorpromazine photosenstized damage to DNA and cell membranes. J Invest Dermatol 77: 59–64
7. Chignell CF, Motten AG, Buettner GR (1985) Photoinduced free radicals from chlorpromazine and related phenothiazines: relationship to phenothiazine-induced photosensitization. Environ Health Perspect 64: 103–110
8. Moan J, Pettersen EO, Christensen T (1979) The mechanism of photodynamic inactivation of human cells in vitro in the presence of haematoporphyrin. Br J Cancer 39: 398–407
9. Ljunggren B, Bjellerup M (1986) Systemic drug phootoxicity. Photodermatol 3: 26–35
10. Moore DE, Chappins PP (1988) A comparative study of the photochemistry of the non-steroidal anti-inflammatory drugs, naproxen, benoxaprophen and indomethacin. Photochem Photobiol 47: 173–180
11. Li ASW, Chignell CF (1987) Spectroscopic studies of cutaneous photosensitizing agents. IX. A spin trapping study of the photolysis of amiodarone and desethylemiodarone. Photochem Photobiol 45: 191–197
12. Ferguson J, Addo HA, Jones S, Johnson BE, Frain Bell W (1985) A Study of cutaneous photosensitivity induced by amiodarone. Br J Dermatol 113: 537–549

13. Takashima A, Yamamoto K, Kimura S, Takakuwa Y, Mizuno N (1991) Allergic contact and photocontact dermatitis due to psoralens in patients with psoriasis treated with topical PUVA. Br J Dermatol 124: 37–42

14. Epling GA, Wells JL, Ung Chan Yoon (1988) Photochemical transformations in salicylanilide photoallergy. Photochem Photobiol 47: 167–171

15. Li ASW, Chignell CF (1987) Spectroscopic studies of cutaneous photosensitizing agents. XII. A spin-trapping study of the free radicals generated during the photolysis of photoallergens bithionol and fentichlor. Photochem Photobiol 46: 445–452

16. Morison WL, Kochevar IE (1983) Photoallergy. In: Parrish JA, Kripke M, Morrison WL (eds) Photoimmunology. Plenum, New Yok, pp 227–253

17. Takigawa M, Miyachi Y (1982) Mechanisms of contact photosensitivity in mice: T-cell regulation of contact photosensitivity to tetrachlorosalicylanilide under the genetic restrictions of the major histocompatibility complex. J Invest Dermatol 78: 108–115

18. Miyachi Y, Takigawa M (1982) Mechanisms of contact photosensitivity in mice: II. Langerhans cells are required for successful induction of contact photosensitivity to TCSA. J Invest Dermatol 78: 363–365

19. Giudici PA, Maguire HC (1985) Experimental photoallergy to systemic drugs. J Invest Dermatol 85: 207–210

20. Giovinazzo VJ, Ichikawa H, Kochevar IE, Armstrong RB, Harber LC (1981) Photoallergic contact dermatitis to musk ambrette: action spectrum in guinea pigs and man. Photochem Photobiol 33: 773–777

21. Diffey BL, Farr PM (1988) The action spectrum in drug induced photosensitivity. Photochem Photobiol 47: 49–53

22. Hjorth N, Roed-Petersen J, Thomsen K (1976) Airborne contact dermatitis from Compositae oleoresins stimulates photodermatitis. Br J Dermatol 95: 613–620

23. Wilkinson DS (1962) Patch test reactions to certain halogenated salicylanilides. Br J Dermatol 74: 302–306

24. Wojnarowska F, Calnan CD (1986) Contact and photocontact allergy to musk ambrette. Br J Dermatol 114: 667–675

25. Hölzle E, Plewig G, Lehmann P (1987) Photodermatoses – diagnostic procedures and their interpretation. Photodermatol 4: 109–114

26. Norris PG, Hawk JLM (1990) Chronic actinic dermatitis: a unifying concept. Arch Dermatol 126: 376–378

27. Norris PG, Smith NPS, Chu AC, Hawk JLM (1989) Chronic actinic dermatitis: an immunohistological and photobiological study. J Am Acad Dermatol 21: 966–971

28. Wolf CH, Hönigsmann H (1988) Persistent light reaction – actinic reticuloid. Hautarzt 39: 635–641

29. Kochevar IE, Harber LC (1977) Photoreactions of 3,3',4',5-tetrachlorosalicylanilide with proteins. J Invest Dermatol 68: 151–156

30. Norris P, Hawk JLM, White IR (1988) Photoallergic contact dermatitis from fentichlor. Contact Dermatitis 18: 318–320

31. Murphy GM, White IR, Hawk JLM (1990) Allergic airborne contact dermatitis to Compositae with photosensitivity – chronic actinic dermatitis in evolution. Photodermatol Photoimmunol Photomed 7: 38–39

32. Benezra C, Ducombs G, Sell Y, Foussereau J (1985) Plant contact dermatitis. Mosby, London, p 11

33. Maurer T (1983) Contact and photocontact allergens. Dekker, New York, p 132

34. Smith AG (1989) Drug-induced photosensitivity. Adverse Drug React Bull 136: 1–3

35. Nater JP, De Groot AC (1985) Unwanted effects of cosmetics and drugs used in dermatology, 2nd edn. Elsevier. Amsterdam

36. Mozzanica N, Pucci M. Pigatto PD (1989) Contact and photoallergic dermatitis to topical nonsteroidal antiiflammatory drugs (Proprionic acid derivatives): a study of eight cases. In: Frosch PJ, Dooms-Goossens A, Lachapelle LM, Rycroft RJG,

Scheper RJ (eds) Current toipcs in contact dermatitis. Springer, Berlin Heidelberg New York, pp 499–506
37. Dooms-Goossens A, Chrispeels MT, de Veylder II, Roelands R, Willems L, Degreef H (1987) Contact and photocontact sensitivity problems associated with thiourea and its derivatives: a review of the literature and case reports. Br J Dermatol 116: 573–579

Chapter 3
Histopathological
and Immunohistopathological
Features of Irritant and
Allergic Contact Dermatitis

Histopathological and Immunohistopathological Features of Irritant and Allergic Contact Dermatitis

JEAN-MARIE LACHAPELLE

Contents

3.1 Introduction

A detailed description of the histopathological features of allergic contact dermatitis can be found in most textbooks of dermatopathology. Surprisingly, however, the histopathological signs of irritant contact dermatitis are scarcely mentioned or even omitted. The best way to fill this gap is to describe the lesions observed at the sites of positive patch test reactions (allergic or irritant). This choice has two advantages: (a) the histopathological signs reflect a practical situation, encountered daily in the patch test clinic; (b) a positive patch test reaction is a clear-cut, unmodified reaction: the direct consequence of the application of a substance on previously intact skin. This is quite different from clinical situations, in which many additional parameters can play a confounding role, such as: (a) unknown duration of the disease, (b) lesions in relation to scratching, (c) infections, and (d) lichenification. The only possible drawback to using patch test reactions is the role played by occlusion. This might be especially true for allergic reactions and is the reason for this description also based on open (unoccluded) reactions, the use of which is becoming commoner in many clinics.

This description will be a 'freeze-frame photograph' of the situation at 48h; it does not take into account the chronology of events, starting at time 0 (with application of the substance) and continuing for instance every 6 h until 48 or 72 h. This dynamic view has been achieved in previous research studies [1], but it does not fit within the practical scope of the present review.

3.2 Histopathological Features of Positive Allergic Patch Test Reactions

The histopathological picture of a positive allergic patch test reaction (read at 48 h) is a typical example of a spongiotic dermatitis [2]. Features are very similar in all cases.

3.2.1 Epidermal Changes

In the epidermis, spongiosis is an almost constant sign, resulting from the accumulation of fluid around individual keratinocytes (exoserosis) and the consequent stretching of intercellular desmosome complexes (or 'prickles').

Spongiosis is focally or evenly distributed along the length of the epidermis; it is either limited to the lower layers or extends from the basal to the granular layer. In some but not all cases, it spares the cells of the sweat duct unit. Hair follicles are usually involved by the spongiotic process. A more plentiful accumulation of fluid results in rupture of the intercellular prickles and the formation of vesicles. Thus, in allergic contact dermatitis, spongiotic vesiculation can be defined as an intra-epidermal cavity with ragged walls and surrounding spongiosis. There is migration of inflammatory cells into the epidermis (exocytosis). These cells, mainly lymphocytes and occasionally polymorphonuclear neutrophils and eosinophils, accumulate in the spongiotic vesicles. Some vesicles are rounded and tense; they are located in the stratum spinosum, whereas others are flat and located in the stratum corneum. They finally rupture at the surface of epidermis, and vertical channels of fluid discharge are occasionally seen on serial sections. These channels are sometimes described colourfully as 'Devergie's eczematous wells'. Intracellular oedema of keratinocytes also occurs, with accumulation of glycogen. At the electron microscopic level, dissolution of interdesmosomal areas, or 'microacantholysis', can be demonstrated; remaining desmosomes show tension and alignment of tonofilament bundles.

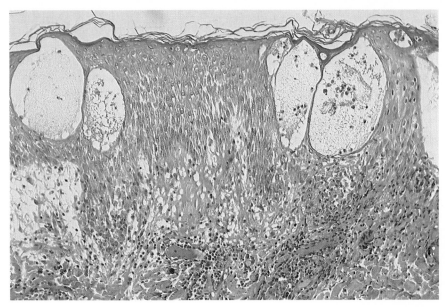

Fig. 3.1. Allergic positive patch test reaction to balsam of Peru at 2 days: spongiotic vesiculation in epidermis with exocytosis of mononuclear cells, dermal oedema. Haematoxylineosin-saffron stain (× 150)

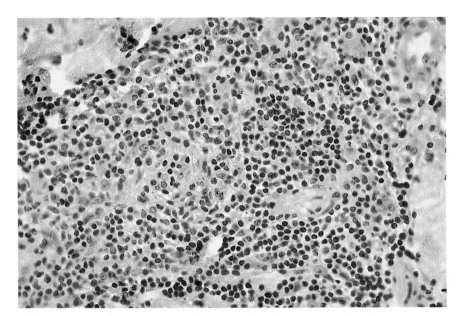

Fig. 3.2. Allergic positive patch test reaction to wool alcohols at 2 days: dense perivascular infiltrate of mononuclear cells. Haematoxylin-eosin-saffron stain (× 250)

3.2.2 Dermal Changes

Papillary blood capillaries are often congested and dilated; dilatation of lymphatic vessels is very conspicuous in some but not all cases. Dermal oedema is prominent, with deposits of acid mucopolysaccharides. A dense mononuclear cell infiltrate is usually present around blood vessels of the lower dermis, and even in the subcutaneous tissue. The cells of the infiltrate migrate from the perivascular spaces to the epidermis and are found throughout the dermal tissue, either isolated or grouped in small clumps. It is not uncommon to see dermal infiltration of inflammatory cells around and within hair sheaths and sebaceous ducts, which show some degree of spongiosis and cellular degeneration. This picture could partly be due to direct penetration of the allergens through the pilosebaceous unit. The infiltrate is of the lymphohistiocytic type, composed almost exclusively of mononuclear cells varying in form and size. As early as 1971 [3, 4], the existence of intimate contact between the cell surfaces of lymphocytes and the cell processes of macrophages was demonstrated at the ultrastructural level. It was emphasized that, in delayed hypersensitivity, macrophages were thought to play an important role, together with lymphocytes [4]. This view was later confirmed and broadened by the discovery of the role played by Langerhans cells (see below). Polymorphonuclear neutrophils are usually absent. Some eosinophils can be found in the oedematous tissue of the upper dermis, migrating towards the epidermis. The histopathological picture is very similar when the biopsy is taken 72 or 96h after application of the allergen. The dermal infiltrate around blood vessels is usually more pronounced. At this later stage, eosinophils are sometimes numerous, but not in all cases. The role of the mast cell in allergic contact hypersensitivity remains controversial. Some studies showing histological evidence of mast cell degranulation suggest that early mast cell activation occurs [5].

In recent years, Hannuksela's repeated open application test (see Sect. 10.1.15) has become popular for confirming the clinical relevance of positive allergic patch test reactions [6]. In the last few months, we have taken biopsies from positive allergic open test reactions on the volar aspect of the forearm or the cubital fossa, 48, 72 or 96 h after application of the allergen. In all cases, the histopathological picture was quite similar to that observed in positive allergic patch test reactions (Lachapelle, unpublished data). The histopathological signs of photoallergic patch test reactions are very similar [7].

3.3 Histopathological Features
of Positive Irritant Patch Test Reactions

The histopathological picture of positive allergic patch test reactions has been shown to be very similar ('monotonous and uniform') in most cases (see above). When irritants are applied – under occlusion – on the skin, a wide range of different lesions can be seen. This kaleidoscope of lesions concerns

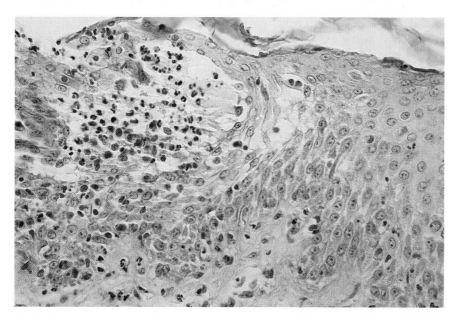

Fig. 3.3. Irritant positive patch test reaction to croton oil at 2 days: spongiotic vesiculation in epidermis with exocytosis of mononuclear cells. This picture is indistinguishable from an allergic reaction. Masson's trichrome blue stain (× 150)

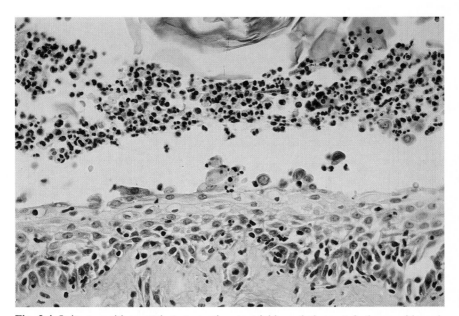

Fig. 3.4. Irritant positive patch test reaction to trichloroethylene at 2 days: epidermal necrosis with acantholytic keratinocytes, exocytosis of inflammatory cells. Masson's trichrome blue stain (× 150)

mainly epidermal alterations. Various factors play a role in the formation of lesions: (a) the nature of the irritant agent and consequently its mode of deleterious action on the cells; (b) the concentration of the irritant applied on the skin; (c) the ways of penetration into the skin; and (d) the individual reactivity of the skin to a well-defined irritant. It is therefore possible that the same irritant chemical can produce different types of lesions in different patients, even when it is applied for the same duration of time and under the same conditions. There is no general rule in this respect.

3.3.1 Epidermal Changes

Various alterations of epidermal cells can be observed. In some cases, these alterations are limited to the superficial layers of the epidermis, the stratum granulosum and the upper part of the stratum spinosum; in others they extend to the dermo-epidermal junction, invading all layers of the epidermis. At first, cells become karyopyknotic and lose their cytoplasmic staining properties on

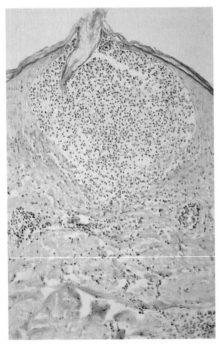

Fig. 3.5. Irritant positive patch test reaction to croton oil at 2 days: a follicular pustule is filled with neutrophils and lymphoid cells. There is a perivascular infiltrate of mononuclear cells. Masson's trichrome blue stain (× 75)

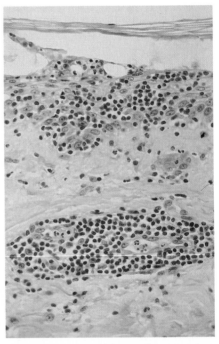

Fig. 3.6. Irritant positive patch test reaction to sodium lauryl sulphate at 2 days: the epidermis is partly necrotic with infiltration of mononuclear cells. There is a dermal perivascular infiltrate of mononuclear cells. Haemotoxylin-eosin stain (× 150)

haematoxylin and eosin sections. These changes are known as 'Bandmann's achromasia' [8]. When the irritation process becomes more severe, complete necrosis (or cytolysis) of epidermal cells occurs, leading to the formation of intra- or subepidermal vesicles and bullae. 'Chemical acantholysis' of epidermal cells can be seen mainly, but not exclusively, with certain irritants such as cantharidin and trichloroethylene [9]. Polymorpho-nuclear neutrophils accumulate in the damaged epidermis, leading to the formation of subcorneal or intra-epidermal pustules. In some cases, the formation of pustules is preferentially limited to the hair follicles. Follicular pustules are preferentially provoked by some irritants, such as croton oil ('croton oil effect') or metal salts such as chromates, and those of mercury and nickel. Pustules due to metals are observed mainly, but not exclusively, in atopics. As already noted many years ago [10], some irritant reactions do not show any of the aforementioned histopathological signs; they are exclusively spongiotic (with or without vesicles). Such observations can be made: (a) with weak irritants; (b) with strong irritants, applied on the skin at low concentration; (c) in the 'excited' (or irritable) skin syndrome. Examples of epidermal lesions classically observed with certain categories of irritants are given in Table 3.1.

Many years ago, ultrastructural studies threw some light on the mode of action of certain irritants, including croton oil [11], sodium hydroxide and hydrochloric acid [12]. More recently, Willis et al. [13, 14] completed an extensive study comparing the action of several categories of irritants, using semi-thin section technology. They noted in particular that various kinds of detergents damaged epidermal cells in different ways when applied at low concentration. For instance, the major response to the anionic detergent sodium lauryl sulphate was parakeratosis, indicating increased epidermal cell turnover, whilst benzalkonium chloride, a cationic detergent, caused a different type of reaction, spongiosis and exocytosis with spotty necrotic damage [13, 14]. Phototoxic reactions are characterized by the presence of eosinophilic necrotic keratinocytes ('sunburn cells').

Table 3.1. Epidermal lesions observed in relation to certain common irritants

Irritants	Epidermal lesions
Nonchlorinated organic solvents (i.e. alkanes, such as *n*-hexane; toluene; xylene; white spirit; turpentine, etc.)	Achromasia; superficial necrosis; karyopyknosis; very occasional acantholysis; subepidermal vesicles and/or bullae
Chlorinated organic solvents (i.e. trichloroethane; trichloroethylene; carbon tetrachloride; etc.)	Acantholysis + +; karyopyknosis; complete necrosis of epidermal cells; intraepidermal vesicles and/or bullae
Acids, alkalis, surfactants, detergents, aldehydes	Achromasia; superficial or complete necrosis of epidermal cells; subepidermal vesicles and/or bullae; no acantholysis

3.3.2 Dermal Changes

Dermal changes are also related to the mechanisms involved in the mode of action of each individual irritant. Dermal oedema is absent or slight. Blood capillaries and lymphatics are discretely dilated, but usually to a lesser extent than in positive allergic patch test reactions. In some cases, there is an important inflammatory response distributed around the blood vessels of the upper- and mid-dermis. It is either homogeneously mononuclear or mixed (polymorphonuclear neutrophils and lymphocytes/histiocytes). Eosinophils are absent. In cases of severe irritation, it is usual to find pyknotic remnants of neutrophils in the upper part of the dermis.

3.4 Histopathological Criteria for Distinguishing Between Allergic and Irritant Patch Test Reactions in Man

In the preceding paragraphs, the various histopathological signs encountered in allergic and irritant patch test reactions have been reviewed in detail [8, 15, 16]. We must remember that this description refers to 'typical' cases: irritant (without allergic component) or allergic (without irritant component). Comparative signs are presented in Table 3.2. These distinctive criteria are of limited value in practice for many reasons: (a) most criteria are present in irritant as well as in allergic positive patch test reactions; (b) other criteria are

Table 3.2. Distinctive histopathological criteria between allergic and irritant patch test reactions in man. (Modified from [8])

	Allergic Reactions	Irritant Reactions
Epidermis		
Spongiosis	+ to + + +	+ or −
Exocytosis	+ to + + +	+ + +
Vesicles	+ (spongiotic)	+ (rarely spongiotic)
Formation of bullae	Facultative (spongiotic)	Facultative (rarely spongiotic)
Pustules	−	+ or −
Necrosis of epidermal cells	−	+ to + + +
Acantholysis of epidermal cells	−	+ or −
Distribution of the infiltrate in epidermis	Focal [17]	Diffuse [17]
Dermis		
Perivascular infiltrate	Mononuclear	Mononuclear or mixed (mononuclear + neutrophils)
Eosinophilic leucocytes	+ or −	−
Dilatation of lymphatic vessels	+ or −	−
Dilatation of blood capillaries	+ or −	+ or −
Oedema	+ or −	Very unusual

predominant either in irritant or in allergic reactions, but they lack specificity; (c) most allergens also have irritant properties. Even when allergens are patch tested at a concentration below the level of clinical irritancy to avoid 'mixed' pictures, it is just possible that subclinically, at the microscopic level, they might show a mixed picture of irritation and allergy. In practice, when a positive patch test reaction is clinically doubtful (irritant? – allergic?), the help of a biopsy is minimal, due to the differential bias which has been explained above.

Avnstorp et al. [17] conducted a semiquantitative histological study of individual morphological parameters in allergic and irritant patch test reactions. Their conclusions were as follows: statistical analysis by correlation of 17 selected variables gives a diagnostic specificity of 87% and a sensitivity of 81% for allergic reactions. For irritant reactions, the specificity is 100% and the sensitivity 46%. By multiple regression analysis, an index was calculated for the differentiation of allergic and irritant reactions. If this index were to be used in cases of allergic patch test reactions, all would be reported as allergic reactions while half of the irritant reactions would also be reported as allergic. Although this study has shed some light on the problem of the histopathological differentiation of allergic and irritant contact dermatitis, many difficulties remain in making such a differentiation [17].

In conclusion, though conventional histopathology of positive patch test reactions can provide some useful information, it is of little help in separating allergic from irritant or mixed reactions. Drawing such a conclusion at the end of this section might appear to be negativistic, since a different view has prevailed for decades in so many European clinics. Nevertheless, it is based on a careful review of the literature and a reappraisal of our own material. It coincides with the views of the basic scientists and must be considered by practising dermatologists as reflecting reality.

3.5 Comparative Immunohistochemical and Immunocytochemical Characteristics of Allergic and Irritant Patch Test Reactions in Man

3.5.1 Introduction

An explosion in knowledge concerning the mechanisms involved in contact dermatitis has been occurring in the past ten years; the discovery of the key role played by the Langerhans cell and the ability to identify subpopulations of lymphocytes by the use of monoclonal antibodies must be considered as major advances. This has raised the question as to whether the use of new immunocytopathological techniques might help in distinguishing between irritant and allergic patch test reactions.

3.5.2 Epidermal Langerhans Cells in Irritant and Allergic Positive Patch Test Reactions

Semiquantitative studies related to the number of Langerhans cells (LC;CD1 or T_6 dendritic cells) in the epidermis have been conducted in positive irritant and allergic patch test reactions. These studies have revealed a statistically significant decrease in LC 48 at 72 h after the application of various types of irritants: sodium lauryl sulphate, mercuric chloride, benzalkonium chloride, croton oil or dithranol. There was also a significant reduction in dendritic length. These changes in density were unrelated to the intensity of the inflammatory response [18].

Similar studies in positive allergic patch test reactions showed an early transitory increase in LC in the first few hours [19] following the application of allergens, but a similar response occurred at the sites of petrolatum application [19]. This phenomenon may therefore lack specificity. Later on, at 24, 48 or 72h after application of the allergen, the number of LC is unchanged or decreased when compared with normal skin. It may also be reduced at the site of negative patch test reactions [20]. The current studies indicate that allergic and irritant patch test reactions cannot be differentiated reliably by counting the LC, in spite of the small differences observed [21]. Moreover, lymphocyte/LC apposition is observed in both types of reactions [22, 23]. The presence of HLA-DR antigens on keratinocytes in allergic reactions could reflect an immunological response [24].

3.5.3 Cells of the Infiltrate in Irritant and Allergic Positive Patch Test Reactions: Immunophenotypic Studies

In the various studies conducted so far, the composition of the infiltrates is similar in allergic and irritant reactions, and consists of T lymphocytes of helper/inducer types in association with T-cell accessory cells, that is, LC and HLA-DR positive macrophages [25]. No differences in expression of T cells or macrophage-associated antigens are seen in early, as opposed to late, biopsies. The proportion of cells positive for markers associated with activation (interleukin-2 receptor) or proliferation (transferrin receptor, K_i 67 nuclear antigen) of lymphoid cells is found to increase with time in both types of reactions [25]. Immunophenotypical analysis of infiltrating cells has been expanded, in relation to the availability of new monoclonal antibodies (see Sect. 2.1.1.4). Using these panels of antibodies, Brasch et al. [20] showed an early accumulation of memory T cells in positive patch test reactions.

It is therefore possible that in coming years new techniques will allow a more precise distinction between irritant and allergic patch test reactions.

3.6 Conclusions

In spite of certain differences in the histopathological lesions observed in allergic and irritant patch test reactions, there is as yet no reliable diagnostic tool (either morphological or immunophenotypic) to 'label' specifically each type of reaction.

3.7 References

1. Kerl H, Burg G, Braun-Falco O (1974) Quantitative and qualitative dynamics of the epidermal and cellular inflammatory reaction in primary toxic and allergic dinitrochlorobenzene contact dermatitis in guinea pigs. Arch Dermatol Forsch 249: 207–226
2. Ackerman AB, Ragaz A (1982) A plea to expunge the term "eczema" from the lexicon of dermatology and dermatopathology. Arch Dermatol Res 272: 407–411
3. Braun-Falco O Wolff HH (1971) Zur Ultrastruktur der menschlichen Epidermis bei der allergischen Epicutantestreaktion. Arch Dermatol Forsch 240: 23–37
4. Wolff HH, Braun-Falco O (1971) Zur Ultrastruktur dermaler Veränderungen bei der allergischen Epicutantestreaktion des Menschen. Arch Dermatol Forsch 240: 219–236
5. Angelini G, Vena GA, Filotico R, Tursi A (1990) Mast cell participation in allergic contact sensitivity. Contact Dermatitis 23: 239
6. Hannuksela M, Salo H (1986) The repeated open application test (ROAT). Contact Dermatitis 14: 221–227
7. Thune P, Eeg-Larsen T (1984) Contact and photocontact allergy in persistent light reactivity. Contact Dermatitis 11: 98–107
8. Lachapelle JM (1973) Comparative histopathology of allergic and irritant patch test reactions in man. Current concepts and new prospects. Arch Belg Dermatol 28: 83–92
9. Mahmoud G, Lachapelle JM (1985) Evaluation expérimentale de l'efficacité de crèmes barrière et de gels antisolvants dans la prévention de l'irritation cutanée provoquée par des solvants organiques. Cah Med Trav 22: 163–168
10. Achten G, Oleffe J (1966) Tests épicutanés et dermatoses professionnelles. Etude histologique. Bull Soc Fr Dermatol 73: 49–52
11. Metz J (1972) Elektronenmikroskopische Untersuchungen in allergischen und toxischen Epicutantestreaktionen des Menschen. Arch Dermatol Forsch 245: 125–146
12. Nagao S, Stroud JD, Hamada T, Pinkus H, Birmingham DJ (1972) The effect of sodium hydroxide and hydrochloric acid on human epidermis. An electronmicroscopic study. Acta Derm Venereol (Stockh.) 52: 11–23
13. Willis CM, Stephens CJM, Wilkinson JD (1989) Epidermal damage induced by irritants in man: a light and electron microscopic study. J Invest Dermatol 93: 695–699
14. Willis CM, Stephens CJM, Wilkinson JD (1989) Preliminary findings on the patterns of epidermal damage induced by irritants in man. In: Frosch PJ, Dooms-Goossens A, Lachapelle JM, Rycroft RJ, Scheper RJ (eds) Current topics in contact dermatitis. Springer, Berlin Heidelberg New York, pp 42–45
15. Medenica M, Rostenberg A (1971) A comparative light and electron microscopic study of primary irritant contact dermatitis and allergic contact dermatitis. J Invest Dermatol 56: 259–271
16. Nater JP, Hoedemaeker PHJ (1976) Histopathological differences between irritant and allergic patch test reactions in man. Contact Dermatitis 2: 247–253
17. Avnstorp C, Balslev E, Thomsen HK (1989) The occurrence of different morphological parameters in allergic and irritant patch test reactions. In: Frosch PJ, Dooms-Goossens A, Lachapelle JM, Rycroft RJ, Scheper RJ (eds) Current topics in contact dermatitis. Springer, Berlin Heidelberg New York, pp 38–41

18. Ferguson J, Gibbs JH, Beck JS (1985) Lymphocyte subsets and Langerhans cells in allergic and irritant patch test reactions: histometric studies. Contact Dermatitis 13: 166–174
19. Christensen OB, Daniels TE, Maibach HI (1986) Expression of OKT6 antigen by Langerhans cells in patch test reactions. Contact Dermatitis 14: 26–31
20. Brasch J, Mielke V, Künne N, Weber-Matthiesen V, Bruhn S, Sterry W (1990) Immigration of cells and composition of cell infiltrates in patch test reactions. Contact Dermatitis 23: 238
21. Kanerva L, Ranki A, Lauharanta J (1984) Lymphocytes and Langerhans cells in patch tests. An immunohistochemical and electron microscopic study. Contact Dermatitis 11: 150–155
22. Willis CM, Young E, Brandon DR, Wilkinson JD (1986) Immunopathological and ultrastructural findings in human allergic and irritant contact dermatitis. Br J Dermatol 115: 305–316
23. Willis CM, Wilkinson JD (1990) Changes in the morphology and density of epidermal Langerhans cells (CD1$^+$ cells) in irritant contact dermatitis. Contact Dermatitis 23: 239
24. Scheynius A, Fischer T (1986) Phenotypic difference between allergic and irritant patch test reactions in man. Contact Dermatitis 14: 297–302
25. Avnstorp C, Ralfkiaer E, Jorgensen J, Lange Watzin G (1987) Sequential immunophenotypic study of lymphoid infiltrate in allergic and irritant reactions. Contact Dermatitis 16: 239–245

Chapter 4
Molecular Aspects of Allergic Contact Dermatitis

Molecular Aspects
of Allergic Contact Dermatitis

JEAN-PIERRE LEPOITTEVIN, CLAUDE BENEZRA[†],
CAROLINE C. SIGMAN, DONYA BAGHERI, ROSSANA FRAGINALS[†]
and HOWARD I. MAIBACH

Contents

4.1 Molecular Approach to Allergic Contact Dermatitis

It is now generally accepted that contact allergens (haptens) must have special properties in order to be sensitizing. Among these properties, the most important appears to be the faculty of reacting with epidermal proteins, giving a complete allergen [1, 2]. The most economical way of looking at the nature of the carrier protein is to consider that membrane-embedded proteins are the most likely candidates. Protein groups capable of forming strong covalent bonds with a hapten are nucleophilic groups, -Nu-H, where Nu (= nucleophile) stands for S- or NH-. They can react with electrophiles to produce the antigen, a modified protein:

protein-Nu-H + hapten → protein-Nu-hapten.

4.1.1 Electrophilic Haptens

Electrophilic properties of haptens can be estimated by their ability to react with nucleophiles. There is, unfortunately, no quantitative data allowing one to build a scale measuring electrophilicity. General organic chemistry knowledge allows one to have a qualitative 'feeling' for this reactivity.

Attempts to use the reaction of a number of electrophiles (haptens) with a standard nucleophiles such as *n*-butylamine have been made [3], but there are no available data for a large selection of electrophiles.

When no electrophilic properties are apparent, it is believed that the compounds must undergo in vitro or in vivo modification to become truly haptenic. These compounds are called prohaptens [2]. This concept was first proposed by Landsteiner [1]. As an example of these prohapten or proelectrophilic compounds, pentadecylcatechol (PDC), one of the poison ivy allergens, is inactivated if the two phenolic groups are blocked by methyl substituents, thus preventing the transformation of a nonelectrophilic catechol into a potent electrophile, an *o*-quinone (Fig. 4.1).

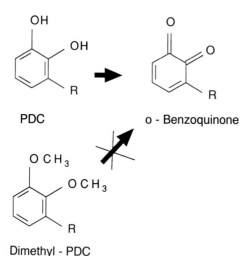

Fig. 4.1. Oxidation of pentadecylcat-echol (PDC) gives an *o*-quinone. When methylated (dimethyl-PDC), PDC cannot be oxidized further

4.1.2 Lipophilic Haptens

Among the most potent haptens known, poison ivy and poison oak play a dominant role in the United States [4, 5]. The haptens, called urushiols, are nonelectrophilic compounds, catechols, equipped with a long straight hydro-carbon chain, hydrophobic and able to insert into membranes. Lipophilic properties enhance sensitizing power. Are they able to explain alone the allergenic effects? In the case of alkyl catechols it is probable that proelec-trophilic (= prohaptenic) as well as lipophilic properties are in operation. One can imagine, for instance, that, once inserted into a cell membrane (or once bound by hydrophobic attraction onto the cell surface), the pyrocatechols undergo oxidation, allowing attack by a nearby protein.

We have, however, shown [6] that truly nonelectrophilic, nonproelec-trophilic compounds, saturated analogues of catechols (i.e. 3-alkyl-1,2-cyclohexanediols; Fig. 4.2), were capable of sensitizing guinea pigs, provided

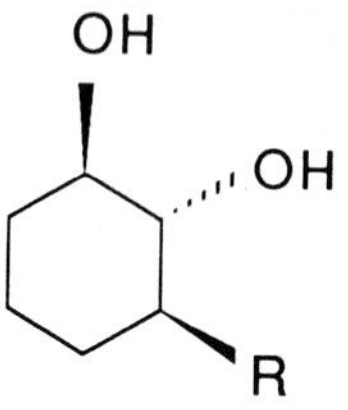

Fig. 4.2. Structure of *all-trans*-3-alkyl-1,2-cyclohexanediol

that the alkyl chain was long enough ($>C_{10}$). This could be a true example of a hydrophobic hapten. In lanolin, long-chain saturated alcohols are also thought to be allergenic.

4.1.3 Are there Nucleophilic Haptens?

It does not seem that proelectrophilic properties (prohaptens) can always explain the sensitizing power of substances. Little is known about the skin metabolism of haptens. Oxidation and radical formation are likely reactions in the epidermis, but no study has been devoted entirely to this problem.

In principle, because of the presence of disulphide bridges in proteins, a nucleophilic hapten could still form covalent bonds with carrier proteins. Thus, a well-known reaction of thiols is the replacement of one of the two sulphurs (Fig. 4.3).

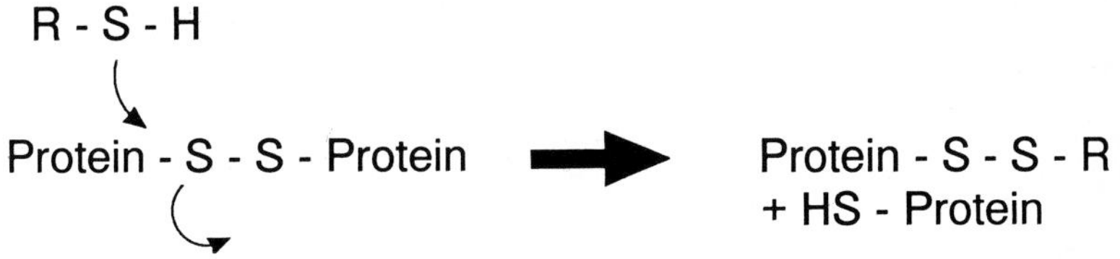

Fig. 4.3. A nucleophilic thiol group: R–S–H can attack a disulphide bridge, giving rise to an antigen

Thus, 2-mercaptoethanol ($HSCH_2CH_2OH$) is classically used to reduce S–S linkages. It is unlikely that nucleophiles other than thiols are as efficient in this respect as the newly formed bonds; for instance N–S or O–S bonds are not very stable.

The well-known allergens, the mercaptobenzothiazoles, are typical nucleophilic allergens (Fig. 4.4).

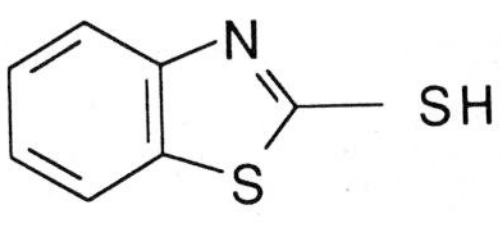

Fig. 4.4. Chemical structure of mercaptobenzothiazole (MBT)

4.2 Use of a Data Base of Skin Allergens: Example of Aminophenols

We described in 1985 the creation of a data base of contact allergens [7]. This data base has been used to look for structure-activity relationships (SAR) of some functional groups such as benzoquinones and gallic acid esters [7] and *p*-phenylenediamine (PPD) derivatives [8]. We have explained our approach in detail in the two papers just cited and, in particular, the concept of 'degree of confidence', a figure from 1 to 5 assessing the reliability of data, 5 being the maximum. This degree of confidence scale, summarized in Table 4.1, is based on objective criteria such as the number of described cases, the presence of controls, the relevance of the tests, the purity of compounds, etc. [8]. After adding together the different numbers assigned to these criteria, degrees of confidence are assigned according to Table 4.2. Three other degrees of confidence are used: 0 for reviews (only the title of the review is recorded), 6 for standard allergens (i.e. allergens present in the European standard series) and 7 for data extracted from textbooks which generally lack detailed information.

Table 4.1. Criteria used to assess degree of confidence. (Reproduced by permission of *Seminars in Dermatology*)

Criteria	Score
No. of cases	2, Significant; 0, not significant
Controls	2, Adequate; 0, inadequate no. or none
Relevance of test	2, Relevant; 0, irrelevant or consecutive patient testing
Induction (sensitization) route	1, Appropriate or known; 0, inappropriate or unknown
Vehicle	1, Appropriate; 0, inappropriate
Purity of test substance	1, Adequate; 0, inadequate
Concentrations	1, Adequate; 0, inadequate
Statistics	1, Yes; 0, no
Dilution series	1, Yes; 0, no
Use test	1, Yes; 0, no

Table 4.2. Interpretation of criteria scores as degrees of confidence. (Reproduced by permission of *Seminars in Dermatology*)

Total score	Degree of confidence
11–13	5
8–10	4
6–7	3
4–5	2
0–3	1

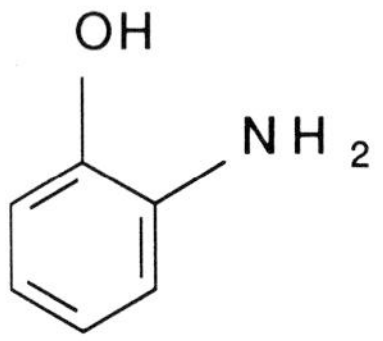

1   o - Aminophenol

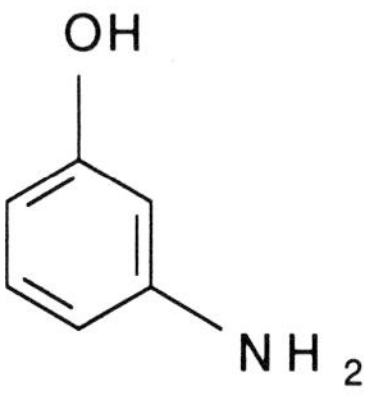

2   m - Aminophenol

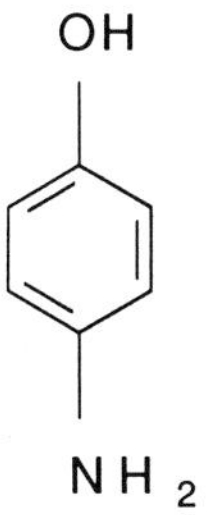

3   p - Aminophenol

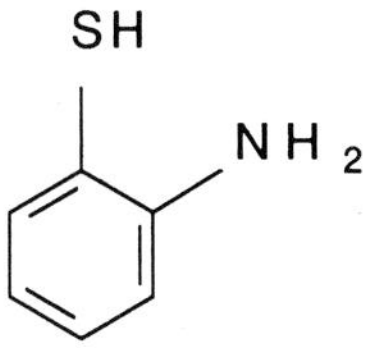

4   o - Aminothiophenol

Fig. 4.5. Structures of *o*-, *m*-, and *p*-aminophenols (*1–3*) and of *o*-aminothiophenol (*4*)

We have now applied this approach to the search for SAR among aminophenols. The compounds studied were *o*-, *m*- and *p*-aminophenols and *o*-aminothiophenol (compounds 1–4, Fig. 4.5). An example of printouts obtained when aminophenols are recalled as primary sensitizers and cross-reactants is shown in Table 4.3. Table 4.4 is the printout obtained when compounds cross-reacting with aminophenols are recalled. All of the items from any of the columns can be recalled, for instance, vehicles, methods of sensitization and concentration. These printouts allow one to look for the sensitizing activity of aminophenols and SAR from cross-sensitivity studies.

4.2.1 Sensitizing Capacity of Aminophenols

Among the different aminophenols, sensitization rates varied from 19% to 40%. Of the three unsubstituted aminophenols, *p*-aminophenol was the most efficient sensitizer (32%–40% sensitization rate). This is quite in line with the Mayer quinone theory [9]: *p*-aminophenol is the most likely to undergo an in vivo oxidation-hydrolysis set of reactions, leading to an excellent electrophile, benzoquinone (5), as shown in Fig. 4.6.

The second most sensitizing compound is *m*-aminophenol (3) (21%–32% sensitization rate). This finding is quite surprising, especially in view of

Table 4.3. Contact allergens data base: aminophenols as primary sensitizers and cross-reactants

Reactant	Type of reactant	No. of cases	No. positive	Type of cases	Type of Test/animal	Conc./ vehicle	No. of controls	Degree of confidence	Reference code
p-Aminophenol (123-30-8)	X [o-Diaminobenzene (95-54-5)]	12 or 24	0	3	OET GP FCA	0.09 mmol/l, H_2O	Yes?	4	CODE85130226
p-Aminophenol (123-30-8)	X [m-Diaminobenzene (108-45-2)]	12 or 24	0	3	OET GP FCA	0.09 mmol/l, H_2O	Yes?	4	CODE85130226
p-Aminophenol (123-30-8)	P	12 or 24	40%	3	OET GP FCA	0.09 mmol/l, H_2O	Yes?	4	CODE85130226
p-Aminophenol (123-30-8)	P	12 or 24	0	3	OET GP GP Topical	0.09 mmol/l, H_2O	Yes?	4	CODE85130226
p-Aminophenol (123-30-8)	X [p-Phenylenediamine (106-50-3)]	10	3	3	PT MSIAT	5%, H_2O/ace-tone	Yes?	4–5	CODE88190248
p-Aminophenol (123-30-8)	X [o-Aminophenol (95-55-6)]	9	1	3	PT MSIAT	5%, H_2O/ace-tone	Yes?	4–5	CODE88190248

Aminophenols acting as primary sensitizers and cross-reactants were recalled. Successively are shown: *column 1*, name of compound with Chemical Abstracts Service (CAS) number; *column 2*, the type of reaction (*P*, primary sensitizer; *X*, cross-reactant; in brackets, the name and CAS number of the corresponding primary sensitizer); *column 3*, the number of the recorded cases; *column 4*, number of positive tests; *column 5*, type of cases (1, contact dermatitis; 2, other diseases; 3, normal humans or naive animals); *column 6*, type of test and animal (GP, guinea pigs; MO, mouse; HU, human) with method of sensitization used (FCA, Freund's complete adjuvant technique; OET, open epicutaneous test; topical sensitization; MSIAT, modified single injection adjuvant test; PT, patch test; *column 7*, concentration in % or millimoles per litre and solvent; *column 8*, number of controls; *column 9*, degree of confidence; *column 10*, reference code with 4 letters for the journal, e.g. CODE = *Contact Dermatitis*, year and volume number (four digits in all), and first page number.

Table 4.4. Contact allergens data base: Chemicals that cross-react with aminophenols (see Table 4.3 for explanation)

Reactant	Type of reactant	No. of cases	No. positive	Type of cases	Type of Test/animal	Conc./ vehicle	No. of controls	Degree of confidence	Reference code
Benzoquinone (106-51-3)	X [o-Aminophenol (95-55-6)]	9	4	3	PT GP MSIAT	25%, ace-tone/p EG400	Yes?	4–5	CODE88190248
Benzoquinone (106-51-3)	X [m-Aminophenol (591-27-5)]	10	6	3	PT GP MSIAT	25%, ace-tone/p EG400	Yes?	4–5	CODE88190248
Benzoquinone (106-51-3)	X [p-Aminophenol (123-30-8)]	10	9	3	PT GP MSIAT	25%, ace-tone/p EG400	Yes?	4–5	CODE88190248
Benzoquinone (106-51-3)	X [p-Aminophenol (123-308)]	10	0	3	PT GP CCET	2.5%, ace-tone/p EG400	Yes?	4–5	CODE88190248
m-Diaminoben-zene (108-45-2)	X [o-Aminophenol (123-30-8)]	12 or 24	0	3	OET GP GP Topical	0.09 mmol/l, H_2O	Yes?	4	CODE85130226
m-Diaminoben-zene (108-45-2)	X [m-Aminophenol (591-27-5)]	12 or 24	0	3	OET GP GP Topical	0.09 mmol/l, H_2O	Yes?	4	CODE85130226

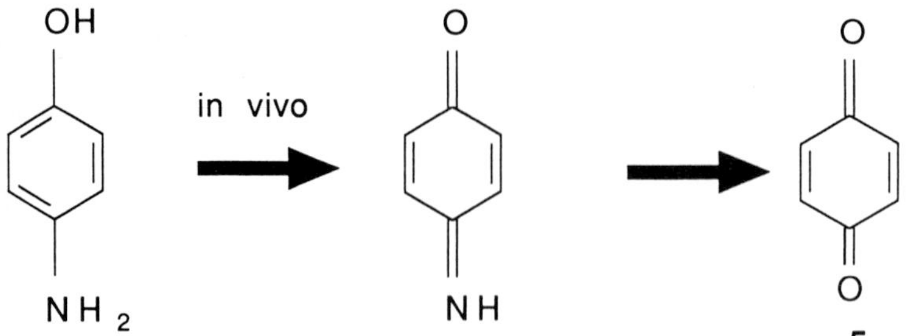

Fig. 4.6. Oxidation of *p*-aminophenol into a quinone-imine and hydrolysis of the latter into *p*-benzoquinone (*5*)

the fact that this compound cannot be transformed as easily as the *para* derivative (3) into an electrophile. There can always, however, be some in vivo hydroxylation, either *ortho* or *para* to the phenol, which would eventually lead to an *o*- or a *p*-quinone (6 and 7, respectively), with an amine function. Figure 4.7 shows an *ortho*-hydroxylation and Fig. 4.8 a *para*-hydroxylation, while Fig. 4.9 shows an in vivo *para*-hydroxylation of *o*-aminophenol, leading to the same aminobenzene metabolite as in Fig. 4.8.

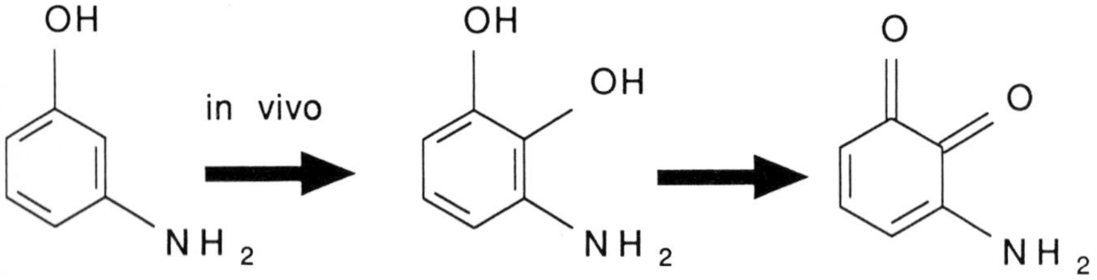

Fig. 4.7. *ortho*-Hydroxylation of *m*-aminophenol gives an *o*-benzoquinone (*6*)

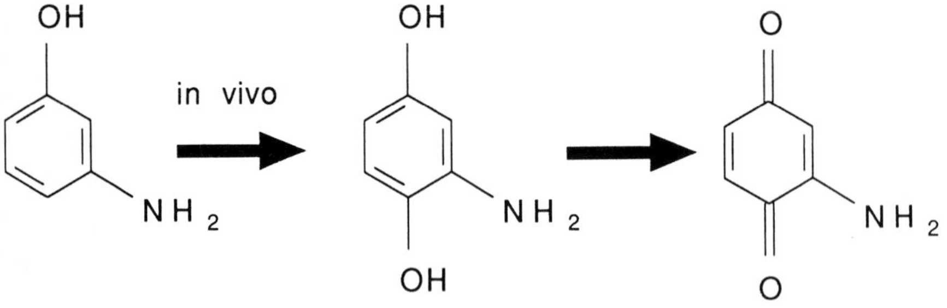

Fig. 4.8. *para*-Hydroxylation of *m*-aminophenol gives an amino-*p*-benzoquinone (*7*)

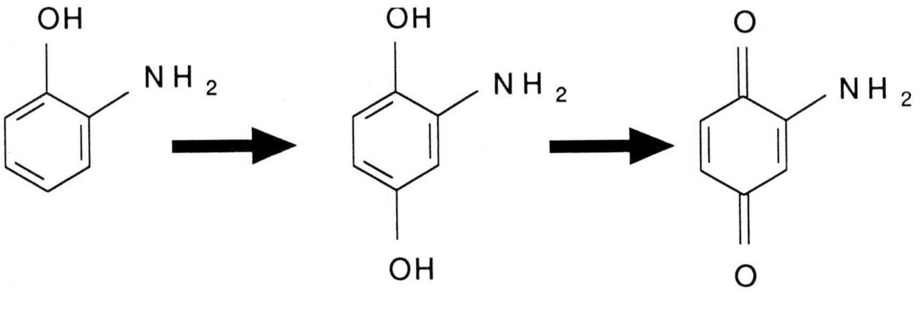

Fig. 4.9. *para*-Hydroxylation of *o*-aminophenol gives an amino-*p*-benzoquinone (*7*)

The third compound, *o*-aminophenol (1) (19%–25% sensitizing power), can be oxidized in vivo into an *o*-quinone (8), a potent electrophile (Fig. 4.10).

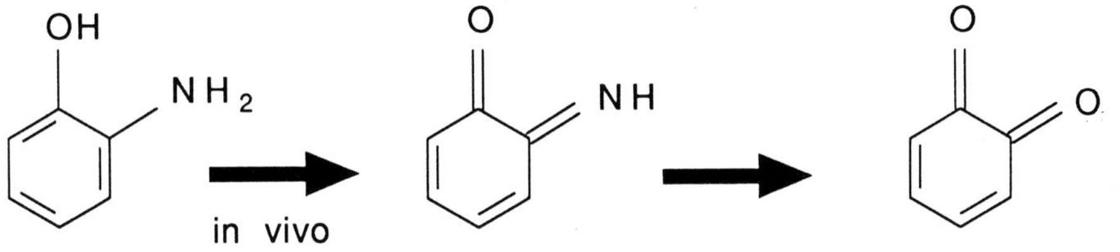

Fig. 4.10. Oxidation and hydrolysis of *o*-aminophenol gives the *o*-benzoquinone (*8*)

These results, however, must be interpreted with caution. The studies concerning *m*-aminophenol (2) [10] were conducted with concentrations 5000 times higher than that where *m*-aminophenol was found to be a nonsensitizer [11]!

4.2.2 Cross-reactions with Aminophenols

In *p*-aminophenol (3)-sensitized guinea-pigs (Table 4.4), there was no cross-reaction with either *m*- or *o*-aminophenols (2 or 1, respectively). There was, however, a reaction to benzoquinone (9 out of 10 animals giving a positive test) in guinea pigs sensitized using the modified single injection adjuvant test (MSIAT), but not with the animals sensitized using the cumulative contact enhancement test (CCET) [10]. These animals also reacted to *o*-diaminobenzene (*o*-phenylenediamine) (9) and to *p*-diaminobenzene (PPD) (10). The latter is also believed to be metabolized into benzoquinone [2], while the *o*-derivative would be transformed into *o*-benzoquinone.

In m-aminophenol-sensitized guinea-pigs, cross-reactions to p-benzoquinone were observed in 6 out of 10 animals. The reaction depicted in Fig. 4.8 (transformation of m-aminophenol into amino-p-benzoquinone) could explain this reaction, through the formation of a common metabolite. A cross-reaction with PPD, again supposed to be biotransformed into p-benzoquinone [2], could also explain the cross-reaction observed.

In o-aminophenol-sensitized guinea pigs, there was cross-sensitization with p-benzoquinone and PPD. These results are more difficult to rationalize, unless o-aminophenol, like m-aminophenol, could first be *para* hydroxylated as depicted in Fig. 4.9, giving a metabolite identical to the one coming from m-aminophenol (Fig.4.8). However, there was no cross-reaction between o- and m-aminophenol, a result which is not quite compatible with this hypothesis.

4.2.3 Other Information obtained from the Allergen Data Base

The data base contains information about many other parameters concerning aminophenols. For instance, the vehicles used for testing were petrolatum, acetone, water and water/acetone. Concentrations varied between 0.09 molal (0.09 mole per 1000 g solvent) and 1%–5% (from 1000 to 5000 times higher). Methods of sensitization included the open epicutaneous test (OET), Freund's complete adjuvant (FCA), MSIAT and CCET. The efficiency of these tests was variable. Thus, in p-aminophenol-sensitized animals, cross-reaction with p-benzoquinone was observed only in MSIAT-sensitized guinea pigs.

4.2.4 Discussion and Conclusions

The prohapten theory [1, 2] explains nicely some of the results observed in data from the literature in the data base. The cross-reactions between *para*-substituted compounds can be interpreted through the formation of a common metabolite, p-benzoquinone. Reactions with *ortho*-substituted derivatives and, even more, *meta*-derivatives of phenols or amines are more difficult to explain, but are again consistent with a quinone formation theory.

4.3 Skin Allergens that are also Carcinogens

Contact allergens are reactive chemicals capable of reacting with cellular macromolecules, nucleic acids and proteins. The reaction may be nucleophilic, electrophilic, free radical or electrostatic. Presumably, reactions with carrier proteins mediate the immunogenicity of contact allergens. Because they are biologically reactive, contact allergens also have other pharmacological and toxicological effects.

Many carcinogens are also reactive chemicals. In particular, they are electrophiles that react with DNA bases. Carcinogenic N-nitroso compounds, for example, alkylate guanosine residues of DNA. These reactions damage DNA, causing mutations and ultimately neoplastic cells. To examine the possibility that some contact allergens could also be carcinogens, we compared the chemicals in the contact allergens data base with those in a data base of well-documented carcinogenicity test results. One should exercise care in interpreting these results, as carcinogenic activity has been for the most part studied in animal models.

The carcinogenicity data base was compiled first in 1979–1984 by SRI International for the National Cancer Institute (NCI, under contracts NO1-CP-33285 and NO1-CP-95607). It has been maintained by SRI International since then. This data base covers the NCI and National Toxicology Program *Carcinogenesis Bioassay Technical Reports,* the International Agency for Research on Cancer (IARC) *Monographs on the Evaluation of the Carcinogenic Risk of Chemicals to Humans* and the primary literature from 1965 to 1987. It includes chemical names, Chemical Abstracts Service (CAS) registry numbers, information on the test protocol, target site and tumor types, an evaluation of the test, and full literature citations. Like the contact allergens data base, it is maintained in dBASE for IBM-PC/XT/AT and compatible computers.

Chemicals in the contact allergens data base with demonstrated sensitizing activity were compared with chemicals in the carcinogenicity data base with demonstrated tumorigenic activity. For this preliminary study, we chose to review a specific subset of contact allergens, i.e. those capable of reacting directly with cellular protein without enzymatic modification. Therefore, this comparison excludes a large group of well-known contact allergens that require enzymatic activation. For example, aromatic amines such as p-phenylenediamine and amino-substituted dyes are not covered. These allergens will be the subject of future reviews.

The chemicals that have shown both allergenic and carcinogenic activity are listed in Table 4.5. This table includes summaries of the chemicals' activities as contact allergens and as carcinogens, as they are cited in the data bases. The indication of allergenicity provided is the lowest concentration at which sensitization was observed in human patch tests cited in the contact allergens data base. The indication of carcinogenicity is the species and sites in which tumors were observed in tests cited in the carcinogenicity data base.

Although the data are limited, some tentative conclusions may be drawn from them. First, many direct-acting contact allergens are also carcinogens. The allergens are potent. Except for acetaldehyde, all the contact allergens cited in Table 4.5 have activity at less than molar concentrations. The tumor sites observed suggest that these allergens are also primarily direct-acting carcinogens. That is, tumors are observed at sites close to the carcinogen's route of administration where it should not be affected by systemic metabolism. For example, benzoyl peroxide causes skin tumors

Table 4.5. Contact allergens with demonstrated carcinogenic activity

Chemical	Allergenicity[a]	Carcinogenicity	References
Acetaldehyde	4.5 mmol/l in water	Hamster: larynx Rat: nasal Mucosa	14, 15
Benzoyl peroxide	0.04 mmol/l in paraffin	Mouse: skin	12, 16, 17
Butylated hydroxyanisole	0.11 mmol/l in petrolatum	Hamster: forestomach Rat: forestomach	18–20
Captafol	0.001 mmol/l in petrolatum	Mouse: forestomach, harderian gland, heart, intestines, liver, spleen	21, 22
Captan	0.08 mmol/l in petrolatum	Mouse: duodenum	23–25
Chlorothalonil	0.1 mmol/l in petrolatum	Rat: kidney	26, 27
Coumarin	0.34 mmol/l in petrolatum	Rat: bile Duct	28, 29
Epichlorohydrin	0.11 mmol/l in ethanol	Mouse: injection site, skin Rat: forestomach	30–32
Ethyl acrylate	0.1 mmol/l in petrolatum	Mouse: forestomach Rat: forestomach	13, 33
Ethylene thiourea	0.1 mmol/l in petrolatum	Mouse: liver, lymphatic system Rat: thyroid gland	22, 34–36
Formaldehyde	0.67 mmol/l in water	Rat: nasal turbinates	37–39
Hydrazine	0.08 mmol/l in petrolatum (as sulphate)	Mouse: liver, lung	40, 41
Phenoxybenzamine hydrochloride	0.03 mmol/l in water	Mouse: peritoneal cavity Rat: peritoneal cavity	42–44
o-Phenylphenol	0.06 mmol/l in petrolatum	Rat: urinary bladder	45, 46
Propylene Oxide	0.17 mmol/l in 70% ethanol	Mouse: nasal cavity Rat: forestomach, injection site, mammary glands	47–49, 50, 51
Styrene	0.01 mmol/l in ethanol	Mouse: lung	52, 53
Thiourea	0.001 mmol/l in petrolatum	Rat: liver	54, 55
Ziram	0.03 mmol/l in petrolatum	Rat: thyroid gland	56, 57

[a] The allergenicity activities listed are the lowest concentrations at which sensitization was observed in human patch tests are currently cited in the contact allergens data base. The species and tumor sites are listed for studies cited in the carcinogenicity data base.

when administered topically [12] and ethyl acrylate causes forestomach tumors when administered by gavage [13].

4.4 References

1. Landsteiner K, Jacobs JL (1936) Studies on the sensitization of animals with simple chemicals. III. J Exp Med 64: 625–639
2. Dupuis G, Benezra C (1982) Allergic contact dermatitis to simple chemicals: a molecular approach. Dekker, New York
3. Roberts DW, Williams DL (1982) The derivation of quantitative correlations between skin sensitization and physico-chemical parameters for alkylating agents and their application to experimental data for sultones. J Theor Biol 99: 807–825
4. Kligman AM (1958) Poison ivy (Rhus) dermatitis. Arch Dermatol 77: 149
5. Benezra C, Ducombs G, Sell Y, Foussereau J (1985) Plant contact dermatitis. St Louis Decker/Mosby, Toronto/V, pp 72–79
6. Lepoittevin JP, Benezra C (1986) Saturated analogs of poison ivy allergens. Synthesis of trans, trans- and cis, trans-3-alkyl-1,2-cyclohexanediols and sensitizing properties in allergic contact dermatitis. J Med Chem 29: 287–291
7. Benezra C, Sigman CC, Perry LR, Helmes CT, Maibach HI (1985) A systematic search for structure-activity relationships of skin contact sensitizers: methodology, J Invest Dermatol 85: 351–356
8. Benezra C, Sigman CC, Bagheri D, Helmes CT, Maibach HI (1989) A systematic search for structure-activity relationships of skin contact sensitizers. II. *Para*-phenylenediamines. Semin Dermatol 8: 88–93
9. Mayer RL (1950) Compounds of quinone structures as allergens and cancerogenic agents. Experiential 6: 241–280
10. Basketter DA, Goodwin BFJ (1988) Investigation of the prohapten concept. Cross-reactions between 1,4-benzene derivatives in the guinea pig. Contact Dermatitis 19: 248–253
11. Dossou KG, Sicard C, Kalopissis G, Schaefer H (1985) Methods for assessment of experimental allergy in guinea-pigs adapted to cosmetic ingredients. Contact Dermatitis 13: 226–234
12. Haustein UF, Tegetmeyer L, Ziegler V (1985) Allergic and irritant potential of benzoyl peroxide. Contact Dermatitis 13: 252–257
13. National Toxicology Program (NTP) (1986) Carcinogenesis Studies of ethyl acrylate (CAS 140-88-5) in F344 rats and B6C3F1 mice (Gavage studies). Public Health Service, National Institutes of Health, U.S. Department of Health and Human Services, Washington (Technical report 259)
14. International Agency for Research on Cancer (IARC) (1985) IARC monographs on the evaluation of the carcinogenic risk of chemicals to humans: allyl compounds, aldehydes, epoxides, and peroxides, vol 36. IARC, Lyon, pp 101–132
15. Stotts J, Ely J (1977) Induction of human skin sensitization to ethanol. J Invest Dermatol 69: 219–222
16. Foussereau J, Benezra C, Maibach HI (1982) Occupational contact dermatitis: clinical and chemical aspects, Munksgaard, Copenhagen, pp 229–230
17. Kurokawa Y, Takamura N, Matsushima Y, Imazawa T, Hayashi Y (1984) Studies on the promoting and complete carcinogenic activities of some oxidizing chemicals in skin carcinogenesis. Cancer Lett 24: 299–304
18. Ito N, Hagiwara A, Shibata M, Ogiso P, Fukushima S (1982) Induction of squamous cell carcinoma in the forestomach of F344 rats treated with butylated hydroxyanisole. Jpn J Cancer Res 73: 332–334

19. Ito N, Fukushima S, Hagiwara A, Shibata M, Ogiso T (1983) Carcinogenicity of butylated hydroxyanisole in F344 rats. J Natl Cancer Inst 70: 343–352
20. Meynadier J-M, Meynadier J, Colmar A, Castelain PI, Ducombs G, Chabeau G, LaCroix M, Martin P, Ngangu Z (1982) Allergie aux conservateurs. Acta Dermatol Venereol (Stockh) 109: 1017–1023
21. Ito N, Ogiso T, Fukushima S, Shibata M, Hagiwara A (1984) Carcinogenicity of captafol in B6C3F1 mice. Gann 75: 853–65
22. Lisi P, Caraffini S, Assalve D (1987) Irritation and sensitization potential of pesticides. Contact Dermatitis 17: 212–218
23. De Groot AC, Bos JD, Jagtman BA, Bruynzeel DP, van Joost T, Weyland JW (1986) Contact allergy to preservatives II. Contact Dermatitis 15: 218–222
24. Lisi P, Caraffini S, Assalve D (1986) A test series for pesticide dermatitis. Contact Dermatitis 15: 266–269
25. National Cancer Institute (NCI) (1977) Bioassay of captan for possible carcinogenicity. Public Health Service, National Institutes of Health, Department of Health, Education, and Welfare, Washington (Technical report no 15)
26. Bruynzeel DP, van Ketel WG (1986) Contact dermatitis due to chlorothalonil in floriculture. Contact Dermatitis 14: 67–68
27. National Cancer Institute (NCI) (1978) Bioassay of chlorothalonil for possible carcinogenicity. Public Health Service, National Institutes of Health, Department of Health, Education, and Welfare, Washington (Technical report no 41)
28. International Agency for Research on Cancer (IARC) (1976) IARC monographs on the evaluation of the carcinogenic risk of chemicals to humans: some naturally occurring substances, vol 10. IARC, Lyon, pp 113–119
29. Foussereau J, Benezra C, Maibach HI (1982) Occupational contact dermatitis: clinical and chemical aspects. Munksgaard, Copenhagen, p 40
30. Foussereau J, Benezra C, Maibach H (1982) Occupational contact dermatitis: clinical and chemical aspects. Munksgaard, Copenhagen, p 221
31. International Agency for Research on Cancer (IARC) (1976) IARC monographs on the evaluation of the carcinogenic risk chemicals to humans: cadmium, nickel, some epoxides, miscellaneous industrial chemicals and general consideration on volatile anesthetics, vol 11. IARC, Lyon, pp 131–140
32. Wester PW, Van der Heijden CA, Bisschop A, Van Esch GJ (1985) Carcinogenicity study with epichlorohydrin (CEP) by gavage in rats. Toxicology 36: 325–339
33. Fregert S (1978) Allergic contact dermatitis from ethylacrylate in a window sealant. Contact Dermatitis 4: 56
34. International Agency for Research on Cancer (IARC) (1974) IARC monographs on the evaluation of the carcinogenic risk of chemicals to humans: some anti-thyroid and related substances, nitrofurans and industrial chemicals, vol 7. IARC, Lyon, pp 45–52
35. Innes JRM, Ulland B, Valerio MG, Petrucelli L, Fishbein L, Hart ER, Pallotta AJ, Bates RR, Falk HL, Gart JJ, Klein M, Mitchell I, Peters J (1969) Bioassay of pesticides and industrial chemicals for tumorigenicity in mice: a preliminary note. J Natl Cancer Inst 42: 1101–1114
36. Weisburger EK, Ulland BM, Nam J-M, Gart JJ, Weisburger JH (1981) Carconogenicity tests of certain environmental and industrial chemicals. J Natl Cancer Inst 67: 75–88
37. Albert RE, Sellakumar AR, Laskin S, Kuschner M, Nelson N, Snyder CA (1982) Gaseous formaldehyde and hydrogen chloride induction of nasal cancer in the rat. J Natl Cancer Inst 68: 597–603
38. International Agency for Research on Cancer (IARC) (1982) IARC monographs on the evaluation of the carcinogenic risk of chemicals to humans: some industrial chemicals and dyestuffs, vol 29. IARC, Lyon, pp 345–390
39. Ormerod, AD, Main RA (1985) Sensitisation to "sensitive teeth" toothpaste. Contact Dermatitis 13: 192–193

40. International Agency for Research on Cancer (IARC) (1974) IARC monographs on the evaluation of the carcinogenic risk of chemicals to humans: some aromatic amines, hydrazine and related substances, N-nitroso compounds and miscellaneous alkylating agents, vol 4. IARC, Lyon, pp 127–136
41. Wrangsjo K, Maartensson A (1986) Hydrazine contact dermatitis from gold plating. Contact Dermatitis 15: 244–245
42. International Agency for Research on Cancer (IARC) (1980) IARC monographs on the evaluation of the carcinogenic risk of chemicals to humans: some pharmaceutical drugs, vol 24. IARC, Lyon, pp 185–194
43. Mitchell JC, Maibach HI (1975) Allergic contact dermatitis from phenoxybenzamine hydrochloride: cross-sensitivity to some related haloalkylamine compounds. Contact Dermatitis 1: 363–366
44. National Cancer Institute (NCI) (1980) Bioassay of phenoxybenzamine hydrochloride for possible carcinogenicity. Public Health Service, National Institutes of Health, Department of Health, Education, and Welfare, Washington (Technical report no 72)
45. Hiraga K, Fujii T (1984) Induction of tumours of the urinary bladder in F344 rats by dietary administration of o-phenylphenol. Food Chem Toxicol 22: 865–870
46. Van Hecke E (1986) Contact sensitivity to o-phenylphenol in a coolant. Contact Dermatitis 15: 46
47. Dunkelberg H (1982) Carcinogenicity of ethylene oxide and 1,2-propylene oxide upon intragastric administration to rats. Br J Cancer 46: 924–933
48. International Agency for Research on Cancer (IARC) (1976) IARC monographs on the evaluation of the carcinogenic risk of chemicals to humans: some anti-thyroid and related substances, nitrofurans and industrial chemicals, vol 7. IARC, Lyon, pp 191–200
49. Kuper CF, Reuzel PG, Feron VJ, Verschuuren H (1988) Chronic inhalation toxicity and carcinogenicity study of propylene oxide in Wistar rats. Food Chem. Toxicol 26: 159–167
50. Van Ketel WG (1979) Contact dermatitis from propylene oxide. Contact Dermatitis 5: 191–192
51. National Toxicology Program (NTP) (1985) Carcinogenesis studies of propylene oxide (CAS no 75-56-9) in F344 Rats and B6C3F1 mice (inhalation studies). Public Health Service, National Institutes of Health, U.S. Department of Health and Human Services, Washington (Technical report no 267)
52. International Agency for Research on Cancer (IARC) (1979) IARC monographs on the evaluation of the carcinogenic risk of chemicals to humans: some monomers, plastics and synthetic elastomers, and acrolein, vol 19. IARC, Lyon, pp 231–284
53. Sjoborg S, Fregert S, Trulsson L (1984) Contact allergy to styrene and related chemicals. Contact Dermatitis 10: 94–96
54. International Agency for Research on Cancer (IARC) (1974) IARC monographs on the evaluation of the carcinogenic risk of chemicals to humans: some anti-thyroid and related substances, nitrofurans and industrial chemicals, vol 7. IARC, Lyon, pp 95–110
55. Kellett JK, Beck MH, Auckland G (1984) Contact sensitivity to thiourea in photocopy paper. Contact Dermatitis 11: 124
56. Estlander T, Jolanki R, Kanerva L (1986) Dermatitis and urticaria from rubber and plastic gloves. Contact Dermatitis 14: 20–25
57. National Toxicology Program (NTP) (1983) Carcinogenesis studies of ziram (CAS no 137-30-4) in F344 rats and B6C3F1 mice. Public Health Service, National Institutes of Health, U.S. Department of Health and Human Services, Washington (Technical report no 238)

Chapter 5
Individual Predisposition
to Contact Dermatitis

Individual Predisposition to Contact Dermatitis

TORKIL MENNÉ and JOHN D. WILKINSON

Contents

5.1 Introduction

Contact dermatitis is a consequence of environmental factors and a susceptible host. Although the individual propensity to develop both sensitization
and irritation of the skin is well known to the dermatologist working with
occupationally related problems, systematic studies in the field have been
relatively sparse. Even under extreme exposure some individuals continue
to remain unaffected whereas others develop either contact sensitization or
irritation.

5.2 Contact Sensitization

5.2.1 Genetic Factors

Breeding experiments combined with sensitization testing have shown that
contact sensitivity among inbred laboratory animals is genetically controlled

[1]. In humans, the importance of genetic influence in the development of contact allergy has been evaluated by epidemiological, family and twin studies, or a combination of all these approaches. Because susceptibility to contact allergy does not seem to follow simple Mendelian inheritance with complete penetrance, all of the methods may provide useful information [2].

Sulzberger and coworkers [3,4], in human sensitization experiments with p-nitroso-dimethylaniline (NDMA) and 2,4-dinitrochlorobenzene (DNCB), established an individual variation in susceptibility to contact sensitization, and further showed that some persons who were highly susceptible to sensitization with one chemical showed little or no susceptibility to sensitization with other chemicals. More recent studies suggest that individual susceptibility occurs by a non-antigen-specific amplification of the immune response [5].

Twin studies on allergic contact sensitization are sparse and partly contradictory. One study including nickel-sensitive female twins suggests that genetic influence over contact sensitization to nickel is likely [6].

Numerous studies of the HLA genes in contact sensitization have not disclosed any consistent pattern [2]. The lack of association between the HLA genes and contact sensitization does not exclude the importance of genetic factors. Hitherto unknown HLA genes might be associated with allergic contact dermatitis, there might be genetic heterogeneity in allergic contact dermatitis and/or allergic contact dermatitis might not be associated or linked to the HLA region.

In conclusion, it appears that some persons are more easily sensitized than others to common haptens due to their genetic background, but the total number sensitized in the population depends upon the degree of cutaneous exposure.

5.2.2 Sex

Women have in general superior immune capability compared to men. They have higher immunoglobulin levels of IgM and IgG and stronger cell-mediated immune responses than men [7]. Both in animal studies and in man there is a preponderance of autoimmune disease in women compared to men [8].

Walker et al. [9] found men more susceptible to DNCB sensitization compared to women in a large well-controlled study. A similar study on patch test sensitization from p-amino-diphenylamine and isopropyl-p-diphenylamine disclosed a significantly increased number of women sensitized as compared to men [10]. The authors held the position that the results did not reflect a true difference in liability to contact sensitization between the sexes, but rather that women have more frequent contact with para substances than men and thus achieve subclinical sensitization. Leyden and Kligman [11] support this opinion, as the overall male and female sensitization rates obtained by maximization testing of 185 substances were 9.9% and 9.2%, respectively. For some allergens, mainly fragrances, there was a female predominance. Rees et al. [12], however, found an increased reactivity to challenge with DNCB in DNCB-sensitized women as compared to DNCB-sensitized men.

Allergic contact dermatitis and irritant contact dermatitis are more frequent in women as compared to men. This might be a consequence of different exposure patterns between women and men [13].

The main reason for the female preponderance in clinical patch test studies is the high number of nickel- and cobalt-sensitive women [14]. Most see this difference as a consequence of different exposure, although a recent study discloses a low frequency of nickel allergy in men with pierced ears as compared to women with pierced ears [15].

The influence of sex hormones on induction and elicitation of contact allergy is largely unknown. In a pilot study the response to DNCB was enhanced in women receiving oral contraceptive hormones [16]. Another preliminary report indicates that the cutaneous reactivity to patch testing differs within the menstrual cycle [17]. The limited knowledge in this field is inconclusive and deserves further systematic evaluation.

5.2.3 Age

The most frequently recognized causes of contact sensitivity in children are nickel, balsam of Peru and rubber chemicals [18–20] and, in the United States, poison oak/ivy. Although there is an increasing body of publications on patch testing in children, the interpretation of these data is difficult as appropriate concentrations need to be established in each age group. Particularly the metal salts and formaldehyde may give irritant reactions in children when used in the recommended concentrations.

The ability to become contact sensitized to DNCB is largely unchanged with increasing age [21]. Patch testing with *Rhus* oleoresins in different age groups in persons with a history of poison ivy dermatitis showed a diminished inflammatory response in the elderly [22].

A number of long-term follow-up studies have tried to ascertain the rate of loss of sensitivity by repeating patch testing after some years. The claimed 20%–50% loss is doubtful, as none of the studies (in the primary data) considered the possibility of the excited-skin syndrome [23].

More important than age-dependent immunological reactivity is that each age group has a different exposure to environmental chemicals. Younger people are exposed more to industrial and cosmetic chemicals and the elderly to topical medicaments, as for instance in treatment of leg ulcers. Senior citizens may have one or more cutaneous sensitivities reflecting exposure 30–40 years earlier, with the positive patch test being of historical interest only. In epidemiological studies on contact allergy, whether these are population-based or clinical patch test studies, age is an important confounding factor and should be handled adequately, for example, by stratification or multivariate statistical analysis [14].

5.2.4 Race

Judging from experimental sensitization studies with poison ivy and DNCB, blacks are less susceptible to contact sensitization as compared to whites [24,25]. Whether this has any clinical implication is unknown.

5.2.5 Regional Factors

Sensitivity is most easily acquired if the allergen is applied to demaged skin. In both animal and human sensitization studies, the frequency of sensitization is increased by traumatizing the skin with sodium lauryl sulphate, repeated freezing or stripping of the skin. The increased risk of sensitization might be ascribed to increased absorption or a change in the immunopresenting capabilities of the skin.

Occlusion promotes precutaneous absorption and undoubtedly contributes to the high incidence of medicament dermatitis in stasis eczema, eczema following traumatic injury, otitis externa and perianal eczema [26].

Reactivity to diagnostic patch testing differs greatly according to the anatomical site of the test. As skin responsiveness on the back is more pronounced than on the arms and thighs, only the upper back is recommended for routine diagnostic patch testing [27]. These regional differences in reactivity have great practical implications, as topical medicaments or cosmetics that might give rise to allergic contact dermatitis in one region may be tolerated in another [28].

5.2.6 Coincidental Disease

Atopics have a downregulation of the Th1 cells, which may explain their tendency to severe viral infections, particularly with herpes simplex virus [29, 30, 52]. Because of this Th1 cell downregulation a decreased propensity to contact sensitization is expected. Clinical studies addressing this problem are contradictory, but most find a decreased tendency to contact sensitization [14, 31–35]. One study suggests that only patients with severe atopic dermatitis have a diminished tendency to DNCB sensitization [36]. The presence of respiratory symptoms may also be of importance. So subgroups of atopic patients with different propensities to contact sensitization may exist. Another source of error is the increased number of irritant patch test results in atopic patients, especially when testing with metals, e.g. nickel, cobalt and chromate [37], although recent studies indicate that atopics seem to have an increased frequency of nickel sensitization [38, 39]. Because of these uncertainties, patch test results should specify the number of patients included with atopy, based on well-defined criteria.

Patients with acute or debilitating diseases, such as cancer (Hodgkin's disease and lymphoma) have impaired capacity for contact sensitization.

5.2.7 Medication

Systemic prednisolone treatment in a dose exceeding 15 mg a day and topical corticosteriod treatment suppresses an allergic contact dermatitis reaction. Some patients, however, may react with a positive patch test even during treatment with prednisolone doses exceeding 15 mg a day. Antihistamines and disodium cromoglycate appear to have only a minor effect on the allergic contact dermatitis reaction.

Azathioprine in doses of 100–150 mg a day is used in dermatology for a number of skin diseases including chronic allergic contact dermatitis and chronic actinic dermatitis due to ubiquitous or airborne allergens. How this drug influences the outcome of patch testing in contact-sensitized individuals is unexplored. Nonsteroidal antiinflammatory drugs are now widely used, and new compounds in this family are currently being developed. Their possible interference with patch testing needs evaluation. Recent exposure to ultraviolet light (UVB, PUVA) and X-rays may temporarily diminish the ability to mount allergic reactions in sensitized individuals, although these effects seem to play only a minor role in the outcome of clinical patch testing [40].

5.3 Individual Susceptibility to Irritants

The considerable interindividual susceptibility to irritants is well known but poorly understood [41–43]. It is well established that patients with ongoing contact dermatitis are more reactive to irritants as compared to controls, but hitherto it has been impossible using any skin irritation model actually to predict irritant contact dermatitis. This may be explained by the difficulties in clearly defining the concept of irritant contact dermatitis. The introduction of noninvasive bioengineering methods such as transepidermal water loss (TEWL) measurement, laser Doppler flowmetry and ultrasound scanning, combined with irritation testing, might improve the value of predictive testing [44, 53–55]. Those with a past history of irritant hand eczema, atopics and nonatopics, have an increased risk of later developing recurrent hand eczema when exposed to wet work [45].

5.3.1 Genetic Factors

Holst and Möller [46] studied the reactivity to benzalkonium chloride, sodium lauryl sulphate and sapo kalinus in twins. A statistically significant difference between the concordance rate among the monozygotic twins compared with dizygotic twins suggests that genetic factors influence the outcome of skin irritation.

Black skin develops skin irritation less frequently than white skin. Marginal irritant reactions on Negro skin may be overlooked by visual scoring because faint erythema is more difficult to quantify. Bioengineering techniques evaluating erythema, vasodilatation and damage to the skin barrier function demonstrate clear differences between black and white skin in response to irritants [47]

5.3.2 Sex

In population-based epidemiological studies, women outnumber men with respect to irritant contact dermatitis [13] Agner et al. [56] found a similar skin irritation to sodium lauryl sulphate in males and females. The skin response to an irritant stimulus in healthy women was found to be statistically significantly stronger at day 1 in the menstrual cycle than at days 9 through 11.

5.3.3 Atopy

Patients with atopic dermatitis have a higher basal transepidermal water loss than controls. The skin response to sodium lauryl sulphate was found to be increased in atopic patients compared with controls [57]. Individuals with previous or present atopic dermatitis have an increased susceptibility later to develop irritant contact dermatitis [45, 48–50], possibly caused by defective stratum corneum function in this disease, present even in normal-looking skin [51].

5.4 References

1. Parker D, Sommer G, Turk JL (1975) Variation in guinea pig responsiveness. Cell Immunol 18: 233–238
2. Menné T, Holm NV (1986) Genetic Susceptibility in human allergic contact sensitization. Semin Dermatol 5: 301–306
3. Sulzberger MB, Rostenberg A Jr (1939) Acquired specific hypersensitivity (allergy) to simple chemicals. J Immunol 36: 17–27
4. Landsteiner K, Rostenberg A Jr, Sulzberger MB (1939) Individual differences in susceptibility to eczematous sensitization with simple chemical substances. J Invest Dermatol 2: 25–29
5. Moss C, Friedmann PS, Shuster S, Simpson JM (1985) Susceptibility and amplification of sensitivity in contact dermatitis. Clin Exp Immunol 61: 232–241
6. Menné T, Holm NV (1983) Nickel allergy in a female twin population. Int J Dermatol 22: 22–28
7. Ansar Ahmed S, Penhale WJ, Talal N (1985) Sex hormones, immune responses, and autoimmune diseases. Am J Pathol 121: 531–551
8. Kalman B, Olsson O, Linto H, Kam-Hansen S (1989) Estradiol potentiates poke-weed mitogen-induced B cell stimulation in multiple scleroisis and healthy subjects. Acta Neurol Scand 79: 340–346

9. Walker FB, Smith PD, Maibach HI (1967) Genetic factors in human allergic contact dermatitis. Int Arch Allergy 32: 453–462
10. Schønning L, Hjorth N (1969) Sex difference in capacity for sensitization. Contact Dermatitis Newslett 5: 100
11. Leyden JJ, Kligman AM (1977) Allergic contact dermatitis. Sex differences. Contact Dermatitis 3: 333–336
12. Rees JL, Friedmann PS, Matthews JNS (1989) Sex difference in susceptibility to development of contact hypersensitivity to dinitrochlorobenzene (DNCB). Br J Dermatol 120: 371–374
13. Meding B (1990) Epidemiology of hand eczema in an industrial city. Acta Derm Venereol Suppl (Stockh) 153
14. Christophersen J, Menné T, Tanghøj P, Andersen KE, Brandrup F, Kaaber K, Osmundsen PE, Thestrup-Pedersen K, Veien NK (1989) Clinical patch test data evaluated by multivariate analysis. Contact Dermatitis 5: 291–300
15. Widström L, Erikssohn I (1989) Nickel allergy and ear piercing in young men. In: Frosch PJ, Dooms-Goosens A, Lachapelle JM, Rycroft RJ, Scheper RJ (eds) Current topics in contact dermatitis. Springer, Berlin Heidelberg New York, pp 188–190
16. Rea TH (1979) Quantitative enhancement of dinitrochlorobenzene responsivity in women receiving oral contraceptives. Arch Dermatol 115: 361–362
17. Alexanader S (1988) Patch testing and menstruation. Lancet ii: 751
18. Hjorth N (1981) Contact dermatitis in children. Acta Derm Venereol Suppl (Stockh) 95: 36–39
19. Veien NK, Hattel T, Justesen O, Nørholm A (1982) Contact dermatitis in children. Contact Dermatitis 8: 373–375
20. Balato N, Lembo G, Patruno C, Ayala F (1989) Patch testing in children. In: Frosch PJ et al. (eds) Current topics in contact dermatitis. Springer, Berlin Heidelberg New York, pp 73–79
21. Schwartz M (1953) Eczematous sensitization in various age groups. J Allergy 24: 143–148
22. Lejman E, Stoudemayer T, Grove G, Kligman AM (1984) Age differences in poison ivy dermatitis. Contact Dermatitis 11: 163–167
23. Keczkes K, Basheer AM, Wyatt EH (1982) The persistence of allergic contact sensitivity: 10 year follow-up in 100 patients. Br J Dermatol 107: 461–464
24. Kligman AM (1966) The identification of contact allergens by human assay. II. Factors influencing the induction and measurements of allergic contact dermatitis. J Invest Dermatol 47: 375–392
25. Andersen KE, Maibach HI (1979) Black and white human skin differences. J Am Acad Dermatol 1: 276–282
26. Meneghini CL (1985) Sensitization in traumatized skin. Am J Ind Med 8: 319–321
27. Magnusson B, Hersle K (1965) Patch test methods. II. Regional variations of patch test responses. Acta Derm Venereol (Stockh) 45: 257–261
28. Maibach HI, Prystowsky SD (1977) Glutaraldehyde (pentanedial). Allergic contact dermatitis. Usage test on sole and antecubital fossa: regional variations in response. Arch Dermatol 113: 170–171
29. Hanifin JM (1983) Clinical and basic aspects of atopic dermatitis. Semin Dermatol 2: 9–19
30. Clark RAF (1989) Cell-mediated and IgE-mediated immune responses in atopic dermatitis. Arch Dermatol 125: 413–416 (editorial)
31. Cronin E, Bandmann HJ, Calnan CD, Fregert S, Hjorth N, Magnusson B, Maibach HI, Malten K, Meneghini CL, Pirilä V, Wilkinson DS (1970) Contact dermatitis in the atopics. Acta Derm Venereol (Stockh) 50: 1983–1987
32. Marghescu S (1985) Patch test reactions in atopic dermatitis. Acta Derm Venereol Suppl (Stockh) 114: 113–116

33. Blondeel A, Achten G, Dooms-Goossens A, Buekens P, Broeckx W, Oleffe J (1987) Atopic et allergie de contact. Ann Dermatol Venereol 114: 203–209

34. von Huber A, Fartasch M, Diepgen TL, Bäurle G, Hornstein OP (1987) Auftreten von Kontaktallergien beim atopischen Ekzem. Dermatosen 35: 119–123

35. de Groot AC (1990) The frequency of contact allergy in atopic patients with dermatitis. Contact Dermatitis 22: 273–277

36. Uehara M, Sawai T (1989) A longitudinal study of contact sensitivity in patients with atopic dermatitis. Arch Dermatol 125: 366–368

37. Möller H, Svensson Å(1986) Metal sensitivity: positive history but negative test indicates atopy. Contact Dermatitis 14: 57–60

38. Diepgen TL, Fartasch M, Hornstein OP (1989) Evaluation and relevance of atopic basic and minor features in patients with atopic dermatitis and in the general population. Acta Derm Venereol Suppl (Stockh) 144: 50–54

39. Ring J, Braun-Falco O (1991) Atopy and contact allergy. In: Ring J (ed) New trends in allergy. Springer, Berlin Heidelberg New York

40. Dooms-Goossens A, Lasaffre E, Heidbuchel M, Dooms M, Degreef H (1988) UV sunlight and patch test reactions in humans. Contact Dermatitis 19: 36–42

41. Björnberg A (1968) Skin reactions to primary irritants in patients with hand eczema. Thesis, Göteborg

42. Frosch P (1985) Hautirritation und empfindliche Haut. Grosse, Berlin (Grosse Scripta 7)

43. Lammintausta K, Maibach HI (1988) Exogenous and endogenous factors in skin irritation. Int J Dermatol 27: 213–222

44. Pinnagoda J, Tupker RA, Coenraads PJ, Nater JP (1989) Prediction of susceptibility to an irritant response by transepidermal water loss. Contact Dermatitis 20: 341–346

45. Nilsson E, Bäck O (1986) The importance of anamnestic information of atopy, metal-dermatitis and earlier hand eczema for the development of hand dermatitis in woman in wet hospital work. Acta Derm Venereol (Stockh) 66: 45–50

46. Holst R, Möller H (1975) One hundred twin pairs patch tested with primary irritants. Br J Dermatol 93: 145–149

47. Berardesca E, Maibach HI (1988) Racial differences in sodium lauryl sulphate induced cutaneous irritation: black and white. Contact Dermatitis 18: 65–70

48. Rystedt I (1985) Hand eczema in patients with history of atopic manifestations in childhood. Acta Derm Venereol (Stockh) 65: 305–313

49. Rystedt I (1985) Factors influencing the occurrence of hand eczema in adults with a history of atopic dermatitis in childhood. Contact Dermatitis 12: 185–191

50. Nilsson E, Mikaelsson B, Andersson S (1986) Atopy, occupation and domistic work as risk factors for hand eczema in hospital workers. Contact Dermatitis 13: 216–223

51. Berardesca E, Fideli D, Borroni G, Rabbiosi G, Maibach M (1990) In vivo hydration and water-retention capacity of stratum corneum in clinically uninvolved skin in atopic and psoriatic patients. Acta Derm Venereol (Stockh) 70: 400–404

52. Bos JO, Wierenga EA, Smitt JHS, van der Heijden FL, Kaspenberg ML (1992) Immune dysregulation in atopic eczema. Arch Dermatol 128: 1509–1512

53. Agner T, Serup J (1990) Sodium lauryl sulphate for irritant patch testing – a dose-response study using bioengineering methods for determination of skin irritation. J Invest Dermatol 95: 543–547

54. Agner T (1991) Skin susceptibility in uninvolved skin of hand eczema patients and healthy controls. Br J Dermatol 125: 140–146

55. Frosch PJ, Kligman AM (eds) (1993) Noninvasive methods for the quantification of skin functions. Springer, Berlin Heidelberg New York

56. Agner T, Damm P, Skouby SO (1991) Menstrual cycle and skin reactivity. J Am Acad Dermatol 24: 566–570

57. Agner T (1991) Susceptibility of atopic dermatitis patients to irritant dermatitis caused by sodium lauryl sulphate. Acta Derm Venereol 71: 296–300

Chapter 6
Epidemiology

Epidemiology

PIETER-JAN COENRAADS and JET SMIT

Contents

6.1 Introduction

The epidemiology of contact dermatitis is concerned with describing the distribution of contact dermatitis in human populations and with identifying factors that affect this distribution. A basic activity in epidemiology involves counting the number of diseased persons (cases) in a specified population and recording relevant characteristics of these diseased persons and of the study population. From this information, the frequency of disease among the study population can be calculated and associations between the disease frequency and the presence or absence of relevant characteristics suggest whether these characteristics may cause contact dermatitis.

In the first part of this chapter, some general epidemiological concepts are applied to the study of contact dermatitis. In the context of these concepts, several sources of available data on the distribution of contact dermatitis in population groups will be discussed. Subsequently, the prevalence and incidence of contact dermatitis among the general population and the working population will be discussed. Very few truly epidemiological studies have been published which were aimed at the identification of risk factors for the development of contact dermatitis. Therefore, this chapter concludes with some methodological considerations for the design of such epidemiological studies.

6.2 Basic Concepts

The epidemiological concepts discussed in this section are important for interpreting and comparing results from epidemiological studies and from routinely registered data.

6.2.1 Measures of Disease Frequency

Measures of disease frequency consist of the number of cases in the numerator and the size of the population under study in the denominator. Measures of disease frequency that are commonly used in epidemiology are *incidence* and *prevalence*. The incidence of contact dermatitis refers to the number of new cases of contact dermatitis during a defined period in a specified population. Commonly, the *incidence rate* is defined as the number of nondiseased persons who become diseased within a certain period of time, divided by the number of person-years in the population. Person-years are contributed only by those who are not ill at the beginning of the study. From the point in time at which a person becomes diseased, he or she also no longer contributes to the total number of person-years in the denominator. Even when a subject becomes nondiseased again, person years are no longer contributed. The *cumulative incidence* is the proportion of a fixed population that becomes ill in a specific period of time. The difference between the two measures of incidence is small when the proportion of people that becomes ill in a specific period is small, but it can be sizable when many people become ill in a short period of time. The incidence of contact dermatitis can be measured by periodic screening to detect all new cases in the study population over a certain period of time.

The *prevalence* of contact dermatitis is the number of persons with contact dermatitis at a certain point in time or during a certain (usually short) period of time. The *point prevalence* refers to the proportion of subjects having active contact dermatitis at the time of data collection and the *period prevalence* includes, in addition to these active cases, those cases that have occurred during a specified short period of time prior to the investigation. When comparing prevalences between studies, the time period to which the prevalence refers should be taken into account. It is likely that the point prevalence of contact dermatitis is lower than a period prevalence because symptoms are not continuously present. In theory, the period prevalence of contact dermatitis over a period of several years should be higher than the period prevalence over a period of months. However, the difference may be small due to the fact that in many patients contact dermatitis is a condition with an unfavourable prognosis and a high rate of recurrence. In addition, the accuracy of recall will decrease with time, and it is conceivable that those persons who did not have symptoms recently will more often forget to report their earlier symptoms.

6.2.2 Case Definition

Counting the number of diseased persons in a population requires the explicit statement of diagnostic criteria to judge whether a person is considered to have the disease or not. In many publications, diagnostic criteria for the definition of contact dermatitis are not explicity stated, and several authors reserve this term to denote allergic contact dermatitis. Since contact dermatitis refers to eczematous symptoms due to exposure of the skin to irritant or sensitizing agents, it can be considered as a subcategory of eczema. Other categories of eczema are, for example, dyshidrotic eczema, nummular eczema and atopic eczema. In practice, the distinction into categories of eczema is often difficult because the classifications are based upon a combination of morphological, aetiological, constitutional and other factors. This leads to inconsistent terminology and overlapping categories. In some publications the terms 'contact dermatitis' and 'eczema' (especially of the hands) are used interchangeably, assuming that irritant or sensitizing agents often play a role in the causation of (hand) eczema. The descriptive epidemiology of contact dermatitis presented in this chapter mostly refers to eczema, unless contact dermatitis is mentioned explicitly.

Another aspect of case definition, apart from diagnostic criteria, is the *localization* of eczema. In theory, the prevalence of contact dermatitis on one site should be lower than the prevalence on all sites. When restricted to the hands and forearms, the difference is often minimal because contact dermatitis occurs on the hands in the majority of patients [1].

The ambiguity in diagnostic criteria also plays a role in the further distinction between allergic and irritant contact dermatitis. Detailed investigation (for example, patch testing) is necessary to determine whether sensitization to certain agents has occurred, but even then it is sometimes not certain whether the contact dermatitis is of allergic origin. In many instances, simultaneous exposure to irritant factors plays an essential part in the development of allergic contact dermatitis. Therefore, the distinction between allergic and irritant contact dermatitis should be interpreted with care in those publications where this distinction is made.

6.2.3 Source Population

The population in which the cases arise (source population) is the denominator of the measure of disease frequency (incidence or prevalence). A common feature of observational studies is the occurrence of nonresponders in the population that was invited to participate in the study. The denominator then refers to the responders only. Whether generalizations can be made to the source population as a whole depends on the extent to which the nonresponders were different in relevant characteristics from the source population.

To describe patterns in the distribution of contact dermatitis in the population according to characteristics like age, gender and occupation, these characteristics should be recorded not only among cases, but also among the population from which the cases originated.

6.2.4 Case Ascertainment

The case ascertainment refers to the methods used to let cases come to the attention of the investigator. It depends largely on the sources of data that are used, such as mortality statistics, morbidity statistics or observational studies. It may have major consequences on the magnitude of the disease frequency which one obtains. In mortality or morbidity statistics, case ascertainment usually involves registration of persons with eczema or dermatitis who fulfil additional criteria for registration, like hospital admission or sickness leave. This restriction in the definition of a 'case' will probably result in selective inclusion of the more severe cases, since a large proportion of individuals suffering from contact dermatitis do not come to medical attention [2–5]. In general, the diagnostic criteria for eczema are not clear in these morbidity statistics, since the information is compiled from diagnoses made by many different physicians who were not usually instructed to use a standardized set of criteria.

In observational studies, active case ascertainment usually involves screening of the study population by clinical examination, by questionnaire or by a combination of both. The advantage of observational studies is that case ascertainment can be performed using uniform criteria (chosen by the investigators) for the definition of cases. However, the frequency of cases obtained by questionnaire may be quite different from those ascertained by clinical examination. Problems in defining diagnostic criteria in a clinical examination were mentioned before. The case definition in questionnaire surveys depends on the phrasing of the questions and on the responders' perception of the disease. For example, the question "Have you had hand eczema in the past 12 months?" requires that the responders compose their own criteria for judging whether they have (had) hand eczema or not. The comparison of results of questionnaire surveys is hampered by the lack of standardized and adequately validated questionnaires.

6.2.5 Observational Studies

The three most important types of observational study in the epidemiology of contact dermatitis are follow-up studies, case-control studies and cross-sectional studies. Important measures of association are the *relative risk*, the *rate ratio*, the *rate difference* and the *odds ratio*.

In follow-up studies, selection of subjects is based upon exposure to the factor of interest. For example, the *relative risk* of having an atopic constitution (relative to not having it) for developing contact dermatitis can be studied in a follow-up study. This implies that a population of atopics and nonatopics is selected before the disease has developed and that they are followed over a certain period of time. The *rate ratio* (RR) is a basic measure of association between exposure and disease. This is the ratio of the incidence rates in exposed and unexposed persons. Another measure of association is the *rate difference* (RD), being the difference between the incidence rates in exposed and unexposed subjects.

In case-control studies, the subjects are selected according to their disease status. Information is collected on the past exposure of the diseased persons (cases) and the nondiseased persons (controls). The odds of exposure among cases is compared to the odds of exposure among controls. This can be expressed in an odds ratio (OR): when 40 cases (out of 100 cases) are exposed and 60 are not exposed, the exposure odds are 40:60. When the exposure odds among controls are 20:80, the odds ratio is 2.7. A case-control study can be seen as a study among a defined population in which all diseased persons, and only a sample of the nondiseased persons, are studied. This design is especially efficient in the study of a rare disease. In this situation, the majority of the population does not have the disease, and it is not necessary to study all nondiseased persons. For reasons of interpretability, it is necessary to make an effort to select a population of controls in such a way that they reflect the exposure distribution among the nondiseased part of the source population from which the cases originated. Case-control studies can be based on incident cases or on prevalent cases. A study of incident cases includes as cases only those that develop the illness during a specified time period. In a case-control study of prevalent cases, all existing cases of illness at a point in time are selected.

In cross-sectional studies, a study population is selected regardless of exposure status or disease status (in contrast to case-control and follow-up studies). Usually, the information on exposure and disease in cross-sectional studies refers to the time of data collection. In cross-sectional studies, it is not possible to draw conclusions with regard to the relationship between previous exposure and disease, because current exposure may be different from the exposure in the past which caused the disease.

Cross-sectional studies are especially suitable to study the prevalence of a disease in a population in relation to characteristics that do not change much over time.

6.2.6 Examples of Use and Misuse of Terms

Suppose a publication in which the authors state that "The incidence of nickel contact dermatitis at hospital X was 18/120 = 15%." They imply that, out of 120 patients seen, 18 were found to have this disease. In this common example the use of the term 'incidence' is wrong and term 'prevalence' should be used. If the authors had followed a group of 120 healthy nurses without contact dermatitis in their hospital over a certain time period, and at the end of that period had found 18 to have developed nickel dermatitis during that period, then they could use the term 'cumulative incidence'.

The term 'incidence rate' (often abbreviated to 'incidence') could only be used if this group of 120 nurses were examined at the beginning of the study, to ascertain that nobody had nickel dermatitis, and if this group were continuously monitored during follow-up (e.g. 5 years). This design would yield exact information about the point in time that anybody becomes diseased and would allow calculation of the number of person-months that each person contributes. A person no longer contributes after he or she becomes diseased. The number of months of follow-up until he or she shows dermatitis, or the total amount of months of follow-up (5×12 months) if no dermatitis appears, will be known at the end of the study. Suppose that the 18 persons who became diseased had a total of 300 months of follow-up without disease (e.g. one person 10 months until dermatitis appeared, another 14 months, etc.). The remaining 102 were followed for the total period of 5 years, contributing $102 \times 5 \times 12 = 6120$ months of follow-up. Thus, for the whole group, we have $300 + 6120 = 6420$ months of follow-up with a yield of 18 cases. This implies an incidence rate of $18/6420 = 0.0028$ cases per person-month of follow-up. If necessary, this can be converted to 0.034 cases per person-year of follow-up, and often this can be regarded as 0.034 cases per person-year exposure to nursing work.

Unfortunately, in contact dermatitis research, there are very few publications based on this more sophisticated design. The advantage of such a design is that it permits comparison with a different, unexposed group, provided it is followed up in the same way (e.g. clerical staff). The comparison can be expressed as a ratio of the two incidence rates, the rate ratio (RR), or as a difference between the two incidence rates, the rate difference (RD), which tells us about the association between exposure and dermatitis risk.

Suppose the incidence rate of dermatitis was 0.017 per person-year of follow-up in clerical staff, then the RR (sometimes called 'relative risk') of $0.034/0.017 = 2$ would quickly tell us that the risk of developing dermatitis during nursing work is twice as high compared to low-risk clerical work. The RR and the RD are also amenable to further statistical elaboration, which could tell us more about, for example, the importance of soaps or gloves as specific exposure factors, or the role of nickel allergy.

6.3 Sources of Data

6.3.1 Morbidity Statistics

Morbidity statistics which provide information on the occurrence of skin diseases, and eczema or contact dermatitis specifically, are, for example, hospitalization records, case records from dermatology clinics and data on sickness leave and occupational diseases. As mentioned before, it is likely that morbidity statistics include mainly the more severe cases of skin disease.

Data on hospital admissions show that contact dermatitis is a rare cause of hospitalization. Johnson [6] estimated that 1%–2% of patients admitted to hospitals in the United States were admitted for conditions of the skin. In the Netherlands, the hospital admission rate for contact dermatitis as a primary diagnosis was approximately 9 persons per 100 000 inhabitants per year, which is 6% of the rate for all skin diseases, and less than 1% of all hospital admissions in 1988 [7].

There are several publications on the number and characteristics of patients visiting dermatology clinics and/or patch testing units [8–10]. However, no information on the incidence or prevalence of contact dermatitis can be derived from these publications, because information on the size of the source population from which the cases originated is usually lacking. It is difficult to interpret the distribution of occupations, age or sex in a patient population without knowing the distribution of these characteristics among the source population. Also, information on type and severity of skin disease in patient populations is difficult to interpret, because of selection mechanisms that play a role before a dermatology clinic is consulted.

Occupational disease statistics provide useful information on the incidence of occupational skin diseases among the working population. Registers of occupational diseases are kept in several European countries and in the United States [11–16]. Although most of these registers concern all types of skin disease, and no distinction is made with regard to eczema or contact dermatitis, it is estimated that eczema or contact dermatitis accounts for 85%–98% of all occupational skin diseases [17, 18]. The registration of occupational diseases in Sweden, Federal Republic of Germany and Finland is based upon the notification of diseases caused by exposure to factors associated with employment. Usually only those cases are notified for which compensation is payable. Criteria for compensation, and thus criteria for notification of occupational diseases, depend on the legislation on occupational diseases in each country. Evidently, this influences the comparability of the incidence figures between countries. In the United States the occupational disease statistics are based upon annual surveys by the Bureau of Labor Statistics (BLS) among a random sample of approximately 280 000 employers in private industry [16]. All illnesses should be reported, whether or not time is lost from work. Consequently, the less severe cases should be included in the incidence figures. However, it has been suggested that the incidence of occupational skin diseases in the United States is being underestimated by 10 to 50 times [18], the milder cases of skin disease not being registered at all. Some of the occupational disease statistics give a breakdown by sex and occupation or branch of industry (usually not by age). Depending on whether the distributions are known in the working population as a whole, the occupation- or industry-specific figures can be calculated. Unfortunately, information on the actual cause of contact dermatitis and predisposing factors is not available in most statistics.

6.3.2 Observational Studies

Publications of true follow-up studies are virtually nonexistent, with a retrospectively designed study among Danish women [19] being one of the exceptions. Thus, incidence figures are hard to obtain. An eczema incidence of 7.9 new cases per 1000 persons per year has been derived from two consecutive cross-sectional studies in the general population [20]. Very high occupation-specific incidence rates were found in a follow-up study among apprentice hairdressers and nurses: 145 per 1000 persons per year and 328 per 1000, respectively [21].

Information on the prevalence of eczema in the general population can be obtained from six major cross-sectional studies that were performed in the last 20 years in the Netherlands [4], Sweden [2, 22], England [3], the United States [5] and Norway [23]. In all studies, a geographically defined population or a sample thereof was screened. In some of the studies all skin disorders were recorded, others focused on eczema only. In this chapter, only the data on eczema will be discussed. In most of the studies the term 'eczema' included allergic contact dermatitis, irritant contact dermatitis, seborrhoeic eczema, nummular eczema, atopic eczema, dyshidrotic eczema and unclassified eczema. In the Dutch study [4], 'eczema' referred to the presence of eczematous symptoms for a period longer than 3 weeks, or to recurrent eczematous symptoms. The American [5] and the Dutch [4] studies provide information on contact dermatitis explicitly. Relevant characteristics of the studies, like the method of case ascertainment, localization of eczema and the period to which the prevalence refers, are summarized in Table 6.1. Four of the studies allow calculation of age and sex specific prevalence figures. Because Rea et al.[3] do not present the distribution of eczema by age, and Agrup [2] does not provide the age and sex distribution of the source population in the denominator, it is not possible to calculate age- and sex-specific rates in those two studies. Occupation-specific rates can be obtained from the Dutch cross-sectional study [4].

6.4 Prevalence in the General Population

Table 6.1 summarizes the results of the prevalence studies. The estimated point prevalence of eczema varied from 1.7% to 6.3%. The estimated prevalence over a period of 1–3 years varied from 6.2% to 10.6%. As was to be expected, the estimated point prevalence was lower, on average, than the period prevalence. However, it is difficult to interpret the differences in point prevalence or period prevalence between studies. They may arise from a combination of true differences in prevalence between the studies, but also from differences in diagnostic criteria and aspects of methodology, like the method of case ascertainment. As mentioned before, clinical examination of the study population is probably a more reliable method for case ascertainment then the use of a self-administered questionnaire. In the American [5] and Dutch [4] studies, the complete study populations underwent clinical examination. In contrast, cases in the study in Norway [23] were ascertained by a self-administered mail questionnaire. The validity of the questionnaire is unknown. The other studies used combinations of these methods, where a first screening by questionnaire was followed by a clinical examination of a subpopulation. Agrup [2] performed a clinical examination on a subsample of her study population consisting of 1819 persons. 1.8% has responded affirmatively to the question: "Do you have any skin changes on the hands (apart from common warts)?". In the clinical examination of the positive and negative responders, the diagnosis of skin disease was confirmed in 32 out of 33 positive responders and in addition, another 33 persons (1.8%) among the negative responders were found to have skin disorders. Consequently the prevalence of skin disorders by clinical examination was almost twice as high due to false-negative answers in the questionnaire. A comparable result was obtained for eczema: 15 of the positive responders were diagnosed as eczema, while another 16 persons among the negative responders were found to have eczema. The prevalence of eczema in the subsample was thus estimated to be 1.7% (31 out of 1819 persons).

Rea et al. [3] examined a stratified subsample of the study population consisting of three-quarters of the positive responders to a question on the presence of any skin disorder and one-fifth of the negative responders. They found that 86% of the positive responders had a skin disorder and that another 13% of the negative responders had skin disorders. The estimate of the prevalence rate of eczema made by the authors was based on the findings in the stratified sample and took into account the distribution of age, sex and occupation and the disproportionate sampling fraction in the subsample.

Meding and Swanbeck [22] performed a clinical examination on 70.7% of the positive responders to a question about symptoms of eczema in the previous 12 months. The diagnosis of eczema was confirmed in 89.4% of the positive responders. Based on these results they estimated that the prevalence of eczema was 10.6% in the study population. However, since negative

Table 6.1. Prevalence of all skin disorders, eczema and contact dermatitis in the general population

Author(s)	Area and population	Year of study	No. of responders	Method of case escertainment	Localization of disorder	Measure of prevalence	Prevalence of eczema (%)
Agrup [2]	South Sweden; 10 years and older	1964–1965	107 206 1 819	Questionnaire clinical exam.	Hands Hands	Point Point	1.7
Rea et al. [3]	London, England; 15–74 years Subsample	1967–1969	1 979 614	Questionnaire Clinical exam.	All sites All sites	Point Point	6.1
Johnson and Roberts [5]	USA; 1–74 years	1971–1974	20 749	Clinical exam.	All sites	Point	2.0 4.2
Coenraads et al. [4]	Urban and rural areas (1983), Netherlands; 28–71 years	1979, 1981	3 140	Clinical exam.	Hands	3 years	6.2
Kavli and Förde [23]	Tromsø, Norway; 20–54 years	1979	14 667	Questionnaire	Hands	12 months	8.9
Meding and Swanbeck [22]	Gothenburg, Sweden; 28–63 years	1982	16 587	Questionnaire, verified by clinical exam.	Hands	12 months Point	10.6 6.3

responders were not examined, this may be an underestimate due to false-negative answers in the questionnaire.

Table 2 shows the prevalences of eczema for men and women separately. In the Netherlands, Norway and Sweden, the prevalence was higher among women, in London the prevalence was higher among men, while there was no difference between sexes in the United States. No unanimous conclusion can be drawn from these data. It is possible that the differences are obscured by differences in age distribution of the populations. Figure 6.1a, b shows the age-specific prevalence of hand eczema in men and women. Figure 6.2 represents the age-specific prevalence of contact dermatitis by sex in the study by Johnson and Roberts [5]. There was no clear trend in age distribution in men. The prevalence in women was especially high in the younger age groups (under 30 years). One possible explanation is that many of the women have high exposure to 'wet work' in household activities and child care [4, 23].

In the United States, the prevalence seems to increase with age, while according to the publication from the Netherlands, Sweden and Norway, the prevalence seems to decrease slightly in the age groups above 50 years. The Dutch study [4] analysed the relative contribution of age and occupation to the prevalence of eczema and found that the relationship with age disappeared after controlling for occupation. The same phenomenon was described in a population of Australian rubber and cement industry workers: the prevalence of dermatitis was relatively high in workers under 45 years, but the age effect also disappeared after controlling for job classification [24].

The only study reporting on socioeconomic status of the population in relation to the prevalence of skin disorders is the community study in London [3]. No significant trend was seen, but the prevalence in the socioeconomic class IIIM (skilled occupations, manual) was relatively high. The authors suggest that persons in this socioeconomic class are more frequently occupationally exposed to industrial chemicals. So, once again the suggestion is that there are underlying factors responsible for higher prevalences of contact dermatitis found in some subgroups in these studies.

The major risk factor for contact dermatitis is considered to be exposure to irritant or sensitizing factors. This exposure is common during household

Table 6.2. Prevalence of eczema among males and females

Country	n	Prevalence of eczema (%) Males	Females
England [3]	1979	8.0	4.3
USA [5]	20 749	1.9	1.9
Netherlands [4]	3140	4.6	8.0
Sweden [22]	16 587	8.8	14.6
Norway [23]	14 667	4.9	13.2

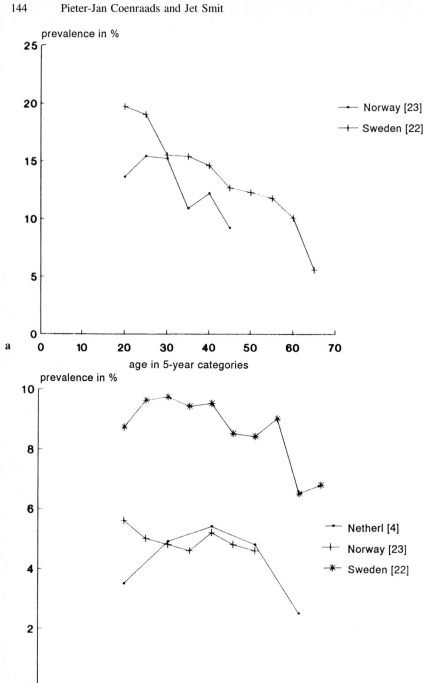

Fig. 6.1. Prevalence of hand eczema by age in **a** females and **b** males

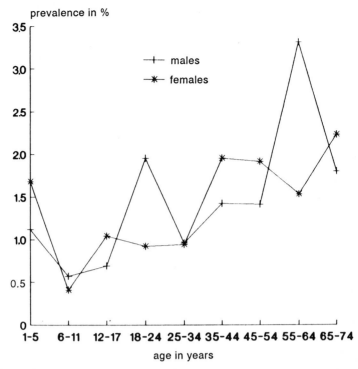

Fig. 6.2. Prevalence of contact dermatitis in the United States by age and gender [5]

activities and in certain occupations. This was evident in a study, using a validated questionnaire, which compared the general population with certain occupations, and which obtained a prevalence of 5.2% for men and 10.6% for women [25]. Several cross-sectional studies have been performed among very specific occupational groups, for example in metal [26] and construction workers [27], hospital workers [28] and painters [29]. These studies will not be reviewed in this chapter (see Chap. 11).

In conclusion, the prevalence studies strongly suggest that age and sex are not risk factors for contact dermatitis in themselves, but that these characteristics are associated with exposure in occupational and household activities. In a review of the epidemiology of allergic contact sensitization, where similar phenomena were seen, Menné et al. [30] concluded that the age-dependent immunological reactivity was less important than differences in exposure between age groups, and that differences in sensitization pattern between sexes seem to be caused by different exposures. The dissimilarity was considered to be so obvious that patch test results were always given for men and women separately.

Table 6.3. Occupational skin diseases as a percentage of all registered occupational diseases in six countries

Country	Year	Cases of occupational diseases			Rank order among all occupational diseases
		Total	Skin diseases		
			(n)	(%)	
Netherlands [11]	1984	527	159	30.2	1
Finland [12]	1982	5365	1132	21.1	3
Sweden [13]	1981	17 107	2271	13.0	2
FRG [14]	1971–1976	81 255	unknown	24.6	2
GDR [15]	1971–1975	unknown	unknown	20.3	2
USA [16]	1984	unknown	42 500	34.0	?

6.5 Incidence in the Working Population

Table 6.3 shows the incidence of occupational skin diseases in five European countries and the United States [11–16]. As mentioned earlier, eczema or contact dermatitis accounts for 85%–98% of all causes of occupational skin diseases [17, 18]. In spite of the differences between legal criteria for the registration of occupational diseases in the six countries, it appears that the incidence of occupational skin disease in these countries is of the same order of magnitude, with 0.5–0.7 cases per 1000 workers per year. In these recent figures, skin diseases constitute 9%–34% of all occupational diseases. Occupational skin diseases either take the first rank among all occupational diseases, or they follow musculoskeletal disorders and/or hearing damage closely. An even higher proportion was mentioned in many older publications. However, the proportion of occupational skin diseases has declined in recent years, although the incidence rates remained approximately the same. This can be explained by the fact that the criteria for the definition of occupational diseases in some countries were broadened in the last few years. As a consequence, the total number of notified occupational diseases has increased, and the proportion of occupational skin diseases has decreased.

Table 6.4 shows the highest incidences of occupational diseases in several branches of industry in Finland [12], the United States [16] and the Federal Republic of Germany [31]. The Swedish publication [13] presents a breakdown by occupation only of the occupational diseases. The distribution of occupations among the total working population is not mentioned. The incidence in the construction industry was 0.7 cases per 1000 workers per year in all three countries.

The incidence of occupational skin diseases by sector of industry is hard to compare because of the differences in classification of industries. The highest incidence rates were recorded in the leather, metal, food, chemical and rubber industries. High incidence rates, including very mild cases, were also found in a follow-up study of apprentice hairdressers and nurses [21].

Table 6.4. Incidence of occupational skin diseases by division of industry per 1000 workers per year [12, 16, 31]

United States		Finland		Federal Republic of Germany	
Construction	0.7	Construction	0.7	Construction	0.7
Manufacturing	1.2	Manufacturing	1.0		
leather	2.7	textile and leather	0.6		
metal products	1.8	metal and machinery	1.0	iron and steel	0.6
machinery	1.4				
electrical products	1.4				
rubber	1.9	rubber and chemical	1.3	chemical	0.6
chemical	1.3				
food	1.7	food	1.1	food	0.6
miscellaneous	2.6	miscellaneous	1.9		
Health service	0.8	sanitary services	1.3	Health service	2.8
Agriculture	2.8	Agriculture	0.4		
Total	0.6		0.5		0.5

6.6 Methodological Considerations in the Design of Epidemiological Studies on Contact Dermatitis

The following characteristics of contact dermatitis may affect the choice of study design in the planning of an epidemiologic study:

1. Contact dermatitis is a multifactorial disease: Apart from exposure to irritating or sensitizing agents there are many factors that may influence the development of contact dermatitis, such as weather conditions, humidity, psychological factors and atopic constitution. These factors may act as confounders in studies if they are not properly controlled for either in the design of the study or in the analysis. In the design of the study these factors can be controlled for by matching cases and controls (or exposed and unexposed) so that they are equal with respect to the distribution of confounders, or by restriction to subjects within certain confounder categories only. In the analysis of the study, several statistical methods (e.g. multivariate analysis) can be used to adjust for the influence of confounders on the estimated rate ratios, rate differences or odds ratios.

2. Persons suffering from contact dermatitis do not necessarily exhibit symptoms continuously, although they are often recurrent: In follow-up studies, where the incidence is measured, this implies that cases are only those persons who exhibit symptoms for the first time. In case-control studies and cross-sectional studies different definitions of a case may be used, as long as it is clear which definition was used. Thus, a prevalent case may be defined as a person exhibiting symptoms at the time of the examination, or as a person who has had symptoms during a specified period of time prior to the investigation.

3. The exposure of interest may vary over time: In some situations the change of exposure status will be determined by the fact that the person has contact dermatitis. Persons who are susceptible to the development of eczematous symptoms are often aware of this. So they may change their habits or use medications to suppress symptoms. In that case, when current exposure (as opposed to past exposure) is recorded in a case-control study or a cross-sectional study, the results will show that cases use medications more often than controls. Obviously the use of medications is a result of being a case and not a cause. In many situations this type of distortion is less obvious. It is therefore preferable to record exposure with reference to the time prior to the first occurrence of eczematous symptoms. However, in practice it may be difficult to obtain reliable information on past exposure. In follow-up studies this poses less of a problem, because exposure is recorded before the symptoms of eczema become manifest.

4. Contact dermatitis is not extremely rare among the general population: The incidence of contact dermatitis in the general population is not known. In follow-up studies a rough idea about the incidence of contact dermatitis in the population to be studied is necessary to determine the size of the exposed and unexposed populations. The prevalence figures suggest that a relatively large population needs to be followed to obtain enough cases at the end of follow-up. However, the majority of the population remains free of contact dermatitis, contributing little information to the study. A follow-up study will in this respect be less efficient than a case-control study. In situations where the effect of a factor is studied that changes over time, and cannot be determined in retrospect, it may be necessary to perform a follow-up study.

5. Not many people stop working because of skin disease: This suggests that, in studies of occupational populations, selection bias (in case-control studies and cross-sectional studies) and bias due to loss of follow-up (in follow-up studies) is small.

6. The time interval between exposure and onset (induction period) of contact dermatitis is virtually unknown: This average period of time elapsed from the start of exposure until the disease becomes manifest is a result of cumulative toxic damage in irritant contact dermatitis. The time course of this process is different from the induction of sensitization in allergic contact dermatitis, but little information is available on the exact duration of the induction period. Rothman [32] stresses that the issue of induction period must nevertheless be addressed, because inaccurate assumptions cause a type of misclassification that tends to reduce the magnitude of associations and underestimate effects. If the duration of follow-up in a prospective study is shorter than the induction period, the cases will not have enough time to become manifest. As a result, the incidence rate among the exposed population will be underestimated, and thus the relative risk will be underestimated. A prospective study among apprentice

hairdressers showed that the incidence rate was high during the first 6 months after the start of exposure, and decreased thereafter [21].

6.7 References

1. Meneghini CL, Angelini G (1984) Primary and secondary sites of occupational contact dermatitis. Dermatosen 32: 205–207
2. Agrup G (1969) Hand eczema and other dermatoses in South Sweden. Acta Derm Venereol Suppl (Stockh) 49: 61
3. Rea JN, Newhouse ML, Halil T (1976) Skin diseases in Lambeth. A community study of prevalence and use of medical care. Br J Prev Soc Med 30: 107–114
4. Coenraads PJ, Nater JP, van der Lende R (1983) Prevalence of eczema and other dermatoses of the hands and arms in the Netherlands. Association with age and occupation. Clin Exp Dermatol 8: 495–503
5. Johnson MLT, Roberts J (1978) Skin conditions and related need for medical care among persons 1–74 years. Vital Health Stat 11
6. Johnson MLT, Burdick AE, Johnson KG, Klarman HE, Krasner M, McDowell AJ, Roberts J (1979) Prevalence morbidity and cost of dermatological disease. J Invest Dermatol 73: 395–401
7. LMR, National Medical Registration (1987) LMR yearbook 1987 (in Dutch). SIG, Utrecht
8. Wilkinson DS (1980) A 10-year review of an industrial dermatitis clinic. Contact Dermatitis 6: 11–17
9. Fregert S (1975) Occupational dermatitis in a 10-year material. Contact Dermatitis 1: 96–107
10. Calnan CD, Bandmann HJ, Cronin E, Fregert S, Hjort N, Magnussen B, Malten K, Meneghini CL, Pirilä V, Wilkinson DS (1970) Hand dermatitis in housewives. Br J Dermatol 82: 543–548
11. Central Bureau of Statistics (CBS) (1985) Statistics of occupational accidents 1984 (in Dutch). Staatsuitgeverij, The Hague
12. Vaaranen V, Vasama M, Alho J (1983) Occupational diseases in Finland in 1982. Institute of occupational health, Publication office, Vantaa
13. Arbetar Skyddsstyrelsen (1984) Occupational injuries 1981. Statistics Sweden, Stockholm
14. Eggeling F (1980) Zur Epidemiologie der Berufskrankheiten. Eine Analyse der von den Staatlichen Gewerbeärzten dokumentierten Berufskrankheiten Meldungen 1971–1976 in der Bundesrepublik Deutschland. BAU, Dortmund (Forschungsbericht no 254)
15. Laubstein H, Mönnich HT (1980) Zur Epidemiologie der Berufsdermatosen (III). Dermatol Monatsschr 166: 369–381
16. Mathias CGT, Morrison JH (1988) Occupational skin diseases. United States results from bureau of Labor Statistics annual survey of occupational injuries and illnesses, 1973 through 1984. Arch Dermatol 124: 1519–1524
17. Mathias CGT (1985) The cost of occupational skin disease. Arch Dermatol 121: 332–334
18. Emmet EA (1984) The skin and occupational disease. Arch Environ Health 39: 144–149
19. Menné T, Bogan O, Green A (1982) Nikkel allergy and hand dermatitis in a stratified sample of the Danish female population: an epidemiological study including a statistic appendix. Acta Derm Venereol (Stockh) 62: 35–41
20. Lantinga H, Nater JP, Coenraads PJ (1984) Prevalence, incidence and course of eczema on the hands and forearms in a sample of the general population. Contact Dermatitis 10: 135–139

21. Smit HA, van Rijssen A, Vandenbroucke J, Coenraads PJ (1994) Individual susceptibility and the incidence of hand dermatitis in a cohort of apprentice hairdressers and nurses. Scand J Work Environ Health 20: 113–121
22. Meding BE, Swanbeck G (1987) Prevalence of hand eczema in an industrial city. Br J Dermatol 116: 627–634
23. Kavli G, Förde OH (1984) Hand dermatoses in Tromsö. Contact Dermatitis 10: 174–177
24. Varigos GA, Dunt DR (1981) Occupational dermatitis. An epidemiological study in the rubber and cement industries. Contact Dermatitis 7: 105–110
25. Smit HA, Burdorff A, Coenraads PJ (1993) Prevalence of hand dermatitis in different occupational groups. Internat J Epidemiol 22: 288–293
26. De Boer EM, van Ketel WG, Bruynzeel DP (1989) Dermatoses in metal workers. Contact Dermatitis 20: 212–218
27. Coenraads PJ, Nater JP, Jansen HA, Lantinga H (1984) Prevalence of eczema and other dermatoses of the hands and forearms in construction workers in the Netherlands. Clin Exp Dermatol 9: 149–158
28. Lammintausta K, Kalimo K, Aanton S (1982) Course of hand dermatitis in hospital workers. Contact Dermatitis 8: 327–332
29. Högberg M, Wahlberg JE (1980) Health screening for occupational dermatoses in housepainters. Contact Dermatitis 6: 100–106
30. Menné T. Christoffersen J, Maibach HI (1987) Epidemiology of allergic contact sensitization. Monogr Allergy 21: 132–161
31. Fabry H (1981) Statistik der Berufskrankheiten der Hautgefährdungskataster. Dermatosen 29: 42–44
32. Rothman KJ (1986) Modern epidemiology. Little Brown, Boston

Chapter 7
Clinical Features

Clinical Features

NIELS K. VEIEN

Contents

7.1 Introduction

A diagnosis of contact dermatitis can be made only after the careful consideration of many variables. A thorough knowledge of the clinical features of the skin's reactions to various contactants is important in making a correct diagnosis of contact dermatitis.

While an eczematous reaction is the most commonly encountered adverse reaction to contactants, other clinical manifestations are also seen. These include erythema multiforme, purpura, lichenoid eruptions, exanthems, erythroderma, allergic contact granuloma, toxic epidermal necrolysis, pigmented contact dermatitis and photosensitive reactions. Generalized symptoms have also been described in association with contact sensitivity, and contact urticaria may become anaphylactoid [1] and life-threatening [2].

The emphasis in this chapter will be on eczemas as a manifestation of contact dermatitis.

7.2 The Medical History of the Patient

7.2.1 History of Hereditary Diseases

The family and personal history of a patient with contact dermatitis should be taken in as much detail as possible, especially with regard to atopy. Patients who have suffered from severe atopic dermatitis in childhood are likely to experience irritant contact dermatitis later in life [3]. A history of contact urticaria, particularly of the lips and hands, due to uncooked food items is common among atopics [3]. Contact urticaria due to animal dander may aggravate atopic dermatitis of the arms and the periorbital area. It is important to note the results of prick tests carried out, for example, in previous attempts to discover the cause of respiratory allergy.

Patients with recurrent vesicular hand eczema are often atopics [4], and Schwanitz [5] coined the term 'das atopische Palmoplantarekzem' after a study of the literature and having seen 58 patients with recurrent vesicular hand eczema. Edman, however [6], found no statistical correlation between atopy and this type of hand dermatitis. Details concerning the relationship between atopy and contact sensitization are given in Sect. 7.3.5.4.

It is unusual for a patient to have a family history of contact dermatitis. Although hereditary factors were seen to have some significance among twins with nickel allergy, these were found to be less important than environmental factors [7].

A family history of psoriasis is important as it may be difficult to distinguish psoriasis from contact dermatitis. Likewise, Koebner reactions on the hands may show a striking resemblance to hyperkeratotic hand eczema. Both these conditions can be aggravated by physical trauma from various tools and handles.

7.2.2 General Medical History

Eczematous lesions sometimes occur when there is zinc depletion due to malnutrition or acrodermatitis enteropathica, as well as when metabolic disorders like phenylketonuria are seen.

In order to make a diagnosis of systemically induced dermatitis it is important to take a complete history of drug intake. Cutaneous sensitization to a drug may give rise to symmetrical dermatitis when the same drug, or a chemically related drug, is taken orally or is injected [8]. Drug intake can also play a significant role in a number of photodermatoses.

Obesity is an important factor in the development of intertriginous dermatoses and mechanical contact dermatitis due to friction; the latter may be seen, for example, on the inner surfaces of the thighs.

7.2.3 History of Previous Dermatitis

A firm history of previous allergic contact dermatitis from, for example, nickel, fragrances or topical remedies would be reason to suspect inadvertent contact with the same haptens if an otherwise unexplained eruption of contact dermatitis occurs. Further details on the relationship between the history of nickel allergy and atopy are given in Sect. 7.3.5.4.

A history of previous dermatitis near leg ulcers should lead to a suspicion of topical remedies being the cause of current or possible future eruptions of dermatitis in this area or elsewhere. A history of dermatitis where adhesive tape has been applied should lead the physician to inquire about colophony sensitivity and, keeping in mind the known cross-sensitivities, also sensitivity to fragrances. It should be mentioned, however, that most modern adhesive tapes contain no colophony, as the adhesive substance is usually an acrylate.

7.2.4 Time of Onset

For long-standing contact dermatitis, the exact time of onset is usually ill-defined and is not useful in establishing the final diagnosis. The cause of contact dermatitis with recent abrupt onset may be established by taking a careful history of contactants during the days immediately preceding the onset of dermatitis. The history should include occupational exposures and exposures during leisure time and while working in the home or with hobbies, as well as any changes in clothing or personal cosmetics, including soaps and detergents. Topical remedies used for the treatment of the dermatitis, both prescription and over-the-counter products, should be recorded, as well as any recent changes in systemic drug therapy.

7.2.5 History of Aggravating Factors

For chronic contact dermatitis, the history should include information about contactants in relation to aggravation of the dermatitis rather than to its onset. Two types of flares of chronic dermatoses should be considered: those eruptions which appear suddenly and without warning, and those which show seasonal variation. Seasonal variations may help to establish the type of dermatitis and possibly also the specific cause, a point which is illustrated in Fig. 7.1.

The sudden aggravation of chronic dermatitis or recurrences at short intervals may help to establish the cause of the dermatitis or, if this is not possible, those factors which aggravate it. Recurrent vesicular eczema of the hands provides a typical example of how such help can be obtained.

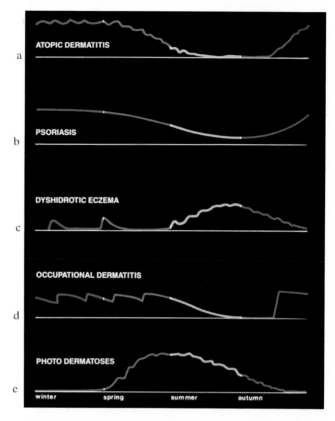

Fig. 7.1a–e. Seasonal variation in dermatitis. *a Atopic dermatitis:* fluctuates, severely pruritic, improves during the summer months. *b Psoriasis:* no pruritus, slow or no fluctuations, improves during the summer months. *c Dyshidrotic eczema:* eruptive throughout the year, often especially active during the summer months. *d Occupational dermatitis:* slow improvement seen over several consecutive days away from the workplace, fades during long periods of vacation, typically during the summer months; prompt recurrence upon resumption of work. *e Photodermatoses:* sudden onset during the spring, fluctuates during the summer months, fades during late summer; there is increased sun tolerance as pigmentation and epidermal thickness increase during the summer months

Although a definite cause of this type of dermatitis is rarely established, a number of factors may cause the eruption of a crop of vesicles. The time period between exposure to aggravating factors and the eruption of vesicles is 1 to 3 days, and with proper instruction a patient is often able to recall exposures which occurred up to 3 days prior to the onset of dermatitis and thus identify aggravating factors.

There are certain fundamental causes of chronic eczemas such as atopic dermatitis, seborrhoeic dermatitis, allergic contact dermatitis and irritant contact dermatitis. Possible aggravating factors include contact allergens, contact irritants (chemical, physical), contact urticaria, extreme variations in temperature, low or high humidity, ingestion of certain foods, smoking (controversial), psychological stress, sweating, drug intake, sun exposure, infections (local, systemic; dermatophytes and yeasts, bacteria, herpes simplex virus).

When discussing sun exposure with the patient, it should be stressed that the offending ultraviolet irradiation may penetrate window glass both in the home and in an automobile. It should also be stressed that aggravation during outdoor activities is not necessarily related to the sun. Dermatitis in areas of the body normally exposed to the sun can also be caused by airborne irritants and allergens such as dust particles, pollen and other plant material [9].

7.2.6 Course of the Dermatitis

In dealing with chronic dermatoses it is important to record treatment response as well as response to the elimination of suspected causative substances. Seborrhoeic dermatitis, for example, is easily suppressed by means of topical treatment, but recurrence is common. Contact dermatitis usually requires intensive treatment and recurs after discontinuation of therapy if the causative substance is not removed.

While allergic contact determatitis usually recurs very quickly after reexposure to the causative agent, irritant contact dermatitis tends to recur more slowly [10]. This difference can be useful in making the diagnosis.

The response to vacation periods and sick leave is of particular importance when occupational contact dermatitis is suspected. The result of reexposure to the suspected causative agent is equally important.

7.2.7 Types of Symptoms

Pruritus is the fundamental symptom of contact dermatitis. The onset is usually during the first day of contact with the offending item. The intensity of symptoms varies greatly and depends on the type of dermatitis and also on various individual factors. Some persons with irritant contact dermatitis have practically no symptoms, while some adults with atopic dermatitis suffer so much from itching that it is impossible for them to carry out everyday tasks.

Subtle symptoms of insidious onset include the stinging sensation felt in some cosmetic reactions in which there is no visible physical symptom. Stinging can be caused by a number of substances and is elicited on very sensitive skin. This symptom does not necessarily represent irritancy in general [11]. Pain rather than itching is frequent in phototoxic dermatitis like that caused by giant hogweed.

Symptoms of contact urticaria are often noticed seconds to minutes after contact with the causative substance. Characteristically, the symptoms include stinging and smarting in addition to pruritus. Such symptoms are often caused by uncooked foods or animal dander. In many patients, the symptoms fade quickly if the causative substance is rinsed off the skin.

Mayonnaise preserved with sorbic acid caused an epidemic of perioral contact urticaria in a group of kindergarten children. The careful histories which were taken proved to be the most important tool in arriving at the correct diagnosis [12].

Patients who suffer from hay fever in the birch pollen season often have a history of contact urticaria of the oral mucosa caused by hazelnuts [13]. Birch pollen may cause cellular immune reactions and contact dermatitis with an airborne pattern [14]. An association has also been found between birch pollen allergy and reactions to apple, carrot, pear and cherry and between grass pollen and tomato and certain types of melon [15, 16]. The taking of a careful history is, therefore, very important in the diagnostic work-up of patients with stomatitis and contact urticaria.

7.3 Clinical Features of Eczematous Reactions

7.3.1 Acute and Recurrent Dermatitis

Spongiosis of the epidermis is one of the histological hallmarks of eczematous reactions. Confluence of spongiosis can lead to vesicles and even bullae [17] (see Chap. 3)

The vesicular response is associated with acute and recurrent contact dermatitis and is best visualized on the palms (Figs. 7.2, 7.3), the sides of the fingers, around the fingernails (Fig. 7.4) and on the soles of the feet. Vesicular eruptions on the palms and the plantar aspects of the feet often occur simultaneously [18]. Vesicular palmar eruptions are not specific for eczema, as discussed in Sect. 7.6.

Vesicular eruptions at other than the above-mentioned sites are uncommon. Hyperacute dermatitis may present with vesicular eruptions (Fig. 7.5) or even bullae (Fig. 7.6). The vesicular or bullous reaction may be seen in allergic as well as in irritant reactions and cannot be used to distinguish between these two types of dermatitis. A typical irritant, bullous, contact dermatitis is the dermatitis seen after the application of cantharidin in the treatment of warts (Fig. 7.7).

The onset of an eczematous reaction can be more subtle. On the face and on the dorsa of the hands, the initial symptoms may be 'chapping' (Fig. 7.8) [10]. Irritants may subsequently cause the chapping to progress to frank eczema. The environmental temperature and humidity are of significance for the development of dermatitis from low-grade irritants [19–22].

The distinction between allergic and irritant contact dermatitis is difficult. A distinction can sometimes be made at the site of 'experimental' contact dermatitis, for example, a patch test site. Minimal itching occurs when a primary irritant is placed on the skin and subsequently occluded, and erythema

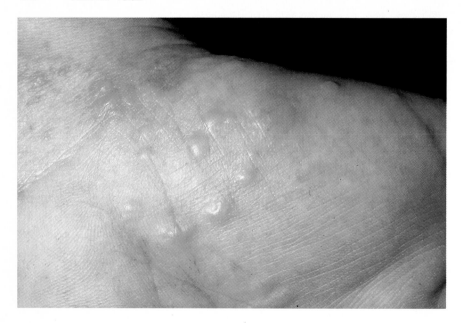

Fig. 7.2. Confluent vesicles on the palm

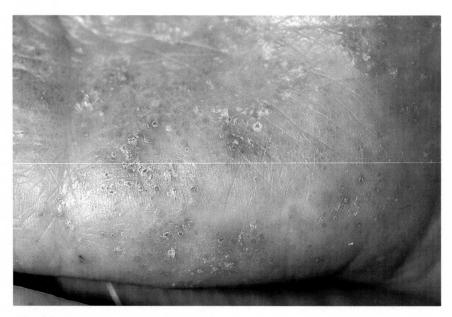

Fig. 7.3. Deep-seated vesicles on the palm

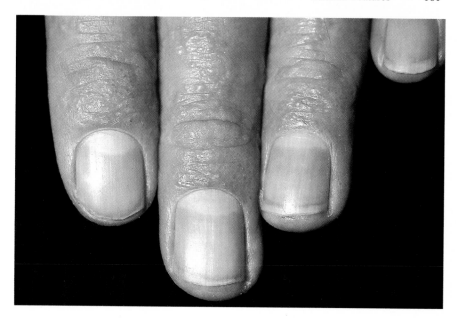

Fig. 7.4. Periungual vesicles

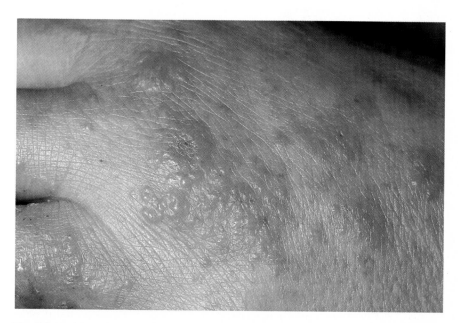

Fig. 7.5. Vesicular dermatitis on the dorsum of the hand

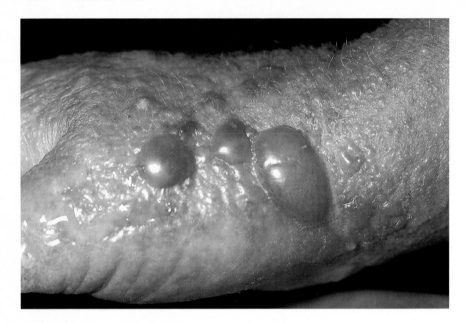

Fig. 7.6. Bullous dermatitis

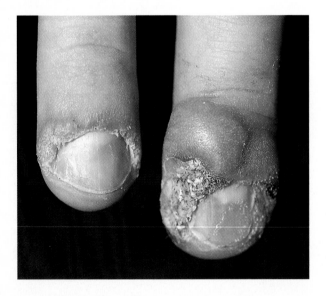

Fig. 7.7. Bullous periungual dermatitis
caused by cantharidin

and slight infiltration will be strictly limited to the area of the patch. Strong
irritants may produce bullous or pustular reactions (Fig. 7.9), but these will
also be limited to the occluded area. Similar occlusive testing with a substance
to which the patient has a cellular immune reaction tends rather to give
a markedly pruritic, infiltrated, papular or vesicular reaction which extends
beyond the rim of the occluding disc (Fig. 7.10).

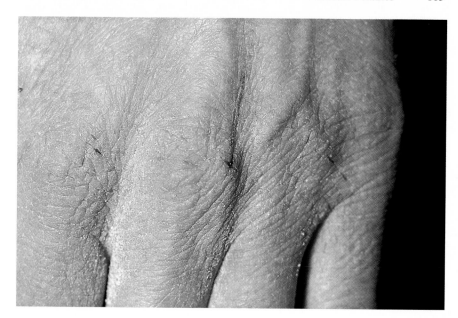

Fig. 7.8. Chapping on the dorsum of the hand

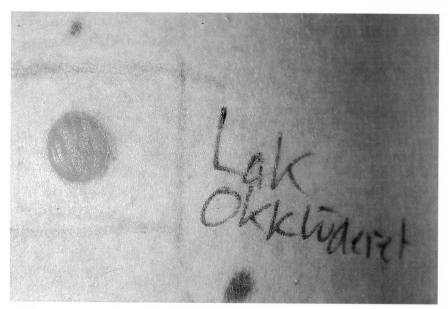

Fig. 7.9. A bullous irritant patch test reaction

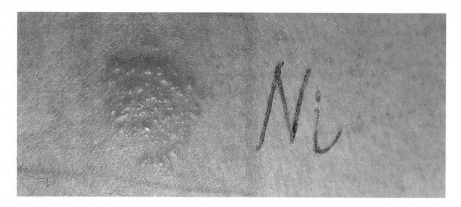

Fig. 7.10. A vesicular allergic patch test reaction

One possible explanation for this difference in the periphery of the test area may be that it is necessary to have a higher concentration of the offending substance to elicit an irritant reaction than to elicit an allergic reaction. The concentration of the substance used for a patch test will ordinarily be quite low outside the occluded area and will thus be less than the amount necessary to elicit an irritant reaction, even though an allergic reaction may still occur.

The vesicular response is often seen as recurrent vesicular dermatitis of the palms and soles. If frequent acute eruptions occur, this type of eruption will tend to become a chronic eczematous reaction. Careful inspection will often reveal a purely vesicular reaction, particularly at the periphery of the area of skin involved.

7.3.2 Chronic Dermatitis

If contact with an offending item persists, chronic dermatitis may eventually develop. The characteristic features of chronic dermatitis are pruritus, lichenification, erythema, scaling, fissures and excoriations (Fig. 7.11). Histologically, spongiosis becomes less pronounced, and psoriasiform features supervene. The clinical correlate to this histological transition is lichen simplex chronicus (neurodermatitis) (Fig. 7.12).

7.3.3 Nummular (Discoid) Eczema

The term 'nummular' (or 'discoid') eczema is based on the morphology or coin shape of the lesions (Fig. 7.33). This type of dermatitis may be of endogenous origin, but it may be confused with contact dermatitis from soluble oils [23, 24] (see Chap. 11).

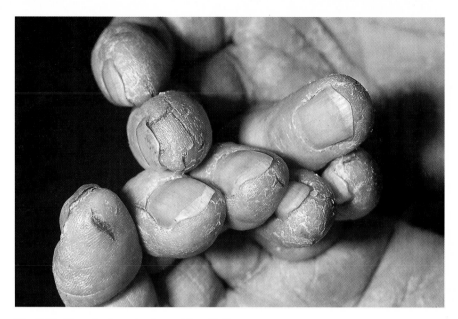

Fig. 7.11. Chronic fingertip dermatitis with fissures

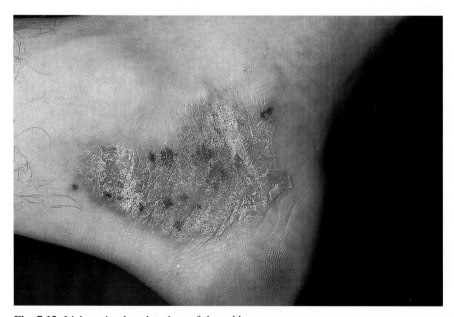

Fig. 7.12. Lichen simplex chronicus of the ankle

7.3.4 Secondarily Infected Dermatitis

When, as in chronic dermatitis, the epidermal barrier is no longer intact, secondary infection often develops at the site of the dermatitis. In fact, chronic dermatitis is often the result of cumulative insults by irritants, microorganisms and allergens to which the patient has become sensitized. Frank bacterial infection of contact dermatitis is common (Figs. 7.13, 7.14), and the possibility of pathogenic bacteria being present should therefore be considered before initiating treatment of chronic contact dermatitis.

Secondary infection should be distinguished from pustular irritant contact dermatitis caused by croton oil [25] or fluorouracil [26].

7.3.5 Clinical Features of Contact Dermatitis in Specific Groups of Persons

The clinical features of contact dermatitis may vary between specific groups of persons.

7.3.5.1 Children

Children have been thought to develop allergic contact dermatitis less often than adults. However, Weston and Weston [27] reviewed recent literature and concluded that allergic contact dermatitis was common in children and that the clinical pattern of the dermatitis provided an important clue to the specific diagnosis.

7.3.5.2 Elderly Persons

Elderly persons frequently develop allergic contact dermatitis from substances in topical medicaments. Inflammatory reactions are more subtle in elderly persons, and their contact dermatitis therefore often has a scaly appearance and is less vesicular than in younger individuals.

7.3.5.3 Dark-Skinned Persons

Black individuals and others with dark skin tend to develop hyperpigmentation and infiltration, particularly in chronic contact dermatitis, to a greater degree than those with light-coloured skin. Contact dermatitis in dark-skinned persons therefore frequently has the appearance of lichen simplex chronicus.

7.3.5.4 Atopics

Patients with atopic dermatitis who develop allergic contact dermatitis from a given substance often react with both aggravation of their atopic dermatitis and a pattern of allergic contact dermatitis. There is some question as to

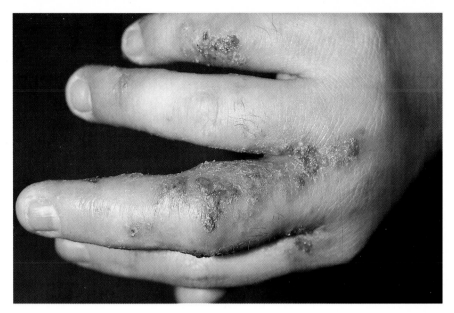

Fig. 7.13. Hand eczema with secondary bacterial infection

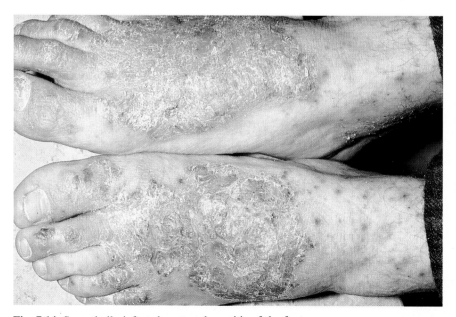

Fig. 7.14. Secondarily infected contact dermatitis of the foot

the exact relationship between atopy and contact sensitization. It has been suggested that atopics become contact sensitized less often than nonatopics [28]. In a population of patients with eyelid dermatitis, positive patch tests were significantly less common among atopics than among nonatopics [29]. In another study, 23% of a group of 130 adults who had moderate atopic dermatitis in childhood had positive patch tests to one or more allergens in a standard series, whereas 17% of 159 adults who had severe atopic dermatitis in childhood had similar positive patch tests [30]. These results support the theory that atopics experience fewer delayed-type sensitizations.

Christophersen et al. [31] carried out a multivariate statistical analysis of various parameters in 2166 patch-tested patients and found that nickel allergy was significantly less common among atopics than among nonatopics. This difference could not be demonstrated for other common contact allergens. Since nickel is a ubiquitous environmental allergen, atopics and nonatopics are equally exposed to this allergen. This type of study overlooks the fact that there may be a true impairment among atopics in developing contact sensitivity to allergens in topical remedies such as lanolin and the hydroxyquinolines, patients with atopic dermatitis being more often exposed to these than nonatopics. It is difficult to carry out valid statistical studies on such relatively uncommon allergens.

Negative nickel patch tests in patients with a history of nickel allergy have been linked to atopy [32], but no agreement has as yet been reached on the relevancy of such findings [33].

7.4 Identifying the Cause of Contact Dermatitis from the Clinical Pattern

It is often difficult to trace the substance which has caused the skin to react to contact, particularly if the patient has chronic lesions. Reactions to substances which are not a part of everyday life, such as dinitrochlorobenzene or infrequently used topical drugs, usually present little diagnostic difficulty, while the cause of reactions to ubiquitous allergens like nickel and fragrances may be much more difficult to trace. Certain patterns of skin disease can, however, point in the direction of particular groups of substances, or even towards one specific causative substance.

7.4.1 Clinical Patterns Indicating General Causes of Contact Dermatitis

7.4.1.1 Contact Pattern

In the most obvious cases, an eczematous reaction is seen at the exact site of contact with the offending item. This type of reaction is frequently recognized by the patient and will commonly not be brought to the attention of a physician.

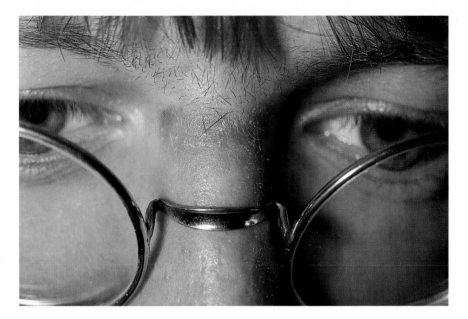

Fig. 7.15. Allergic nickel contact dermatitis

A typical example of contact-pattern dermatitis is allergic nickel contact dermatitis (Fig. 7.15). Historically, the most characteristic nickel contact sites have changed with changes in women's fashions. While, in the 1930s, most of Bonnevie's [34] patients had dermatitis at the site of contact with nickel-plated stocking suspender clasps, later the metal hooks on brassieres became a common offender. In the 1970s, sites of contact with metal buttons and studs in blue jeans became the most common sites of nickel dermatitis. At present, the earlobes, particularly if the patient has pierced ears [35], and sites of contact with nickel-plated watch bands and clasps are the most common primary sites of nickel dermatitis. Gawkrodger et al. [36] examined 134 patients with positive patch tests to nickel and found the following prevalence of sites: palm 49%, dorsum of the hands 39%, wrist 22%, face 20%, arm 16%, neck 14% and periorbital area 12%.

A study carried out in Singapore showed the most common sites to be the wrist, the ears and the waist [37]. The contact pattern of nickel dermatitis is also dependent on cultural tradition and on the groups of patients studied, as well as on climatic factors. For example, sweating caused by high temperatures increases the release of nickel from nickel-plated items [38]. Nickel is also released by plasma, a fact which may explain the high rate of nickel sensitization after ear piercing [39].

In 1969, Kanan [40] described the typical site of nickel dermatitis among males in Kuwait as the sites of contact with metal studs in undergarments. Fisher [41] noted that the most common sites of nickel dermatitis in males were under blue jeans' buttons and under watch bands.

More unusual sites of nickel contact dermatitis seen by the author include a small eczematous patch at the entry site of a venepuncture needle or a patch of eczema caused by the small nickel-plated part of a rubber stopper used to make a prosthesis airtight. Nickel dermatitis has also developed at sites of Dermojet injection [42] and at sites of the closure of surgical wounds with skin clips [43].

Irritant contact dermatitis occurring under objects which occlude the skin, such as the metal case of a watch or a plastic watch strap, may mimic nickel dermatitis.

The rubber in the elastic used in undergarments, for example brassieres, may produce characteristic patterns of dermatitis. Contact-pattern dermatitis may also be caused by the chemicals in rubber used in the manufacture of shoes.

Topical medicaments may also produce eczematous contact-pattern reactions, and these often have a biphasic course. Improvement initially seen following the use of a certain medicament applied to relieve an existing problem may be followed by aggravation in the area of application.

If a contact allergen – typically a topical drug – repeatedly applied to the legs of a sensitized person results in severe dermatitis, this will tend to spread in an id-like manner to the arms and possibly to the entire body. This pattern of spreading is also seen in severe stasis dermatitis, and it has been suggested that in patients with stasis dermatitis such spreading is caused by cell-mediated autoimmunity [44].

Since dermatitis caused by topical medicaments is most common in occluded areas and at sites where the skin is particularly delicate, this cause should be suspected if there is aggravation of existing dermatitis of the anogenital area, on the lower leg, on the ear or on the eyelids [45–47].

Treatment with caustic agents may produce ulcerations at the sites of application. Severe reactions may follow the erroneous use of topical wart remedies applied to nevi on parts of the body which are normally occluded.

Certain contact allergens can produce contact-pattern dermatitis which does not appear at the actual site of contact. Nail polish is such an allergen, and typical sites of allergic contact dermatitis caused by nail polish are the eyelids, neck and genitalia, rather than the skin around the fingernails [48].

7.4.1.2 Streaked Dermatitis in Exposed Areas

Dermatitis may appear in streaks if it has been caused by liquids allowed to run down the skin. Caustic substances such as those used by farmers to clean milking equipment can cause such reactions. Dermatitis caused by plant juices or the toxins from jellyfish like the Portuguese man-of-war often appears in a bizarre streaked pattern [49]. Dermatitis caused by juices from Umbelliferae is often phototoxic. Upon resolution, a streaked bullous dermatitis can be followed by marked hyperpigmentation which may last for many months (Figs. 7.16, 7.17).

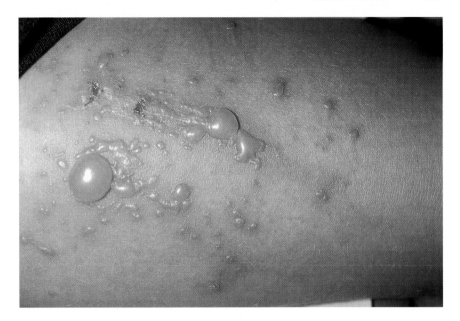

Fig. 7.16. Phototoxic dermatitis caused by giant hogweed

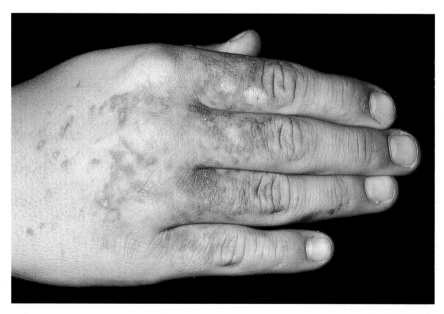

Fig. 7.17. Postinflammatory hyperpigmentation following resolution of phototoxic dermatitis caused by giant hogweed

7.4.1.3 Airborne Contact Dermatitis

Airborne contact dermatitis may be caused by
1. Fibrous materials such as glass fibre, rock wool and grain dust, which give rise to mechanical dermatitis [50]
2. Wood and cement dust, which cause irritant reactions [51]
3. Dust containing particles from plants like *Parthenium hysterophorus*, ragweed or certain types of wood or medicaments to which the patient has delayed-type sensitivity [52–55]

Particles of medicaments in the dust from, for example, pigsties can cause dermatitis if the patient has contact allergy to the medicament in question. Airborne contact dermatitis appears on areas of the skin where the dust or fibres can be trapped, for example on the eyelids, neck (under a shirt collar), forearms (under cuffs) or lower legs (inside trouser legs) [9]. Chronic airborne contact dermatitis tends to mimic photocontact dermatitis [56].

Dermatitis from wood dust and dust from plant particles often cause lichenified dermatitis at the sites of contact. Various cutaneous symptoms, including pruritus and paraesthesia, have been described after long-term exposure to computer screens, but few patients exhibit diagnostic skin lesions [57]. Similar problems may be associated with the handling of large amounts of carbonless copy paper and laser printed paper. In one study an increased level of plasma histamine was documented after exposure to carbonless copy paper [58].

7.4.1.4 Mechanical Dermatitis

Friction can cause both hyperkeratosis and dermatitis. Acute lesions may appear as actual abrasions of the skin (Fig. 7.18), while chronic mechanical dermatitis is often more subtle and therefore more difficult to diagnose. Mechanical trauma is particularly important as an occupational disorder. Many different aspects of this type of dermatitis were detailed at a conference on the cutaneous effects of repeated mechanical trauma to the skin [59].

The handling of large quantities of paper, for example computer printouts, may eventually lead to hyperkeratosis on the involved fingers. Eczematous dermatitis may develop after long-term, often unconscious, manipulation of the skin (Fig. 7.19). Some popular sports activities have given rise to new dermatological entities caused by physical trauma. These include 'rower's rump', 'jogger's nipples' and 'black heel' [60, 61].

Mechanical dermatitis on the inner aspects of the thighs may mimic inter-trigo. Bizzare patterns of dermatitis and purpura may result from curious cultural habits, such as coin rubbing. Unusual patterns of skin lesions can also be seen in the victims of physical or electrical torture.

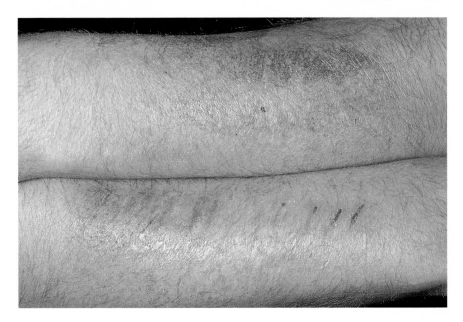

Fig. 7.18. An abrasion caused by contact with rough fibres in a sack made of jute

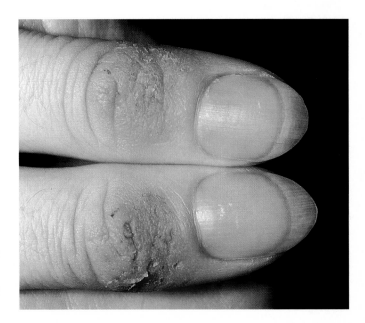

Fig. 7.19. Mechanical contact dermatitis caused by manipulation of the skin

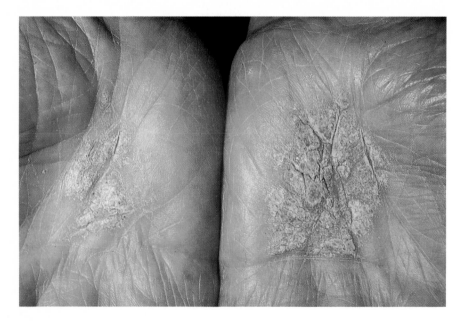

Fig. 7.20. Hyperkeratotic palmer eczema

7.4.1.5 Hyperkeratotic Eczema

Symmetrical, hyperkeratotic plaques on the central parts of the palms and/or pressure areas of the soles represent an entity which is clinically distinct from other types of eczema, because no vesicles are seen. At the onset of the eruption, this dermatitis is often pruritic, while pruritus is uncommon in chronic lesions (Fig. 7.20). Histologically, this type of eczema is also distinct from psoriasis [62]. The aetiology is unknown, but the condition is aggravated by mechanical trauma.

7.4.1.6 Ring Dermatitis

Dermatitis which occurs under tight-fitting jewellery such as finger rings can be due to allergic reactions to constituents of the jewellery. If a ring is made of relatively pure gold or of plastic, this type of eczema is most commonly due to sweat retention and the accumulation of occluded irritants from detergents (Fig. 7.21). Interestingly, ring dermatitis may spread to the corresponding area on the opposite hand, even though no ring is worn on this hand.

7.4.1.7 Follicular Reactions

Folliculitis of acneiform appearance may develop following cutaneous contact with or the absorption of certain polyhalogenated aromatic hydrocarbons, such as dioxin, or following skin contact with crude oil or its derivatives. Exposed

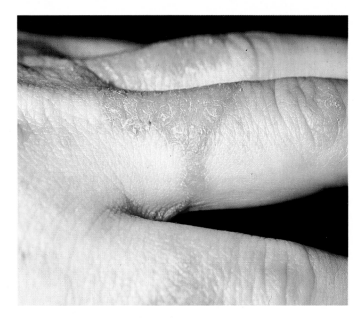

Fig. 7.21. Irritant contact dermatitis under a finger ring

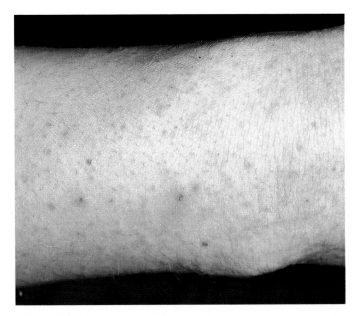

Fig. 7.22. Folliculitis caused by oil

areas of the body are most commonly involved (Fig. 7.22), but chloracne caused by the inhalation of chlorinated compounds can appear on parts of the body which are normally covered, and oil folliculitis may occur on the thighs if a patient has worn trousers which have become soaked in oil. Pomade acne of the forehead caused by oils applied to the hair is usually found only on the forehead and the temples, while cosmetic acne is most often distributed over the entire face [63].

Allergic contact dermatitis may appear as a pustular dermatosis. Pustular reactions have been described in allergic contact dermatitis caused by mercaptobenzothiazoles [64]. A galvanizer was seen to have occupational contact folliculitis [65]. Pustular patch test reactions, interpreted as nonallergic, were seen in 2% of 853 persons tested with sodium tungstate. The reactions were often reproducible [66]. This type of contact dermatitis is described in greater detail in Chap. 9.

7.4.1.8 Connubial Dermatitis

Contact with rubber condoms can cause genital eczema in women. Allergic contact urticaria may occur following contact with semen, and such contact can also cause systemic symptoms [67]. Males can develop dermatitis of the penis after contact with contraceptive cream. Connubial dermatitis is not confined solely to the genitals, as witnessed by the fact that some women develop allergic contact dermatitis on the face after contact with a partner's aftershave lotion [68].

7.4.1.9 Recurrent Vesicular Hand and/or Foot Dermatitis

This common pruritic dermatosis occurs as eruptions of crops of vesicles on the palms, on the sides of fingers, on the central part of the soles or on the sides of the toes (Figs. 7.2–7.4). The eruptions heal with subsequent scaling, but repeated frequent eruptions may lead to chronic hand and/or foot eczema. Recurrent vesicular dermatitis is a nonspecific clinical reaction pattern which may be caused by external agents, but it is commonly considered to be an example of an endogenous dermatosis [18].

7.4.1.10 Fingertip Eczema

Dermatitis of the fingertips, particularly on the thumb and index fingers, is a common ailment among chefs due to their repeated contact with irritants or allergens found in plants such as garlic. Dental technicians can also develop fingertip eczema, due to contact with the acrylic substances used to make dental prostheses (Fig. 7.23).

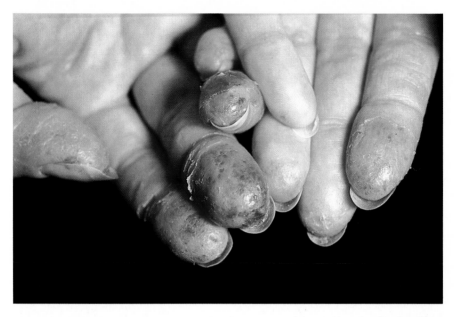

Fig. 7.23. Fingertip eczema in a patient with allergic contact dermatitis caused by handling acrylic materials

7.4.1.11 Eczema Nails

A characteristic pattern of transverse grooves and ridges may be seen in the nail plates of patients with eczema on the dorsal aspects of the fingers. There is usually also involvement of the nail cuticle. The number of grooves on the nail often corresponds to the number of episodes of flare of the eczema (Fig. 7.24). Subungual vesicular dermatitis under the periphery of the nail plate is less common (Fig. 7.25) [69]. This pattern of subungual dermatitis has been seen, however, following work with anaerobic acrylic sealants [70]. Allergic contact dermatitis to formaldehyde-based nail hardening resins and acrylates used to build up artificial nails has caused severe nail damage, including irreversible nail dystrophy [71].

7.4.1.12 Papular and Nodular Excoriated Lesions

Practically all reported cases of delayed hypersensitivity to aluminium have occurred following deposition in the dermis or subcutis of vaccines used for childhood immunizations or following hyposensitization procedures. Pruritic, excoriated, deeply infiltrated lesions at injection sites are characteristic [72, 73]. Intolerance to antiperspirants which contain aluminium salts has been described, but such cases appear to be rare [74].

Infiltrated papular lesions have also been seen at the sites of injection of zinc-bound insulin. The patients in question had zinc hypersensitivity, as

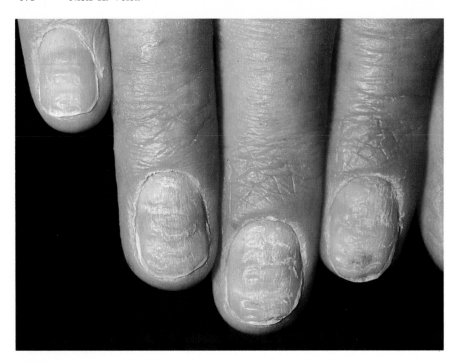

Fig. 7.24. Transverse ridges and grooves in the nail plates of a patient with eczema on the dorsal aspects of the fingers

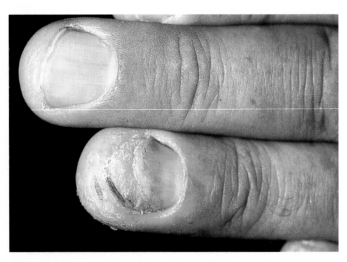

Fig. 7.25. Subungual eczema

demonstrated by intracutaneous testing and lymphocyte transformation studies [75]. A similar morphology of contact sensitization is seen if tattoo pigment causes sensitization. Chromium, cobalt and mercury salts used to be common sensitizing tattoo pigments [76]. Modern tattoo pigments are, however, rare sensitizers. See also Sect. 7.5.7.

7.4.1.13 Contact Urticaria of the Hands and Lips Caused by Foods

Contact urticaria should be suspected if dermatitis or intermittent urticaria is seen on the lips and/or the hands, particularly if an itching or a burning sensation has arisen seconds to minutes after contact with uncooked food items. The symptoms on the hands sometimes disappear when the hands are rinsed: in some cases hand eczema develops or, more commonly, an existing hand eczema is aggravated [77, 78]. This problem is particularly common among atopics [3]. Allergens in foods may penetrate eczematous skin, but the same allergens usually cannot penetrate intact skin (see Sect. 2.3.2.1).

7.4.1.14 Clinical Patterns of Systemically Induced Contact Dermatitis

If a substance to which a person has developed cellular immunity due to contact with the skin is subsequently ingested or otherwise absorbed, a variety of cutaneous reactions may occur [79, 80]. Vesiculation of the hands, for example, may be seen in patients who have not previously experienced this reaction pattern. A patient who suffers from recurrent vesicular hand eczema may experience a flare of dermatitis after experimental oral challenge with the substance to which he or she is sensitive. One nickel-sensitive patient developed palmar vesicles and small bullae a few days after beginning a weight-reducing diet which called for the ingestion of vegetables rich in nickel. Nickel-sensitive patients may have dermal lesions with evidence of vasculitis, which can be reproduced by placebo-controlled oral challenge [81]. A keratotic eruption of the elbows has been described as accompanying a systemically induced dermatitis [82].

So-called secondary eruptions were noted by Calnan [83] when he described the clinical features of large groups of nickel-allergic patients. These secondary eruptions consisted of erythematous flares in skin folds such as the antecubital fossae and on the sides of the neck, the eyelids and the inner thighs. Widespread oedematous erythemas in the skin folds of the anogenital area has been termed the baboon syndrome [84], and oedematous lesions of this type have also been observed in nickel-sensitive patients following oral challenge with nickel [85].

If patients who have positive patch tests to a specific substance such as gentamicin are given this substance intravenously, widespread symmetrical eczematous lesions may occur after a few hours [86].

Sensitization from the topical application of drugs is common. If a drug to which a patient is sensitized is taken orally, a variety of reactions can be seen, ranging from recurrence of the dermatitis in its original site to widespread dermatitis. Such widespread dermatitis may be accompanied by fever and toxic epidermal necrolysis, which may be life-threatening [8, 87, 88].

Fixed drug eruption is a distinct nummular eruption occurring repeatedly in the same location after the ingestion of the drug in question [89]. It may be, but is not necessarily, associated with topical sensitivity to the drug. In one study, a fixed eruption could be reproduced in 18 of 24 patients after topical application of the drug. The study showed topical sensitivity to phenazones to be especially common [90].

Flares of old patch test sites and sites of previous nickel contact dermatitis may be seen after experimental oral challenge with nickel. An example of this seen by the author was a flare of dermatitis seen at sites of contact with garter belt clasps despite the patient not having worn a garter belt for 20 years.

Other examples of specific clinical features associated with systemically induced contact dermatitis include the symptoms following oral hyposensitization treatment of patients allergic to poison ivy, which have been described in detail. These patients characteristically developed widespread, symmetrical, oedematous, erythematous, eruptions, as well as symmetrical vesicular eruptions of the hands and feet, flares of patch test sites and anal and vulvar pruritus [91, 92].

7.4.2 Characteristic Clinical Patterns of Dermatitis Associated with Specific Substances

7.4.2.1 Cement Ulcerations

Caustic reactions at the site of prolonged contact with wet cement are sometimes seen under the tops of socks or on other parts of the lower leg which are normally occluded. The alkalinity of the cement and prolonged skin contact with wet cement are the most likely cause of this dermatitis [93, 94] (Fig. 7.26).

7.4.2.2 Pigmented Contact Dermatitis

Optical brighteners were originally described by Osmundsen and Alani [95] as the cause of severely pruritic, purpuric, allergic contact dermatitis which caused little or no discernible change in the epidermis. In Japan, pigmented contact dermatitis is relatively common. A resin commonly used in the dyeing of cotton fabrics (naphthol AS) can cause pigmented allergic contact dermatitis which is typically seen on the neck and upper arms [96] (see Chap. 15).

7.4.2.3 Caterpillar Dermatitis

Spicules hidden among the hairs of certain caterpillars contain a toxin which can cause persistent pruritic vesicles or papules at sites of contact with the skin. This is a characteristic clinical finding among children who have played

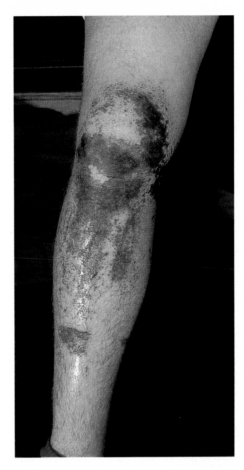

Fig. 7.26. Caustic reaction caused by cement (Courtesy of T. Menné)

with these caterpillars [97]. Sun worshippers may come in contact with this toxin on beaches where large numbers of this species of caterpillar have wandered in procession. Similar toxic substances are found in sea urchins and in various plants. Mechanical injuries from thorns and similar projections on plants or fish may mimic this dermatosis.

7.4.2.4 Head and Neck Dermatitis

Adults with atopic dermatitis and persistent pruritic dermatitis of the face, the sides of the neck and the shoulders may have immediate-type sensitivity to the saprophytic fungus *Pityrosporum ovale* [98, 99]. The dermatitis probably represents contact urticaria caused by the yeast.

7.4.2.5 Dermatitis from Transcutaneous Delivery Systems

Eczematous lesions as well as general cutaneous reactions and systemic symptoms sometimes occur where transcutaneous drug delivery systems have been applied [100, 101]. Continuous percutaneous drug delivery systems are used for such drugs as clonidine, nitroglycerin, scopolamine, oestradiol, nicotine and testosterone [102]. Studies of why the drugs applied in this manner sometimes cause cutaneous reactions have revealed that a limited number of patients have allergic contact dermatitis from the active drug or from ingredients in the delivery system itself [103]. Oral ingestion of the drugs in question has been seen to produce widespread dermatitis in a few patients [102].

7.4.2.6 Berloque Dermatitis

The application of perfumes on the sides of the neck may give rise to oedematous dermatitis and subsequent pigmentation at the exact sites of application of the perfume.

7.4.2.7 Stomatitis due to Mercury Allergy

Greyish streaks on the oral mucous membranes at sites of contact with amalgam dental fillings indicate contact stomatitis to the mercury in the amalgam fillings. This entity is discussed in detail in Sect. 7.5.6.

7.5 Regional Contact Dermatitis

The diagnosis of contact dermatitis is facilitated by a thorough knowledge of substances which characteristically cause dermatitis of specific areas of the skin. Computer analysis of the relationship between eczema sites and contact allergens have shown statistically significant correlations between, for example, nickel and cobalt and various sites on the fingers and palms, between chromate and the upper back, and between lanolin and the lower legs. Fragrance mix was shown to correlate with dermatitis of the axillae, balsam of Peru with dermatitis of the face and the lower legs, and neomycin and '-caine' mix with dermatitis of the lower leg [104]. Other examples of substances which cause dermatitis in specific areas of the body are presented in the following sections.

7.5.1 Dermatitis of the Scalp

Allergic contact dermatitis of the scalp itself is surprisingly rare in view of the fact that the level of percutaneous absorption of the skin of the scalp is high compared with other areas of the body. While sensitization to leave-on products such as pomades does occur, they commonly cause dermatitis on adjacent areas such as the ears, the forehead and sides of the neck rather than on the scalp itself [105, 106].

Contact sensitizers applied to the scalp such as thioglycolates in permanent wave solutions or dyes used to colour the hair more frequently cause hand eczema in the persons who apply the substances than contact dermatitis in the person to whom they are applied [107].

Nickel in hairpins and decorative items of nickel used near the scalp may cause dermatitis at the sites of contact.

Rinse-off products such as shampoos may cause allergic contact dermatitis of the scalp, but such reactions are rare in view of the amounts used [108]. Patients who have previously become sensitized to preservatives may react to similar compounds in shampoos and other hair-care products. Medicated shampoos, for example those containing tar, may cause irritant contact dermatitis of the scalp or aggravation of the seborrhoeic dermatitis or psoriasis they were intended to improve.

Microorganisms like *Pityrosporum ovale* may aggravate existing diseases of the scalp, and seborrhoeic dermatitis of the scalp has been seen to improve following treatment with ketoconazole shampoo. Bacterial infection may aggravate atopic dermatitis of the scalp and cause folliculitis as well as exudative dermatitis.

Discoloration of the hair due to external contactants may be due to the copper salts found in swimming pool water (green colour), anthralin preparations used on the scalp (reddish colour) or hydroxyquinoline preparations (brownish-yellow colour).

7.5.2 Dermatitis of the Face and Neck

The face and neck, like the backs of the hands, are the areas of the body most heavily exposed to the sun. These areas are, therefore, the prime targets for photocontact dermatitis. In typical cases the symptoms of this dermatitis are burning, stinging and itching. There is a sharp delineation along the collar and no dermatitis under the chin or behind the earlobes. Less typical cases may include symptoms similar to the above but with little to be seen on physical examination. The pigmentation seen following some types of photo-toxic contact dermatitis is caused by furocoumarins, and such pigmentation is in itself almost diagnostic.

Photocontact dermatitis following contact with tar products commonly appears where drops of, for example, wood preservatives have fallen on the skin. Hyperpigmentation is more commonly seen after photocontact dermatitis caused by furocoumarins than by tar.

Photocontact dermatitis which remains undiagnosed, or which is caused by substances which are difficult to avoid, may eventually become what is known as the actinic reticuloid syndrome [109]. The aetiology of this entity is not clear, and airborne contact dermatitis may also be a causative factor.

Even when the substance causing this dermatitis has been removed, some patients remain permanently light sensitive (see Sect. 2.4.6)

The face and neck are also typical sites of airborne contact dermatitis, which in its early phases may be distinguished from photocontact dermatitis by the presence of dermatitis in submental areas and behind the ears. Airborne contact dermatitis is commonly most intense where dust is trapped under the shirt collar, while light-induced dermatitis is seen only above the collar. A typical mechanical dermatitis in this area is the classic fiddler's neck caused by long-term contact with the chin rest on a violin.

Allergic contact dermatitis of the neck is commonly caused by nickel in jewellery, but jewellery made of exotic woods can also be the cause. Plastics rarely cause dermatitis on the neck. Nurses in intensive-care units who wear a stethoscope for many hours a day may develop nickel dermatitis on the sides of the neck.

In a study by Hausen and Oestmann [110], 50% of 64 flower vendors with contact dermatitis caused by plants had dermatitis of the face. The most common causative plants were chrysanthemums, tulips and alstroemeria, while daffodils and primulas were rarely the cause.

Facial dermatitis is commonly caused by cosmetics. Of 119 patients with cosmetic dermatitis, 63% had involvement of the face, while 26% had involvement of the hands and arms [111]. Of 13216 patients with contact dermatitis seen by members of the North American Contact Dermatitis Group over a 5-year period, 713 had dermatitis caused by cosmetics. Interestingly, neither patient nor physician had suspected cosmetics as the cause of the contact dermatitis on the basis of the clinical features. The diagnoses were not made until the results of patch testing were known. 81% of the patients had a dermatitis which could be described as allergic contact dermatitis; irritation accounted for the reactions of 16% of the patients and phototoxic and photoallergic reactions each accounted for less than 1% of the reactions. Fragrances, preservatives, hair-colouring agents and permanent wave solutions accounted for most of the cases of allergic contact dermatitis seen in this study [112].

The use of soap containing chromium is a rare cause of pigmented contact dermatitis of the face [113]. Depigmentation may also be seen following the use of cosmetic products such as toothpaste containing cinnamic aldehyde [114] and incense [115].

Ammonium persulphate used to bleach hair is a peculiar substance in that it may produce symptoms in both the hairdresser and the customer, following either contact with the solution used to treat the hair or with airborne particles of it. The substance can cause histamine release, leading to severe respiratory symptoms and urticaria. It may also produce irritant contact dermatitis and allergic reactions which may be either immediate-type or delayed-type [116].

Cosmetic acne presenting as discrete poral occlusion is common. An acneiform folliculitis of the forehead known as pomade acne is occasionally seen after the long-term use of oily hair-care products [63]. A transient

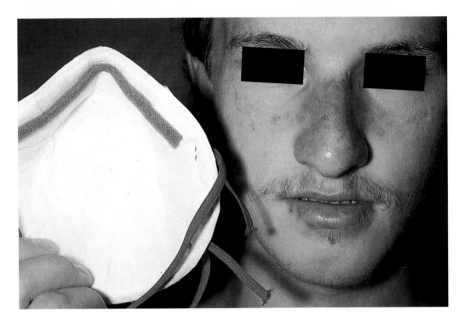

Fig. 7.27. Allergic contact dermatitis due to formaldehyde in a protective mask

stinging sensation on the face, with no apparent dermatitis, following the application of cosmetic preparations is common [11]. The stinging sensation may in some cases be due to contact urticaria. Individuals with fair, freckled skin are probably more likely to develop irritation from cosmetics than others. A questionnaire study of 90 student nurses revealed contact dermatitis from cosmetics in 29, while 25 others had rhinitis caused by cosmetic preparations [117]. Sunscreen preparations may produce allergic as well as photoallergic contact dermatitis at the sites of application.

Facial dermatitis can also be caused by allergens and irritants in face masks (surgical masks, scuba-diving masks and masks worn to filter out dust or used to supply fresh air while working with dangerous substances) [118]. The contact pattern of the dermatitis characteristically follows the outline of the mask worn (Fig. 7.27). Nickel dermatitis, as illustrated in Fig. 7.15, is usually located at the site of specific contact with, for example, metal spectacle frames.

Particular attention should be paid to three specific locations on the face and neck, as discussed below.

7.5.2.1 The Lips

On the lips, dermatitis may be caused both by cosmetics and by foods which make contact with the lips. Contact urticaria is commonly the cause when contact with certain foods results in cheilitis. The characteristic symptoms include stinging, burning, tingling and itching of the lips seconds to minutes after contact with the offending item [119]. Similar symptoms may occur on the oral mucosa.

7.5.2.2 The Eyes and Eyelids

The skin of the eyelid is very thin and delicate, but in spite of this it is covered by a coat of water-fast make-up by a large proportion of the female population. The cosmetic products used for this purpose are often based on oils which are considered primary irritants.

Many people rub the eyelids frequently and substances otherwise found on the hands are thereby transported to the eyelids. The eyelids are also a common site of airborne and systemic contact dermatitis. It is therefore not surprising that eyelid dermatitis is common and that it can have a multitude of causes [29] (Fig. 7.28). The very loosely bound subcutis of the eyelid makes marked oedema a characteristic feature of eyelid dermatitis.

Eyelid dermatitis has been used as a model for various enhanced patch test techniques such as patch testing on tape-stripped skin and patch testing on scarified skin. These techniques are recommended for the detection of weak sensitizers such as eye medications used for a prolonged period of time [120].

Atopics frequently have fissured dermatitis of the upper eyelids, probably due to mechanical irritation from rubbing the eyes and from airborne fibres from carpets, animal hair and other sources. In patients sensitized to house

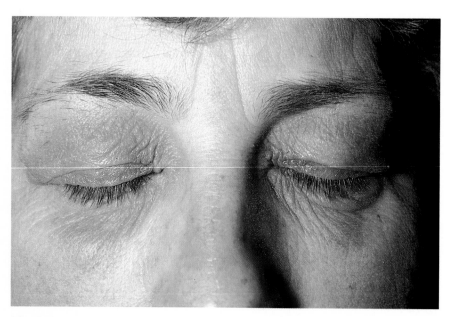

Fig. 7.28. Eyelid eczema

dust mites and animal dander, contact urticaria on the eyelids may also be caused by these allergens.

Nickel dermatitis of the eyelids may be due to nickel contamination of the fingers or to the systemic administration of nickel, as evidenced by the flares seen after oral challenge with nickel.

Topical ophthalmic products and preparations used in the care of contact lenses can cause contact dermatitis of the eyelids [121, 122]. Irritant contact conjunctivitis has been seen after the use of acrylic monomers found in printing inks [123], and after contact with crystals from plants of the genus *Dieffenbachia* [124].

7.5.2.3 The Ear

There are three common causes of dermatitis of the ear. One of these is seborrhoeic dermatitis. This condition frequently recurs after periods of quiescence and may require long-term or intermittent treatment. Such treatment may result in sensitization and cause allergic contact dermatitis [45–47].

A second major cause of dermatitis of the ear is objects put into the ear. Hairpins containing nickel used to relieve itching in the ear canal may cause allergic contact dermatitis. Matches containing chromate or phosphorus sesquisulphide may likewise cause allergic contact dermatitis of the external ear. Hearing aids rarely produce allergic contact dermatitis but do sometimes cause dermatitis as a result of occlusion, particularly in patients with seborrhoeic dermatitis.

The third type of dermatitis commonly found on the ear is earlobe dermatitis caused by nickel sensitization. In fact, today's most commonly described cause of nickel sensitization is earrings used in pierced ears [35]. There is sometimes a discrepancy between a history of dermatitis at sites which have been in contact with cheap jewellery and patch test results, which may be negative in spite of the repeated appearance of a rash after such jewellery is worn. One explanation for this discrepancy could be that nickel sensitization has not actually occurred and that the dermatitis is caused by irritancy or is some other nonimmunological reaction. Other possibilities are that only local sensitization has taken place, or that the patch test results were false negative [125]. Nickel-plated spectacle frames may cause dermatitis at the site of contact on the ear and nose, while dermatitis from plastic frames is rare.

7.5.3 Dermatitis of the Trunk

The principal sensitizers causing dermatitis of the trunk are
1. Nickel in brassiere straps, zippers and buttons
2. Rubber in the elastic of undergarments and other clothing (rubber items may cause contact urticaria as well as allergic contact dermatitis)
3. Fragrances used in soaps, skin-care products and detergents
4. Formaldehyde and other textile resins and dyes

Textile fibre dermatitis is usually most pronounced at sites of intense contact with the fibres and at typical sweat retention sites such as the axillary folds, the sides of the neck, the inner aspects of the thighs and the gluteal folds [126, 127]. In addition to the fibres themselves, the chemicals used to improve the appearance of textiles may also cause dermatitis at the above-mentioned sites. The incidence of textile dermatitis caused by the release of formaldehyde has decreased over the past several years [128].

New, unwashed, permanent-press sheets caused moderately pruritic or burning papules of the helices and lobes of the ears, the cheeks and the sides of the neck in 25 patients. An irritant reaction to textile resins was thought to have caused the dermatitis [129]. Irritant contact dermatitis may be caused by detergents which have not been thoroughly rinsed out of clothing after washing. Children with atopic dermatitis are particularly susceptible to irritation from detergent residues.

Mechanical dermatitis caused by rough woollen fibres and various artificial fibres is common, particularly among atopics, who may also suffer from sweat retention dermatitis on the trunk. The pressure exerted by tight-fitting items of clothing such as girdles and brassieres can lead to dermatitis and hyperpigmentation.

One distinct type of mechanical dermatitis of the upper back is a patch of excoriated dermatitis seen at the site of a label in a blouse. This condition is very common among patients with atopic dermatitis, but it also occurs in adults with no history of atopic dermatitis. The label causing the dermatitis is often made of stiff artificial fibres which cause pruritus in atopic patients and others with sensitive skin [130].

Another distinct type of clothing dermatitis is seen in patients who wear undergarments which have been machine washed together with textiles containing glass fibre, for example curtains, or work clothes contaminated with rock wool or glass fibre. The fibres bound in the undergarments may cause an intensely pruritic mechanical dermatitis at the sites of contact.

Rare causes of dermatitis of the trunk include contact with the electrode jelly used for electrocardiograms.

7.5.3.1 The Axillary Region

There are certain types of dermatitis which are peculiar to the axillary region.

In view of the extensive use of antiperspirant products containing aluminium, aluminium allergy is rare. Aluminium sensitization has been seen largely as a consequence of the injection of vaccines precipitated with aluminium hydroxide, while dermatitis elicited by aluminium in antiperspirants is uncommon.

Five of 20 patients with cosmetic dermatitis had axillary dermatitis due to the perfume in their deodorant or antiperspirant [131]. Fragrance dermatitis caused by deodorants and antiperspirants is characteristically seen in the entire axillary region. Dermatitis due to textile resins, on the other hand, is most intense in the axillary folds and often does not affect the central area of the axilla. Dermatitis of the axillary folds caused by friction between clothes and the skin is common in patients with atopic dermatitis. It is possible that in the past the diagnosis of perfume dermatitis was obscured by the fact that a corticosteroid preparation used to suppress axillary eczema once contained perfume [132].

A form of contact dermatitis commonly seen in both the axillary and the genital areas is caused by irritant reactions to chemical depilatory agents or various mechanical means of hair removal. The shaving off of the curly hair in the genital region may cause pseudofolliculitis when regrowth occurs.

7.5.3.2 The Anogenital Region

The anogenital area is a common site of contact dermatitis. This is due, among other things, to the fact that allergens and irritants can easily penetrate the delicate skin of this normally occluded area.

Age plays an important role in the development of anogenital contact dermatitis, as witnessed by the irritant contact dermatitis caused by urine and faeces during the first years of life and also in older incontinent individuals [133]. Diapers themselves may cause mechanical dermatitis as well as irritant contact dermatitis, but they rarely cause allergic contact dermatitis. In baby girls dermatitis at the top of the vulvar folds is often considered to be evidence of dermatitis caused by diapers (W pattern) (Fig. 7.29), while dermatitis which is most intense in the vulvar creases is more likely to be caused by microorganisms.

Mothers tend to exchange disposable paper diapers for old-fashioned cloth diapers when diaper rash appears. This change is unnecessary and is, in fact, potentially harmful. A 26-week double-blind study of various diaper types used for infants with atopic dermatitis showed that the use of disposable diapers gave rise to diaper dermatitis less often than the use of conventional cloth diapers [134] (see Sect. 12.2.1).

In older incontinent persons, rubber uridoms may cause allergic contact dermatitis. A dermatitis with a peculiar pattern was seen in a group of faeces-incontinent persons treated for constipation with Dianthon, a drug which releases anthralin in the intestine. A burn-like irritant contact dermatitis appeared on the thighs where the faeces had made contact with the skin.

Among sexually active individuals, connubial dermatitis may occur in the vulvar area and on the penis and scrotum. One characteristic of this dermatitis is that its activity fluctuates with the sexual activity of the patient. If connubial dermatitis in the male can be relieved by the use of a condom, this suggests that it is caused by substances applied to the vulva or the vagina. Such substances include spermicidal creams, jellies or suppositories, the fragrances in creams and cleansing agents and the rubber in diaphragms. Microorganisms in the vagina such as *Candida albicans* commonly cause transient balanitis in the male.

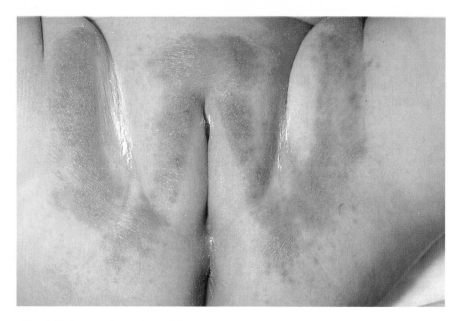

Fig. 7.29. Irritant diaper dermatitis

Vulvitis is less frequently relieved by the use of a condom. Females have been observed to suffer from contact urticaria caused by semen. This is an important entity, as anaphylactoid reactions have been seen [67].

Other dermatological problems associated with sexual activity include traumatic lesions such as fissures, erosions or even ulcers caused by the friction of intense sexual activity, lack of lubrication or bizarre habits. In both sexes a mechanical Koebner phenomenon may cause eruptions or aggravation of psoriasis lesions on the genitals. Lichen planus is common on the penis, and the Koebner phenomenon may delay clearing of this disease. Neurodermatitis of the vulva may remain active due to sexual activity. A particular problem in males is sclerosing lymphangitis of the penile lymph vessels. This condition is commonly considered to be traumatic.

In addition to problems related to sexual activity, dermatitis on the genitals may be caused by substances normally found on the hands which have been transferred to the genitals. In males this type of dermatitis may present as allergic contact dermatitis caused, for example, by sawdust or preservatives in paints [52].

Females may develop irritant or allergic contact dermatitis of the vulva due to contact with nail polish.

Widespread pruritus and dermatitis with features similar to those of systemically induced contact dermatitis have appeared following the introduction of intrauterine contraceptive devices made of copper [135]. Sensitivity to copper is unusual, and this may not be the sole explanation for these symptoms.

Another curious eruption in the anogenital and bikini area is the baboon syndrome described earlier in Sect. 7.4.1.14. The accumulation of an irritant substance, for example seaweed, in swim suits may cause irritant contact dermatitis in the bikini area, and a similar type of dermatitis may occur if a wet swim suit is worn for prolonged periods.

Allergic and/or irritant contact dermatitis in the anogenital area is often caused by the topical application of various medicaments. A wide range of compounds can cause such reactions, including antifungal agents used to combat dermatophyte infections and candidiasis, haemorrhoid remedies and agents used to relieve anogenital pruritus. Some of the sensitizing agents commonly used in this area of the body are benzocaine, neomycin, the hydroxyquinolines and bufexamac [45–47, 136].

Ingested irritants and sensitizers may cause pruritus and contact dermatitis in the perianal region. The mechanism here may be the deposition of the suspected substance on perianal skin. In some situations, however, systemically induced contact dermatitis or other systemic mechanisms may be to blame, as in the case of coffee drinkers' rash [137]. The anal pruritus seen after oral challenge with nickel or balsam of Peru may be due to unabsorbed substances in the faeces present in higher concentrations than those normally experienced [80].

7.5.3.3 Stoma Dermatitis

Excretions from a stoma may cause dermatitis when irritant substances come into contact with skin which is not suited for such contact. This is particularly true in the case of ileostomies, where the faeces are rather liquid and may contain enzymes and other irritants which would normally be degraded during passage through the colon and rectum. The materials used for the stoma appliances themselves, or their adhesive surfaces, are today so well researched and carefully selected that they rarely cause sensitization or irritation [138]. An important exception was noted by Beck et al. [139], who discovered low molecular weight epoxy resin in a type of ostomy bag which sensitized six patients. A similar patient was described by Mann et al. [140].

Dermatological problems in connection with the use of ostomy bags are, however, commonly due to the leakage of secretions under incorrectly attached bags or to sweat retention in the area of the stoma or under the bag itself if this makes direct contact with the skin [141]. Rothstein [142] has provided a detailed review of the problems associated with stoma care and their management.

7.5.4 Dermatitis of the Legs and Feet

Dermatitis of the thighs may be clinically characterized by patches of eczema at sites where pockets make contact with the skin. Persons who normally carry nickel-plated items, 'strike-anywhere' matches containing phosphorus sesquisulphide, or matches with heads containing chromium in their pockets may suffer from dermatitis of this type. Follicular dermatitis on the anterior aspects of the thighs is a typical consequence of wearing trousers which have become soaked with splashing cutting oil or caked with oil rubbed off the hands.

The dermatitis occasionally seen on the stump of a femur amputee has several possible causes. Among the most common are friction and pressure exerted on specific skin areas due to an ill-fitting prosthesis or insufficient tissue under the distal tip of the femur bone. In such situations there may also be trophic disturbance of the skin overlying the bone. Irritant contact dermatitis and dermatitis due to sweat retention under the prosthesis may also occur, even when it is well-fitting [143]. Allergic contact dermatitis may be caused by materials in the prostheses themselves or by antibacterial agents used under them [144].

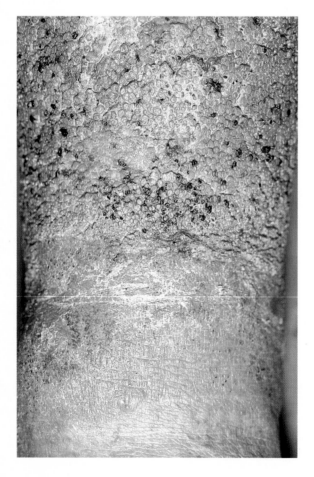

Fig. 7.30. Chronic   stasis dermatitis

Dermatitis at the site of, or in close proximity to, varicose veins is an early indication of stasis dermatitis. This type of dermatitis tends to spread, and eventually the pattern of dermatitis becomes less characteristic (Fig. 7.30). Trophic disturbance, often aggravated by the oedema of the lower leg typical of patients with varicose veins, is probably an aetiological factor. Patients with stasis dermatitis may develop venous leg ulcers.

The chronicity of leg ulcers and stasis dermatitis, in combination with the occlusive bandages applied to afflicted legs, makes this area a rival to the anogenital region as the most common site of allergic contact dermatitis caused by topical medicaments. Unless a short course of treatment can be anticipated, the selection of agents for the topical treatment of stasis dermatitis should be made with emphasis on substances which rarely cause sensitization.

Stocking dermatitis is, as the name implies, seen in those areas which have the most intense contact with stockings or socks [145]. Rubber dermatitis due to the elastic in men's socks occurs in a limited area of the lower legs, while nylon stocking dermatitis may appear on the medial aspects of the thighs as well as in the popliteal fossae and on the feet, where pressure from shoes provides intense contact. Interestingly, shoe dermatitis may mimic stocking dermatitis on the feet, and mercaptobenzothiazole leached from shoes has been shown to accumulate in socks [146]. Children with atopic dermatitis often develop irritant contact dermatitis from synthetic fibres in tights (pantyhose) or wool in leggings and obese children, in particular, may also develop friction dermatitis on the medical aspects of the thighs.

Dermatitis of the feet presents with specific characteristic clinical patterns at, for example, the points of shoe contact, primarily on the dorsal aspects of the feet and toes and on the sides of the feet. This dermatitis rarely appears in the interdigital spaces or in the plantar flexure creases of the toes. Frictional dermatitis on the dorsal aspects of the toes, usually on the big toes, may be seen in children with atopic dermatitis.

One type of dermatitis which is specific to children is juvenile plantar dermatosis. Although the aetiology of this dermatitis is unknown, friction and pressure probably play significant roles in the pathogenesis, as illustrated in Fig. 7.31 [147–149]. In this patient the dermatitis appeared only on the weight-bearing aspects of the soles. There are two characteristic morphologies of plantar dermatoses in addition to juvenile plantar dermatitis. These are recurrent, pruritic, vesicular plantar dermatitis and hyperkeratotic eczema.

7.5.4.1 Recurrent, Pruritic, Vesicular, Plantar Dermatitis

This dermatitis consists of crops of vesicles in the central part of the sole and sometimes also between the toes. If frequent eruptions occur, this dermatitis may become a chronic eczematous condition. This plantar eruption is less common than an eruption of similar morphology which appears on the hands [19]. It is not usually possible to identify the aetiology of the dermatitis,

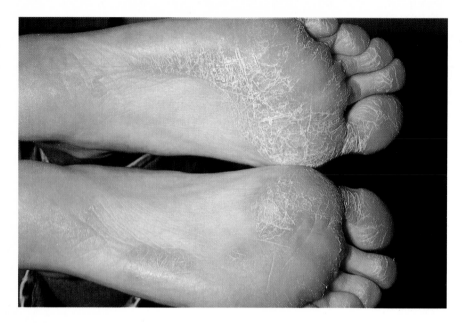

Fig. 7.31. Juvenile plantar dermatitis in pressure areas on the soles

although it has been reproduced by oral challenge with metal salts in some patients with positive patch tests to the same substances, and even in some patch-test-negative patients [18].

7.5.4.2 Hyperkeratotic Eczema

Hyperkeratotic eczema consists of well-demarcated plaques of hyperkeratosis, often with painful fissures. For further details, see Sect. 7.4.1.5.

7.5.5 Dermatitis of the Arms

There are two main sites of dermatitis of the arms. One is the antecubital fossa, which is a typical site of sweat retention dermatitis, atopic dermatitis and secondary nickel dermatitis. The other is the forearm, to which hand dermatitis frequently spreads. Eczema of the forearm with no involvement of the hands can be seen in occupational eczema caused by dust, detergents and the juices of meat and fish.

7.5.6 Contact Stomatitis

The metals used in dentistry may cause allergic contact stomatitis. Lichenplanus-like lesions and erosion of the oral mucosa have been linked to mercury allergy elicited by mercury in amalgam dental fillings. Greyish streaks on the buccal mucosa at the sites of contact with amalgam dental fillings in patients who have positive patch tests to mercury salts certainly suggest a causative relationship.

Of a group of 67 patients with an atrophic-erosive type of oral lichen planus 17% had positive patch tests to mercury compounds, compared with 8% of a reference group [150]. In another group of 29 patients with similar symptoms, 18 patients (62%) had contact allergy to mercury compared with 3.2% of a control group. For three of the patients, the symptoms disappeared after removal of all amalgam dental fillings [151]. Sensitization to mercury and systemic toxicity of amalgam dental restorations are subjects which are still open to discussion [152].

It has been suggested that dental braces made of steel and containing nickel, cobalt and/or chromium are sometimes responsible for systemic contact dermatitis [153]. Gold crowns on teeth have also been reported to cause contact stomatitis of the oral mucosa [154]. In view of the common use of dental plates and their intense contact with the oral mucosa, sensitization to such plates is rare. Dental technicians who manufacture the uncured dental plates may, however, become sensitized to the acrylic materials they handle.

Flavourings added to toothpaste may also cause contact stomatitis. Common causes of contact stomatitis and cheilitis have been reviewed by Fisher [155]. Foodstuffs rarely cause allergic contact stomatitis, but contact urticaria of the oral mucosa caused by foods is common. Sonnex et al. [156] described a patient with contact stomatitis to coffee. The term "oral allergy syndrome" has been proposed to describe immediate-type reactions which include irritation of the oral mucosa shortly after the ingestion of certain foods [15, 16]. The burning mouth syndrome is a poorly understood entity which may be caused by a number of factors including systemic diseases, psychological stress and, occasionally, contact sensitivity [157].

Mechanical stomatitis may be caused by the uneven surfaces of dental fillings or sharp edges of the teeth.

7.5.7 Dermatitis Caused by Items Within the Body

Implanted items such as pacemakers have been blamed for widespread pruritic dermatitis and for eczema and bullous eruptions on the skin overlying the pacemaker. The aetiology of such dermatitis is uncertain, but traces of metals, and in some cases epoxy resin, released from the case of the pacemaker have been suggested as a cause [158, 159]. Copper intrauterine devices have been blamed for similar types of dermatitis [135] as have metal orthodontic braces (see Sect. 7.5.6).

Nickel wiring left in the tissues following surgery may give rise to dermatitis of the skin overlying these tissues or to vesicular hand eczema. Such dermatitis has also been seen in sensitized individuals whose fractures have been set with metal plates and screws, and in a patient who had bits of shrapnel left in the tissues [160].

Artificial hip joints are now primarily of the metal-to-plastic type and rarely give rise to allergic reactions [160].

Widespread dermatitis and vesicular hand eczema have been seen in patients who have swallowed coins containing nickel. The dermatitis faded when the coins were removed [161].

The tattoo pigments used today rarely lead to sensitization, but one recent study described a granulomatous reaction in a tattoo caused by aluminium [162].

Metals in the oral cavity are dealt with in Sect. 7.5.6.

7.6 Differential Diagnosis

Two main groups of diseases should be considered in the differential diagnoses when dealing with possible contact dermatitis, namely
1. Other types of eczema
2. Noneczematous dermatoses which have clinical features similar to those of contact dermatitis

Atopic dermatitis may have a number of features in common with contact dermatitis and contact dermatitis is commonly superimposed on atopic dermatitis. One example of this is 'head and neck dermatitis' which has already been described as a contact urticaria reaction caused by *Pityrosporum ovale*. Lichen simplex chronicus (neurodermatitis) and nummular eczemas are morphological terms used to describe eczema which may be endogenous or caused by mechanical stimuli (Fig. 7.32) [23].

Seborrhoeic dermatitis is usually so characteristic that it presents no diagnostic difficulty but, when there is facial and anogenital involvement, seborrhoeic dermatitis can be difficult to distinguish from contact dermatitis. Low-humidity dermatoses may have clinical features which are similar to those of seborrhoeic dermatitis of the face [21]. Eczematous eruptions associated with rare metabolic diseases such as acrodermatitis enteropathica, other zinc deficiency syndromes or phenylketonuria may also mimic contact dermatitis.

Pityriasis alba may be mistaken for contact dermatitis, but is morphologically characteristic with dry patches of eczema on the cheeks and/or upper arms. Asteatotic eczema is seen mainly in elderly persons due to xerosis of the skin. Hailey-Hailey disease, as well as intertrigo, may mimic contact dermatitis and acrodermatitis Hallopeau and palmoplantar pustulosis may have clinical features similar to those of contact dermatitis.

Most cases of psoriasis and hyperkeratotic eczema are easily recognized as distinct entities, but psoriasis on the hands may be difficult to distinguish from contact dermatitis (Fig. 7.33). Koebner-induced psoriasis at the site of nickel contact in a nickel-sensitive person is another difficult differential diagnosis.

Collagenoses such as lupus erythematosus of the palms may have eczematous features similar to those of contact dermatitis.

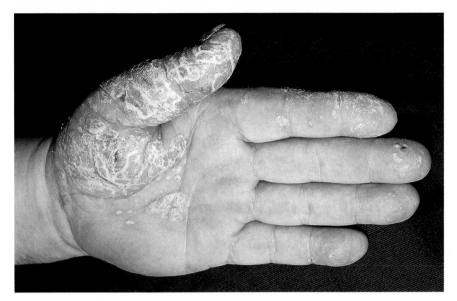

Fig. 7.32. Nummular (discoid) eczema on the hand (Courtesy of P.J. Frosch)

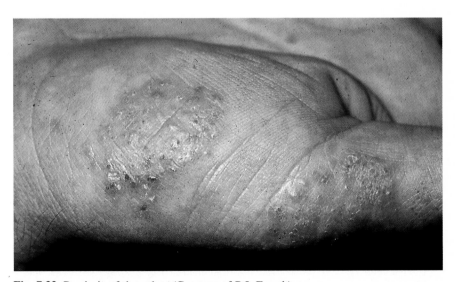

Fig. 7.33. Psoriasis of the palms (Courtesy of P.J. Frosch)

It calls for a high degree of suspicion to make a correct diagnosis of Norwegian scabies, which, clinically, can mimic contact dermatitis.

Another important differential diagnosis is dermatophytosis, particularly when there is involvement of the feet or when *T. rubrum* has infected the skin of the hands. The diagnostic problems increase if the dermatophytosis has been treated with topical steroids. Dermatophytids on the fingers resulting from plantar dermatophytosis are clinically indistinguishable from vesicles associated with other causes, such as systemically induced contact dermatitis. This supports the view that a vesicular eruption of the fingers is a nonspecific reaction pattern which may have a number of different causes. One of these could be lichen planus [163], and palmar lichen planus can have a striking resemblance to hand eczema.

Dysplasias such as actinic keratoses and tumours resulting, for example, from Bowen's disease may also have certain features in common with contact dermatitis.

A diagnosis of contact dermatitis cannot be made by means of histological examination of a biopsy specimen. Nonetheless, a biopsy may be a useful tool in making this diagnosis, as it will enable the exclusion of a number of the above-mentioned diseases which have specific histological features.

7.7 *References*

1. Fisher AA (1987) Contact urticaria and anaphylactoid reaction due to corn starch surgical glove powder. Contact Dermatitis 16: 224–235
2. Van der Meeren HLM, Van Erp PEJ (1986) Life-threatening contact urticaria from glove powder. Contact Dermatitis 14: 190–191
3. Rystedt I (1985) Hand eczema and long-term prognosis in atopic dermatitis. Dissertation, Department of Occupational Dermatology, National Board of Occupational Safety and Health and Karolinska Hospital, Karolinska Institute, Stockholm
4. Thelin I, Agrup G (1985) Pompholyx – a one year series. Acta Derm Venereol (Stockh) 65: 214–217
5. Schwanitz HJ (1986) Das Atopische Palmoplantarekzem. Springer, Berlin Heidelberg New York
6. Edman B (1988) Palmar eczema: a pathogenetic role for acetylsalicylic acid, contraceptives and smoking? Acta Derm Venereol (Stockh) 68: 402–407
7. Menné T (1983) Nickel allergy. Dissertation, University of Copenhagen
8. Menné T, Veien NK, Maibach HI (1989) Systemic contact-type dermatitis due to drugs. Semin Dermatol 8: 144–148
9. Dooms-Goosens AE, Debusschere KM, Gevers DM et al. (1986) Contact dermatitis caused by airborne agents. J Am Acad Dermatol 15: 1–11
10. Malten KE (1981) Thoughts on irritant contact dermatitis. Contact Dermatitis 7: 238–247
11. Frosch PJ, Kligman AM (1977) A method for appraising the stinging capacity of topically applied substances. J Soc Cosmet Chem 28: 197–209
12. Clemmensen O, Hjorth N (1982) Perioral contact urticaria from sorbic acid and benzoic acid in a salad dressing. Contact Dermatitis 8: 1–6
13. Andersen KE, Løwenstein H (1978) An investigation of the possible immunological relationship between allergen extracts from birch pollen, hazelnut, potato and apple. Contact Dermatitis 4: 73–79

14. Murphy GM, Rycroft RJG (1989) Allergic contact dermatitis from silver birch pollen. In: Frosch PJ, Dooms-Goosens A, Lachapelle J-M, Rycroft RJG, Scheper RJ (eds) Current topics in contact dermatitis. Springer, Berlin Heidelberg New York, pp 146-148

15. Amlot PL, Kemeny DM, Zachary C, Parkes P, Lessor MH (1987) Oral allergy syndrome (OAS): symptoms of IgE-mediated hypersensitivity to foods. Clin Allergy 17: 33-42

16. Ortolani C, Ispano M, Pastorello E, Bigi A, Ansaloni R (1988) The oral allergy syndrome. Ann Allergy 61: 47-52

17. Ackerman AB (1978) Histological diagnosis of inflammatory skin diseases. Lea and Febiger, Philadelphia, p 863

18. Menné T, Hjorth N (1983) Pompholyx – dyshidrotic eczema. Semin Dermatol 2: 75-80

19. Frosch PJ (1989) Irritant contact dermatitis. In: Frosch PJ, Dooms-Goossens A, Lachapelle J-M, Rycroft RJG, Scheper RJ (eds) Current topics in contact dermatitis. Springer, Berlin Heidelberg New York, pp 385-403

20. Rothenborg HW, Menné T, Sjølin K-E (1977) Temperature dependent primary irritant dermatitis from lemon perfume. Contact Dermatitis 3: 37-48

21. Rycroft RJG (1985) Low humidity and microtrauma. Am J Ind Med 8: 371-373

22. Rycroft RJG (1987) Low-humidity occupational dermatoses. In: Gardner AW (ed) Current approaches to occupational health, 3rd edn. Wright, Bristol, pp 1-13

23. Hellgren L, Mobacken H (1969) Nummular eczema – clinical and statistical data. Acta Derm Venereol (Stockh) 49: 189-196

24. Rycroft RJG (1981) Soluble oil dermatitis. Clin Exp Dermatol 6: 229-234

25. Torinuki W, Tagami H (1987) Pustular irritant dermatitis due to croton oil. Acta Derm Venereol (Stockh) 68: 257-260

26. Sevadjian CM (1985) Pustular contact hypersensitivity to fluorouracil with rosacealike sequelae. Arch Dermatol 121: 240-242

27. Weston WL, Weston JA (1984) Allergic contact dermatitis in children. Am J Dis Child 138: 932-936

28. Jones HE, Lewis CW, McMarlin SL (1973) Allergic contact sensitivity in atopic patients. Arch Dermatol 107: 217-222

29. Svensson A, Möller H (1986) Eyelid dermatitis: the role of atopy and contact dermatitis. Contact Dermatitis 15: 178-182

30. Rystedt I (1985) Contact sensitivity in adults with atopic dermatitis in childhood. Contact Dermatitis 12: 1-8

31. Christophersen J, Menné T, Tanghøj P, Andersen KE, Brandrup F, Kaaber K, Osmundsen PE, Thestrup-Pedersen K, Veien NK (1989) Clinical patch test data evaluated by multivariate analysis. Contact Dermatitis 21: 291-299

32. Möller H, Svensson A (1986) Metal sensitivity: positive history but negative test indicates atopy. Contact Dermatitis 14: 57-60

33. Todd DJ, Burrows D, Stanford CF (1989) Atopy in subjects with a history of nickel allergy but negative patch tests. Contact Dermatitis 21: 129-133

34. Bonnevie P (1939) Aethiologie und Pathogenese der Eczemkrankheiten (Dissertation). Nyt Nordisk, Copenhagen

35. Larsson-Stymne B, Widström L (1985) Ear piercing – a cause of nickel allergy in schoolgirls? Contact Dermatitis 13: 289-293

36. Gawkrodger DJ, Vestey JP, Wong W-K, Buxton PK (1986) Contact clinic survey of nickel-sensitive subjects. Contact Dermatitis 14: 165-169

37. Moorthy TT, Tan GH (1986) Nickel sensitivity in Singapore. Int J Dermatol 25: 307-309

38. Hemingway JD, Molokhia MM (1987) The dissolution of metallic nickel in artificial sweat. Contact Dermatitis 16: 99-105

39. Emmett EA, Risby TH, Jiang L, Ng SK, Feinman S (1988) Allergic contact dermatitis to nickel: bioavailability from consumer products and provocation threshold. J Am Acad Dermatol 19: 314–322
40. Kanan MW (1969) Contact dermatitis in Kuwait. J Kuwait Med Assoc 3: 129–144
41. Fisher AA (1985) Nickel dermatitis in men. Cutis 35: 424–426
42. De Corres LF, Garrastazu MT, Soloeta R, Escayol P (1982) Nickel contact dermatitis in a blood bank. Contact Dermatitis 8: 32–37
43. Oakley AMM, Ive FA, Car MM (1987) Skin clips are contraindicated when there is nickel allergy. J R Soc Med 80: 290–291
44. Kasteler JS, Petersen MJ, Vance JE, Zone JJ (1992) Circulating activated T lymphocytes in autoeczematization. Arch Dermatol 128: 795–798
45. Andersen KE, Maibach HI (1983) Drugs used topically. In: de Weck AL, Bundgaard H (eds) Allergic reactions to drugs. Springer, Berlin Heidelberg New York, pp 313–377
46. Wilkinson JD, Hambly EM, Wilkinson DS (1980) Comparison of patch test results in two adjacent areas of England. II. Medicaments. Acta Derm Venereol (Stockh) 60: 245–249
47. Edman B, Möller H (1986) Medicament contact allergy. Derm Beruf Umwelt 34: 139–143
48. Avnstorp C, Hamann K (1981) Neglelakeksem. Ugeskr Laeger 143: 2504–2505
49. Burnett JW, Calton GJ (1987) Jellyfish envenomation syndromes updated. Ann Emerg Med 16: 1000–1005
50. Hogan DJ, Dosman JA, Li KYR et al. (1986) Questionnaire survey of pruritus and rash in grain elevator workers. Contact Dermatitis 14: 170–175
51. Lachapelle JM (1986) Industrial airborne irritant or allergic contact dermatitis. Contact Dermatitis 14: 137–145
52. Beck MH, Hausen BM, Dave VK (1984) Allergic contact dermatitis from *Machaerium scleroxylum* Tul. (Pao ferro) in a joinery shop. Clin Exp Dermatol 9: 159–166
53. Ippen H, Wereta-Kubek M, Rose U (1986) Haut- und Schleimhautreaktionen durch Zimmerpflanzen der Gattung Dieffenbachia. Dermatosen 34: 93–101
54. Hausen BM (1982) Häufigkeit und Bedeutung toxischer und allergischer Kontaktdermatitiden durch *Machaerium scleroxylum* Tul. (Pao ferro), einem Ersatzholz für Palisander (*Dalbergia nigra* All.). Hautarzt 33: 321–328
55. Møller NE, Nielsen B, von Würden K (1986) Contact dermatitis to semisynthetic penicillins in factory workers. Contact Dermatitis 14: 307–311
56. Hjorth N, Roed-Petersen J, Thomsen K (1976) Airborne contact dermatitis from Compositae oleoresins simulating photodermatitis. Br J Dermatol 95: 613–619
57. Berg M (1988) Skin problems in workers using visual display terminals. Contact Dermatitis 19: 335–341
58. LaMarte FP, Merchant JA, Casale TB (1988) Acute systemic reactions to carbonless copy paper associated with histamine release. JAMA 260: 242–243
59. Kligman AM, Klemme JC, Susten AS (eds) (1985) The chronic effects of repeated mechanical trauma to the skin. Am J Ind Med 8: 253–513
60. Powell FC (1994) Sports dermatology. J Eur Acad Dermatol Venereol 3: 1–15
61. Tomecki KJ, Mikesell JF (1987) Rower's rump. J Am Acad Dermatol 16: 890–891
62. Hersle K, Mobacken H (1982) Hyperkeratotic dermatitis of the palms. Br J Dermatol 107: 195–202
63. Plewig G, Fulton JE, Kligman AM (1970) Pomade acne. Arch Dermatol 101: 580–584
64. Pecegueiro M, Brandao M (1984) Contact plantar pustulosis. Contact Dermatitis 11: 126–127
65. Andersen KE, Sjølin KE, Solgaard P (1989) Acute irritant contact folliculitis in a galvanizer. In: Frosch PJ, Dooms-Goossens A, Lachapelle J-M, Rycroft RJG,

Scheper RJ (eds) Current topics in contact dermatitis. Springer, Berlin Heidelberg New York, pp 417–418

66. Rystedt I, Fischer T, Lagerholm B (1983) Patch testing with sodium tungstate. Contact Dermatitis 9: 69–73
67. Freeman S (1986) Woman allergic to husband's sweat and semen. Contact Dermatitis 14: 110–112
68. Held JL, Ruszkowski AM, Deleo VA (1988) Consort contact dermatitis due to oak moss. Arch Dermatol 124: 261–262
69. Rycroft RJG, Baran R (1984) Occupational abnormalities and contact dermatitis. In: Baran R et al. (eds) Diseases of the nails. Blackwell, London, pp 267–287
70. Mathias CGT, Maibach HI (1984) Allergic contact dermatitis from anaerobic acrylic sealants. Arch Dermatol 120: 1202–1205
71. Cronin E (1982) "New" allergens of clinical importance. Semin Dermatol 1: 33–41
72. Clemmensen O, Knudsen HE (1980) Contact sensitivity to aluminium in a patient hyposensitized with aluminium precipitated grass pollen. Contact Dermatitis 6: 305–308
73. Veien, NK, Hattel T, Justesen O, Nørholm A (1986) Aluminium allergy. Contact Dermatitis 15: 295–297
74. Fischer T, Rystedt I (1982) A case of contact sensitivity to aluminium. Contact Dermatitis 8: 343
75. Feinglos MN, Jegasothy BV (1979) "Insulin" allergy due to zinc. Lancet 1: 122–124
76. Cronin E (1980) Contact dermatitis. Churchill Livingstone, Edinburgh
77. Hjorth N, Roed-Petersen J (1976) Occupational protein contact dermatitis in food handlers. Contact Dermatitis 2: 28–42
78. Von Krogh G, Maibach HI (1981) The contact urticaria syndrome–an updated review. J Am Acad Dermatol 5: 328–342
79. Menné T, Veien N, Sjølin K-E, Maibach HI (1994) Systemic contact dermatitis. Am J Contact Dermatitis 5: 1–12
80. Veien NK (1989) Systemically induced eczema in adults. Acta Derm Venereol Suppl (Stockh) 147 (Dissertation, University of Copenhagen)
81. Veien NK, Krogdahl A (1989) Is nickel vasculitis a clinical entity? In: Frosch P, Dooms-Goossens A, Lachapelle J, Rycroft RJG, Scheper RJ (eds) Current topics in contact dermatitis. Springer, Berlin Heidelberg New York, pp 172–177
82. Kaaber K, Sjølin KE, Menné T (1983) Elbow eruptions in nickel and chromate dermatitis. Contact Dermatitis 9: 213–216
83. Calnan CD (1956) Nickel dermatitis. Br J Dermatol 68: 229–236
84. Andersen KE, Hjorth N, Menné T (1984) The baboon syndrome: systemically-induced allergic contact dermatitis. Contact Dermatitis 10: 97–100
85. Christensen OB (1981) Nickel allergy and hand eczema in females. Dissertation, University of Lund, Malmö
86. Ghadially R, Ramsay CA (1988) Gentamicin: systemic exposure to a contact allergen. J Am Acad Dermatol 19: 428–430
87. Lechner T, Grytzmann B, Bäurle G (1987) Hämatogenes allergisches Kontaktekzem nach oraler Gabe von Nystatin. Mykosen 30: 143–146
88. Bernard P, Rayol J, Bonnafoux A et al. (1988) Toxidermies apres prise orale de pristinamycine. Ann Dermatol Venereol 115: 63–66
89. Sehgal VN, Gangwani OP (1987) Fixed drug eruption. Int J Dermatol 26: 67–74
90. Alanko K, Stubb S, Reitamo S (1987) Topical provocation of fixed drug eruption. Br J Dermatol 116: 561–567
91. Shelmire B (1941) Cutaneous and systemic reactions observed during oral poison ivy therapy. J Allergy 12: 252–271
92. Kligman AM (1958) Poison ivy (Rhus) dermatitis. AMA Arch Dermatol 77: 149–180
93. Rycroft RJG (1980) Acute ulcerative contact dermatitis from Portland cement. Br J Dermatol 102: 487–489

94. Rycroft RJG (1980) Acute ulcerative contact dermatitis from ready mixed cement. Clin Exp Dermatol 5: 245–247
95. Osmundsen PE, Alani MD (1971) Contact allergy to an optical whitener, "CPY", in washing powders. Br J Dermatol 85: 61–66
96. Hayakawa R, Matsunaga K, Kojima S, Kaniwa M, Nakamura A (1985) Naphthol AS as a cause of pigmented contact dermatitis. Contact Dermatitis 13: 20–25
97. Schmidt H, Barfred T (1979) Caterpillar dermatitis of the palm associated with osteitis of finger bones. Acta Derm Venereol (Stockh) 59 [Suppl 85]: 157–159
98. Waersted A, Hjorth N (1985) Pityrosporum orbiculare – a pathogenic factor in atopic dermatitis of the face, scalp and neck? Acta Derm Venereol Suppl (Stockh) 114: 146–148
99. Kieffer M, Bergbrant IM, Faergemann J et al. (1990) Immune reactions to Pityrosporum ovale in adult patients with atopic dermatitis and seborrhoeic dermatitis. J Am Acad Dermatol 29: 739–742
100. Maibach HI (1987) Oral substitution in patients sensitized by transdermal clonidine treatment. Contact Dermatitis 16: 1–8
101. Harari Z, Sommer I, Knobel B (1987) Multifocal contact dermatitis to nitroderm TTS 5 with extensive postinflammatory hypermelanosis. Dermatologica 174: 249–252
102. Holdiness MR (1989) A review of contact dermatitis associated with transdermal therapeutic systems. Contact Dermatitis 20: 3–9
103. Weickel R, Frosch PJ (1986) Kontaktallergie auf Glyceroltrinitrat (Nitroderm TTS). Hautarzt 37: 511–512
104. Edman B (1985) Sites of contact dermatitis in relationship to particular allergens. Contact Dermatitis 13: 129–135
105. Näher H, Frosch PJ (1987) Contact dermatitis to thioxolone. Contact Dermatitis 17: 250–251
106. Tosti A, Guerra L, Bardazzi F (1991) Contact dermatitis caused by topical minoxidil: case reports and review of the literature. Am J Contact Dermatitis 2: 56–59
107. Storrs FJ (1984) Permanent wave contact dermatitis: contact allergy to glyceryl monothioglycolate. J Am Acad Dermatol 11: 74–85
108. Andersen KE, Roed-Petersen J, Kamp P (1984) Contact allergy related to TEA-PEG-3 cocamide sulfate and cocamidopropyl betaine in a shampoo. Contact Dermatitis 11: 192–193
109. Frain-Bell W, Lakshmipathi T, Rogers J, Willock J (1974) The syndrome of chronic photosensitivity dermatitis and actinic reticuloid. Br J Dermatol 91: 617–634
110. Hausen BM, Oestmann G (1988) Untersuchungen über die Häufigkeit berufsbedingter allergischer Hauterkrankungen auf einem Blumengroßmarkt. Dermatosen 36: 117–117
111. de Groot AC, Bruynzeel DP, Bos JD et al. (1988) The allergens in cosmetics. Arch Dermatol 124: 1525–1529
112. Adams RM, Maibach HI (1985) A five-year study of cosmetic reactions. J Am Acad Dermatol 13: 1062–1069
113. Mathias CGT (1982) Pigmented cosmetic dermatitis from contact allergy to a toilet soap containing chromium. Contact Dermatitis 8: 29–31
114. Mathias CGT, Maibach HI, Conant MA (1980) Perioral leukoderma simulating vitiligo from use of a toothpaste containing cinnamic aldehyde. Arch Dermatol 116: 1172–1173
115. Hayakawa R, Matsunaga K, Arima Y (1987) Depigmented contact dermatitis due to incense. Contact Dermatitis 16: 272–274
116. Fisher AA, Dooms-Goossens A (1976) Persulfate hair bleach reactions. Arch Dermatol 112: 1407–1409
117. Guin JD, Berry VK (1980) Perfume sensitivity in adult females. J Am Acad Dermatol 3: 299–302

118. Brandrup F, Hansen NS, Schultz K (1987) Ansigtseksem fremkaldt af gummi i åndedraetsvaern. Ugeskr Laeger 149: 968
119. Hannuksela M, Lahti A (1977) Immediate reactions to fruits and vegetables. Contact Dermatitis 3: 79–84
120. Frosch PJ, Weickel R, Schmitt T, Krastel H (1988) Nebenwirkungen von ophthalmologischen Externa. Z Hautkr 63: 126–136
121. Grundmann H, Wozniak K-D, Tost M (1981) Zum allergischen Kontaktekzem im Lid- und Augenbereich. Folia Ophthalmol 6: 258–261
122. Valsecchi R, Imberti G, Martino D, Cainelli T (1992) Eyelid dermatitis: an evaluation of 150 patients. Contact Dermatitis 27: 143–147
123. Nethercott JR (1978) Skin problems associated with multifunctional acrylic monomers in ultraviolet curing inks. Br J Dermatol 98: 541–551
124. Ottosen C-O, Irgens-Møller L (1984) øjenskader kan skyldes stueplanten Dieffenbachia. Ugeskr Laeger 146: 3927–3928
125. Kieffer M (1979) Nickel sensitivity: relationship between history and patch test reaction. Contact Dermatitis 5: 398–401
126. Hatch KL, Maibach HI (1985) Textile fiber dermatitis. Contact Dermatitis 12: 1–11
127. Hatch KL, Maibach HI (1986) Textile chemical finish dermatitis. Contact Dermatitis 14: 1–13
128. Andersen KE, Hamann K (1982) Cost benefit of patch testing with textile finish resins. Contact Dermatitis 8: 64–67
129. Tegner E (1985) Sheet dermatitis. Acta Derm Venereol (Stockh) 65: 254–257
130. Veien NK, Hattel T, Laurberg G (1992) Can 'label dermatitis' become 'creeping neurotic excoriations'? Contact Dermatitis 27: 272–273
131. Larsen WG (1977) Perfume dermatitis. Arch Dermatol 113: 623–626
132. Larsen WG (1979) Allergic contact dermatitis to the perfume in Mycolog cream. J Am Acad Dermatol 1: 131–133
133. Longhi F, Carlucci G, Bellucci R, di Girolamo R, Palumbo G, Amerio P (1992) Diaper dermatitis: a study of contributing factors. Contact Dermatitis 26: 248–252
134. Seymour JL, Keswick BH, Hanifin JM, Jordan WP, Milligan MC (1989) Clinical effects of diaper types on the skin of normal infants and infants with atopic dermatitis. J Am Acad Dermatol 17: 988–997
135. Romaguera C, Grimalt F (1981) Contact dermatitis from a copper-containing intrauterine contraceptive device. Contact Dermatitis 7: 163–164
136. Frosch PJ, Raulin C (1987) Kontaktallergie auf Bufexamac. Hautarzt 38: 331–334
137. Veien NK, Hattel T, Justesen O, Nørholm A (1987) Dermatoses in coffee drinkers. Cutis 40: 421–422
138. Heskel NS (1987) Allergic contact dermatitis from stomadhesive paste. Contact Dermatitis 16: 119–121
139. Beck MH, Burrows D, Fregert S, Mendelsohn S (1985) Allergic contact dermatitis to epoxy resin in ostomy bags. Br J Surg 72: 202–203
140. Mann RJ, Stewart E, Peachey RDG (1983) Sensitivity to urostomy pouch plastic. Contact Dermatitis 9: 80–81
141. Fisher AA (1986) Contact dermatitis, 3rd edn. Lea and Febiger, Philadelphia, pp 341–346
142. Rothstein MS (1986) Dermatologic considerations of stoma care. J Am Acad Dermatol 15: 411–432
143. Fisher AA (1986) Contact dermatitis, 3rd edn. Lea and Febiger, Philadelphia, pp 349–352
144. van Ketel WG (1977) Allergic contact dermatitis of amputation stumps. Contact Dermatitis 3: 50–61
145. Hausen BM, Schulz (1984) Strumpffarben-Allergie. Dtsch Med Wochenschr 109: 1469–1475
146. Rietschel RL (1984) Role of socks in shoe dermatitis. Arch Dermatol 120: 398

147. Möller H (1972) Atopic winter feet in children. Acta Derm Venereol (Stockh) 52: 401–405
148. Jones SK, English JSC, Forsyth A, Mackie RM (1987) Juvenile plantar dermatosis: an 8-year follow-up of 102 patients. Clin Exp Dermatol 12: 5–7
149. Ashton RE, Griffiths WAD (1986) Juvenile plantar dermatosis: atopy or footwear? Clin Exp Dermatol 11: 529–534
150. Mobacken H, Hersle K, Sloberg K, Thilander H (1984) Oral lichen planus: hypersensitivity to dental restoration material. Contact Dermatitis 10: 11–15
151. Finne K, Göransson K, Winckler L (1982) Oral lichen planus and contact allergy to mercury. Int J Oral Surg 11: 236–239
152. Burrows D (1989) Mischievous metals – chromate, cobalt, nickel and mercury. Clin Exp Dermatol 14: 266–272
153. Hensten-Pettersen (1989) Nickel allergy and dental treatment procedures. In: Maibach HI, Menné T (eds) Nickel and the skin: immunology and toxicology. CRC, Boca Raton, pp 195–205
154. Izumi AK (1982) Allergic contact gingivostomatitis due to gold. Arch Dermatol 272: 387–391
155. Fisher AA (1987) Reactions of the mucous membrane to contactants. Clin Dermatol 5: 123–136
156. Sonnex TS, Dawber RPR, Ryan TJ (1981) Mucosal contact dermatitis due to instant coffee. Contact Dermatitis 7: 298–300
157. Guerra L, Vincenzi C, Peluso AM, Tosti A (1993) Role of contact sensitizers in the burning mouth syndrome. Am J Contact Dermatitis 4: 154–157
158. Peters MS, Schroeter AL, Van Hale VM, Broadbent JC (1984) Pacemaker contact sensitivity. Contact Dermatitis 11: 214–218
159. Romaguera C, Grimalt F (1981) Pacemaker dermatitis. Contact Dermatitis 7: 333
160. Wilkinson JD (1989) Nickel allergy and orthopedic prostheses. In: Maibach HI, Menné T (eds) Nickel and the skin: immunology and toxicology. CRC, Boca Raton, pp 187–193
161. Lacroix J, Morin CL, Collin P-P (1979) Nickel dermatitis from a foreign body in the stomach. J Pediatr 95: 428–429
162. McFadden N, Lyberg T, Hensten-Pettersen A (1989) Aluminium-induced granulomas in a tattoo. J Am Acad Dermatol 20: 903–908
163. Feuerman EJ, Ingber A, David M, Weissman-Katzenelson V (1982) Lichen ruber planus beginning as a dyshidrosiform eruption. Cutis 30: 401–404

Chapter 8
Hand Eczema

8 Hand Eczema

ETAIN CRONIN

Contents

8.1 Introduction

The terms 'eczema' and 'dermatitis' are used here interchangeably and do not imply an identified aetiology. The diagnosis 'eczema' has been criticized on the grounds that it is not definable [1], but as a clinical concept it is useful, understood and irreplaceable for many inflammatory dermatoses of the hands. The term 'hand eczema' may not be precise but the condition is common. For the patient it is a misery which is often chronic and sometimes disabling. For the dermatologist it means application, time spent and trouble taken to elucidate its aetiology. In general dermatology, a glance and a diagnosis may sometimes coincide, but for hand eczema speedy glances rarely suffice.

8.2 Incidence

The incidence of hand eczema in the general population is difficult to determine but has been studied. In the 1960s, during a health survey of a mainly rural population in the south of Sweden, it was estimated that 4% had hand dermatoses of various kinds other than warts [2]. The offer of an examination was accepted by 1659 subjects and Agrup [2] found the changes to be eczema in 50%, acrovesiculatio recidivans in 3%, psoriasis in 7% and fungal infection in 1.4%. She assessed the overall prevalence of hand eczema in this community to be about 2%. In contrast, in the Swedish industrial city of Gothenburg, a population study by Meding and Swanbeck [3] in the mid – 1980s estimated, after extrapolation, that the prevalence of hand eczema was 5.4%. In the Netherlands [4], a survey of the adult population found eczema of the hands and arms in 4.6% of men and 8% of women.

Patients coming to a contact clinic were studied by Goh in Singapore [5] and, in over 2000 patients, 34% had hand eczema, amongst whom men (56%) outnumbered women (44%) and the cause was occupational in 30%. During the 3-year period 1987–1989, 2262 men and 3170 women attended the Contact Clinic at St John's Hospital for Diseases of the Skin in London. The hands were recorded as the only or initial site of eczema in 37% of the men and 30% of the women.

8.3 Patterns of Hand Eczema

It is probably correct that there are few correlations between clinical patterns of hand eczema and their aetiology [6]. Increased markings on the palmar sides of the hands may indicate an associated ichthyosis [7] or atopic dermatitis [8] but these are both markers of a clinical background rather than diagnostic criteria for categorizing an existing hand eczema. The only difference Svensson [8] found between the hand eczema of those with and without atopic dermatitis was that among the atopics there was a greater frequency of eczema of the hypothenar eminences. In food handlers, Fisher [9] considered oedema, erythema and fissuring to be characteristic of an irritant contact dermatitis, and vesiculation and severe itching of an allergic contact dermatits.

In one study [6], the distribution of hand eczema in women was divided into four clinical patterns, palmar (palms and fingers), dorsal (dorsa and fingers), fingers only, and all over the hands. So divided, the palmar pattern was the commonest (44%), the dorsal pattern was seen in 15%, fingers only in 19%, and all over the hands in 22%. Sensitizers, including nickel, affected the four groups equally. Irritants were considered relevant in each group, especially the dorsal (75%), fingers only (71%), and all over the hands groups (54%), but of less importance in the palmar pattern (42%). Atopic hand eczema was not thought to be clinically distinctive. Two patterns were proposed as being endogenous. One, the 'apron pattern' (C.D. Calnan, 1970, personal communication), more common in women than men, is a patch of eczema on the distal palm contiguous with eczema of the associated web space or proximal finger (s) (Fig. 8.1). The form of the patch is that of a half circle and it resembles a small waist apron. Svensson [8] had three such patients, all

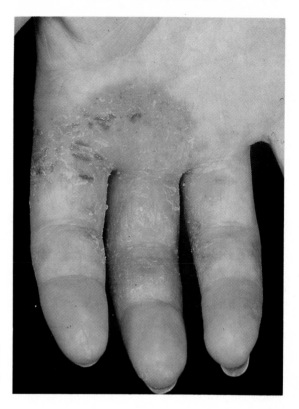

Fig. 8.1. 'Apron pattern': the patch of eczema on the distal palm is like an upside-down apron

women, each atopic, and each with negative patch tests. The second pattern suggested as being endogenous [6] was a localized eczema of the centre of the palm, spreading proximally to the base or heel of the hand. This distribution is not always endogenous, however, as a central palmar eczema may also be caused by the friction and pressure of holding a tool.

8.3.1 Allergic

Characteristic patterns for allergens do occur, but rather infrequently. Occasionally, a rubber glove dermatitis is obvious when it presents as a sheeted eczema of the dorsa of the hands, with a sharply cut off border on the lower forearms. Much commoner is a deteriorating hand eczema in a patient wearing rubber gloves on medical advice, when the rubber sensitivity is often as big a surprise to the clinician as it is to the patient. A fissured eczema of the palms and palmar sides of the fingers is usually endogenous but it may be allergic, as proved by patch testing in a patient sensitized to his rubber motorcycle handle grips [10]. Itchy isolated blisters on the fingers and painful pulps of the dominant fingers and thumb is likely to be a plant dermatitis. In the United Kingdom it is usually a primula dermatitis. However, this pattern is

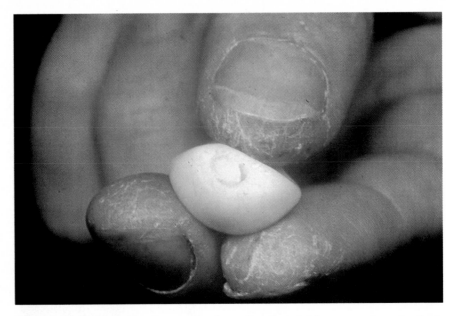

Fig. 8.2. Garlic dermatitis: the way the clove of garlic is held corresponds to the distribution of the dermatitis

frequently unrecognized and, without patch testing, the diagnosis also remains unrecognized. It is well known that garlic causes a fissured eczema of the thumb and finger pulps (Fig. 8.2), but so can chromate in match heads and, without patch testing, who would incriminate them? [11]. Most allergens are unsuspected not only by the patient but also by the clinician and they are likely to remain so without patch testing.

8.3.2 Irritant

When irritants cause direct damage to the skin, the clinical changes produced are readily recognizable as a destructive effect. When irritants induce eczema, the clinical appearance is the same as eczema from any other cause.

Irritants vary in their toxic effect. Concentrated acids and alkalis produce burns, an obvious clinical diagnosis, but knowledge of the injurious nature of the substance implicated is required to link cause and effect. It took 20 years for cement burns to be recognized and they can be of second or third degree in severity. Strong irritants cause recognizable damage, weak irritants cause more subtle changes not so readily appreciated.

Asteatosis. Asteatosis may be caused by climatic conditions, the physical effect of clothing, or even some topical cream formulations, in those constitutionally predisposed.

The cutaneous effects of low humidity have been described by Rycroft [12]. Irrespective of the temperature, a low relative humidity causes asteatosis or chapping. When the relative humidity becomes low, moisture is slowly drawn out of the skin, causing it to become dry, scaly and sometimes superficially fissured. This asteatosis may gradually worsen to become an asteatotic eczema (eczema craquelée), especially in the elderly. Low relative humidity at work may cause an occupational asteatosis of the face [13, 14].

Asteatosis is seen on the fronts of the shins of elderly patients in hospital wards. The changes are attributed to frequent washing of the patient and possibly friction from frequently changed sheets. Gradually, the skin of the lower legs dries and cracks. The regular use of an emollient prevents the condition.

Irritant Reaction. This same low-grade, chronic, irritant, asteatotic effect, which is not eczema but dryness and cracking of the skin, has been named 'irritant reaction' by Fregert (1980, personal communication). This is not established nomenclature but it seems to me to be a useful term for this distinctive and recognizable change, and emphasizes that it is not eczematous (Fig. 8.3). Irritant reactions occur particularly over the dorsal surfaces of the metacarpophalangeal joints in those doing wet work, especially when in combination with detergents. Young hairdressers doing many shampoos each day are particularly vulnerable. Avoidance of wet work, the wearing of gloves and the use of emollients is curative. Topical corticosteroids are unnecessary.

Irritant Dermatitis. Irritant contact dermatitis on the hands often begins under rings and may then spread over the fingers to the hands and the forearms. It is usually thought of as affecting the dorsa of the hands and

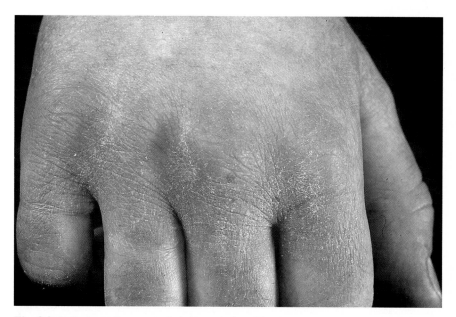

Fig. 8.3. Irritant reaction over a hairdresser's knuckles.

fingers, but irritants can also cause eczema of the palmar sides of the fingers and hands. This distribution occurs in caterers [15] and, described as a dyshidrotic eczema, it has been reported in metal workers with an irritant contact dermatitis from soluble oils [16].

Pulpitis. A dry scaly fissured change on the pulps of the fingers of young women is not uncommon but little reported. Among my patients, it nearly always occurs in young housewives doing an unaccustomed amount of domestic work, especially those with young children. However, this is not always the case, as I have seen it in a secretary, who denied all such activities. The dryness and scaling begin on the pulps of the dominant fingers and may spread to affect most of the fingers. The pulps are always painful, extremely so when the skin cracks and bleeds. It is most disabling, interfering with housework and the care of children; in particular the doing-up of buttons becomes a nightmare. It seems reasonable to assume that it is an irritant degreasing effect of household cleaners, but, unlike asteatosis, it responds very poorly to all forms of treatment, including emollients and topical corticosteroids. Maybe the avoidance of housework is impossible for these young women and so the cause and effect continue, but it does seem that, once established, the change is difficult to reverse.

Probably an identical condition, designated dermatitis palmaris sicca, has been reported from Singapore [17], where it is not uncommon and occurs even in children. Irritants were thought to be an unlikely cause as the patients were not sufficiently exposed. It was suggested that the humidity of their climate and air conditioning made the skin more vulnerable to friction.

8.3.3 Pompholyx

The term 'pompholyx' had become almost obsolete in many clinics, but it regained popularity when used to describe the vesicular response on the hands to nickel ingestion in nickel-sensitive women. The features of pompholyx have been reviewed by Menné and Hjorth [18]. It is erroneous to consider pompholyx as a dyshidrosis, because it is not a disease of sweat glands or sweat ducts. Pompholyx is a recurrent vesicular eczema of the palmar sides of the hands and sometimes the soles of the feet. Its appearance is modified by the structure of the site. It is characterized by the eruption of small vesicles on the palms, palmar and lateral sides of the fingers, and distal dorsal fingers around the nail folds. Not every site may be involved and occasionally the vesicles are large rather than small. Involvement of the nail fold causes ridging of the nail.

Sixty-eight patients with pompholyx were studied by Thulin and Agrup [19]. In this group it was disabling and had caused 56 to lose time from work. Of those patch tested, 28% had a positive test but in none could a correlation be found with their hand eczema.

Although contact sensitizers identified by patch testing may appear irrelevant, such allergens given orally, particularly nickel, to sensitized subjects may cause a pompholyx-like eruption on the hands. Similarly, the implantation of a nickel-containing pacemaker evoked a pompholyx-type eruption on the hands of a nickel-sensitive woman [20]. Other allergens so described are neomycin, chromate and cobalt [21].

In a survey of 286 metal workers, 39 were found to have dermatitis and in 21 the pattern was termed a dyshidrotic eczema [16]. In these 21, the relationship to work was strong: in 11 the dermatitis was considered entirely occupational, and in 10 partly but not entirely so. Only one was an atopic and only three had positive patch tests, one to nickel and two to formaldehyde releasers. It was therefore concluded that it was the irritant effect of the soluble oils which was of major importance in causing this palmar pattern of hand dermatitis. Cactus spines penetrated the skin and caused a 'dyshidrotic' dermatitis in a worker in a plant nursery. Histological examination identified cactus spines in the vesicles [22].

Some patients blame their 'nerves' as the cause of their pompholyx and they may be right, but in the majority the cause is quite unknown. Using the name pompholyx implies that the eczema is endogenous; therefore it is a diagnosis which should be used with discretion, so as to avoid missing an identifiable cause of a palmar pattern of hand eczema.

8.4 Endogenous Hand Eczema

An endogenous hand eczema, regardless of whether its initiation is known or unknown, is one which always was, or has become, self-perpetuating. Although many hand eczemas are primarily, or have become, essentially endogenous, they are frequently worsened by irritants or sometimes by sensitizers. Irritants, allergens and infection should be considered in all patients with hand eczema. Their removal helps greatly in the patient's management.

While an absolute marker for atopy awaits recognition, the diagnosis must rest on clinical features. A positive history of flexural eczema, asthma or hay fever in the patient or in a close (first-degree) relative are the fundamental criteria for labelling the patient as atopic. In children, other patterns of atopic eczema occur. It may be distributed on the extensor aspects of the joints and, in young children, the face is often affected. The diagnosis of atopic dermatitis is important because of its implications.

In her study of atopic dermatitis, Rystedt [23] established that it is atopic eczema in childhood which predisposes to adult hand eczema, and the worse the preceding eczema the more likely is hand eczema to occur. Among those who as children had atopic eczema severe enough to have required hospital admission, the incidence of subsequent adult hand eczema was 51%; among those with childhood atopic eczema of moderate severity and treated as outpatients the incidence was 35%; among those patients with mucosal atopic allergy the number was 9%; and in the control group with no personal or family history of atopy the number with hand eczema at some time was 7%.

A history of hand eczema in children before the age of 15 years carried a particularly bad prognosis, in that 76% had adult hand eczema, whereas in children with atopic eczema but clear hands only 31% subsequently developed hand eczema as adults [24]. In contrast, childhood asthma or hay fever carried no such implications and the incidence of hand eczema in such patients was similar to its frequency in nonatopic controls [23]. She also found that the patient's inherent tendency to develop hand eczema was more important than contact with irritants [24].

Advice about careers is most important for children with atopic eczema and should be proffered even if not sought by patient or parent. For all children with atopic eczema, especially if it was severe, the best course is for them to avoid careers involving wet work, particularly hairdressing, nursing and catering. For those with hand eczema as children this is imperative.

8.5 Contact Dermatitis

A hand eczema may be entirely endogenous, entirely irritant or entirely allergic, but it is more likely to be a combination of two or even three of these aetiologies. Perhaps it is the clinician's skill in deciding these priorities which determines success in treatment.

An endogenous background and contact with irritants are elicited in the history. Allergens are identified by patch testing and their relevance is determined by the clinician's application and success in persuading the patient of their significance. This is often difficult.

In Singapore, Goh [5] found in a study of patients with hand eczema that over half (55%) had a contact dermatitis, which was more often irritant (nearly 60%) than allergic (about 40%).

8.5.1 Allergic

Any allergen may cause or complicate a hand eczema. Even nail varnish very occasionally causes dermatitis of the nail folds in a messy user. Ubiquitous allergens, such as perfumes, may not be the entire cause of a hand eczema but may be a significant aggravating factor.

Chromate in cement is a good example of the great influence and relevance of an allergen in the precipitation and chronicity of hand eczema. Fregert et al. [25] showed that ferrous sulphate added to cement reduced the water-soluble hexavalent chromate to the water-insoluble trivalent form which is precipitated. In Denmark in 1981, their only cement manufacturer adopted the procedure, and 2 years later legislation was passed prohibiting the use of cement with a chromate content higher than 2 ppm. Workers in contact with wet cement in the manufacture of prefabricated concrete components for the building industry were studied by Avnstorp [26]. In 1981, the prevalence of hand eczema was 11.7% and of chromate allergy, 10.5%. In 1987 the prevalence of hand eczema was 4.4% and of chromate sensitization, 2.6%. No such change occurred in irritation from cement, which was 5.6% in 1981 and 3.9% in 1987. Facilities for the workers were unaltered during this 6-year period. The fall in chromate sensitivity in construction workers may or may not be due to the addition of ferrous sulphate to cement, because in some countries automation may be responsible. Whatever its cause, the Danish study has shown that a reduction in chromate sensitivity is paralleled by a profound fall in the numbers with hand eczema. Avnstorp [27] also found that hand eczema was much more likely to become chronic in a worker allergic to chromate than in a man who was not so sensitized.

Allergens are usually significant and the benefit of avoiding them should be believed by the clinician and stressed to the patient.

8.5.2 Irritant

Common irritants include wet work, detergents, soaps, organic solvents, cutting fluids, acids, alkalis, foods, domestic cleaners, soil (earth) and plants. Physical injury may contribute, as do abrasions, friction or penetration of the skin by spicules as in glass fibre dermatitis.

Studies show that the prognosis for irritant hand dermatitis is remarkably bad. A postal survey of patients previously diagnosed as having irritant hand dermatitis found that in nearly 70% the eczema continued. Irrespective of whether or not they changed their jobs, the prognosis was bad [28]. Soluble oil dermatitis carries a remarkably similar bad prognosis [29]. Two years after this diagnosis being made, of those who continued to work with soluble oil 78% had not recovered, and of those who stopped 70% had not recovered. Nevertheless, early cessation of contact was beneficial in some, and their skin healed within 3 months. This indicates that, although a change of jobs is not realistic for established workers, it should seriously be considered for young trainees and apprentices. Similarly in caterers, irritants are of major importance. In one investigation of 12 who had to give up catering because of their dermatitis, the hands healed in only four and in eight the eczema continued [15].

These studies show that, in those who are predisposed, irritants may precipitate an endogenous hand eczema, which may continue regardless of the patient's work. However, on clinical grounds it is reasonable to advise young patients to change to a clean dry job. In older patients established in their work such advice may not be economically feasible, and avoidance of irritants and protective clothing must be stressed.

Complete healing of a hand eczema away from the initiating irritant exposure cannot be required as a criterion for making the diagnosis of an irritant contact dermatitis. Not all hand eczemas heal when the original precipitating factors are removed.

8.6 Post-Traumatic Eczema

It is generally accepted that eczema may follow trauma to the skin. However, the clinical criteria for post-traumatic eczema are not well established and the mechanism is not understood, so the diagnosis has to rest 'on the grounds of reasonable probability' [30]. The interval between injury and the development of eczema at the site is important. Calnan [31] gave it as being normally 2 weeks. Wilkinson [30] described two patients. In one a caustic soda burn on the hand was followed in 1 week by the appearance of a patch of discoid eczema. The discoid lesions spread and were present 15 months later. A liquid hardener splashed on the leg of the second patient, and it was 3 weeks later that the site became eczematous. A year later discoid lesions spread to other sites.

On the basis of his personal experience, Mathias [32] divided post-traumatic eczema into two types. The first type, the isomorphic reaction, he equated with a Koebner reaction and subdivided it into primary and secondary groups: a primary isomorphic reaction was an initial traumatic eczema subsequently followed by eczema elsewhere; and a secondary isomorphic reaction was trauma precipitating eczema at its site, but in a person with an already existing endogenous eczema. The second main type he called the idiopathic reaction, in which the eczema remained localized to the site of trauma and was neither associated with a coexistent eczema nor followed by eczema for 1 year, this time interval being his own criterion. These divisions may be valid but are not generally used; in particular eczema following injury in an eczematous patient is not usually categorized as a post-traumatic eczema. Mathias [32] described 13 patients, the time from injury to the onset of eczema being 3 weeks in 12 patients and 4 weeks in only one. He emphasized the significant observation of his patients that, following the injury, their skin never completely healed. In several patients their post-traumatic eczema persisted for several years.

These case reports confirm that post-traumatic eczema does occur. Any type of injury may be implicated, including chemical or thermal burns, lacerations, abrasions or chemical injury. The interval between the trauma and the appearance of the eczema varies from 1 to 3 weeks and the local eczema may persist for years. When the eczema spreads it appears to do so as discoid (nummular) patches, as described by both Wilkinson [30] and Mathias [32].

8.7 Lymphangitis and Lymphoedema

Occasionally, patients are seen with a triad of hand eczema, recurrent lymphangitis and lymphoedema, a combination which is very difficult to treat. The patients present with attacks of vesicular eczema of the palms and fingers, associated with streptococcal lymphangitis and lymphoedema of the hands. In most patients the initial episodes are intermittent and resolve, but slowly the eczema and lymphoedema become established and worsen with each successive attack of lymphangitis. The hands become permanently eczematous and swollen with a woody oedema which spreads up the arms. The condition is progressively disabling. Patch tests are usually negative or noncontributory but the two patients described by Lynde and Mitchell [33] did have relevant patch tests, one to *Frullania* and the other to thiurams and carbamates in rubber gloves.

This condition occurs only in those with a primary defect of their lymphatics, and lymphangiograms have shown lymphatic hypoplasia [34]. Never common, lymphoedema and hand eczema seems to have become very rare.

Secrétan's syndrome is a self-inflicted lymphoedema of the dorsum of the hand, effected by the patient through the application of a tourniquet or by repeated trauma. Its inadvertent production occurred in four fishing divers in Italy as an occupational disease [35]. It was caused by the constricting effect of the tight sleeves of their diving suits. Repeated pricks from the spines of sea urchins contributed and caused sea urchin granulomas on the hands of two of the men. Lymphangiograms were normal in three men and slightly abnormal in the fourth. These men did not have hand eczema.

8.8 Differential Diagnosis

The commonest differential diagnosis of a hand eczema is a fungus infection or psoriasis. The presence of fungus is easily established, whereas psoriasis of the hands is a clinical opinion frequently disputed. Even the same clinician may label the patient as having psoriasis on one occasion and eczema on the next. Examining the whole patient is surprisingly helpful.

8.9 References

1. Ackerman AB, Ragaz A (1982) A plea to expunge the word "eczema" from the lexicon of dermatology and dermatopathology. Am J Dermatopathol 4: 315–326
2. Agrup G (1969) Hand eczema and other hand dermatoses in South Sweden. Acta Derm Venereol (Stockh) 49 [Suppl 61]: 73, 84, 74
3. Meding B, Swanbeck G (1987) Prevalence of hand eczema in an industrial city. Br J Dermatol 116: 627–634
4. Coenraads PJ, Nater JP, Lende van der R (1983) Prevalence of eczema and other dermatoses of the hands and arms in the Netherlands. Association with age and occupation. Clin Exp Dermatol 8: 495–503
5. Goh CL (1989) An epidemiological comparison between occupational and non-occupational hand eczema. Br J Dermatol 120: 77–82
6. Cronin E (1985) Clinical patterns of hand eczema in women. Contact Dermatitis 13: 153–161
7. Uehara M, Hayashi S (1981) Hyperlinear palms. Association with ichthyosis and atopic dermatitis. Arch Dermatol 117: 490–491
8. Svensson Å(1988) Hand Eczema: an evaluation of the frequency of atopic background and the difference in clinical pattern between patients with and without atopic dermatitis. Acta Derm Venereol (Stockh) 68: 509–513

9. Fisher AA (1982) Contact dermatitis of the hands due to foods. Part 1. Cutis 30: 21, 22, 24
10. Goh CL (1987) Hand dermatitis from a rubber motorcycle handle. Contact Dermatitis 16: 40–41
11. Sinclair PA, Nurse DS (1985) Finger tip dermatitis. Australas J Dermatol 26: 137–138
12. Rycroft RJG (1984) Low-humidity occupational dermatoses. In: Storrs FJ (ed) Dermatologic clinics, vol 2. Saunders, Philadelphia, pp 553–559
13. Rycroft RJG, Smith WDL (1980) Low humidity occupational dermatoses. Contact Dermatitis 6: 488–492
14. White IR, Rycroft RJG (1982) Low humidity occupational dermatosis–an epidemic. Contact Dermatitis 8: 287–290
15. Cronin E (1987) Dermatitis of the hands in caterers. Contact Dermatitis 17: 265–269
16. De Boer EM, Bruynzeel DP, van Ketel WG (1988) Dyshidrotic eczema as an occupational dermatitis in metal workers. Contact Dermatitis 19: 184–188
17. Lim KB, Tan T, Rajan VS (1986) Dermatitis palmaris sicca–a distinctive pattern of hand dermatitis. Clin Exp Dermatol 11: 553–559
18. Menné T, Hjorth N (1983) Pompholyx–dyshidrotic eczema. Semin Dermatol 2: 75–80
19. Thelin I, Agrup G (1986) Pompholyx–a one year series. Acta Derm Venereol (Stockh) 65: 214–217
20. Landwehr AJ, van Ketel WG (1983) Pompholyx after implantation of a nickel-containing pacemaker in a nickel-allergic patient. Contact Dermatitis 9: 147
21. Menné T, Hjorth N (1982) Reactions from systemic exposure to contact allergens. Semin Dermatol 1: 15–24
22. Vassileva S, Stransky L (1987) Beruflich bedingte dyshidrosiforme Dermatitis der Hände nach Kontakt mit Kakteen. Dermatosen 35: 204–205
23. Rystedt I (1985) Hand eczema in patients with history of atopic manifestations in childhood. Acta Derm Venerol (Stockh) 65: 305–312
24. Rystedt I (1985) Factors influencing the occurrence of hand eczema in adults with a history of atopic dermatitis in childhood. Contact Dermatitis 12: 185–191
25. Fregert S, Gruvberger B, Sandahl E (1979) Reduction of chromate in cement by iron sulfate. Contact Dermatitis 5: 39–42
26. Avnstorp C (1989) Prevalence of cement eczema in Denmark before and since addition of ferrous sulfate to Danish cement. Acta Derm Venereol (Stockh) 69: 151–155
27. Avnstorp C (1989) Follow up of workers from the prefabricated concrete industry after the addition of ferrous sulphate to Danish cement. Contact Dermatitis 20: 365–371
28. Keczkes K, Bhate SM, Wyatt EH (1983) The outcome of primary irritant hand dermatitis. Br J Dermatol 109: 665–668
29. Pryce DW, Irvine D, English JSC, Rycroft RJG (1989) Soluble oil dermatitis: a follow-up study. Contact Dermatitis 21: 28–35
30. Wilkinson DS (1979) Letter to the editor. Contact Dermatitis 5: 118–119
31. Calnan CD (1968) Eczema for me. Trans St John's Hosp Dermatol Soc 54: 54–64
32. Mathias CGT (1988) Post-traumatic eczema. In: Taylor JS (ed) Dermatologic clinics. Saunders, Philadelphia, pp 35–42
33. Lynde CW, Mitchell JC (1982) Unusual complication of allergic contact dermatitis of the hands–recurrent lymphangitis and persistent lymphoedema. Contact Dermatitis 8: 279–280
34. Borrie P, Taylor GW (1962) Lymphoedema presenting in the skin department. Br J Dermatol 74: 403–413
35. Angelini C, Vena GA, Meneghini CL (1990) Occupational traumatic lymphedema of the hands. In: Adams RM, Nethercott JR (eds) Dermatologic clinics, vol 8. Saunders, Philadelphia, pp 205–208

Chapter 9
Noneczematous
Contact Reactions

Noneczematous Contact Reactions

CHEE LEOK GOH

Contents

9.1 Introduction

Skin contact reactions usually present as an eczematous eruption, but some are noneczematous. There are different types of noneczematous contact reaction, including:

- Erythema-multiforme-like eruption or urticarial papular and plaque eruption
- Pigmented purpuric eruption
- Lichen-planus-like or lichenoid eruption
- Bullous eruption
- Papular and nodular eruption
- Granulomatous eruption
- Pustular eruption
- Erythematous and exfoliative eruption
- Scleroderma-like eruption
- Pigmented contact dermatitis (see Chap. 15)

9.2 Erythema-Multiforme-like Eruption or Urticarial Papular and Plaque Eruption

Some skin allergens, e.g. metals, medicaments, woods and industrial chemicals, can cause an erythema-multiforme-like eruption (see Table 9.1).

Table 9.1. Reported causes of UPPE

Woods and plants
  Dalbergia nigra (Brazilian rosewood)
  Machaerium scleroxylon (pao ferro)
  Eucalyptus saligna (gum)
  Toxicodendron radicans (poison ivy)
  Primula obconica
  Artemisia vulgaris (common mugwort)

Topical medicaments
  Ethylenediamine
  Pyrrolnitrin
  Sulphonamide
  Promethazine
  balsam of Peru
  p-Phenylenediamine
  Mafenide acetate
  Proflavine
  vitamin E

  Sulphanilamide

  Furazolidone
  Nifuroxime
  Scopolamine hydrobromide
  Clioquinol (Vioform)
  Diaminodiphenylmethane
  Mephenesin
  Econazole
  Nitrogen mustard

Metals and chemicals
  Nickel
  Cobalt
  9-Bromofluorene precursors
  Phenylsulphone derivatives
  Epoxy resin
  p-Chlorobenzene sulphonylglycolic acid nitrile
  Formaldehyde
  Trichloroethylene
  Trinitrotoluene
  Dimethoate

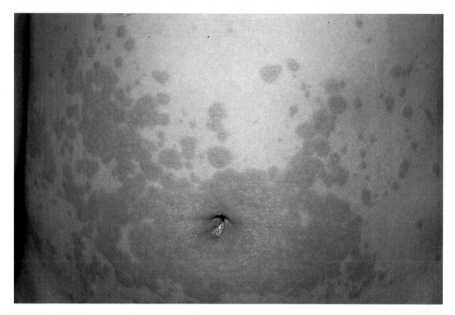

Fig. 9.1. Erythema-multiforme-like eruption (UPPE) from contact allergy to trinitrotoluene. Note urticarial papular and plaque eruption

Such as eruption appears to be a manifestation of a delayed allergic reaction and is usually associated with a positive patch test reaction in the patient. The morphology of such eruptions has been described as target-like, erythematovesicular or urticarial.

9.2.1 Clinical Features

The characteristic presentation of an erythema-multiforme-like eruption from a contact allergen usually begins about 1–14 days after an episode of allergic contact dermatitis. The primary contact site may be eczematous but becomes urticarial after a few days. Erythematous urticarial papular and/or plaque eruptions (Fig. 9.1) then begin to appear around the primary contact site and also often at distant sites. The eruptions, some of which are target-like, usually persist longer than the primary eczematous lesion and may appear after the clearance of the initial dermatitis. They are usually pruritic.

9.2.2 Patch Test

A positive patch test reaction to the causative allergen can usually be obtained in patients with such eruptions. The patch test reaction is often vesiculobullous and occasionally urticarial.

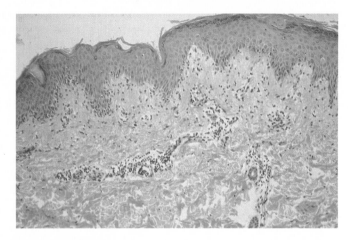

Fig. 9.2. Histology of an UPPE lesion from the patient in Fig. 9.1. Mild upper dermal oedema and lymphohistiocytic infiltrates with normal epidermis. Note absence of changes typical of erythema multiforme

9.2.3 Histology

The histology in the erythema-multiforme-like eruption of contact allergy is usually nonspecific. The epidermis is normal or shows minimal spongiosis. There is mild upper dermal oedema and mild perivascular lymphohistiocytic infiltration. Vacuolar degeneration of the basal cells is rarely present. There is no epidermal necrosis or interface infiltration, as are present in erythema multiforme (Fig. 9.2).

9.2.4 Differentiation from Classical Erythema Multiforme

Besides the occasional target-like lesions, the morphology, clinical course and histology of erythema-multiforme-like eruptions of contact allergy are not characteristic of classical erythema multiforme. Lesions of erythema multiforme tend to have an acral distribution, appear in crops and are almost all target-like. The term 'urticarial papular and plaque eruption' (UPPE) of contact allergy was suggested to describe such an eruption [1]. UPPE will be used synonymously with erythema-multiforme-like eruption in the rest of this chapter. The exact mechanism of UPPE is unknown, but appears to represent an immune complex reaction.

9.2.5 Causes

Contact allergens known to cause of UPPE include (a) woods and plants, (b) topical medicaments and (c) chemicals. Table 9.1 lists the known causes of UPPE.

9.2.5.1 Woods and Plants

Several types of tropical woods are known to cause UPPE. Three different tropical woods, Brazilian rosewood (*Dalbergia nigra*), pao ferro (*Machaerium scleroxylon*) and *Eucalyptus saligna,* were reported to cause occupational UPPE in three carpenters [2]. The allergen in pao ferro is *R*-3,4-dimethoxy-dalbergione. A wooden bracelet [3] and a pendant [4] made from *Dalbergia nigra* were also reported to cause UPPE in patients wearing the items. The specific chemical antigen was identified as the quinone *R*-4-methoxydalbergione [5]. Irvine et al. reported similar eruptions from pao ferro (*Machaerium scleroxylon*) in a hobbyist who used the wood to make boxes [6].

Plants reported to cause UPPE include poison ivy (*Toxicodendron radicans*) [7, 8], primula (*Primula obconica*) [9] and common mugwort (*Artemisia vulgaris*) [10]. Kurz and Rapaport [10] reported a patient who treated his poison ivy dermatitis with 'mugwort brew' and later developed an erythema multiforme eruption after drinking the brew.

9.2.5.2 Topical Medicaments

Numerous topical medicaments have been reported to cause UPPE, most of them topical antimicrobials. Topical medicaments reported to cause UPPE as a manifestation of contact allergy include pyrrolnitrin, sulphonamide, promethazine, balsam of Peru, clioquinol (Vioform) and ethylenediamine [11, 12]. Some of these patients had vasculitic or purpuric lesions. Yaffe et al. reported two patients who developed generalized UPPE after a mafenideacetate-containing cream was applied on a skin burn [13]. Mephenesin was suspected to be the cause of UPPE in five patients who used a mephenesin-containing ointment for burns, four of the patients having positive patch test reactions to mephenesin [14]. Proflavine was reported to cause purpura and UPPE. Two patients developed purpura and UPPE after applying proflavine for a skin abrasion and both had strong positive patch test reactions to proflavine [15]. Other medicaments reported to cause UPPE as a manifestation of contact allergy include econazole [16] and vitamin E [17].

Medicaments which are applied to mucosae are rapidly absorbed systemically and may enhance the skin and systemic sensitization process. UPPE occurred in a patient who applied sulphanilamide cream for vulvovaginitis; she had a positive patch test reaction to the sulphanilamide cream and also developed UPPE after ingesting sulphanilamide [18]. UPPE was also described in contact allergy to furazolidone- and nifuroxine-containing suppositories in another patient. A flare-up of the eruption developed when she was patch tested to the suppository. UPPE was also reported from contact allergy to eyedrops. Two case reports of Stevens-Johnson syndrome from contact allergy to sulphonamide-containing eyedrops were described [19, 20]. Another patient developed UPPE from scopolamine hydrobromide eyedrops; his eruption recurred on rechallenge to the eyedrops [21].

9.2.5.3 Metals and Chemicals

Metals. UPPE may be a manifestation of contact allergy to some metals and industrial chemicals. Calnan first described UPPE in the secondary spread of nickel dermatitis [22]. Cook reported UPPE in a 13-year-old girl following allergic contact dermatitis from nickel and cobalt in the metal studs of her jeans [23]. A similar eruption was reported in a garment worker who developed nickel dermatitis on her hands from nickel-plated scissors; she had a vesiculopapular patch test reaction to nickel salt and during patch testing her hand dermatitis and UPPE reappeared [24]. UPPE was also reported in a patient with nickel dermatitis due to a metallic necklace [25].

Laboratory Chemicals. UPPE from laboratory chemicals was first described by Cavendish in 1940 in a student who developed recurrent eruptions after 9-bromofluorene exposure. During patch testing, one of the control patients became sensitized to the chemical and developed UPPE 13 days after the patch test [26]. Powell also reported a student with a similar eruption due to 9-bromofluorene and, similarly, one control patient became sensitized to the chemical [27]. De Feo also described how, out of 250 chemistry students, 24 developed localized acute contact eczema followed by generalized UPPE, while synthesizing 9-bromofluorene in the laboratory. They had positive patch tests to the chemical [28]. Roed-Petersen reported a chemistry student who developed UPPE on the exposed skin from a phenyl sulphone derivative which he was synthesizing. He had a strong positive reaction to the compound [29].

Industrial Chemicals. Several industrial chemicals have been suspected to cause UPPE. Nethercott et al. reported UPPE in four workers handling printed circuit boards. Liver involvement was documented in three of the workers. Two of the workers had a positive reaction to formaldehyde and formaldehyde was implicated as the cause of the eruptions [30]. Phoon et al. described five workers who developed UPPE and Stevens-Johnson syndrome after exposure to trichloroethylene in an electronics factory. Three workers had hepatitis and one died of hepatic failure. A patch test to trichloroethylene on one worker was negative. The eruption was suspected to be due a hypersensitivity reaction to trichloroethylene from percutaneous and/or transrespiratory absorption of trichloroethylene [31].

UPPE was also reported in a worker with allergic contact dermatitis from trinitrotoluene; the patient had a strong eczematous patch test reaction to trinitrotoluene [32]. It was recently reported in a warehouseman allergic to dimethoate, an organophosphorus insecticide and acaricide [33].

9.3 Pigmented Purpuric Eruption

Purpuric eruption is an uncommon manifestation of contact allergy. The eruption is usually asymptomatic, macular and purpuric, with or without preceding itch or erythema (Fig. 9.3). The purpuric eruption then becomes

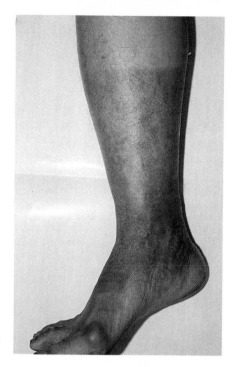

Fig. 9.3. Pigmented purpuric dermatitis from IPPD in rubber boots

brownish and fades away. The exact mechanism of the reaction is unknown. Causes of contact pigmented purpuric eruption include rubber chemicals, dyes, raw wool and medicaments.

Isopropyl-N-phenyl-p-phenylenediamine (IPPD) is the commonest reported cause of contact purpuric eruption. IPPD present in rubber clothing [34], rubber boots [35], rubber diving suits, elasticized shorts, a rubberized support bandage [36] and a rubberized brassiere [37] was reported to cause such an eruption.

p-Phenylenediamine present in hat dye caused contact purpuric eruptions in a saleswomen handling black hats [38]. Raw wool was also reported to cause a contact purpuric eruption [39].

Contact allergy to balsam of Peru [40] and proflavine [15] in medicaments, and the azo dye Disperse Blue 85 [41] in naval uniforms, may also manifest as a purpuric eruption.

9.4 Lichen-Planus-like and Lichenoid Eruption

Lichen-planus-like and lichenoid eruptions are another uncommon manifestation of contact allergy to some chemicals.

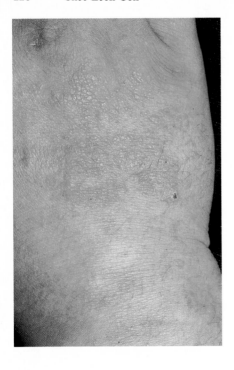

Fig. 9.4. Lichenoid eruption on back of hand from colour developer (CD 4) (Courtesy of P.J. Frosch)

9.4.1 Clinical Features

The eruptions appear as itchy dusky or violaceous papules or plaques on areas of skin exposed to the allergen (Fig. 9.4). The eruptions may also appear at distant sites.

9.4.2 Causes

Contact allergy to colour developers is the commonest cause of contact lichenoid eruption. Several colour developers have been implicated (Fig. 9.5), including Kodak CD2 (4-$\underline{N}$, $\underline{N}$-diethyl-2-methylphenylenediamine monohydrochloride), Kodak CD3 (4-(N-ethyl-N-2-methanesulphonylaminoethyl)-2-methyl-phenylenediamine sesquisulphate monohydrate), Agfa TSS(4-amino-N-diethylaniline sulphate), Ilford MI 210(N-ethyl-N(5-hydrocy-amyl) p-phenylenediamine hydrogen sulphate) and Kodak CD4 (2-amino-5-N-ethyl-N-(β-hydroxyethyl)-aminotoluene sulphate) [42]. Mandel reported that 9 out of 11 workers with contact allergy to colour developer showed lichen-planus-like eruptions [43], but Fry reported a lower rate of 7 out of 20 patients, the remainder presenting with eczematous reactions [44].

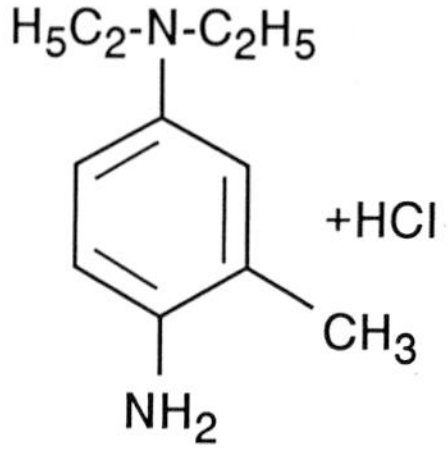

H_5C_2-N-C_2H_5

+HCl

CH_3

NH_2

CD2

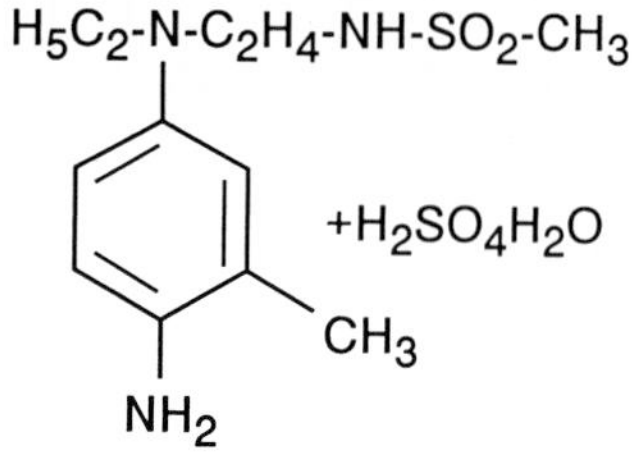

H_5C_2-N-C_2H_4-NH-SO_2-CH_3

+$H_2SO_4H_2O$

CH_3

NH_2

CD3

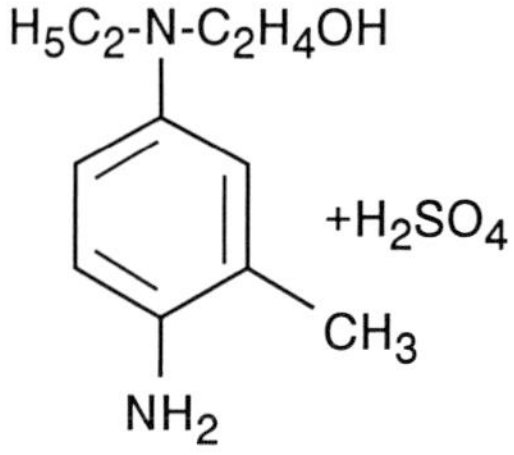

H_5C_2-N-C_2H_4OH

+H_2SO_4

CH_3

NH_2

CD4

H_5C_2-N-C_2H_5

+H_2SO_4

NH_2

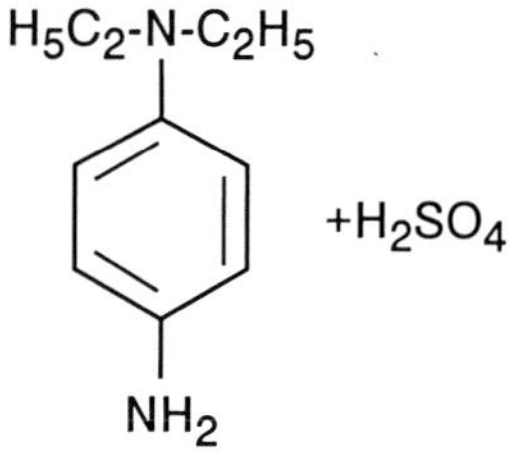

TSS

Fig. 9.5. Contact Sensitizing colour developers

9.4.3 Histology

The histology of lichen-planus-like eruptions from colour developers may show features compatible with lichen planus or a nonspecific chronic superficial perivascular dermatitis. Some reports indicate that the histology in the majority of patients shows changes compatible with lichen planus [45–47], but others indicate that a nonspecific chronic dermatitis change is more common [42, 44]. In Fry's report, out of seven patients with lichenoid lesions biopsied, one showed changes of eczema, two showed lichenoid dermatitis and two showed lichen planus changes [44].

9.4.4 Mechanism

There is controversy about the aetiology of the lichen-planus-like eruption from colour developers. Lichenoid eruptions may be due to direct contact with the chemicals on the skin producing allergic contact dermatitis, but may also represent eruptions resulting from systemic absorption of the allergen [44, 46]. A combination of both mechanisms may be responsible.

Other allergens reported to cause lichenoid eruptions include metallic copper [48] and mercury [49] from dental amalgam. These patients presented with lichen-planus-like lesions on the buccal mucosa. Both had positive patch test reactions to the respective allergen. Nickel salts were also reported to cause lichenoid dermatitis [50, 51]. Lembo et al. reported a chronic lichenoid eruption in a schoolboy from aminoglycoside-containing creams. Biopsy showed a band-like mononuclear upper dermal infiltrate. Patch tests showed a lichenoid reaction to neomycin [52]. A lichenoid reaction has also been reported to epoxy resin [53].

9.5 Bullous Eruption

Bullous eruptions mimicking bullous pemphigoid have been reported as a manifestation of contact allergy to cinnamic aldehyde and cinnamic alcohol [54]. The patient developed bullous eruptions after applying cinnamon powder to treat scars on her legs. The morphology and histology of the eruption resembled bullous pemphigoid but direct immunofluorescence studies were negative. She had a strong vesicular patch test reaction to the cinnamon powder, cinnamic aldehyde and cinnamic alcohol. The exact mechanism of the cell-mediated hypersensitivity reaction is unknown. Contact allergy to nickel and its oral ingestion has also been reported to cause dyshidrosiform pemphigoid [55].

9.6 Nodular and Papular Eruption

Contact allergy to gold may present as a nodular or papular eruption. Such eruptions occur particularly on the earlobes in sensitized individuals wearing pierced-type gold earrings and usually persist for months after the patients have avoided contact with metallic gold [56–61]. Patch test reactions to gold and gold salts in these patients are usually strongly positive. Occasionally the patch test may evoke an infiltrative lymphoblastic reaction which persists for months [57, 61, 62]. The histology of these eruptions or its patch test reaction usually shows a dense lymphomonocytic infiltrate mimicking mycosis fungoides, but mycosis fungoides cells are absent. The cellular infiltrate consists mainly of suppressor/cytotoxic T cells [62]. Dental amalgam allergy was reported to cause a nodular eruption mimicking oral carcinoma [63].

9.7 Granulomatous Eruption

Contact reactions to metals and metallic salts can manifest as granulomatous eruptions. Skin injury from zirconium, silica, magnesium, beryllium and collagen may cause granulomas. Some granulomatous reactions are allergic and others nonallergic.

Zirconium salts are known to cause allergic granulomatous reactions. Clinically, such reactions appear 4–6 weeks after skin contact with zirconium salts (e.g. in deodorants) [64–66]. Eczema is usually present but pruritus is minimal. The eruptions are usually confined to the area of application, e.g. the axillae. Patients with the eruptions have associated positive patch test reactions to zirconium compounds. The histology shows epithelioid cells and may be indistinguishable from sarcoid. Allergic granulomatous eruptions were also reported in sensitized patients who use zirconium compounds to treat rhus dermatitis [67–70].

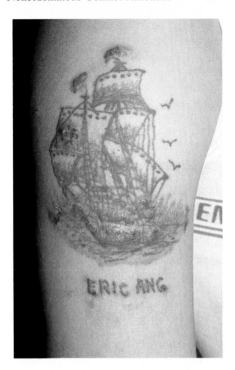

Fig. 9.6. Allergic granulomatous reaction from mercury pigment (red) and cobalt pigment (blue). Note overlying eczematous reactions

Cutaneous granulomas may also occur following immunization with vaccines containing aluminium hydroxide, such patients having positive patch tests to aluminium chloride and/or aluminium Finn Chambers. In one series of 21 children, the granulomas of 11 improved with time [71].

Metallic salts in tattoo pigments are known causes of allergic granulomatous reactions. Mercury (red cinnabar, mercury sulphide–red pigment), chromium (chromium oxide powder–green pigment), cobalt (cobaltous aluminate–blue pigment) and cadmium (cadmium sulphide–yellow pigment) are known causative agents [72]. An unknown substance in purple tattoo pigment has also been reported to cause a granulomatous reaction [73–74]. Granulomatous reactions may be preceded by or associated with eczematous reactions (Fig. 9.6). The lesion is usually non-itchy. Biopsy shows typical granulomas. These patients usually have positive patch test reactions to the respective metallic salts.

9.8 Pustular Eruption

Pustular reactions to contactants were first observed in patch test reactions. These pustules are sterile and transient. Metallic salts, e.g. nickel, copper, arsenic and mercury salts, are the commonest causes of such pustular reactions [75]. The significance of such a pustular reaction remains speculative. Stone and Johnson explained that such reactions may represent an enhanced reaction of prior inflammation rather than an irritant or allergic reaction [76]. Atopics are predisposed to such reactions [77]. Wahlberg and Maibach believe that such reactions are usually irritant in nature but may also be a manifestation of allergic reactions [78].

Allergic contact dermatitis from a nitrofurazone-containing cream manifested as a pustular eruption [79]. Subcorneal pustular eruption may also be a manifestation of allergy to trichloroethylene [80].

9.9 Erythematous and Exfoliative Eruption

Trichloroethylene and methyl bromide exposure have been reported to cause localized or generalized erythema and exfoliation. The eruption presents as localized or generalized erythema with or without papular and vesicular features. Skin exfoliation then follows. The eruption usually takes several weeks to clear. This skin reaction is believed to be a systemic toxic or allergic reaction to a chemical, following its percutaneous or mucosal absorption.

9.9.1 Trichloroethylene

Generalized erythema followed by exfoliation resulting from exposure to trichloroethylene was first described by Schwartz et al. [81] and later by Bauer and Rabens [82]. The reaction was believed to be due to a systemic sensitization to trichloroethylene.

Conde-Salazar reported a patient who developed a generalized erythema and subcorneal pustular eruption from a cutaneous hypersensitivity reaction to trichloroethylene [80]. The allergic reaction was confirmed by a positive erythematous scaly patch test reaction to 5% trichloroethylene. The patient also reacted systemically to a cutaneous challenge test made by exposing his leg to an environment saturated with trichloroethylene. Nakayama et al. also described generalized erythema and exfoliation with mucous membrane ulceration in a patient from cutaneous exposure to trichloroethylene. The patient had positive patch test reactions to trichloroethylene and trichloroethanol (a metabolite of trichloroethylene) [83]. The patient's skin eruption continued to appear after cessation of exposure to trichloroethylene. The prolonged duration of the eruption was believed to be due to the slow release of accumulated trichloroethylene and its metabolites in the patient's fatty tissue.

Cutaneous reaction to inhaled trichloroethylene can also cause a characteristic skin eruption consisting of localized erythematous xerotic plaques which become parched and fissured [84].

9.9.2 Methyl Bromide

Exposure to methyl bromide was described as causing sharply demarcated erythema with vesiculation in six fumigators [85]. Plasma bromide levels in these patients after exposure strongly suggested percutaneous absorption of methyl bromide. The lesions were more prominent on skin that was relatively moist or subject to mechanical pressure, such as the axillae, groins and abdomen. Histologically, the early skin lesions showed keratinocytes, necrosis, severe upper dermal oedema and bullae, and diffuse dermal neutrophilic infiltration. The skin eruptions were believed to be due to the direct toxic effect of methyl bromide as an alkylating agent.

9.10 Scleroderma-like Eruption

Solvents have been reported as predisposing or eliciting factors in some patients with scleroderma-like eruptions [86, 87]. The pathogenic mechanism is unknown. Solvents implicated include aromatic hydrocarbon solvents, such as benzene, toluene and white spirit, and aliphatic hydrocarbons, such as naphtha, n-hexane and hexachloroethane. Unlike chlorinated hydrocarbons, these hydrocarbons do not produce multisystem disease resembling vinyl chloride disease. The associated scleroderma and morphoea-like sclerosis is usually limited to the skin of the hands and feet, where direct contact took place, but occasionally may be widespread.

9.11 References

1. Goh CL (1989) Urticarial papular and plaque eruption. A manifestation of allergic contact dermatitis. Int J Dermatol 28: 172–176
2. Holst R, Kirby J, Magnusson B (1976) Sensitization to tropical woods giving erythema multiforme-like eruptions. Contact Dermatitis 2: 295–296
3. Fisher AA (1986) Erythema multiforme-like eruptions due to exotic woods and ordinary plants. Part I. Cutis 37: 101–104
4. Fisher AA, Bikowski J (1981) Allergic contact dermatitis due to wooden cross made of Dalbergia nigra. Contact Dermatitis 7: 45–46
5. Hausen BM (1981) Woods Injurious to Human Health. De Gruyter, Berlin, p 59
6. Irvine C, Reynolds A, Finlay AY (1988) Erythema multiforme-like reaction to "rosewood". Contact Dermatitis 19: 24–225
7. Mallory SB, Miller OF, Tyler WB (1982) Toxicodendron radicans dermatitis with black lacquer deposit on the skin. J Am Acad Dermatol 6: 363–368
8. Schwartz RS, Downham TF (1981) Erythema multiforme associated with Rhus contact dermatitis. Contact Dermatitis 27: 85–86
9. Hjorth N (1966) Primula dermatitis. Trans St John's Hosp Der Soc 52: 207–219
10. Kurz G, Rapaport MJ (1979) External/internal allergy to plants (Artemesia). Contact Dermatitis 5: 407–4
11. Fisher AA (1986) Erythema multiforme-like eruptions due to topical medications. Part II. Cutis 37: 158–161
12. Meneghini CL, Angelini G (1981) Secondary polymorphic erutpions in allergic contact dermatitis. Dermatologica 163: 63–70
13. Yaffe H, Dressler DP (1969) Topical application of mafenide acetate. Its association with erythema multiforme and cutaneous reactions. Arch Dermatol 100: 277–281
14. Degreef H, Conamie A, van Derheyden D et al. (1984) Mephenesin contact dermatitis with erythema multiforme-like features. Contact Dermatitis 10: 220–223

15. Goh CL (1987) Erythema multiforme-like and purpuric eruption due to contact allergy to proflavine. Contact Dermatitis 17: 53–54
16. Valsecchi R, Foiadelli L, Cainelli T (1982) Contact dermatitis from econazole. Contact Dermatits 8: 422
17. Saperstein H, Rapaport M, Rietschel RL (1984) Topical vitamin E as a cause of erythema multiforme-like eruptions. Arch Dermatol 120: 906–908
18. Goette DK, Odom RB (1980) Vaginal medications as a cause for varied widespread dermatitides. Cutis 26: 406–409
19. Gottschalk HR, Stone OJ (1976) Stevens-Johnson syndrome from ophthalmic sulfonamide. Arch Dermatol 112: 513–514
20. Rubin Z (1977) Ophthalmic sulfonamide-induced Stevens-Johnson syndrome. Arch Dermatol 113: 235–236
21. Guill MA, Goette DK, Knight CG et al. (1979) Erythema multiforme and urticaria. Eruptions induced by chemically-related ophthalmic anticholinergic agents. Arch Dermatol 115: 742–743
22. Calnan CD (1956) Nickel dermatitis. Br J Dermatol 68: 229–232
23. Cook LJ (1982) Associated nickel and cobalt contact dermatitis presenting as erythema multiforme. Contact Dermatitis 8: 280–281
24. Friedman SF, Perry HO (1985) Erythema multiforme associated with contact dermatitis. Contact Dermatitis 12: 21–23
25. Fisher AA (1986) Erythema multiforme-like eruptions due to topical miscellaneous compounds. Part III. Cutis 37: 262–264
26. Cavendish A (1968) A case of dermatitis from 9 bromofluorene and a peculiar reaction to a patch test. Br J Derm 1940; 52: 155–164
27. Powell EW. Skin reactions to 9-bromofluorene. Br J Derm 80: 491–496
28. De Feo CP (1966) Erythema multiforme bullosum caused by 9-bromofluorene. Arch Dermatol 94: 545–551
29. Roed-Petersen J (1975) Erythema multiforme as an expression of contact dermatitis. Contact Dermatitis 1: 270–271
30. Nethercott JR, Albers J, Gurguis S et al. (1982) Erythema multiforme exudativum linked to the manufacture of printed circuit boards. Contact Dermatitis 3: 314–322
31. Phoon WH, Chan MOY, Rajan VS et al. (1984) Stevens-Johnson syndrome associated with occupational exposure to trichloroethylene. Contact Dermatitis 10: 270–276
32. Goh CL (1988) Erythema multiforme-like eruption from trinitrotoluene allergy. Int J Dermatol 27: 650–651
33. Schena D, Barba A (1992) Erythema-multiforme-like contact dermatitis from dimethoate. Contact Dermatitis 27: 116–117
34. Batchvaros B, Minkow DM (1968) Dermatitis and purpura from rubber in clothing. Trans St John's Hosp Derm Soc 54: 73–78
35. Calnan CD, Peachey RDG (1971) Allergic contact purpura. Clin Allergy 1: 287–290
36. Fisher AA (1974) Allergic petechial and purpuric rubber dermatitis. The PPPP syndrome. Gutis 14: 25–27
37. Romaguera C, Grimalt F (1977) PPPP syndrome. Contact Dermatitis 3: 103.
38. Shmunes E (1978) Purpuric allergic contact dermatitis to paraphenylenediamine. Contact Dermatitis 4: 225–229
39. Agarwal K (1982) Contact allergic purpura to wool dust. Contact Dermatitis 8: 281–282
40. Bruynzeel DP, van den Hoogenband HM, Koedijk F (1984) Purpuric vasculitis-like eruption in a patient sensitive to balsam of Peru. Contact Dermatitis 11: 207–209
41. van derm Veen JPW, Neering H, de Haan P, Bruynzeel (1988) Pigmented purpuric clothing dermatitis due to Disperse Blue 85. Contact Dermatitis 19: 222–223
42. Goh CL, Kwok SF, Rajan VS (1984) Cross sensitivity in Colour developers. Contact Dermatitis 10: 280–285

43. Mendel EH (1960) Lichen planus-like eruption caused by a colorfilm developer. Arch Dermatol 70: 516–519
44. Fry L (1965) Skin disease from colour developers. Br J Derm 77: 456–461
45. Buckley WR (1958) Lichenoid eruptions following contact dermatitis. Arch Dermatol 78: 454–457
46. Canizares O (1959) Lichen planus-like eruption caused by colour developer. Arch Dermatol 80: 81–86
47. Hyman AB, Berger Ra (1959) Lichenoid eruption due to colour developer. Arch Dermatol 80: 243–244
48. Frykholm KO, Frithiof L, Fernstorm AI et al. (1969) Allergy to copper derived from dental alloys as a possible cause of oral lesions of lichen planus. Acta Derm Venereol (Stockh) 49: 268–269
49. Bircher AJ, von Schultheiss A, Henning G (1993) Oral lichenoid lesions and mercury sensitivity. Contact Dermatitis 29: 275–276
50. Lombardi F, Campolmi P. Sertoli A (1983) Lichenoid dermatitis caused by nickel salts? Contact Dermatitis 9: 520–521
51. Meneghine CL (1971) Lichenoid contact dermatitis. Contact Dermatitis Newsletter 9: 194
52. Lembo G. Balato N, Patrupo C, Pini D, Ayala F (1987) Lichenoid contact dermatitis due to aminoglycoside antibiotics. Contact Dermatitis 17: 122–123
53. Lichter M, Drury D, Remlinger K (1992) Lichenoid dermatitis caused by epoxy resin. Contact Dermatitis 26: 275
54. Goh CL, Ng SK (1988) Bullous contact allergy from cinnamon. Dermatosen 36: 186–187
55. Atakan N, Tüzün J, Karaduman A (1993) Dyshidrosiform pemphigoid induced by nickel in the diet. Contact Dermatitis 29: 159–160
56. Shelley WB, Epstein E (1963) Contact-sensitivity to gold as a chronic papular eruption. Arch Dermatol 87: 388–391
57. Monti M, Berti E, Cavicchini S, Sala F (1983) Unusual cutaneous reaction after gold chloride patch test. Contact Dermatitis 9: 150–151
58. Petros H, Macmillan AL (1973) Allergic contact sensitivity to gold with unusual features. Br J Dermatol 88: 505–508
59. Young E (1974) contact hypersensitivity to metallic gold. Dermatologica 149: 294–298
60. Fisher AA (1974) Metallic gold: the cause of persistent allergic "dermal" contact dermatitis. Cutis 14: 177–180
61. Iwatsuki K, Tagami H, Moriguchi T, Yamada M (1982) Lymphoadenoid structure induced by gold hypersensitivity. Arch Dermatol 118: 608–611
62. Iwatsuki K, Yamada M, Takigawa M, Inoue K, Matsumoto K (1987) benign lymphoplasia of the earlobes induced by gold earrings: Immunohistologic study on the cellular infiltrates. J Am Acad Dermatol 16: 83–88
63. Zenarola P, Lomuto M, Bisceglia M (1993) Hypertrophic amalgam dermatitis of the tongue simulating carcinoma. Contact Dermatitis 29: 157–158
64. Rubin L (1956) Granulomas of axillae caused by deodorants. JAMA 162: 953–955
65. Sheard G (1957) Granulomatous reactions due to deodorant sticks. JAMA 164: 1085–1087
66. Shelley WB, Hurley HJ (1958) Allergic origin of zirconium deodorant granuloma. Brit J Dermato 70: 75–101
67. Williams RM, Skipworth GB (1959) Zirconium granulomas of glabrous skin following treatment of rhus dermatitis. Arch Dermatol 80: 273–276
68. Epstein WL, Allen JR (1964) Granulomatous hypersensitivity after use of zirconium-containing poison oak lotions. JAMA 190: 162–163
69. Baler GR (1965) Granulomas from topical zirconium in poison ivy dermatitis. Arch Dermatol 91: 145–148

70. LoPresti PJ, Hambrick GW (1965) Zirconium granuloma following treatment of rhus dermatitis. Arch Dermatol 92: 188–189
71. Kaaber K, Nielsen AO, Veien NK (1992) Vaccination granulomas and aluminium allergy: course and prognostic factors. Contact Dermatitis 26: 304–306
72. Levy J, Sewell M, Goldstein N (1979) A short history of tattooing. J Derm Surg Oncol 5: 851–583
73. Nguyen LQ, Allen HB (1974) Reactions to manganese and cadmium in tatoos. Cutis 23: 71–72
74. Schwartz RA, Mathias CGT, Miller CH, Rojas-Corona R, Lamber WC (1987) Granulomatous reaction to purple tattoo pigment. Contact Dermatitis 16: 198–202
75. Fisher AA, Chargrin L, Fleischmayer R et al. (1959) Pustular patch test reactions. Arch Dermatol 80: 742–752
76. Stone OJ, Johnson DA (1967) Pustular patch test–experimentally induced. Arch Dermatol 95: 618–619
77. Hjorth N (1977) Diagnostic patch testing. In: Marzulli F Maibach HI (eds) Dermatoxicology and pharmacology. Wiley, New York, pg 344
78. Wahlberg JE, Maibach HI (1981) Sterile cutaneous pustules–a manifestation of primary irritancy? J Invest Dermatol 76: 381–383
79. Burkhart CG (1981) Pustular allergic contact dermatitis: a distinct clinical and pathological entity. Cutis 27: 630–638
80. Conde-Salazar L, Guimaraens D, Romero LV, Yus ES (1983) Subcorneal pustular eruption and erythema from occupational exposure to trichloroethylene. Contact Dermatitis 9: 235–237
81. Schwartz L, Tulipan L, Birmingham A (1947) Occupational diseases of the skin, 3rd ed. Lea and Febiger, Philadelphia, pg 771
82. Bauer M, Rabens SF (1977) Trichloroethylene toxicity. Int J Dermatol 16: 113–116
83. Nakayama H, Bobayashi M, Takahashi M, Ageishi Y, Takano T (1988) Generalized eruption with severe liver dysfunction associated with occupational exposure to trichloroethylene. Contact Dermatitis 19: 48–51
84. Goh CL, Ng SK (1988) A cutaneous manifestation of trichloroethylene toxicity. Contact Dermatitis 18: 59–60
85. Hezemans-Boer M, Toonstra J, Meulenbelt J, Zwaveling JH, Sangster B, van Vloten WA (1988) Skin lesions due to exposure to methyl bromide. Arch Dermatol 124: 917–921
86. Walder BK (1983) Do solvents cause scleroderma? Int J Dermatol 22: 157–158
87. Yamakage A, Ishikawa H (1982) Generalized morphea-like scleroderma occurring in people exposed to organic solvents. Dermatologica 165: 186–193

Chapter 10
Diagnostic Tests

10.1 Patch Testing

JAN E. WAHLBERG

Contents

10.1.1 Introduction

10.1.1.1 The Purpose of Patch Testing

Patch testing is a well-established method of diagnosing allergic contact dermatitis, a delayed type of hypersensitivity (type IV reaction). Patients with a history and clinical picture of contact dermatitis are reexposed to the suspected allergens under controlled conditions to verify the diagnosis. Besides testing patients with hand, arm, face or leg eczema (stasis dermatitis), testing of other types of eczema (atopic, seborrhoeic dermatitis, nummular eczema) is sometimes indicated, especially when the dermatologist suspects contact allergy to prescribed topical medicaments and their vehicles.

Apart from its use to confirm a suspected allergic contact dermatitis, the patch test procedure can also be used before recommending alternative corticosteroids, skin care products, cosmetics, gloves, etc. in a particular patient. If the patient does not react to the alternatives tested, it is very unlikely that she or he will react to the products in ordinary use.

10.1.1.2 Standardization

The first patch tests according to present principles were carried out in 1895 [1], but were preceded by some preliminary experiments [2] (see Chap. 1). During the last few decades much effort has been put into standardization of allergens, vehicles, concentrations, patch test materials, tapes and the scoring of test reactions 24(a) [3], and the method is today considered accurate and reliable. A series of papers has demonstrated good reproducibility of patch test results [4–10]. Standardization has facilitated comparisons of contact allergy frequency in and between clinics and geographical areas, but some questions still remain, especially concerning the reading and scoring of test reactions. This will be discussed in detail below.

10.1.1.3 Bioavailability

To obtain optimal bioavailability of a hapten one can influence the following five variables:
- Intrinsic penetration capacity
- Concentration
- Vehicle
- Occlusivity of patch test system and tape
- Exposure time

Since it is desirable to remove all test strips at the same time–usually at day 2 (48 h) – four factors remain and can be varied and optimized by the manufacturers of patch test materials and allergen preparations and by the dermatologist responsible for the testing. The penetration capacity depends upon the salts used; for example, there is a big difference between the penetration of nickel achieved by nickel sulphate and nickel chloride [11]. The higher penetration of nickel from the chloride is probably explained by the partitioning between skin and vehicle of the salts, when applied in the same vehicle in equimolar concentration and under occlusion.

10.1.2 Test Systems

One can distinguish two test systems, the original one, where the allergens, patches and tapes are supplied separately, and the modern ready-to-use system, where only a covering material has to be removed before the test is applied.

10.1.2.1 Original System (Allergen – Patch – Tape)

10.1.2.1.1 Patches

Some of the patch test units now commercially available are depicted in Fig. 10.1.1. In two (Al-test and Finn Chamber), the test areas are circular (diameters 10 and 8 mm, respectively), and in van der Bend square chambers they are 10 mm square. The latter are claimed to facilitate distinguishing

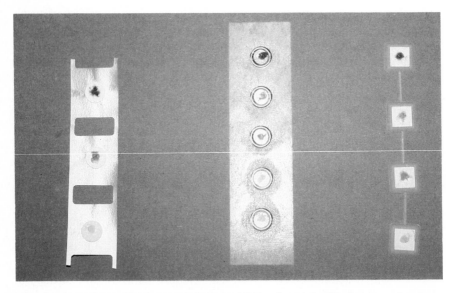

Fig. 10.1.1. Al-test *(left)*, Finn Chambers *(middle)* and van der Bend square chambers *(right)*

allergic reactions from irritant, since an irritant reaction tends to look square, while an allergic reaction tends to look round [12].

10.1.2.1.2 Allergens

The standard patch test allergens sold by Chemotechnique [13] and Hermal [14] can, according to these suppliers' product catalogues, be considered chemically defined and pure. However, the dermatologist responsible for patch testing is recommended repeatedly to request the manufacturers to provide results of chemical analyses.

The test preparations are presented in plastic syringes or bottles of inert material to prevent degradation or other chemical changes due to air, humidity and light. The suppliers' recommendations on storage must be followed in order to minimize these risks. It is suspected that several of the contact allergies reported earlier were due to impurities or degradation products [15]. It has not been possible to confirm the allergenic potential of some claimed 'allergens'.

10.1.2.1.3 Vehicles

Each allergen almost certainly has its own optimal vehicle; it is improbable that just one vehicle (e.g. petrolatum) could be optimal for all allergens. White petrolatum is the most widely used vehicle, but its general reliability may be questioned. It gives good occlusion, keeps the allergens stable and is inexpensive. On the other hand, it can retain the allergen, irritate the skin and even give rise to allergic skin reactions [16]. Liquid vehicles such as water and solvents (acetone, ethanol, methyl ethyl ketone) are recommended since they facilitate penetration into the skin; but they also have some drawbacks. Solvents may evaporate, which does not favour exact dosing, and most test solutions must be freshly prepared. Liquid vehicles are used mainly when testing chemicals and products brought by patients (see Sect.10.1.18), and in research projects.

In the present standard series water is used for formaldehyde and for methylisothiazolinone plus methylchloroisothiazolinone (MI/MCI) (Kathon CG). By using buffer solutions for acid and alkaline products, the test concentration can be raised [17]. A filter paper must be added for liquid allergen preparations when using Finn Chambers. Modern vehicles are hydrophilic gels (cellulose derivates), used, for example, in the TRUE Test [18].

When using more sophisticated vehicles containing salicylic acid, anionic detergents, solvents other than those mentioned above (e.g. dimethyl sulphoxide, DMSO), alkalis, etc. to increase penetration, an extra patch with the vehicle, as is, must be applied to exclude the possibility that the vehicle is irritant. Since the number of test sites is limited, these vehicles cannot be recommended for routine use. However, they might be valuable where the standard preparation has given a negative reaction but the clinical impression of an allergic contact dermatitis remains.

10.1.2.1.4 Concentrations

In textbooks on contact dermatitis and patch testing, and in suppliers' catalogues, the concentration of an allergen is normally given as a percentage. In one catalogue [13] molality (M) is given together with percentage (weight/weight), and in the TRUE Test concentration is given in milligrams per square centimeter. The traditional method of presenting concentrations as a percentage is simple and probably practical, but has been questioned [19, 20], as we do not know if this means weight/weight, volume/volume, volume/weight or weight/volume. Especially when comparing substances and in research projects, it is the number of moles applied that is of interest [21]. The concentration of Ni ions is 20.9% in nickel sulphate ($NiSO_4$ $7H_2O$) compared to 24.7% in nickel chloride ($NiCl_2 \cdot 6H_2O$) [22]. Thus in comparative studies with these salts it is essential to use the same molality [23].

10.1.2.1.5 Tapes

Previously, most tapes were based on colophony and could cause severe and lasting reactions in patients for whom such a sensitivity was not anticipated. By introducing modern acrylate-based adhesive tapes, for example, Scanpor (Norgesplaster, Kristiansand, Norway), the problem has been almost completely eliminated. Finn Chambers on Scanpor tape are commercially available. In cases where loosening can be anticipated (oily or hairy skin, sweating, high humidity) some reinforcing tapes are recommended.

10.1.2.1.6 Application of Test Preparations to the Patches

Commercial test preparations–allergens in petrolatum and kept in syringes–are applied directly into the Finn Chambers, or onto the filter paper discs of the other patches. A small amount, 'a snake', of the mixture is applied across the diameter of the disc. The orifice of the syringe is adjusted to facilitate this.

Liquid test preparations are preferably applied via a digital pipette with disposable plastic tips to allow exact dosing (15 μl). Ordinary glass bottles cannot be recommended until it can be shown that they give adequate and reproducible dosing with different types of allergen mixtures. Bottles introduced by Blohm [24] and Pirilä [25] seem to fulfil these criteria.

10.1.2.1.7 Some Practical Suggestions

Storage. The allergens should be kept in a cool dark place (refrigerator) to minimize degradation. However, wool alcohols to be applied to the patches must be at room temperature, otherwise it is difficult to squeeze them from the syringes. Allergens diluted in liquids (water, solvents) should be kept in dark bottles.

Sequence of Allergens. Adjust the sequence of the allergens so that those frequently causing strong, cross or concomitant reactions are not adjacent. The order given in the catalogues [13, 14] can usually be followed.

Testing in Pregnancy. Do not test pregnant women! There are no indications that the minute amounts of allergens absorbed in patch testing could influence the fetus, but in cases of miscarriage or deformity it is natural to blame several things, including medical investigations.

Test Sites. The preferred site is the upper back. For a small number of allergens, for example at retesting, the outer aspect of the upper arm is also acceptable. False-negative test results can be obtained when testing on the lower back or on the volar forearms (see Sect. 10.1.11.1).

Removal of Hair. On hairy areas of the back it is difficult to get acceptable skin contact, and for this reason clipping is recommended. However, a combination of clipping, petrolatum and tapes sometimes contributes to the irritation seen, which may make reading somewhat difficult.

Degreasing of Test Site. In cases of oily skin, gentle treatment with ethanol or another mild solvent is recommended. The solvent must evaporate before the test strips are applied.

Application of Test Strips. Test strips should be applied from below with mild pressure to remove air pouches, followed by some moderate strokes with the back of the hand to improve adhesion [26].

Marking. Several solutions, inks or marking pens are available [26–28]. If test strips with constant distances between the discs are used, only one mark is needed.

Positive Control. To be sure that the test patches have adhered properly we use nonanoic acid as a positive control at my clinic. This irritant gives a slight, red-to-brown, well-defined reaction which is easy to read [29, 30].

Instructions. We have found it valuable to inform our patients as to the aim of the test; about avoidance of showers, wetting the test site, irradiation and excessive exercise; and about symptoms such as itch, loosening of patches and late reactions. Examples of such written instructions and guidelines for patients are available [12, 28].

Reading. The light should be good when reading the test (sidelighting may be of help) and adjustable. A magnifying lamp or lens is often of help. To facilitate reading, the Finn Chamber system has a special reading plate with punched-out holes corresponding to the test sites.

10.1.2.2 Ready-to-Use System

In a ready-to-use patch test system, all necessary material is prepared in advance and the dermatologist, nurse or technician has only to remove the covering material, apply the test strips and mark. In the TRUE Test system [18], the allergens are incorporated in hydrophilic gels and the patches are 9 mm square (Fig. 10.1.2).

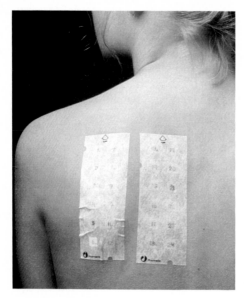

Fig. 10.1.2. TRUE Test system

Some comparative studies have been carried out with TRUE Test versus Finn Chambers 31–35 and other studies are under way.

The accuracy, reliability, simplicity and costs of these new systems must be balanced by the costs, including personnel, of the original systems (Sect. 10.1.2.1).

10.1.3 Allergens

10.1.3.1 Numbers

According to de Groot [36], some 2800 contact allergens are known. New ones are identified each year when carrying out predictive testing and when examining and testing patients with contact dermatitis.

10.1.3.2 Suppliers

The catalogues from the suppliers (Chemotechnique Diagnostics AB [13], Ringugnsgatan 7, S-216 16 Malmö, Sweden; Hermal Kurt Herrman (Trolab) [14], P.O. Box 1228, D-2057 Reinbeck//Hamburg, Germany) contain lists of approximately 300 allergens in alphabetical order, allergens in the European standard series, tables of mixes and lists of screening series. The catalogues also contain information on the occurrence of allergens and cross-reactivity, and also some service items such as test sheets, guides to patch testing, marking pens, questionnaires and advice to patients.

10.1.3.3 Screening Series

To evaluate the significance of special exposures, mainly occupational, a number of screening series are available (Table 10.1.1). They are compiled from the experience gathered at departments of occupational dermatology, and from the literature [37]. Newly defined allergens are added regularly and these series can be considered to cover the present exposure situation.

Table 10.1.1. Commercially available screening series

Chemotechnique [13]	Hermal [14]
Bakery	Antimicrobials, preservatives
Corticosteroid	Dental materials
Cosmetic	Hairdressing
Dental	Local anaesthetics
Epoxy	Medicaments
Fragrance	Metal compounds
Hairdressing	Miscellaneous
Isocyanate	Organic dyes
Medicament	Perfumes, flavours
(Meth)acrylate	Pesticides
Adhesives, dental, other	Photoallergens
(Meth)acrylate	Photographic chemicals
Nails-artificial	Plants, woods
(Meth)acrylate	Plastic, glues
Printing	Rubber chemicals
Oil, cooling fluid	Sunscreen agents
Photographic chemicals	Tars, balsams
Plant	Textile finishes
Plastics, glues	Vehicles, emulsifiers
Rubber additives	
Scandinavian photopatch	
Shoe	
Sunscreen	
Textile colours, finish	
Various allergens	

However, the allergens are pure chemicals and if the original offending agent was an impurity, a degradation product, etc., the cause will be missed. A supplementary test with the patient's own working materials should be done in those cases where the test with the screening series was negative but the suspicion of allergic contact dermatitis remains. A matter of dispute is the ethical question: Should a patient be tested with a number of well-known contact allergens to which he or she has never been exposed and what is the risk of patch test sensitization? (see Sect. 10.1.13).

10.1.3.4 Variations Concerning Concentration and Vehicle

Catalogues [13, 14] and textbooks on contact dermatitis and patch testing [12, 20, 28, 38–40] show slight differences in recommendations on concentrations and vehicles. There are thus no ultimate test preparations that are optimal in all clinics or geographical areas. Patch and tape occlusion, humidity, temperature and other climatic factors, local experience and tradition can motivate deviations from these recommendations. However, the test preparations offered in the catalogues are based on tests of several thousand patients and must be considered very useful guidelines when setting up and running a patch test clinic.

10.1.4 Standard Series

The present European standard series contains 23 items, but six of them are *mixes,* so in fact at least 24 additional allergens are applied. Balsam of Peru, colophony and lanolin are examples of *natural* mixes, where much effort has been spent to identify the allergens [41–44]. The basic idea of using mixes instead of single allergens is to save time and space. Also, the patients are tested with a number of closely related substances, among others, rubber chemicals. The screening capacity of the standard series is thereby greatly increased. However, the value of these mixes is sometimes questioned. It is difficult to find an optimal concentration for each allergen in a common vehicle (usually petrolatum) and do the allergens metabolize or interact to potentiate or quench a reaction [45]?

At my clinic we use the mixes for screening purposes, positive cases being retested with the ingredients. Not unusually, these tests are negative and we then have to ask ourselves whether the initial reaction was an expression of irritancy and/or whether the ingredients have interacted. The opposite has also been noticed. The patient may be negative to a particular mix, but react when retested with its ingredients.

The allergens of the standard series are presented in detail in Chap. 13 and the test concentrations in Chap. 22.

10.1.5 Deciding What to Include in the Standard Series

The original standard series was based on the experience of the members of the International Contact Dermatitis Research Group and mirrored the findings and current situation in different parts of Europe and the United States. The series is evaluated regularly by national and international contact dermatitis groups. Each test clinic is recommended to compile its patch test results yearly. If the frequency of positive reactions to a particular allergen is less than 1%, its presence in a standard series can be questioned and it should probably be replaced by another compound. In these ways, the standard series continually changes in composition and in the total number of substances included.

The new allergens are often preservatives. Methylisothiazolinone + methylchloroisothiazolinone (MI/MCI) (Kathon CG) can be mentioned as a typical recent example. The first cases were observed in southern Sweden in 1980 [46] and isothiazolinone then became an almost universal allergen, with local epidemics in Finland, the Netherlands, Italy and Switzerland [47]. It was included in the Swedish standard series in 1985 and in the European standard series in 1988 [48].

Nowadays, following local epidemics, conference reports and communications in scientific journals, several patch test clinics may choose to include a newly identified allergen in their standard series to investigate the frequency in their geographical area. If the initial reports can be confirmed and the allergen is diffused in many and various products, it is then recommended for inclusion in the standard series.

At a joint meeting of the International and European Environmental and Contact Dermatitis Research Groups [48], it was recommended to include MI/MCI and at the same meeting some other changes in the tray were made: carba mix (three rubber chemicals) was removed and replaced by another rubber chemical (mercaptobenzothiazole); p-phenylenediamine hydrochloride was replaced by the corresponding free base and the concentration was raised from 0.5% to 1.0%. The groups' official recommendations for changes can be read by all interested parties, which also gives opportunities for questions and discussion.

10.1.6 Reading: When and How

The reading should be done by the dermatologist him- or herself, after adequate training.

10.1.6.1 Exposure Time

Most authors advocate an exposure time of 2 days (48 h). A few comparisons of 1-day (24-h) and 2-day (48-h) allergen exposure show some reactions positive only at day 1 (D1) and some positive only at day 2 (D2) [49]. No definite conclusions can be drawn from the studies published so far.

It would be convenient for the patient, and probably for the dermatologist, if the exposure time could be reduced to 1 day (24 h) with retained accuracy. For this, the penetration capacity of the hapten must be increased, among other things by using higher concentrations, more efficacious vehicles and optimal occlusion. Working out these parameters for all existing allergens, however, would be an overwhelming task.

10.1.6.2 Reading When?

Wherever possible, it is strongly recommended that two readings be carried out, the first after removal of the patches (day 2) and the second 2–4 days later [50, 51]. In a recent study, paired readings on days 4 and 7 were found more reliable than those on days 2 and 4 [52]. If the patches are applied for only 1 day, readings should be at days 1, 2 and 3.

If they are removed at the dermatologist's clinic or office, it is possible to check that they have adhered properly and that the marking is adequate. One should wait at least 15–30 min after their removal, since the combination of allergen, vehicle, patches and tape causes a transient increase in skin blood flow, a sign of irritation [53]. At the second reading it is possible to record what reactions have turned negative and what reactions have become apparent and/or increased or decreased in intensity. Neomycin and corticosteroids are examples of allergens with late appearance.

A reaction positive on day 2 and negative on day 4 is usually considered to indicate irritancy. There are some anecdotal examples where such a pattern has been found to be clinically relevant, but the frequency is not known. To contribute to the confusion, a few substances are known to cause 'delayed irritancy' [12].

10.1.6.3 A Compromise

If practical or geographical circumstances permit only one reading, the commonly accepted compromise is at day 3 (72 h), i.e. 1 day after removal of the patches. In a recent paper [52] it was stated that a single reading on day 4 would have been most useful. Patients are instructed to report any late reactions.

10.1.7 Recording of Results

The common method of recording patch test reactions, recommended by the International Contact Dermatitis Research Group [27], is presented in Table 10.1.2. These recommendations are followed worldwide and are referred to in most scientific reports. Typical examples are shown in Fig. 10.1.3.

Table 10.1.2. Recording of patch test reactions according to the ICDRG [27]

?+	Doubtful reaction; faint erythema only
+	Weak positive reaction; erythema, infiltration, possibly papules
++	Strong positive reaction; erythema, infiltration, papules, vesicles
+++	Extreme positive reaction; intense erythema and infiltration and coalescing vesicles
IR	Irritant reaction of different types
NT	Not tested

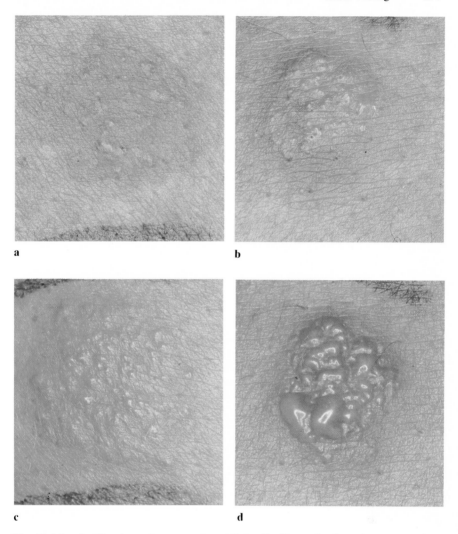

Fig. 10.1.3a–d. Allergic patch test reactions (all day 3) of in reasing intensity. *a* + reaction to nickel sulphate. *b* still a + reaction to *p*-phenylenediamine (PPD). *c* ++ reaction to PPD. *d* + + + reaction to PPD. (Courtesy of P.J. Frosch)

However, this recording system is somewhat simplified and not all types of reaction fit this outline. Irritant reactions (IR) are said [12, 26, 38] to be characterized by: fine wrinkling ('silk paper'), erythema and papules in follicular distribution, petechiae, pustules, bullae and necrosis and with minimal infiltration. Typical examples are shown in Fig. 10.1.4. They smart instead of itch. Extension beyond the defined area exposed to the allergen is used to discriminate between allergic and irritant reactions [12].

It is recommended that forms are used with space for additional notes on the morphological appearance of the test reactions. Especially when repeated

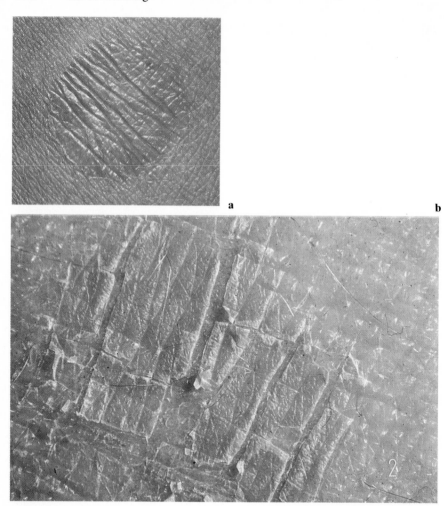

Fig. 10.1.4 a,b. Irritant reactions. *a* Soap effect: typical irritant reaction with glistening of the stratum corneum after a 2-day exposure to a 1% solution of toilet soap. *b* Irritant reaction with redness and scaling after repetitive application of an 8% soap solution over 4 days (soap chamber test according to Frosch and Kligman)

readings are taken, or lesser-known or new substances have been applied, it is essential to follow the appearance and disappearance of the various components of the reactions. Pictures can be of value for documentation, but can rarely replace our traditional aids: inspection and palpation.

10.1.8 Interpretation of Results

Some important and somewhat controversial issues will now be discussed.

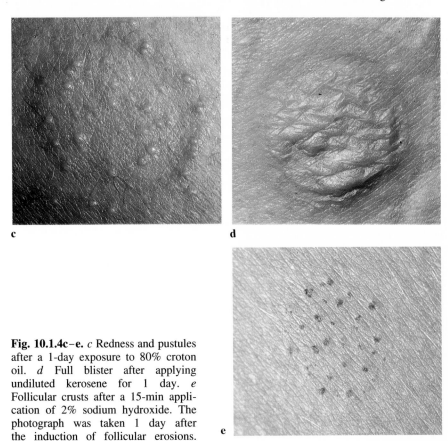

Fig. 10.1.4c–e. *c* Redness and pustules after a 1-day exposure to 80% croton oil. *d* Full blister after applying undiluted kerosene for 1 day. *e* Follicular crusts after a 15-min application of 2% sodium hydroxide. The photograph was taken 1 day after the induction of follicular erosions. (Courtesy of P.J. Frosch)

10.1.8.1 'Positive' Reactions

The word 'positive' merely indicates some kind of change at a test site compared to adjacent, nontested skin: it is not synonymous with 'allergic' or 'relevant'!

10.1.8.2 Discrimination of Allergic Versus Irritant Reactions

To distinguish allergic reactions from irritant reactions on morphological grounds alone is difficult. Fisher [28] frankly states: "There is no morphological way of distinguishing a weak irritant patch test from a weak allergic test." Examples are benzalkonium chloride and MC/MCI, where there has been much discussion concerning the somewhat peculiar features of the test reactions.

In Table 10.1.3 the results from a serial dilution test with nickel sulphate are shown. At dilution step 5(0.01%), a few papules have been recorded and in this case we *know* that the reaction is relevant and that this patient is highly sensitive. However, if "a few papules" are noticed in another patient, where only one concentration of an allergen has been applied, the interpretation is much more difficult, Usually, we have to repeat the test probably to raise the concentration and/or carry out a serial dilution test.

Table 10.1.3. Results of a serial dilution test with nickel sulphate in a patient who had previously reacted to 5.0% $(+++)$

Dilution step		Score
1.	1.0%	$+++$
2.	0.3%	$++$
3.	0.1%	$+$
4.	0.03%	$+$
5.	0.01%	a few papules
6.	0.003%	?
7.	0.001%	$-$
8.	0.0003%	$-$

10.1.8.3 Ring-Shaped Test Reactions

The somewhat peculiar ring-shaped test reactions, the 'edge effect', observed with, among other allergens, formaldehyde, MC/MCI and hydrocortisone in liquid vehicles are in most cases an expression of contact allergy [54].

10.1.8.4 Ultrastructure

For distinguishing between allergic and irritant patch test reactions, traditional light or electronic microscopy has been of minimal help (see Chap. 3). Monoclonal antibody techniques are somewhat more promising [55].

10.1.8.5 'One plus'

When vesicles are present there is rarely any discussion of the allergic nature of the reaction, but the presence or absence of papules is more controversial. As can be seen from Table 10.1.2, "possibly papules" is included in the 1+ reaction. This expression can be interpreted in different ways: Is erythema plus infiltration enough for a reaction to be scored 1+? What about erythema and papules, but no infiltration? According to Cronin [38], 1+ is a palpable erythema. When such a weak reaction has been obtained we recommend, as discussed in Sect. 10.1.8.2, repeating the test, increasing the concentration by a factor of 5 or 10, and carrying out a serial dilution test (Table 10.1.3) and a repeated open application test (Sect. 10.1.15.2).

Consensus on the denomination and interpretation of weak reactions such as ?, ?+ and + would be of great value and would facilitate comparisons between clinics and geographical areas.

10.1.8.6 Cross-Sensitivity

In cross-sensitivity, contact allergy caused by a primary allergen is combined with allergy to other chemically closely related substances. In those patients who have become sensitized to one substance, an allergic contact dermatitis can be provoked or worsened by several other related substances. A patient positive to *p*-phenylenediamine not only reacts to the dye itself, but also to immunochemically related substances which have an amino group in the *para* position, e.g. azo compounds, local anaesthetics and sulphonamides. When studying cross-sensitivity it is essential to use pure test compounds [15].

10.1.9 Relevance

Evaluating the relevance of a reaction is the most difficult and intricate part of the patch test procedure, and is a challenge to both dermatologist and patient. The dermatologist's skill, experience and curiosity are crucial factors.

For standard allergens, detailed lists are available that present the occurrence of each in the environment. The patient and the dermatologist should study the lists together, in order to judge the relevance of a positive patch test reaction, in relation to the exposure, site, course and relapses of the patient's current dermatitis. A positive test reaction can also be explained by a previous, unrelated episode of contact dermatitis (past relevance).

Sometimes the relevance of a positive reaction remains unexplained until the patient brings a package or bottle where the allergen in question is named on the label. In other cases, chemical analyses demonstrate the presence of the allergen, or the manufacturer finally, after many inquiries, admits that the offending substance is present in the product.

In cosmetics, skin care products, detergents, paints, cutting fluids, glues, etc., it is common that new ingredients are added or replace previous ones, but the product keeps its original trade name. Alternatively, well-known allergens are included in new products but with other fields of application than the original. To discover the cause of the patient's dermatitis the dermatologist must sometimes be obstinately determined!

10.1.10 False-Positive Test Reactions

A false-positive reaction is a positive patch test reaction in the absence of contact allergy [56]. The most common causes can be summarized as follows:

---

1. Too high a test concentration for that particular patient
2. Impure or contaminated test substance
3. The vehicle is irritant (especially solvents and sometimes petrolatum)
4. Excess of test preparation applied
5. The test substance, usually as crystals, is unevenly dispersed in the vehicle
6. Current or recent dermatitis at test site
7. Current dermatitis at distant skin sites
8. Pressure effects, mechanical irritation of solid test materials, furniture and garments
9. Adhesive tape reactions
10. The patch itself has caused the reactions
11. Artefacts

Some are self-evident and can be predicted and monitored by the dermatologist carrying out patch testing, while others cannot.

10.1.10.1 The Compromise (Item 1)

While the current recommendations on allergen concentrations in relation to vehicle, patch and tapes are based on long experience, they are nevertheless a compromise! The general problem is that if you lower the concentration to avoid irritancy you will also lose some cases which will be of special occupational and medicolegal importance. Well-known examples are dichromate, formaldehyde, tars, fragrance mix and, previously, carba mix. It is probably better to have a (weak) false-positive reaction than a false-negative reaction because at least with a potentially false-positive reaction one is *alerted* to the possibility of allergy, which one can the confirm or deny, whereas with a false-negative reaction one is never alerted at all and may altogether miss a true allergy. Therefore, most dermatologists seem to prefer the higher concentrations of these marginal irritants, even though they know that nonspecific reactions from them are not uncommon.

10.1.10.2 Excited-Skin Syndrome– 'Angry Back' (Items 6 and 7)

In the excited-skin syndrome, the presence of a strong positive reaction will influence the reactivity at adjacent test sites. When more than one site shows a reaction, this phenomenon must be considered, and retesting of the items one at a time is the usual recommendation. Thanks to Björnberg's [57] important observations, we have always avoided patch testing a patient with current eczema and labile skin, and the excited-skin syndrome is seldom seen in our latitudes [58]. There is an extensive literature on this syndrome [59].

10.1.10.3 The Patch (Item 10)

After receiving intradermal allergen extracts due to pollen allergy, a few patients will develop sensitivity to aluminium. They will then react to Al-test as well as to Finn Chambers. Mercury-containing test preparations can react with aluminium, but nowadays plastic-coated Finn Chambers are available.

10.1.10.4 Artefacts (Item 11)

Sometimes strong necrotic reactions are seen and an artefact is suspected. In medicolegal cases, it is recommended that control patches (empty or containing water or petrolatum) be applied simultaneously and in random order.

10.1.11 False-Negative Test Reactions

10.1.11.1 Common Causes

A false-negative reaction is a negative patch test reaction in the presence of contact allergy [56]. The most common causes can be summarized as follows:

---

1. Insufficient penetration of the allergen
   a) Too low a test concentration for that particular patient
   b) The test substance is not released from the vehicle or retained by the filter paper
   c) Insufficient amount of test preparation applied
   d) Insufficient occlusion
   e) Duration of contact too brief: the test strip has fallen off or slipped
   f) The test was not applied to the recommended site: the upper back
2. The reading is made too early, e.g. neomycin and corticosteroids are known to give delayed reactions
3. The test site has been treated with corticosteroids or irradiated with UV or Grenz rays
4. Systemic treatment with corticosteroids or immunomodulators
5. Allergen is not in active form, insufficiently oxidized (oil of turpentine, rosin compounds) or degraded
6. Compound allergy

Some of these are self-evident and can be predicted and monitored by the dermatologist, while others cannot. Examples of the latter category may arise when testing has been carried out in a refractory or 'anergic' phase; when the test does not reproduce the clinical exposure (multiple applications), where some adjuvant factors are present (sweating, friction, pressure, damaged skin); or when penetration at the test site is lower than that of clinical exposure (eyelids, axillae). A stripped skin technique is recommended in the last case, where the test sites are stripped with tape before application of test preparations.

The differential diagnoses photoallergy and contact urticaria should also be considered.

10.1.11.2 Compound Allergy (Item 6)

The term 'compound allergy' is used to describe the condition in patients who are patch test positive to formulated products, usually cosmetic creams or topical medicaments, but are test negative to all the ingredients tested individually [60]. This phenomenon can sometimes be explained by irritancy of the original formulation, but in some cases it has been demonstrated that reactivity was due to combination of the ingredients to form reaction products [61, 62]. Another reason might be that the ingredients were patch tested at the usage concentrations in petrolatum, which are too low for many allergens (e.g. MI/MCI, neomycin). Pseudo compound allergy, due to faulty patch testing technique, is likely to be commoner than true compound allergy. This topic remains the subject of continuing debate [63, 64].

10.1.12 Effect of Medicaments and Irradiation on Patch Tests

10.1.12.1 Corticosteroids

Treatment of test sites with topical corticosteroids [65] can give rise to false-negative reactions (Sect. 10.1.11.1).

Testing a patient on oral corticosteroids always creates uncertainty. The problem was studied 15–20 years ago [66–68] by comparing the intensity of test reactions before and during treatment with corticosteroids (20–40 mg prednisone). Diminution and disappearance of test reactions were noted in several cases, but not regularly. These findings have been interpreted as allowing us to test patients on oral doses equivalent to 20 mg prednisone without missing any important allergies. However, the test reactions studied were strong (3+, 4+), and fairly weak (1+) and questionable reactions were not evaluated. At my clinic we prefer to defer testing until the patient's dermatitis has cleared. When testing a patient with labile skin there is also the risk of excited-skin syndrome [69]. In selected cases where one or two allergens are strongly suspected, we choose to test for these only, even if the patient is on oral corticosteroids. However, when the dermatitis has cleared, we repeat the test with the whole series to relieve our uncertainty.

10.1.12.2 Antihistamines

In one study [67], the antihistamine Incidal did not influence reactivity, while in another [69] a decrease in intensity was seen in 6 out of 17 patients after cinnarizine had been administered for 1 week. These results also give the dermatologist a feeling of uncertainty, and we prefer either to discontinue anthistamine treatment during testing or to defer testing. However, this contraindication is not universally accepted.

10.1.12.3 Immunomodulators

Topical cyclosporine inhibits test reactions in humans and in animal models [70–72]. There is so far no comparison of test reactions in allergic patients before and during treatment with orally or parenterally administered cytostatic agents.

10.1.12.4 Irradiation

It has been shown that irradiation with UVB [73] and Grenz rays [74, 75] reduces the number of Langerhans cells and the intensity of patch test reactions in man. Repeated suberythema doses of UVB depressed reactivity even at sites shielded during the exposures. This indicates a systemic effect of UVB [73]. Experiments to clarify the mechanism behind these observations have been carried out in experimental animals, but their relevance to man are not yet settled.

From a practical point of view it can be stated that the number of positives is not much influenced by season of the year. However, we recommend avoidance of patch testing on severely tanned persons and that a minimum of 4 weeks after heavy sun exposure should be allowed before testing.

10.1.13 Complications

The most common complications of patch testing are:

1. Patch test sensitization (see below)
2. Irritant reactions from nonstandard allergens or products brought by the patient
3. Flare of previous or existing dermatitis due to percutaneous absorption of the allergen
4. Depigmentation, e.g. phenols
5. Pigmentation, sometimes after sunlight exposure of test sites
6. Scars, keloids

7. Granulomas from beryllium, zirconium
8. Anaphylactoid reactions or shock from, e.g., neomycin, bacitracin
   (regarding penicillin, see below)
9. Infections (bacteria, virus)

Most can be predicted and avoided.

10.1.13.1 Patch Test Sensitization (Item 1)

By definition, a negative patch test reaction followed by a flare-up after 10–20 days, and then a positive reaction after 3 days at retesting, means that sensitization was induced by the patch test procedure. There is a risk of active sensitization from the standard series and common examples are *p*-phenylenediamine, primula extracts and, in recent years, isothiazolinone [46] and a bleach accelerator (PBA-1)[76]. The risk however, is *an extremely low one* when the testing is carried out according to internationally accepted guidelines. Sensitization by a patch test very rarely causes the patient any subsequent dermatitis or affects the course of a previous dermatitis.

It must be emphasized that the overall *risk-benefit* equation of patch testing patients is much in favour of the benefit. On the other hand, we advise against 'prophetic' patch testing of nondermatitic potential employees, because in that case the risk-benefit equation is vey much in favour of the risk of active sensitization.

10.1.13.2 Penicillin (Item 8)

Penicillin can give rise to anaphylactoid reactions or shock and is therefore not recommended for routine patch testing. To minimize the risk, which is also essential from a medicolegal point of view, we recommend radioallergosorbent tests, an oral provocation test with half or one tablet of penicillin and an open test prior to the closed patch test.

10.1.14 Open Tests

'Open test' and 'use test' (see Sect. 10.1.15) are sometimes used as synonyms and no clearcut definitions seem to exist. Open testing usually means that a product, as is or dissolved in water or some solvent (e.g. ethanol, acetone or ether), is dropped onto the skin and allowed to spread freely. No occlusion is used.

An open test is recommended as the first step when testing poorly defined or unknown substances or products, such as those brought by the patient (paints, glues, oils, detergents, cleansing agents based on solvents, etc.). The test site should be checked at regular intervals during the first 30–60 min after application, especially when the history indicates immediate reactions or contact urticaria (Chap. 7). A second reading should be done at 3–4 days.

The usual test site is the volar forearm, but this is less reactive than the back or the upper arms. A negative open test can be explained by insufficient penetration, but indicates that one dares to go on with an occlusive patch test.

10.1.15 Use Tests

10.1.15.1 Purpose

The original (provocative) use (or usage) tests were intended to mimic the actual use situation (repeated open applications) of a formulated product such as a cosmetic, a shampoo, an oil or a topical medicament. A positive result supported the suspicion that the product had caused the patient's dermatitis. The primary goal was not to clarify the nature (allergic or irritant) of the dermatitis – just to reproduce it!

Nowadays these tests are increasingly used to evaluate the clinical significance of ingredient(s) of a formulated product previously found reactive by ordinary patch testing. The concentration of the particular ingredient can be so low that one may wonder whether the positive patch test reaction can explain the patient's dermatitis.

10.1.15.2 Repeated Open Application Test

The repeated open application test (ROAT) in a standardized form was introduced by Hannuksela and Salo [77]. Test substances, either commercial products, as is, or special test substances (e.g. patch test allergen), are applied twice daily for 7 days to the outer aspect of the upper arm, antecubital fossa or back skin (scapular area). The size of the test area is not crucial: a positive result may appear on a 1×1 cm area 1–2 days later than on a larger area. The amount of test substance should be approx. 0.1 ml to a 5×5 cm area and 0.5 ml to a 10×10 cm area [78, 79]. A positive response – eczematous dermatitis – usually appears on days 2–4. The patient is told to stop the application of the test substance(s) when he or she notices the reaction [77].

If a ROAT is carried out with a formulated product, the observed reaction may be due to allergy to an ingredient, but irritancy from other ingredients cannot be excluded. At my clinic we therefore use two coded samples, one containing the allergen and one without it. We instruct the patient to apply one product to the left arm and the other to the right arm, according to a special protocol where the treatments and any observed reaction can be noted. If there is a reaction only at the test site where the allergen-containing product has been applied, we consider the initial patch test reaction relevant. On the other hand, we interpret reactions of the same intensity on both arms as an expression of irritancy. The value of ROAT has been verified both in cases with positive [46] and negative or questionable reactions at initial patch testing.

10.1.16 Noninvasive Techniques

To reduce the well-known interindividual variation when scoring patch test reactions, several attempts have been made to introduce objective bioengineering techniques for assessment. Erythema and skin colour can be assessed by laser Doppler flowmetry (LDF), skin reflectance and colorimeters, and oedema with calipers and ultrasound. The advantages and limitations of these methods have recently been reviewed [80]. These sophisticated techniques cannot replace visual assessment and palpation of test sites by the dermatologist, but are valuable in research work.

A significant correlation between visual scoring of patch test reactions and LDF values was found by Staberg et al. [81]. The method discriminated between negative and positive reactions, but failed to quantify strongly positive reactions. However, it has also been shown that the combination of allergen, vehicle, patch and tape will cause a transient increase in skin blood flow, even in healthy subjects [53]. An increase was noticed for 1–2 days after removal of the patches, without causing any visual changes. Skin blood flow must be increased 3–4 times before the naked eye can detect an erythema [82].

10.1.17 Quality Control of Test Materials

10.1.17.1 Identification and Purity

As pointed out above (Sect 10.1.2.1.2), the dermatologist is recommended to obtain protocols of chemical analyses and data on purity from suppliers of test preparations. Some dermatologists have the laboratory facilities to check the information presented, but most just have to accept it. Especially when 'new' allergens are detected, in cases of unexpected multiple reactivity or suspected cross-reactivity, detailed information on purity and chemical identification of the allergen is indispensable [15]. Some mixes, such as fragrance mix, contain emulsifiers (sorbitan sesquioleate) and a correct retest with ingredients of a mix should thus include the individual frangrances as well as the emulsifier.

10.1.17.2 Test Preparations Under the Microscope

Light microscope examination (magnification $\times$ 100–400 of commercial test preparations with petrolatum as vehicle is usually disappoiting [83–86]. Crystals of different sizes are seen and one wonders how this influences the bioavailability of the allergen. However, in one comparative study no difference in reactivity was found [87].

In the TRUE Test, the allergens are incorporated in hydrophilic gels and are evenly distributed [18].

10.1.17.3 Fresh Samples

In cases of unexpected negative test reactions, the items listed in Sect. 10.1.11.1 should be considered. If the case remains unsolved, it is suggested that a fresh sample of the allergen be purchased from a different supplier.

10.1.18 Tests with Unknown Substances

10.1.18.1 Warning

A word of warning: totally unknown substances of products should never be applied to human skin! Scarring, necrosis, keloids, pigmentation, depigmentation, systemic effects following percutaneous absorption and any other complications listed earlier can appear and the dermatologist may be accused of malpractice.

10.1.18.2 Strategy

When patients bring suspected products or materials from their (work) environment we recommend that product safety data sheets, lists of ingredients, etc. are requested from the manufacturer so that a general impression of the product, ingredients, concentrations, intended use, etc. can be formed. There are usually one or two ingredients that are of interest as suspected allergens, while the rest are well-known substances of proven innocuousness for which detailed information is available. For substances or products where skin contact is unintentional and the dermatitis is a result of misuse or accident, detailed information from the manufacturer is required before any tests are initiated.

10.1.18.3 Test or Not?

The next step is to look for the suspected allergens. If they are available from suppliers of patch test allergens [5, 6], one can rely on the choice of vehicle and concentration. If one suspects impurities or contaminants have caused the dermatitis, this can only be discovered via samples of the ingredient from the manufacturer.

If it is an entirely new substance, where no data on toxicity etc. are available, patient and dermatologist have to decide how to find an optimal test concentration and vehicle, and to discuss the risk of complications. To minimize the risk, one can start with an open test and, if this is negative, continue with occlusive patch testing. Most allergens are tested in the concentration range 0.01%–10% and we usually start with the lowest and raise the concentration when the preceding test is negative. A very practical method is to apply 0.01% and 0.1% for one day in a region where the patient can easily remove the patch her- or himself (upper back or upper arm). If severe stinging or burning occurs, he or she should be instructed to remove it immediately. If the test is negative, the concentration can be raised to 1%. Occasionally, the likely irritant or sensitization potential of a chemical may be such that starting with concentrations of 0.001% and 0.01% is advisable, increasing if negative to 0.1%. An alternative is to start with a higher concentration, but with reduced exposure time (5 h) [88]; but this procedure is not sufficiently standardized.

If the test is positive in the patient, one has to demonstrate in at least 10–20 unexposed controls that the actual test preparation is nonirritant. Otherwise the observed reaction in the particular patient does not prove allergenicity. When testing products brought by the patient, it is essential to use samples from the actual batch to which the patient has been exposed, but when testing, for example, cutting fluids, unused products must be tested for comparison. When testing with dilutions, one runs the risk of overlooking true allergens by using overdiluted materials.

10.1.18.4 Solid Products and Extracts

When a solid product is suspected (textiles, rubber, plants, wood, paper, etc.), these can usually be applied as is. Rycroft [56] recommends that the material be tested as wafer-thin, regular-sided, smooth sheets (e.g. rubber) or as finely divided particulates (e.g. woods). Plants and woods and their extracts constitute special problems, due to variations in the quantity of allergens produced and their availability on the surface. Extracts for testing can be obtained by placing the product or sample in water, synthetic sweat, ethanol, acetone or ether, and heating to 40°–50°C. False reactions to nonstandardized patch tests have been reviewed by Rycroft [56].

10.1.18.5 Cosmetics and Similar Products

For most products intended for use on normal or damaged skin (cosmetics, skin care products, soap, shampoos, detergents, topical medicaments, etc.), detailed predicitve testing and clinical and consumer trials have been performed. The results can usually be obtained from the manufacturer. For this category of products, open tests and use tests probably give more information on the pathogenesis of the patient's dermatitis than an occlusive patch test does. Suggestions on concentrations and vehicles can be found in textbooks [26, 36].

10.1.19 The Future

This section is concluded with the following list of hopes and needs for the future:
- Diversified vehicles to obtain optimal bioavailability of allergens
- Statements in suppliers' catalogues on purity and stability of individual allergens
- Decrease of test exposure times with retained accuracy
- Consensus on the reading, scoring, interpretation and relevance of weak test reactions
- Objective assessment of test reactions
- Further standardization of use tests

10.1.20 References

1. Jadassohn J (1896) Zur Kenntnis der medikamentösen Dermatosen, Verhandlungen der Deutschen Dermatologischen Gesellschaft. Fünfter Congress, Raz, 1895. Braunmuller, Vienna, p 106
2. Foussereau J (1984) History of epicutaneous testing: the blotting-paper and other methods. Contact Dermatitis 11: 219–223
3. Fischer TI, Hansen J, Kreilgård B, Maibach HI (1989) The science of patch test standardization. Immunol Allergy Clin N Am 9: 417–443
4. Belsito DV, Storrs FJ, Taylor JS et al. (1992) Reproducibility of patch tests: a United States multicenter study. Am J Contact Dermatitis 3: 193–200
5. Breit R, Agathos M (1992) Qualitätskontrolle der Epikutantestung – Reproduzierbarkeit im Rechts-Links-Vergleich. Hautarzt 43: 417–421
6. Bousema MT, Geursen AM, van Joost T (1991) High reproducibility of patch tests. J Am Acad Dermatol 24: 322–323
7. Lachapelle JM, Antoine JL (1989) Problems raised by the simultaneous reproducibility of positive allergic patch test reactions in man. J Am Acad Dermatol 21: 850–854
8. Macháčková J, Šeda O (1991) Reproducibility of patch tests. J Am Acad Dermatol 25: 732–733
9. Lindelöf B (1990) A left versus right side comparative study of Finn Chamber™ patch tests in 220 consecutive patients. Contact Dermatitis 22: 288–289
10. Stransky L, Krasteva M (1992) A left versus right side comparative study of Finn Chamber patch tests in consecutive patients with contact sensitization. Dermatosen 40: 158–159
11. Fullerton A, Rud Andersen J, Hoelgaard A et al. (1986) Permeation of nickel salts through human skin in vitro. Contact Dermatitis 15: 173–177
12. Malten KE, Nater JP, van Ketel WG (1976) Patch testing guidelines. Dekker and van de Vegt, Nijmegen
13. Chemo technique Diagnostics (1992) Patch test allergens. Product catalogue. Chemotechnique Diagnostics AB, Malmö
14. Hermal (1991) Patch test allergens. Trolab®. Hermal Kurt Herrmann, Hamburg

15. Fregert S. (1985) Publication of allergens. Contact Dermatitis 12: 123–124
16. Dooms-Goossens A, Degreff H (1983) Contact allergy to petrolatums. I. Sensitizing capacity of different brands of yellow and white petrolatums. Contact Dermatitis 9: 175–185
17. Bruze M (1984) Use of buffer solutions for patch testing. Contact Dermatitis 10: 267–269
18. Fischer T, Maibach HI (1989) Easier patch testing with True test. J Am Acad Dermatol 20: 447–453
19. Magnusson B, Blohm S-G, Fregert S et al. (1966) Routine patch testing II. Acta Derm Venereol (Stockh) 46: 153–158
20. Benezra C, Andanson J, Chabeau C et al. (1978) Concentrations of patch test allergens: are we comparing the same things? Contact Dermatitis 4: 103–105
21. Bruze M (1986) Sensitizing capacity of 2-methylol phenol, 4-methylol phenol and 2,4,6-trimethylol phenol in the guinea pig. Contact Dermatitis 14: 32–38
22. Wall LM, Calnan CD (1980) Occupational nickel dermatitis in the electroforming industry. Contact Dermatitis 6: 414–420
23. Wahlberg JE (1990) Nickel chloride or nickel sulfate? Irritancy from patch test preparations as assessed by laser Doppler flowmetry. Dermatol Clin 8: 41–44
24. Blohm S-G (1960) Storage of epicutaneous test solutions. I. Proposed new type of drop bottle. Acta Derm Venereol (Stockh) 40: 457–459
25. Pirilä V (1989) Droplet bottle. Personal communication
26. Fischer T, Maibach HI (1986) Patch testing in allergic contact dermatitis: an update. Semin Dermatol 5: 214–224
27. Fregert S (1981) Manual of contact dermatitis, 2nd edn. Munksgaard, Copenhagen
28. Fisher AA (1986) Contact dermatitis, 3rd edn. Lea and Febiger, Philadelphia
29. Wahlbeg JE, Maibach HI (1980) Nonanoic acid irritation–a positive control at routine patch testing? Contact Dermatitis 6: 128–130
30. Wahlberg JE, Wrangsjö K, Hietasalo A (1985) Skin irritancy from nonanoic acid. Contact Dermatitis 13: 266–269
31. Gollhausen R, Przybilla B, Ring J (1989) Reproducibility of patch test results: comparison of True test and Finn Chamber test. In: Frosch PJ, Dooms-Goossens A, Lachapelle JM, Rycroft RJ, Scheper RJ (eds) Current topics in contact dermatitis. Springer, Berlin Heidelberg New York, pp 524–529
32. Lachapelle JM, Bruynzeel DP, Ducombs G et al. (1988) European multicenter study of the True test™. Contact Dermatitis 19: 91–97
33. Ruhnek-Forsbeck M, Fischer T, Meding B et al. (1988) Comparative multi-center study with True test™ and Finn Chamber® patch test methods in eight Swedish hospitals. Acta Derm Venereol (Stockh) 68: 123–128
34. Stenberg B, Billberg K, Fischer T et al. (1989) Swedish multicenter study with True test, panel 2. In: Frosch PJ, Dooms-Goossens A, Lachapelle JM, Rycroft RJ, Scheper RJ (eds) Current topics in contact dermatitis. Springer, Berlin Heidelberg New York, pp 518–523
35. Wilkinson JD, Bruynzeel DP, Ducombs G, Frosch PJ, Gunnarsson Y, Hannuksela M, Ring J, Shaw S, White IR (1990) European Multicenter study of TRUE test, panel 2. Contact Dermatitis 22: 218–225
36. de Groot AC (1986) Patch testing. Test concentrations and vehicles for 2800 allergens. Elsevier, Amsterdam
37. Cronin E (1986) Some practical supplementary trays for special occupations. Semin Dermatol 5: 243–248
38. Cronin E (1980) Contact dermatitis. Churchill Livingstone, London
39. Adams RM (1990) Occupational skin disease, 2nd edn. Saunders, Philadelphia
40. Foussereau J, Benezra C, Maibach HI (1982) Occupational contact dermatitis. Clinical and chemical aspects. Munksgaard, Copenhagen

41. Hjorth N (1961) Eczematous allergy to balsams. Allied perfumes and flavouring agents. Munksgaard, Copenhagen
42. Takano S, Yamanaka M, Okamoto K (1983) Allergens of Ianolin: parts I and II. J Soc Cosmet Chem 34: 99–125
43. Fregert S, Dahlquist I, Trulsson L (1984) An attempt to isolate and identify allergens in Ianolin. Contact Dermatitis 10: 16–19
44. Karlberg A-T (1988) Contact allergy to colophony. Chemical identifications of allergens, sensitization experiments and clinical experiences. Thesis, Karolinska Institute, Stockholm, Sweden
45. Hansson C, Agrup G (1993) Stability of the mercaptobenzothiazole compounds. Contact Dermatitis 28: 29–34
46. Björkner B, Bruze M, Dahlquist I et al. (1986) Contact allergy to the preservative Kathon® CG. Contact Dermatitis 14: 85–90
47. de Groot AC (1988) Adverse reactions to cosmetics. Thesis, Rijksuniversiteit Groningen, Netherlands
48. Andersen KE, Burrows D, Cronin E et al. (1988) Recommended changes to standard series. Contact Dermatitis 19: 389–390
49. Kalimo K, Lammintausta K (1984) 24 and 48 h allergen exposure in patch testing. Comparative study with 11 common contact allergens and $NiCl_2$. Contact Dermatitis 10: 25–29
50. Rietschel R, Adams RM, Maibach HI et al. (1988) The case for patch test readings beyond day 2. J Am Acad Dermatol 18: 42–45
51. Shehade SA, Beck MH, Hiller VF (1991) Epidemiological survey of standard series patch test results and observations on day 2 and day 4 readings. Contact Dermatitis 24: 119–122
52. Mac Farlane AW, Curley RK, Graham RM et al. (1989) Delayed patch test reactions at days 7 and 9. Contact Dermatitis 20: 127–132
53. Wahlberg JE, Wahlberg ENG (1987) Quantification of skin blood flow at patch test sites. Contact Dermatitis 17: 229–233
54. Lachapelle JM, Tennstedt D, Fyad A et al. (1988) Ring-shaped positive allergic patch test reactions to allergens in liquid vehicles. Contact Dermatitis 18: 234–236
55. Scheynius A, Fischer T (1986) Phenotypic difference between allergic and irritant patch test reactions in man. Contact Dermatitis 14: 297–302
56. Rycroft RJG (1986) False reactions to nonstandard patch tests. Semin Dermatol 5: 225–230
57. Björnberg A (1968) Skin reactions to primary irritants in patients with hand eczema. An investigation with matched controls. Thesis, Sahlgrenska Sjukhuset, Gothenburg, Sweden
58. Andersen KE, Lidén C, Hansen J, Volund Å (1993) Dose-response testing with nickel sulphate using the TRUE test in nickel-sensitive individuals. Multiple nickel sulphate patch-test reactions do not cause an 'angry back'. Br J Dermatol 129: 50–56
59. Bruynzeel DP (1983) Angry back or excited skin syndrome. Thesis, Vrije Universitet te Amsterdam
60. Kelett JK, King CM, Beck MH (1986) Compound allergy to medicaments. Contact Dermatitis 14: 45–48
61. Aldridge RD, Main RA (1984) Contact dermatitis due to a combined miconazole nitrate/hydrocortisone cream. Contact Dermatitis 10: 58–60
62. Smeenk G, Kerckhoffs HPM, Schreurs PHM (1987) Contact allergy to a reaction product in Hirudoid® cream: an example of compound allergy. Br J Dermatol 116: 223–231
63. McLelland J, Shuster S, Matthews JNS (1991) "Irritants" increase the response to an allergen in allergic contact dermatitis. Arch Dermatol 127: 1016–1019
64. McLelland J, Shuster S (1990) Contact dermatitis with negative patch tests. Br J Dermatol 122: 623–630

65. Sukanto H, Nater JP, Bleumink E (1981) Influence of topically applied corticosteroids on patch test reactions. Contact Dermatitis 7: 180–185
66. O'Quinn SE, Isbell KH (1969) Influence of oral prednisone on eczematous patch test reactions. Arch Dermatol 99: 380–389
67. Feuerman E, Levy A (1972) A study of the effect of prednisone and an antihistamine on patch test reactions. Br J Dermatol 86: 68–71
68. Condie MW, Adams RM (1973) Influence of oral prednisone on patch-test reactions to Rhus antigen. Arch Dermatol 107: 540–543
69. Lembo G, Presti ML, Balato N et al. (1985) Influence of cinnarizine on patch test reactions. Contact Dermatitis 13: 341–343
70. Aldridge RD, Sewell HF, King G et al. (1986) Topical cyclosporin A in nickel contact hypersensitivity: results of a preliminary clinical and immunohistochemical investigation. Clin Exp Immunol 66: 582–589
71. Nakagawa S, Oka D, Jinno Y et al. (1988) Topical application of cyclosporine on guinea pig allergic contact dermatitis. Arch Dermatol 124: 907–910
72. Biren CA, Barr RJ, Ganderup GS et al. (1989) Topical cyclosporine: effects on allergic contact dermatitis in guinea pigs. Contact Dermatitis 20: 10–16
73. Sjövall P (1988) Ultraviolet radiation and allergic contact dermatitis. An experimental and clinical study. Thesis, University of Lund, Sweden
74. Lindelöf B, Lidén S, Lagerholm B (1985) The effect of grenz rays on the expression of allergic contact dermatitis in man. Scand J Immunol 21: 463–469
75. Ek L, Lindelöf B, Lidén S (1989) The duration of Grenz ray-induced suppression of allergic contact dermatitis and its correlation with the density of Langerhans cells in human epidermis. Clin Exp Dermatol 14: 206–209
76. Lidén C, Boman A, Hagelthorn G (1982) Flare-up reactions from a chemical used in the film industry. Contact Dermatitis 8: 136–137
77. Hannuksela M. Salo H (1986) The repeated open application test (ROAT). Contact Dermatitis 14: 221–227
78. Hannuksela M (1991) Sensitivity of various skin sites in the repeated open application test. Am J Contact Dermatitis 2: 102–104
79. Hannuksela A, Niinimäki A, Hannuksela M (1993) Size of the test area does not affect the result of the repeated open application test. Contact Dermatitis 28: 299–300
80. Berardesca E, Maibach HI (1988) Bioengineering and the patch test. Contact Dermatitis 18: 3–9
81. Staberg B, Klemp P, Serup J (1984) Patch test responses evaluated by cutaneous blood flow measurements. Arch Dermatol 120: 741–743
82. Wahlberg JE (1989) Assessment of erythema: a comparison between the naked eye and laser Doppler flowmetry. In: Frosch PJ, Dooms-Goossens A, Lachapelle JM, Rycroft RJ, Scheper RJ (eds) Current topics in contact dermatitis. Springer, Berlin Heidelberg New York, pp 549–553
83. Wahlberg JE (1971) Vehicle role of petrolatum. Acta Derm Venereol (Stockh) 51: 129–134
84. Vanneste D, Martin P, Lachapelle JM (1980) Comparative study of the density of particles in suspension for patch testing. Contact Dermatitis 6: 197–203
85. Fischer T, Maibach HI (1984) Patch test allergens in petrolatum: a reappraisal. Contact Dermatitis 11: 224–228
86. Mellström GA, Sommar K, Wahlberg JE (1992) Patch test preparations of metallic mercury under the microscope. Contact Dermatitis 26: 64–65
87. Karlberg A-T, Lidén C (1988) Comparison of colophony patch test preparations. Contact Dermatitis 18: 158–165
88. Bruze M (1988) Patch testing with nickel sulphate under occlusion for five hours. Acta Derm Venereol (Stockh) 68: 361–364

10.2 Organization of Patch Testing in Office Practice

NIELS K. VEIEN

Contents

10.2.1 Introduction

When used properly, patch testing is a valuable diagnostic procedure. Dermatology departments in which patients with occupational dermatoses are regularly treated ordinarily have extensive supplies of patch test materials and a well-trained staff to carry out the test procedure.

Dermatologists practising alone or in small clinics must have a practical means of patch testing their patients at a reasonable cost. Patch testing with standard series of substances can be carried out in any dermatological practice if the dermatologist is trained to do so. The clinical evaluation of the patch test site requires a skill which can only be acquired through adequate training and extensive experience.

Patch testing with special series or substances which have a very short shelf life and must be made up for each test should be carried out in highly specialized centers.

Some practical suggestions for the dermatologist in private practice are given in the following. For further details of the test procedures please refer to Sect. 10.1.

10.2.2 Equipment Needed

Several patch test systems are currently available. Two of those commonly used in Europe are Finn Chambers and TRUE Test. *Finn Chambers* are available in strips of adhesive tape with ten aluminium chambers attached at regular intervals. The strips can be cut so that any number of additional patches may be applied. Patches for single applications are also available. The *TRUE Test* system, which is described in detail in Sect. 10.1, has several advantages if there is only a limited number of patients to be patch tested or if the dermatologist himself is to apply the patches. In this ready-to-use system, the test substances are dispersed in a gel in a series of ten patches. This means that the amount of the allergen applied, as well as the allergen itself, is well-defined, and the patches can be applied in just a few minutes. Unfortunately, the number of substances available in this system is limited and it is relatively expensive.

10.2.3 Substances for Patch Testing

The shelf life of most patch test material is limited. It is therefore not feasible to stock a wide range of substances for patch testing in a general dermatology practice.

Most cases of allergic contact dermatitis are diagnosed after the use of a standard patch test series, and it is therefore advisable to stock the standard series suggested by the Contact Dermatitis Research Group in the area in which a clinic is located [1–3]. A list of these groups is given in Chap. 21.

It may be useful to stock additional series related to dermatoses commonly associated with specific occupations in the geographical area of a practice. A hairdressers' series and a bakers' series are of value in many metropolitan areas. Cronin [4] has suggested series of test substances for a number of occupations. It may also be helpful to stock test substances for the individual components of fragrances, and wider ranges of preservatives and the components of plastics, than those represented in most standard series. A list of available substances is given in Chap. 22. Such lists can also be obtained from suppliers of patch test materials.

Individual series may also be made up to identify sensitivity to specific sensitizing substances used in local industries [5] or to regularly prescribed topical medicaments, for example in the treatment of leg ulcers [6].

Any dermatologist who engages in patch testing will occasionally need to test with substances brought in by the patients themselves, in addition to ready-to-use patch test materials. Before such testing is carried out, however, a number of pitfalls must be carefully considered. The legal significance of making a correct diagnosis of allergy/nonallergy, particularly in cases of occupational dermatoses, cannot be overemphasized. The results of tests with nonstandard substances must be interpreted with great care to avoid both false-positive and false-negative reactions, and it may also be necessary to test a suitable number of control persons [7, 8].

Generally speaking, topical medicaments, clothing and cosmetic preparations intended to be left on the skin may be tested in the form normally used by the patient. Some plants contain irritants as well as strong sensitizers. It is normally possible to carry out patch testing with pieces of the plant itself, if possible using the stem, the leaf and the flower [9]. In order to avoid patch test sensitization, care should be taken not to patch test with strongly sensitizing plants. Vegetable food items also sometimes contain irritants, including phototoxic substances and sensitizers. Most food items, however, can be used for patch testing 'as is'. Other substances, particularly industrial chemicals, may have to be diluted prior to patch testing, or may require the use of an open patch test [7]. Some chemicals should, of course, not be applied to the skin at all.

Before testing with nonstandard substances, it is important to refer to the existing literature to determine the necessary concentration of the test substance and the best vehicle for the test procedure. Fairly accurate dilutions can be made by using disposable syringes for the determination of volumes and electronic postal scales for the determination of weights. Small porcelain mortars and pestles can be used to pulverize or mix the substances. It is wise to have on hand solvents or bases other than water, such as ethyl alcohol, acetone, methyl ethyl ketone, olive oil and petrolatum.

Some patients experience immediate-type as well as delayed-type reactions to both vegetable and animal foods (see Sect. 10.4). A scratch test, prick test or patch test applied to a previously involved area of the skin, read after 20 min and again after 48 h, may reveal this type of reactivity [10–13]. Patch tests read after 20 min have been found to be positive to spices and balsam of Peru in patients with urticaria and protein contact dermatitis. The relevance and practical value of these test results is as yet not fully determined [14, 15].

The use of the scratch-chamber test with fresh substances brought in by the patient makes it possible to detect both immediate-type and delayed-type reactions. In following this procedure, you will need two sets of test substances. One set should be applied to a site which has been scarified prior to application. This set of tests should be read after 15 min and again after 2 days and 3 days. The other set of test substances should be placed on nonscarified skin and read after 2 days and again after 3 days [16].

For some patients, a rub test with suspected items is a useful method of detecting immediate-type reactions to fresh foods [16]. Some of the allergens in food items are destroyed by heating or freezing. It is therefore important that the patients bring fresh substances for the test procedures.

Cupboards or cabinets designed for the practical storage of patch test materials have been described by Jolliffe [17] and Epstein [18].

10.2.4 Test Procedure

It is advisable to develop your own foolproof system of applying the patches to ensure that you maintain the desired sequence. You can, for example, assign a number to each of the allergens to be applied and then mark a template with these numbers. There is less chance of mistaking one site for another when using the TRUE Test system.

In order to avoid loosening of the patches after application, it is important that the patient stand in a relaxed erect position when they are applied. The patient should be asked to assume the same position for the reading of the patch test sites. Test sites can be distorted by the stretching of the skin when a patient bends over or twists the body.

Marks indicating which allergens have been applied should remain on the skin during the entire test period. Since positive tests may appear after the normal time interval for a reading, it is useful for the markings to remain on the skin for at least a week. Stabilo Boss (fluorescent) (Hermal or Chemotechnique) and TRUE Test marking pens (Pharmacia) are suitable for these purposes.

Photopatch testing may be carried out if a UVA treatment unit or another light source which emits sufficient amounts of UVA light is available [19]. Details of this test procedure are given in Sect. 10.5.

10.2.5 Recording Test Results

If only one reading can be made, this is best done after 72 h [20]. If one 72-h reading is to be made, the patient should remove the patches him- or herself after 48-h, and at that time note whether any of them have become loosened. After the test sites have been read by a dermatologist, the patient may be given a drawing of the application sites to enable him or her to read possible late reactions. The patients should be urged to have late reactions read by a dermatologist if this is at all possible. No definite conclusions can be based on the results of patch tests read by somebody other than a dermatologist or a person equally well-trained and experienced in patch testing.

The relevance of the test result should be recorded when the tests are read. This information may otherwise be difficult to retrieve at a later date when insurance forms are to be completed. The determination of relevance is particularly important for occupational dermatoses. Bruynzeel [21] found nonrelevant reactions among 43% of 157 patients who had strongly positive reactions and concomitant weakly positive reactions to substances in the standard patch test series. He suggests that all patch tests resulting in weakly positive reactions should be repeated.

Although entering data via a computer keyboard is time-consuming, the statistical analysis of patch test results is facilitated by storing the results in a computer. Various systems for the storage of such information are available [22].

One simple way to store patch test data manually is to make a rubber stamp on which the substances in the standard patch test series, or other commonly used series, are listed. The list can then easily be printed in a patient's chart, or in correspondence with referring physicians, and be used to record patch test data. It can also be used to provide the patient with information about the tests applied and to compile a card file for the study of patch test data. The cards thus made can be divided into two groups, one with negative and one with positive test results. The latter group will be the smaller of the two, thus making it relatively easy to locate interesting patients and/or patch test results in this file.

10.2.6 Informing the Patient

The significance of both positive and negative patch test results should be made clear to the patient [23]. For some allergens, the determination of the relevance of the test result is no simple matter. For common allergens it is useful to have lists of where certain substances may be present to give to the patients [24]. This will give the patient an opportunity to think about possible means of exposure to the substance in question and make the follow-up discussion of the relevance of the test more fruitful.

When it has been determined that a patch test result is relevant, the patient should also be informed about possible cross-reactions and about allergen substitutes. It saves time to have lists of such substitutes on hand for some of the more common allergens. A list of contact allergen alternatives has been provided by Adams [25].

The use of product directories makes it easier to provide the patient with complete information, but such directories vary from country to country and, unfortunately, in most countries they are not yet available in computerized form.

10.2.7 Should Dermatologists in Private Practice Hesitate to Patch Test for Legal Reasons? (Is a Patch Test Ever Too Risky?)

Contact dermatitis may occasionally flare after patch testing. Ideally, the patch test procedure should, therefore, only be carried out if the dermatitis is in a quiescent phase. Flares of dermatitis which occur following patch testing usually fade quickly. If the dermatitis persists, it can be controlled by a short course of corticosteroids given orally. Patch test sensitization should be suspected if a positive patch test occurs more than a week after application of an allergen [26]. If standard patch test series are used, and substances other than those in the standard series are properly diluted, patch test sensitization is, however, rare.

The risk associated with correctly performed patch testing are so few and insignificant that neglecting to patch test, if it is indicated, creates a much greater problem than any arising from the test itself [27].

10.2.8 Literature

Certain reference works should be readily available to anyone who engages in patch testing. These are necessary both in order to follow the correct patch test procedure when using nonstandard substances and to inform the patient of the relevance of patch test results. In addition to the present volume, major texts include:

Adams RM (1990) *Occupational skin disease,* 2nd edn. Saunders, Philadelphia

Benezra C, Ducombs G, Sell Y, Foussereau JV (1985) *Plant contact dermatitis.* Decker, Toronto

Cronin E (1980) *Contact dermatitis.* Churchill Livingstone, Edinburgh

De Groot AC (1994) *Patch testing: Test concentrations and vehicles for 3700 allergens,* 2nd edn. Elsevier, Amsterdam

Fisher AA (1986) *Contact dermatitis,* 3rd edn. Lea and Febiger, Philadelphia

Fregert S (1981) *Manual of contact dermatitis,* 2nd edn. Munksgaard, Copenhagen

Hausen BM (1988) *Allergiepflanzen – Pflanzenallergene: Handbuch und Atlas der Allergieinduzierenden Wild-und Kulturpflanzen.* Ecomed, Landsberg

Hausen BM, Brinkmann J, Dohn W (1992) *Lexikon der Kontaktallergene.* Ecomed, Landsberg

Maibach HI (ed) (1987) *Occupational and industrial dermatology,* 2nd edn. Yearbook, Chicago

Mitchell J, Rook R (1979) *Botanical dermatology.* Greengrass, Vancouver

Champion RH, Burton JL, Ebling FJG (1992) *Textbook of dermatology,* 5th edn. Blackwell, Oxford

---

In addition to the above-mentioned books, the periodicals *Contact Dermatitis* (published by Munksgaard, Copenhagen, Denmark), *Dermatosen in Beruf und Umwelt* (published by Editio Cantor, Aulendorf, FRG) and *American Journal of Contact Dermatitis* (published by Saunders, Philadelphia, USA) provide information on new allergens not yet included in the books.

10.2.9 References

1. Lepine EM (1976) Results of routine office patch testing. Contact Dermatitis 2: 89–91
2. Veien NK, Hattel T, Justesen O, Nørholm A (1982) Eksemårsager påvist ved hjaelp af lappeprøver i en dermatologisk speciallaegepraksis. Ugeskr Laeger 144: 1683–1688
3. Veien NK, Hattel T, Justesen O, Nørholm A (1987) Diagnostic procedures for eczema patients. Contact Dermatitis 17: 35–40
4. Cronin E (1986) Some practical supplementary trays for special occupations. Semin Dermatol 5: 243–248
5. Heydenreich G, Larsen PØ (1977) Erhvervseksem på en gummifabrik. Ugeskr Laeger 139: 1021–1027

6. Bajaj AK, Gupta SC (1986) Contact hypersensitivity to topical antibacterial agents. Int J Dermatol 125: 103–105

7. Rycroft RJG (1986) False reactions to nonstandard patch tests. Semin Dermatol 5: 225–230

8. Veien NK (1986) Why test with environmental agents? A review of recent studies concerning the value of routine testing in dermatologic practice. Semin Dermatol 5: 231–242

9. Mitchell J, Rook A (1979) Botanical dermatology. Greengrass. Vancouver

10. Krook G (1977) Occupational dermatitis from *Lactuca sativa* (lettuce) and *Cichorium* (endive). Contact Dermatitis 3: 27–36

11. Temesvåri E, Soos G, Podànyi B, Kovàcs, Nemeth I (1978) Contact urticaria provoked by balsam of Peru. Contact Dermatitis 4: 65–68

12. Veien NK, Hattel T, Justesen O, Nørholm A (1983) Causes of eczema in the food industry. Derm Beruf Umwelt 31: 85–86

13. Hjorth N, Roed-Petersen J (1976) Occupational protein contact dermatitis in food handlers. Contact Dermatitis 2: 28–42

14. Warin RP, Smith RJ (1982) Chronic urticaria investigations with patch and challenge tests. Contact Dermatitis 8: 117–121

15. Forsbeck M, Skog E (1977) Immediate reactions to patch tests with balsam of Peru. Contact Dermatitis 3: 201–205

16. Niinimäki A (1987) Scratch-chamber tests in food handler dermatitis. Contact Dermatitis 16: 11–20

17. Jolliffe DS (1981) A patch test reagent storage cabinet. Contact Dermatitis 7: 171

18. Epstein E (1975) A patch test closet. Contact Dermatitis 1: 177–179

19. Wenerstein G, Thune P, Jansén CT, Brodthagen H (1986) Photocontact dermatitis: current status with emphasis on allergic contact photosensitivity (CPS) occurrence, allergens, and practical phototesting. Semin Dermatol 5: 277–289

20. Rietschel RL, Adams RM, Maibach HI, Storrs F, Rosenthal LE (1988) The case for patch test readings beyond day 2. J Am Acad Dermatol 18: 42–45

21. Bruynzeel DP, Van Ketel WG, Von Blomberg-van der Flier BME, Scheper RJ (1981) The angry back syndrome–a retrospective study. Contact Dermatitis 7: 293–297

22. Dooms-Goossens A (1989) Computers and dermatology. Semin Dermatol 8: 65–133

23. Edman B (1988) The usefulness of detailed information to patients with contact allergy. Contact Dermatitis 19: 43–47

24. Larsen WG (1989) How to instruct patients sensitive to fragrances. J Am Acad Dermatol 21: 880–884

25. Adams RM, Fisher AA (1986) Contact allergen alternatives: 1986, J Am Acad Dermatol 14: 951–969

26. Meneghini CL, Angelini (1977) Behaviour of contact allergy and new sensitivities on subsequent patch tests. Contact Dermatitis 3: 138–142

27. Rycroft RJG (1990) Is patch testing necessary? In: Champion RH, Pye RJ (eds) Recent advances in dermatology, vol 8. Churchill Livingstone, London, pp 101–111

10.3 Spot Tests and Chemical Analyses for Allergen Evaluation

LEON M. WALL

Contents

10.3.1 Introduction

The announcement of a positive patch test can be a confusing affair for a patient if he or she is then told that one cannot explain the relevance of the positive reaction or, alternatively, cannot list *all* possible sources of potential contact with that particular allergen.

This unsatisfactory state of affairs has led to the development of various chemical tests able to detect the presence of contact allergens in both household and occupational situations (Table 10.3.1). Much of this work is due to the tireless efforts of Drs Sigfrid Fregert and Alexander Fisher. Without their knowledge and publications in this field, this chapter would not be possible. The reader is particularly referred to Fregert's review in *Dermatological Clinics,* January 1988 (pp. 97–104).

This is not to say that such tests are available in profusion. Nonetheless, it is now standard procedure in many dermatological departments to have available the resources of chromatographic apparatus, which allows analysis for both content and purity of a number of agents responsible for allergic and irritant contact dermatitis.

For those involved in the detective work of patch testing, it is an invaluable asset to have available simple office procedures which allow demonstration of the presence of chemicals in their patients' environment.

Table 10.3.1. Spot tests and chemical analyses used in allergen evaluation

	Tests for	Chemicals required	Limit of detection	False positives	False negatives
Dimethyl-glyoxime	Nickel	Dimethyl-glyoxime Ammonium hydroxide	0.5 μg/cm^2/week	iron, cobalt	levels below detection limit
Diphenylcar-bazide	Chromate	Diphenyl-carbazide Sulphuric acid			trivalent chromium
Chromo-tropic acid	Formalde-hyde	Formaldehyde Chromotropic acid	2.5 μg/ml		acetone ketones organic matter
Lutidine method	Formalde-hyde	Formaldehyde Acetic acid Acetyl acetone Ammonium acetate	1 μg/g	yellow/green compounds	
Spot tests	Epoxy resins	Sulphuric acid Filter paper		substances which darken with sulphuric acid	
TLC	Epoxy resins	Chloroform Acetonitrile Anisaldehyde Sulphuric acid	0.5 μg	Many chemicals with same R_f value as MW 340	
Spot tests	Atranorin	Acetone Filter paper KOH 20% PPD 2%			
TLC	Textile dyes	Methylene chloride Ethyl acetate Chloroform Reference dyes			

10.3.2 Dimethylglyoxime Test for Nickel

Dimethylglyoxime (DMG) gives a bright, reddish-pink, insoluble salt with nickel salts in neutral, acetic acid or ammoniacal solutions. This test was first described by Feigl [1], later modified by Fisher [2] and subsequently by Shore [3].

Ferrous salts also produce a red colour with DMG whilst, in the presence of considerable amounts of cobalt, DMG is consumed. Thus, possible false-positive tests for nickel may ensue in the presence of ferrous salts or when cobalt is present in high concentration.

False-positive reactions with iron can be eliminated with 10 volumes of hydrogen peroxide. This decolorizes the complexes of iron with DMG, which is not the case for the complexes of nickel with DMG [14].

The *test procedure* is as follows: 1% DMG (alcoholic) is mixed with 10% ammonium hydroxide (aqueous) on a cotton applicator and then rubbed vigorously on the test object (Fig. 10.3.1). Alternatively, a test solution can be placed on filter paper impregnated with the ammoniacal DMG mixture or mixed with the ammoniacal DMG in solution.

The *limit of identification* is indicated by a study in which earrings were tested: the test was only positive when more than 10 μg of nickel was released (as determined by atomic absorption spectrophotometry) [13]. Of course, nickel may be present in too low a concentration to produce a positive DMG test. There has been considerable argument in the literature [8, 9] as to whether a negative DMG test for nickel excludes all possibility of a nickel-sensitive patient's reacting to that particular source of nickel. The evidence is increasing that these low concentrations of nickel may still be responsible for clinical eruptions, even positive patch tests, in nickel-sensitive patients [10–11].

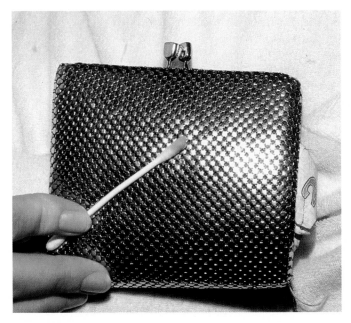

Fig. 10.3.1. Positive dimethylglyoxime test for nickel on a purse

False-negative reactions can be suppressed by the etching of metal with a strong acid (e.g., 3 N hydrochloric acid), followed by neutralization and alkalinization by the ammonia of a normality equal to that of the acid solution prior to the addition of DMG [14].

Some interesting examples of nickel being traced via positive DMG tests lead one to surmise that a more stringent search for sources of external contact with nickel-containing objects in our patient's environment may produce some unexpected, and clinically relevant, sources. Some of these examples include chipped handles on supermarket trolleys; decorative silver mesh of popular purses (Fig. 10.3.1); door and window handles of cars; television dial [3]; wheelchair frame [3]; blow-dry hair brush [4]; pot scourers [5]; chalk [6]; shaving foil of electric shaver [7]; and metallic bracket of blade shaver [7]. In this latter instance, a patient with a rash in the shaving area had been misdiagnosed as having sycosis barbae by several dermatologists before nickel allergy and the source of contact was established.

10.3.3 Diphenylcarbazide Test for Chromate

Strong acid solutions of chromate react with diphenylcarbazide (DPC) to produce a violet coloration, even though only trace amounts may be present [15].

The *test procedure* is as follows: 1 g DPC is mixed with 100 ml absolute alcohol, after initially adding a few drops of concentrated sulphuric acid so that the pH at reaction time is < 2. An ultrasound vibrator may be needed to mix the DPC.

This test does not detect chromic (III) oxide, such as occurs in leather. This can be overcome by converting the trivalent to the hexavalent form via the following process [16]:

A small (less than 1 mg) sample of leather is cut. The sample is ashed in a porcelain microcrucible. A little sodium peroxide is added and heated to complete fusion (caution is required). The chromium is now converted to chromate. After cooling, the mass is dissolved in a few drops of 20% sulphuric acid, and 1 to 2 drops of an alcoholic (about 1%) solution of DPC are added. A deep violet colour appears if chromium is present.

Luck and Jentsch [17] have described a simpler variation of the DPC test in which detection is by a solution consisting of 970 ml ethanol and 30 ml 8 N hydrochloric acid saturated with DPC. A filter paper strip is used to pick up 1 cm of liquid, after which the reactant is applied.

10.3.4 Tests for Formaldehyde

Many positive patch tests with formaldehyde are considered to be of unexplained relevance. However, Fregert et al. [20] made the point that exposure may be occult, especially as formaldehyde may be present as an active ingredient, preservative or contaminant.

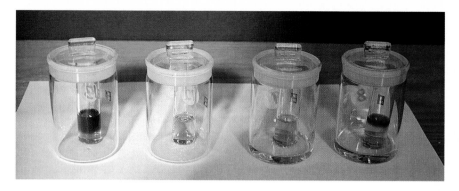

Fig. 10.3.2. Chromotropic acid test for formaldehyde

10.3.4.1 Chromotropic Acid Test [18, 19]

All chemicals used should be of analytical reagent grade. A stock of aqueous formaldehyde (100 μg/l) should be kept in the refrigerator and at the time of testing a substance, concentrations of stock formaldehyde of 2.5 μg/l, 5 μg/l and 10 μg/l prepared. 0.01 g chromotropic acid is weighed out in a glass-stoppered jar and 10 ml concentrated sulphuric acid added.

Test substances are weighed (0.5 g solids; 0.5 ml solutions). 0.5 ml reagent is added to a 12 × 75 mm disposable glass test tube; this is placed in a sample jar and left in complete darkness for 2 days.

All glassware should be carefully washed, rinsed in distilled, deionized water and stored free of dust contamination.

A violet colour develops if formaldehyde is present. Visual comparison of a positive test sample with the working standards will allow an approximate quantitation of formaldehyde concentration (Fig. 10.3.2).

10.3.4.2 Lutidine Method [20]

This is a qualitative method in which formaldehyde reacts with acetylacetone and ammonia to give the yellow compound 3,5-diacetyl-1,4-dihydrolutidine.

The reagent is freshly prepared by dissolving ammonium acetate (15 g), acetylacetone (0.2 ml) and glacial acetic acid (0.3 ml) in 100 ml distilled water. Solid samples (0.5 g), liquid samples (1 ml) and working standards (1 ml) are prepared as described for the chromotropic acid method and placed in a stoppered 10-ml test tube. The described reagent (2.5 ml) is added with vortex mixing to all the tubes, which are then stoppered and heated to 60°C for 10 min.

A yellow colour indicates the presence of formaldehyde. Visual comparison with the working standards gives an approximate concentration of the formaldehyde.

This method is not reliable when the original substance for testing is coloured yellow or green [21], but has been proposed as the best qualitative screening method [31].

10.3.5 Tests for Epoxy Resins

Most epoxy resins are of the bisphenol A type. The oligomer of molecular weight 340 is the sensitizer in this type of epoxy resin [22]. Low molecular weight (average MW < 1000) resins contain up to 95% of this oligomer and high molecular weight resins (average MW > 1000) contain from traces to 10%. When hardened at room temperature, 5%–25% of these epoxy resins remain unhardened for months [23]. Certain objects are coated with varnishes containing epoxy resin that is not completely hardened, e.g. signboards, capsules of bottles, twist-off covers, film cassettes, metal packages and brass door knobs [21, 25].

10.3.5.1 Spot Tests for Epoxy Resins of Bisphenol A Type [26]

This test does not differentiate between cured and uncured resins of bisphenol A type and is used mainly for excluding the presence of epoxy resin of bisphenol A type in materials of unknown composition.

The sample (approximately 0.1 g) is dissolved in 2 ml concentrated sulphuric acid by heating to 40°–50°C in a water bath. If necessary, this is diluted with concentrated sulphuric acid until the colour is orange. With a glass rod, a drop of the epoxy resin solution is streaked across filter paper. A positive result due to the presence of bisphenol A type epoxy resins is indicated by the streak turning purple within 1 min.

Compounds containing bisphenol A other than epoxy resins cannot be distinguished by this test. Confusion with other compounds which darken in concentrated sulphuric acid can be avoided by dilution to a definitive orange colour.

10.3.5.2 Thin-Layer Chromatography [26]

A thin-layer chromatography (TLC) test reveals the presence of uncured, allergenic, low molecular weight oligomers of bisphenol A epoxy resins. Samples may be prepared as a 1% solution in acetone. Alternatively, samples for testing may be cut up into small pieces, placed in dark glass jars and covered (just) in absolute alcohol. Dispersion is obtained using an ultrasound vibrator for 5–10 min. A standard epoxy resin (bisphenol A type) is prepared at 1% in acetone.

The moving phase consists of 90% chloroform ($CHCl_3$) and 10% acetonitrile (CH_3CN) or acetone/ether and methanol/ethanol. Small deposits of each tested substance and the standard epoxy are made on the chromatography

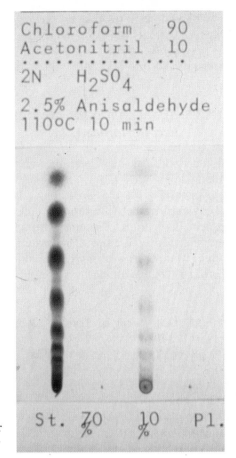

Chloroform   90
Acetonitril   10
· · · · · · · · · · · · · ·
2N   H₂SO₄

2.5% Anisaldehyde
110°C 10 min

St.   70/%   10/%   Pl.

Fig. 10.3.3. Thin-layer chromatography for epoxy resin oligomers (courtesy of S. Fregert)

strip. Solutions are applied with 10-μl micropipettes. A cold air hair-dryer hastens drying and a hand-held Wood's light shows up the epoxy deposits more clearly.

The strips are then placed for 20 min in the moving phase with filter paper lining the sides. These must be kept wet and greased for absolute air tightness. The strips should be taken out using polythene gloves and a mark placed at the point to which the fluid moved.

The strips are sprayed with 10% sulphuric acid (lightly) and then 2.5% anisaldehyde and placed in the oven for 10 min at 110°C. Violet spots appear corresponding to R_f values of the oligomers in the standard (Fig. 10.3.3). The detection limit of the spraying visualization is about 0.5 μg of the MW 340 oligomer.

These tests have uncovered unexpected sources of exposure to uncured epoxy resin, e.g. signboards, door handles, film cassettes, capsules of bottles, twist-off covers and metal packages [25].

It should be noted that the violet colour is not specific for epoxy resin. Many chemicals have the same R_f values as the MW 340 oligomer. For a true positive, there should also be spots corresponding to MW 624 and preferably also to MW 908 oligomers [27].

10.3.6 Spot Testing for Atranorin in Lichens and Perfumes [27]

Contact with oak moss perfumes and lichens in nature may cause atranorin allergy.

Atranorin gives a yellow colour with potassium hydroxide and with *p*-phenylenediamine. One drop of concentrated perfume is applied to 2 filter papers. Two drops of acetone are applied to the perfume spot. On one of the filter papers, 2 drops of potassium hydroxide (20% in water) and, on the other, 2 drops of *p*-phenylenediamine (2% in ethanol) are applied near the perfume spots. If atranorin is present, a yellow colour develops.

10.3.7 Detection of Textile Dyes

Berger et al. [28] described a TLC method for detection of textile dyes. This proved to be of inestimable value in eventually tracking down a new textile dye allergen in a subsequent case investigated by Menezes Brandão et al. [29].

The *method* is as follows: Dyes are extracted by suspending pieces of material (about 2 × 2 cm) in methylene chloride (10 ml) for 1–3 days. The solvent is allowed almost to evaporate at room temperature, and then, using a glass capillary, a drop is deposited 2 cm from the end of a silica gel plate 20 × 20 cm (Merck). The plate is dipped into ethyl acetate-chloroform (1 : 1 v/v) in a glass jar, until the solvent mixture mounts to about 2 cm from the top of the plate. Reference solutions of the various dyes are needed.

10.3.8 References

1. Feigl F (1949) Spot tests in inorganic analysis. Elsevier, Amsterdam
2. Fisher AA (1973) Contact dermatitis, 2nd edn. Lea and Febiger, Philadelphia
3. Shore RN (1977) Dimethylglyoxime stick test for easier detection of nickel. Arch Dermatol 113: 1734
4. Dahlquist I (1982) Nickel itch from a blow-dry hair brush. Contact Dermatitis 8: 217
5. Fernandez de Corres L, Bernaola G, Munoz D, Audicana N, Urrutia I (1988) The innumerable sources of nickel. Contact Dermatitis 19: 386
6. Raith L, Jaeger K (1986) The nickel content of chalk – cause of contact dermatitis? Contact Dermatitis 14: 61
7. Goh CL, Ng SK (1987) Nickel dermatitis mimicking sycosis barbae. Contact Dermatitis 16: 42

8. Fisher AA (1977) Metal dermatitis – some questions and answers. Cutis 19: 170
9. Katz SA, Samitz MH (1975) Leaching of nickel from stainless steel consumer commodities. Acta Derm Venereol (Stockh) 55: 113–115
10. Räsänen L, Lehto M, Mustikkamäki UP (1993) Sensitization to nickel from stainless steel ear-piercing kits. Contact Dermatitis 28: 292–294
11. Wall LM (1980) Nickel penetration through rubber gloves. Contact Dermatitis 6: 461–463
12. Fischer T, Fregert S, Gruvberger B, Rystedt I (1984) Contact sensitivity to nickel in white gold. Contact Dermatitis 10: 23–24
13. Fischer T, Fregert S, Gruvberger B, Rystedt I (1984) Nickel release from ear piercing kits and earnings. Contact Dermatitis 10: 39–41
14. Cavelier C, Foussereau J, Massin M (1985) Nickel allergy: analysis of metal clothing objects and patch testing to metal samples. Contact Dermatitis 12: 65–75
15. Feigl F, Anger V (1972) Spot tests in inorganic analysis, 6th edn. Elsevier, Amsterdam, p 188
16. Feigl F, Anger V (1972) Spot tests in inorganic analysis, 6th edn. Elsevier, Amsterdam, p 615
17. Luck H, Jentsch G (1988) Chromium dermatitis caused by epoxy resin. Contact Dermatitis 19: 154
18. Blohm G (1959) Formaldehyde contact dermatitis. Acta Derm Venerol (Stockh) 39: 450–453
19. Dahlquist I, Fregert S, Gruvberger B (1980) Reliability of the chromotropic acid method for qualitative formaldehyde determination. Contact Dermatitis 6: 357–358
20. Dahlquist I, Fregert S, Gruvberger B (1984) A simple method for the detection of formaldehyde. Contact Dermatitis 10: 132–134
21. Wall LM, Rossi E, Davidson SE, Curnow DH (1985) Qualitative formaldehyde determination in some Australian commerical cleaning and antiseptic products. Aust J Dermatol 26: 77–79
22. Fregert S, Thorgeirsson A (1977) Patch testing with epoxy resin oligomers in humans. Contact Dermatitis 3: 301–303
23. Fregert S (1981) Epoxy dermatitis from the non-working environment. Br J Dermatol 105 (Suppl 21): 63–64
24. Fregert S, Persson K, Trulson L (1979) Allergic contact dermatitis from unhardened epoxy resin in a finished product. Contact Dermatitis 5: 277–278
25. Fregert S, Persson K, Trulson L (1980) Hidden sources of unhardened epoxy resin of bisphenol A type. Contact Dermatitis 6: 446–447
26. Fregert S, Trulson L (1978) Simple methods for demonstrating of epoxy resins of bisphenol A type. Contact Dermatitis 4: 69–72
27. Jenkinson HA, Burrows D (1986) Pitfalls in the demonstration of epoxy resins. Contact Dermatitis 16: 226–227
28. Dahlquist I, Fregert S (1980) Contact allergy to atranorin in lichens and perfumes. Contact Dermatitis 6: 111–119
29. Berger C, Muslmani M, Menezes Brandao F, Foussereau J (1984) Thin layer chromatography search for Disperse Yellow 3 and Disperse Orange 3 in 52 stockings and pantyhose. Contact Dermatitis 10: 154–157
30. Menezes Brandao F, Altermatt C, Pecegueiro M, Bordalo O, Foussereau J (1985) Contact dermatitis to Disperse Blue 106. Contact Dermatitis 13: 80–84
31. Gryllaki-Berger M, Mugny C, Perrenoud D, Pannatier A, Frenk E (1992) A comparative study of formaldehyde detection using chromotropic acid, acetylacetone and HPLC in cosmetics and household cleaning products. Contact Dermatitis 26: 149–154

10.4 Skin Tests
for Immediate Hypersensitivity

MATTI HANNUKSELA

Contents

10.4.1 Introduction

Immediate contact reactions comprise both allergic and nonallergic reactions. In mild reactions, only redness can be seen. In more severe reactions, urticaria on the contact site or eczematous dermatitis are the most common signs. Itching, burning and tingling are the usual symptoms reported by patients.

Skin tests are usually reliable in detecting immediate allergies. Nonimmunological test reactions are more easily suppressed by medication and ultraviolet (UV) light than allergic test reactions. The following describes the skin tests, with their advantages and disadvantages (Table 10.4.1).

10.4.2 Skin Prick Test

The skin prick test (SPT) is usually the most convenient test method for detecting immunoglobulin E (IgE)-mediated immediate allergy. There are large numbers of commercial allergen solutions available, and self-made allergens can also be used.

Drops of allergen solutions are applied to the skin of the back or arm, 3–5 cm apart, and pierced with a special lancet (e.g. the Dome-Hollister-Stier prick test lancet). Histamine hydrochloride 10 mg/ml is used as a positive control and the base solution as a negative control. After 15–20 min the areas

Table 10.4.1. Skin tests for immediate hypersensitivity reactions

Test	Remarks
Skin prick test	For IgE-mediated immediate allergy. Especially for standardized allergen solutions.
Scratch test	For IgE-mediated immediate allergy. Nonstandardized allergens can also be used.
Scratch-chamber test	Especially for testing foodstuffs.
Chamber test	For testing dry materials, such as animal dander, flour and powders.
Open application test	For both immunological and nonimmunological reactions. The test is more sensitive on previously affected skin than on normal kin.
Rub test	A modification of the open application test. Somewhat more sensitive than the open application test.

or diameters of the weals are measured. The result is usually expressed as the mean of the longest diameter and the longest diameter perpendicular to it. Reactions greater than 3 mm and at least half the size produced by histamine are regarded as positive [1–3]. Reactions smaller than those produced by histamine may not be clinically significant.

Lancets with tips containing freeze-dried standardized allergens had recently been developed for easier skin prick testing (Phazet, Pharmacia, Uppsala, Sweden) [4, 5]. Their production, however, has ceased.

10.4.3 Scratch Test

This previously common method for detecting immediate allergy is still used when only nonstandardized allergens are available. If the SPT is used for testing with nonstandardized allergens, e.g. flours, edible roots, vegetables and fruits, skin infections and other untoward inflammatory processes can be produced. A scratch approximately 5 mm long is made with a blood lancet or venepuncture needle, and bleeding is avoided. The back or arms are the preferred test sites. Small amounts of allergen solution are applied to the scratches, and the results are read 15–20 min later. Powdered allergens are mixed with a drop of physiological saline or 0.1 N NaOH on the scratch. Histamine hydrochloride 10 mg/ml is the positive, and saline or 0.1 N NaOH the negative, control. Reactions equal to or greater than that from histamine are usually clinically significant.

10.4.4 Scratch-Chamber Test

Certain foodstuffs, e.g. edible roots, fruits and vegetables, tend to dry out too quickly when applied to a scratch. Covering the scratch with a Finn Chamber

(Epitest, Helsinki, Finland) prevents drying out of the test material [6]. The positive and negative controls and the way the results are read are the same as for the scratch test.

10.4.5 Chamber Test

In addition to the scratch-chamber test, the chamber test has increasingly been used in the diagnosis of immediate contact allergy. There seem to be two types of immediate allergy: that detected by skin prick testing, and that found by occluded epicutaneous testing (chamber test) [7, 8]. There are three kinds of patients: those reacting to SPT only, those reacting to chamber test only, and those reacting to both [7].

The test material is put in an ordinary patch test chamber (e.g., Finn Chamber), moistened with physiological saline or water if needed, and applied to the back or upper arm for 15–20 min. The result is read some min after removal of the test tape. A weal-and-flare reaction is regarded as positive, and erythema without oedema as doubtful. When testing materials of unknown irritancy, tests should also be done in an appropriate number of control persons.

10.4.6 Open Application Test

This test can be used for both immunological immediate contact reactions (IICRs) and nonimmunological immediate contact reactions (NIICRs). IICRs appear on the arms as readily as on the back skin. The ventral aspects of the lower arms are less sensitive than the extensor aspects of the lower arms, the outer aspects of the upper arms and the back skin to substances producing NIICRs [9]. IICRs are usually more readily produced on previously affected skin than on normal-looking skin [10].

Liquids, creams or ointments are tested by applying 0.1 ml to an area of about 5 × 5 cm [11]. After 15–60 min, the test substance is gently wiped off with a soft paper towel or tissue. Dry test materials such as latex gloves [12] and carbonless copy paper [13] are applied as such to the skin, which can be moistened with 2 or 3 drops of water for better contact. The best way to detect latex contact urticaria is to do an SPT with latex extract. The extract can be made from latex milk, from crepe and smoked latex [14], or from latex gloves. The simplest way is to buy the extract from a reputable allergen supply company. A radioallergosorbent test (RAST) is also available from Pharmacia (Uppsala, Sweden). It seems that the SPT is somewhat more reliable than the RAST.

The nonimmunological contact urticaria (NICU) test, known also as the NIICR test, is likewise performed as an open application test. In general 10–30 μl test substance is applied to an area of about 1 × 1 cm. The sensitivity of skin site varies to some extent, but this reactivity is also dependent on the substances tested. The cheek seems to be the most reactive area, at least for benzoic acid [15], but the upper back skin is sensitive enough for routine NICU tests and for screening purposes.

The open application test is also known as the open patch test [16] and as the provocative test [17].

In allergic reactions, an urticarial rash, oedema or at least redness will appear within 15–20 min [18] but may last several hours [12]. Sometimes the very first reaction is not oedema, a weal or a flare but small eczematous vesicles [16, 19].

Nonimmunological reactions tend to appear more slowly than allergic ones. The time of miximal reactivity depends on the substance itself and on the vehicle used [20]. There does not seem to be any one ideal vehicle for testing every substance believed to elicit an immediate type of reaction. A 30-min observation period is usually sufficient, but when substances suspected, but not previously known, to be NIICR-producing agents are tested, a follow-up interval of 1–2 h is advisable.

The results of open application tests can be assesed clinically by recording weals and flares [12], by using scores for oedema and redness [19, 20], or by measuring the change in blood flow with a laser Doppler flowmeter [21].

10.4.7 Rub Test

In this test, the substance suspected of being the cause of current symptoms is gently rubbed into slightly affected or healthy skin [19, 22]. The rub test may be slightly more sensitive than the open application test.

10.4.8 Factors Suppressing Immediate Skin Test Reactivity

Sedating H_1 antihistamines suppress histamine-mediated skin test reactions for up to 1–3 days; the nonsedating H_1 antihistamine astemizole suppresses them for at least 3–4 weeks [23] (Table 10.4.2). Antihistamines have very little or no influence on nonimmunological reactions [7].

Some years ago, Gollhausen and Kligman [24] found that tanned skin reacted to NICU substances much less readily than untanned skin. They assumed that thickening of the barrier layer of the epidermis was the cause of the poorer reactivity. It has recently been shown that not only ultraviolet B (UVB) but also UVA irradiation weakens the reactivity of the skin to NIICR agents for 2 or 3 weeks, and that stripping off the horny layer does not increase the strength of the reactions. This effect is not restricted to the irradiated area only, but some systemic effect can be seen after repeated UVB and UVA irradiation [25–27]. Topical and oral nonsteroidal antiinflammatory drugs also suppress NIICRs, the refractory period being at least 3 days [28, 29].

Table 10.4.2. Factors influencing the results of various skin tests for immediate hypersensitivity

Reaction	Suppressed by
Histamine-mediated	Sedating antihistamines for 1–3 days
	Astemizole for 3 or more weeks
	Other nonsedating antihistamines for 1–4 days
	Over 10 mg prednisolone (or equivalent dose of other steroids)
NIICRs	UV light for 2–3 weeks
	NSAIDs for at least 3 days

NIICR, Nonimmunological immediate contact reaction; NSAID, Nonsteroidal anti-inflammatory drug

10.4.9 Control Tests

When testing patients with nonstandardized allergens, control tests always ought to be done, to detect false-positive, and clinically nonrelevant test results. At least 50 control persons, who should be atopic, are required when testing substances causing IgE-mediated reactions. When testing control persons with NIICR agents, one should remember that antiinflammatory drugs and UV irradiation suppress NIICRs very effectively.

10.4.10 References

1. Basomba A, Sastre A, Pelaez A, Romar A, Campos A, Garcia-Villalmanzo A (1985) Standardization of the prick test. A comparative study of three methods. Allergy 40: 395–399
2. Malling H-J (1985) Reproducibility of skin sensitivity using a quantitative skin prick test. Allergy 40: 400–404
3. Taudorf E, Malling H-J, Laursen LC, Lanner Å, Weeke B (1985) Reproducibility of histamine skin prick test. Allergy 40: 344–349
4. Kjellman N-IM, Dreborg S, Fälth-Magnusson K (1989) Allergy screening including a comparison of prick test results with allergen-coated lancets (Phazet) and liquid extracts. Allergy 43: 277–283
5. Østerballe O, Nielsen JP (1989) Allergen-coated lancets (Phazet) for skin prick testing in children. Allergy 44: 356–362
6. Hannuksela M, Lahti A (1977) Immediate reactions to fruits and vegetables. Contact Dermatitis 3: 79–84
7. Susitaival P, Husman K, Husman L, Hollmen A, Horsmanheimo M, Hannuksela M, Notkola V (1994) Hand dermatoses in dairy farmers. In: McDuffie HH, Dosman JA, Semschuk KM, Olenchock SA, Sendhillselvan A (eds) Human sustainability in agriculture: health, safety, environment. Lewis, Chelsea
8. Morren M-A, Janssens V, Dooms-Goossens A, van Hoyeveld E, Cornelis A, de Wolf-Peeters C, Heremans A (1993) α-Amylase, a flour additive: an important cause of protein contact dermatitis in bankers. J Am Acad Dermatol 29:723–728
9. Lahti A (1980) Non-immunologic contact urticaria. Acta Derm Venereol (Stockh) 60 [Suppl 91]: 1–50

10. Tosti A, Guerra L (1988) Protein contact dermatitis in food handlers. Contact Dermatitis 19: 149
11. Hannuksela M (1987) Tests for immediate hypersensitivity. In: Maibach HI (ed) Occupational and industrial dermatology, 2nd edn. Yearbook Medical, Chicago, pp 168-177
12. Turjanmaa K, Reunala T, Räsänen L (1988) Comparison of diagnostic methods in latex surgical glove contact urticaria. Contact Dermatitis 19: 241-247
13. Hannuksela M, Björksten F (1989) Immediate type dermatitis, contact urticaria, and rhinitis from carbonless copy paper: report of four cases. In: Frosch PJ, Dooms-Goossens A, Lachapelle J-M, Rycroft RJG, Scheper RJ (eds) Current topics in contact dermatitis. Springer, Berlin Heidelberg New York, pp 453-456
14. Köpman A, Hannuksela M (1982) Kumin aiheuttama kosketusurtikaria. Duodecim 98: 39-42.
15. Larmi E, Lahti A, Hannuksela M (1989) Immediate contact reactions to benzoic acid and the sodium salt of pyrrolidone carboxylic acid. Comparison of various skin sites. Contact Dermatitis 20: 38-40
16. Hjorth N, Roed-Petersen J (1976) Occupational protein contact dermatitis in food handlers. Contact Dermatitis 2: 28-42
17. Wrangsjö K, Wahlberg JE, Axelsson IGK (1988) IgE-mediated allergy to natural rubber in 30 patients with contact urticaria. Contact Dermatitis 19: 264-271
18. Krogh G von, Maibach HI (1982) The contact urticaria syndrome - 1982. Semin Dermatol 1: 59-66
19. Niinimäki A (1987) Scratch-chamber tests in food handler dermatitis. Contact Dermatitis 16: 11-20
20. Ylipieti S, Lahti A (1989) Effect of vehicle on non-immunologic immediate contact reactions. Contact Dermatitis 21: 105-125
21. Lahti A, Väänänen A, Kokkonen E-L, Hannuksela M (1987) Acetylsalicyclic acid inhibits non-immunologic contact urticaria. Contact Dermatitis 16: 133-135
22. Hannuksela M (1986) Contact urticaria from foods. In: Roe D (ed) Nutrition and the skin. Liss. New York. pp 178-180
23. Työlahti H, Lahti A (1989) Start and end of the effects of terfenadine and astemizole on histamine-induced wheals in human skin. Acta Derm Venereol (Stockh) 69: 269-271
24. Gollhausen R, Kligman AM (1985) Human assay for identifying substances which induce non-allergic contact urticaria: the NICU-test. Contact Dermatitis 13: 98-106
25. Larmi E (1989) Systemic effect of ultraviolet irradiation on nonimmunologic immediate contact reactions to benzoic acid and methyl nicotinate. Acta Derm Venereol (Stockh) 69: 269-301
26. Larmi E, Lahti A, Hannuksela M (1988) Ultraviolet light inhibits nonimmunologic immediate contact reactions to benzoic acid. Arch Dermatol Res 280: 420-423
27. Larmi E, Lahti A, Hannuksela M (1989) Effect of ultraviolet B on nonimmunologic contact reactions induced by dimethyl sulphoxide, phenol and sodium lauryl sulphate. Photodermatology 6: 258-262
28. Johansson J, Lahti A (1988) Topical non-steroidal anti-inflammatory drugs inhibit non-immunologic immediate contact reactions. Contact Dermatitis 19: 161-165
29. Kujala T, Lahti A (1989) Duration of inhibition of non-immunologic immediate contact reactions by acetylsalicyclic acid. Contact Dermatitis 21: 60

10.5 Photopatch Testing

IAN R. WHITE

Contents

10.5.1 Types of Reaction

Photosensitivity reactions caused by cutaneous exposure or ingestion of certain substances are of four types: contact (topical) photoallergic, contact (topical) phototoxic, systemic photoallergic and systemic phototoxic. The first two types occur when photoreactivity is caused by topical (contact) exposure to an agent and the latter two types by systemic absorption of an agent. Systemic reactivity is most commonly attributable to drug ingestion and topical phototoxicity to plants (phytophototoxic). Photopatch testing is primarily a tool for evaluating reactions caused by contact photoallergens.

In considering photocontact reactions it is important to appreciate the concept of chronic actinic dermatitis (CAD). Patients with CAD presents with chronic eczematous changes on light-exposed areas with or without spread elsewhere. There are abnormal monochromator light tests, with reduced minimal erythema dose (MED) to UV-B irradiation and often to longer wavelenghts. Within the spectrum of CAD are persistent light-related disorders, including those associated with photoallergic contact dermatitis, contact dermatitis, photosensitivity associated with systemic medication and persistent photosensitivity from an endogenous photoallergen [1]. Persistent light reactivity (PLR) is a subgroup of CAD in which there is evidence of hypersensitivity to a relevant photoallergen, but to which there is no apparent current exposure.

10.5.2 Contact Photoallergens

Numerous contact photoallergens have been described, but in most instances reports of these photoallergens causing problems are rare. A comprehensive list of topical photoallergens has been published [2], and this is updated by the list in Sect. 2.4.

10.5.2.1 Photoallergens in Perspective

Some groups of compounds and particular substances have been responsible for causing significant numbers of cases of contact photosensitivity. In the decade before 1975 the halogenated salicylanilides, used as antibacterial agents in soaps, for instance, caused an epidemic of photosensitivity reactions. The problem was first identified by Wilkinson [3]. He described the clinical sign of sparing of a small area of skin behind the ears in those photosensitive individuals with eczematous changes on their faces; this sign is known as 'Wilkinson's triangle'. Once halogenated salicylanilides had been removed from the domestic environment, the epidemic abated, although a very few affected individuals have remained with PLR.

In 1978 musk ambrette, used primarily as a fragrance fixative in toiletries, was identified as a photoallergen by Larsen [4]. During the next few years musk ambrette became an important and common photoallergen, with allergic contact dermatitis also occurring. Again, following the identification of the problem and the lowering of the quantities of musk ambrette used in toiletries, the incidence of new cases of musk ambrette photosensitivity has fallen dramatically.

During more recent years there has been appreciably greater population exposure to a number of UV light screening agents, brought about by the greater awareness of the carcinogenic potential of sunlight and its effect of causing premature aging of the skin. Contact and photocontact sensitivity to these sunscreens has started to become a problem.

10.5.2.2 Musk Ambrette

Musk ambrette has been used extensively as a fragrance enhancer in many perfumed toiletries and in high concentrations (up to 4%) in aftershaves. It is also found in other products such as soaps, hair sprays, furniture polish and in fruit-flavoured foods such as yoghurts and sweets. These various consumables

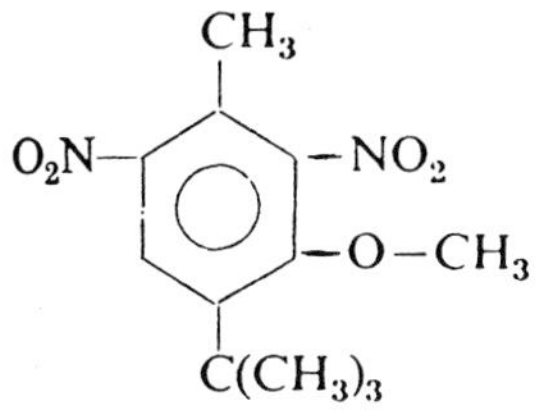

CH$_3$

O$_2$N— [benzene ring] —NO$_2$

—O—CH$_3$

C(CH$_3$)$_3$

Fig. 10.5.1. Musk ambrette

may still contain musk ambrette (Fig. 10.5.1) but under the recommendations of the International Fragrance Research Association the concentrations used, especially in male toiletries, have been reduced. Paralleling this reduction in population exposure, there has been a reduced incidence of musk ambrette photosensitivity. Other musks, musk tibetine, musk xylene, musk ketone and moskene do not seem to be as photosensitizing as musk ambrette and cross-reactions are not the norm [5].

Musk ambrette typically causes photosensitivity in men. Three clinical types of photosensitivity occur [5]. The majority of affected men present with patches of eczema on their faces in the areas on which their aftershaves are patted onto the cheeks and chin. Fewer individuals present with a more widespread eczematous reaction, with a distribution on the light-exposed areas similar to that of CAD.

Although the majority of affected subjects have complete clearing of their skin once obvious contact with musk ambrette ceases, in a few cases, even after carefully removing known sources of musk ambrette from their environment, there is a persistence of photoreactivity. Close evaluation of connubial sources of contact may be important in these cases [6]. Those individuals who have developed PLR have been treated by photoprotection or with PUVA [7], azathioprine [8] or cyclosporin.

10.5.2.3 UV Light Absorbing Agents

The use of UV light absorbing substances has recently increased considerably, and with the consequent increase in skin contact there has been an increase in reports of adverse reactions [9]. The worldwide campaign warning populations of the association of excessive sunlight exposure with the development of malignant melanoma has been one reason for the increased use of these agents. A second reason has been the more frequent incorporation of UV light absorbers into facial toiletries and cosmetics, especially those which claim an anti-wrinkle effect, because of the public's awareness that excessive sunlight exposure is a cause of premature aging of the skin. The third reason has been the incorporation of UV light absorbers into toiletries to increase the shelf-life of the product, by protecting against photodegradation [10].

The main groups of UV absorbers are *p*-aminobenzoic acid (PABA) and its derivatives, cinnamates, benzophenones and dibenzoylmethanes (Fig. 10.5.2). The latter, with excellent long-wave UV light absorbing properties, are being used increasingly in Europe [11–13].

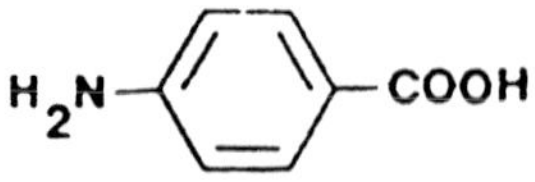

H_2N—⟨benzene⟩—COOH

p-Aminobenzoic acid (PABA)

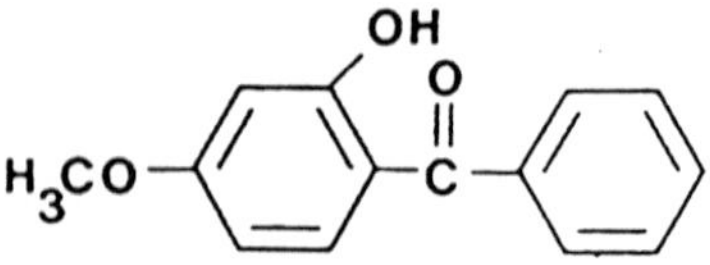

H_3CO—⟨benzene, OH⟩—C(=O)—⟨benzene⟩

Benzophenone-3

H_3CO—⟨benzene⟩—C(=O)—CH_2—C(=O)—⟨benzene⟩—$C(CH_3)(CH_3)CH_3$

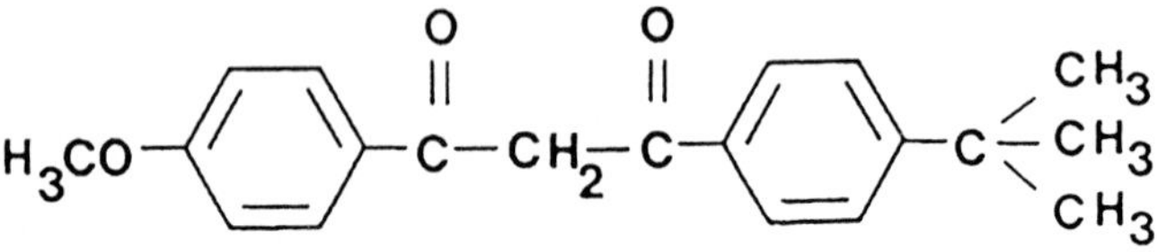

Butyl methoxydibenzoylmethane

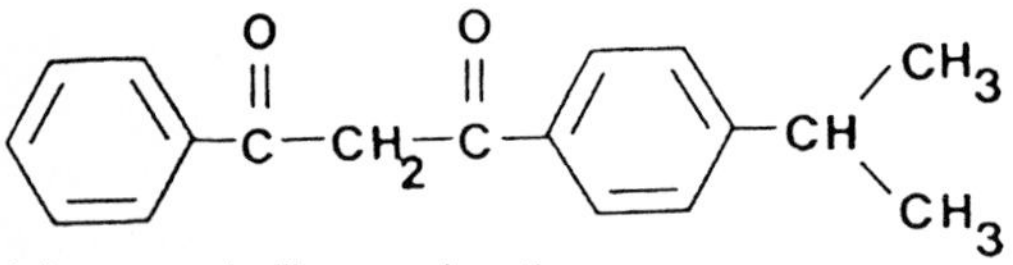

⟨benzene⟩—C(=O)—CH_2—C(=O)—⟨benzene⟩—$CH(CH_3)CH_3$

4-Isopropyl-dibenzoylmethane

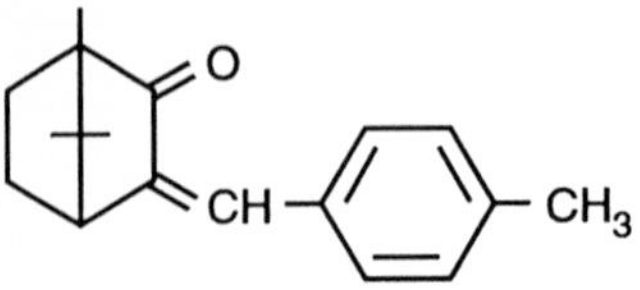

⟨camphor⟩=CH—⟨benzene⟩—CH_3

3-(4′-Methylbenzylidene)-d-1-camphor

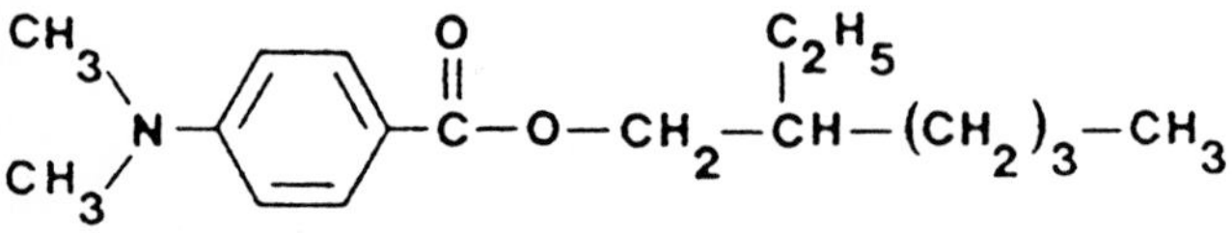

$(CH_3)(CH_3)N$—⟨benzene⟩—C(=O)—O—CH_2—$CH(C_2H_5)$—$(CH_2)_3$—CH_3

Octyl dimethyl PABA

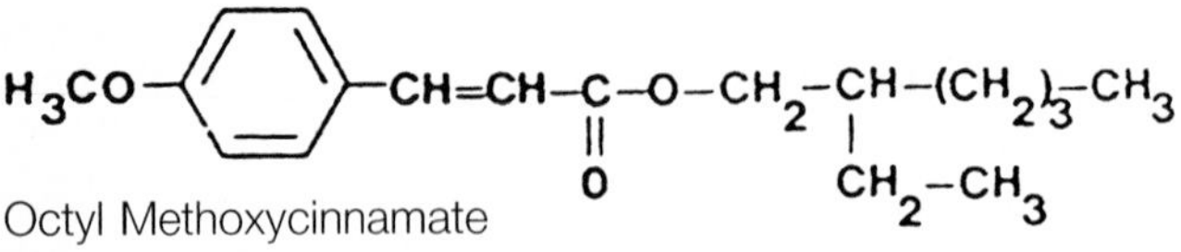

H_3CO—⟨benzene⟩—CH=CH—C(=O)—O—CH_2—CH(CH_2—CH_3)—$(CH_2)_3$—CH_3

Octyl Methoxycinnamate

Fig. 10.5.2. UV light absorbers

UV light absorbing agents can cause an allergic contact dermatitis which may present acutely and have features of an allergic contact dermatitis, similar to those of the more common cosmetic allergens. However, because UV light screening cosmetics are generally applied liberally to the skin before exposure to sunlight, allergic or photoallergic contact reactions to the UV light absorbing substance may be misinterpreted as an idiopathic light sensitivity response. Additionally, some individuals using sunscreens to treat an idiopathic photodermatosis may acquire allergy or photoallergy to the UV light absorbing substance, which may exacerbate the pre-existing condition. An example is photoallergy to 2-ethoxyethyl-p-methoxycinnamate in a Guyanese man, using the screen, who had CAD with negative previous photopatch tests [14]. In such cases the sunscreen may appear to cause 'persistence' of the light-related dermatosis.

Care needs to be taken when evaluating contact and photocontact reactions to some UV light absorbing substances, and especially to PABA and its derivatives. The reactions may be caused by contaminants in the product [15].

10.5.3 Diagnostic Difficulties

Chronic eczema on the light exposed areas may be due to true 'idiopathic' light sensitivity and also to other factors. It has been mentioned that musk ambrette can present with a pattern of photosensitivity identical to such idiopathic light sensitivity. More commonly, however, a chronic eczema on the exposed areas is not due to photosensitivity but is the result of airborne contact allergy. In the United Kingdom this is seen with phosphorus sesquisulphide (P_4S_3) present in some matches, but more globally it occurs with Compositae (see below) dermatitis. Although airborne allergic contact dermatitis characteristically involves the eyelids and extends to involve the skin under the chin and behind the ears, this is not always so; and, conversely, in CAD/PLR there may be involvement of these shaded areas which are typically spared in such light-related conditions.

10.5.3.1 Compositae

Allergic contact dermatitis from Compositae (Asteraceae) can mimic CAD morphologically [16, 17], and, in addition, both are worse in the summer months when there is both increased exposure to sunlight and to Compositae allergens. Further, it is accepted that Compositae sensitivity predisposes to the development of photosensitivity [18], and the clinical evolution of this process has been described [19].

Patch testing with leaves or flowers of Compositae does not always detect Compositae allergy because of ranges in species content of the allergens and seasonal variation. Occlusive patch tests performed with some commercially

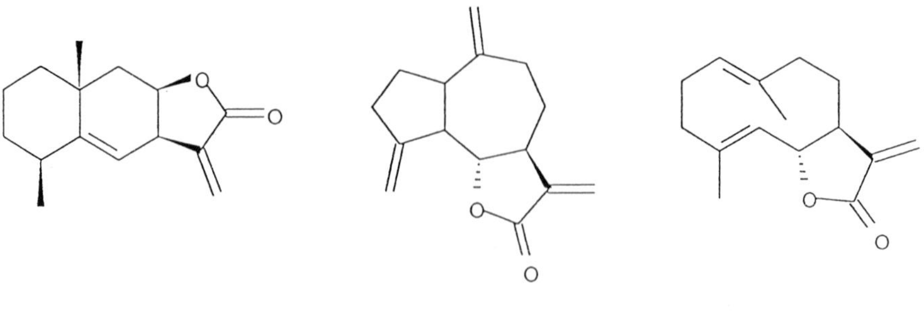

ALANTOLACTONE   DEHYDROCOSTUS LACTONE   COSTUNOLIDE

Fig. 10.5.3. Sesquiterpene lactones

available oleoresin extracts have caused false-positive irritant reactions. Open tests with these oleoresins may give false-negative results in Compositae-sensitive subjects.

The development of a sesquiterpene-lactone mix by Ducombs and Benezra [20] has given increased reliability in the detection of Compositae sensitivity. This mix consists of a 0.1% dilution (pet.) of an equal mixture of alantolactone, costunolide, and dehydrocostuslactone (Fig. 10.5.3). The latter two substances are the more important allergens in the mix (personal observation). This mixture is not irritant, and active sensitization is rare at this concentration. As an alternative to this mix, 1% costus oil may detect the majority of Compositae-sensitive individuals, but the oil contains a variable amount of allergen and may be sensitizing. A Compositae mix developed by Hausen [21] contains the oleoresins of five species of Compositae.

10.5.4 Photopatch Testing

It is clear that there can be diagnostic dilemmas between allergic contact dermatitis, photoallergic contact dermatitis and a photodermatitis of the PLR/CAD type. The purpose of a protocol of photopatch testing is therefore to give an adequate screen of those allergens which can mimic photoallergic reactions as well as being able to detect true photoallergens.

10.5.4.1 Changes in Importance of Photoallergens

There are both temporal and geographical variations in those photoallergens to which an individual is likely to be exposed. New cases of halogenated salicylanilide photosensitivity amongst the general population in the United Kingdom are unlikely to be found, as it has not been exposed to them for nearly two decades. However, these compounds may still be in use in some developing countries, and the possibility remains of contact with them from imported goods (E. Hölzle, personal communication). The incidence of new cases of photoallergy to musk ambrette rapidly decreased as population exposure was reduced. The banning of 6-methylcoumarin from fragrances removed exposure to this photoallergen. In the United Kingdom, photocontact dermatitis to fentichlor has not been reported from domestic exposure to it for more than a decade [22], whilst more recent domestic use in Scandinavia has led to more recent reports of photoallergy to it in these countries. Reactions from UV light absorbing compounds is increasing as population exposure increases. Some UV light absorbing agents are more popular in some countries than others, and the sunscreen formula for a branded product may change seasonally.

Because of these factors, there is no single 'simple' series of allergens which serves as a good screen for photoallergy in all countries, whilst an excessively comprehensive series may be appropriate for use in specialized centres only.

Standard Light Series. The Scandinavians have agreed a series of allergens for use in photopatch testing (Table 10.5.1) which suits their circumstances [23], and results from this series have been published [24]. In Germany the series of allergens in Table 10.5.2 has been developed [25], and in the United States the series in Table 10.5.3 has been recommended [26]. At

Table 10.5.1. The Scandinavian photopatch standard series [23]

Trichlorcarbanilide	1% pet.
Promethazine	1% pet.
p-Aminobenzoic acid	5% pet.
Tribromosalicylanilide	1% pet.
Chlorpromazine	0.1% pet.
Musk ambrette	1% alc.
Tetrachlorosalicylanilide	0.1% pet.
Diphenhydramine	1% pet.
6-Methylcoumarin	1% alc.
Bithionol	1% pet.
Hexachlorophene	1% pet.
Balsam of Peru	25% pet.
Chlorhexidine	0.5% aq.
Wood mix[a]	20% pet.
Lichen mix[b]	16% pet.
Fentichlor	1% pet.
Perfume mix[c]	6% pet.
Compositae mix[d]	3% pet.

[a] Pine, spruce, birch, teak at 5% each
[b] *Parmelia, Hypogymnia, Pseudoevernia, Cladonia, Plasmatica, Physica, Umbilicaria, Cetraria* mixture
[c] Cinnamic alcohol, cinnamaldehyde, hydroxycitronellal, eugenol, isoeugenol, geraniol at 1% each
[d] Oleoresins from *Chrysanthemum, Anthemis, Achillea, Artemisia*

St John's Dermatology Centre in the United Kingdom, the photopatch test series (Table 10.5.4) is reviewed regularly and changed at intervals. Their current series appears to suit the domestic exposure to photoallergens in the United Kingdom, as well as detecting those allergens which may mimic photosensitivity or must be considered in evaluation of an eczema on light-exposed areas. A working party of the European Society of Contact Dermatitis is currently establishing a core list of photoallergens for routine testing.

Table 10.5.2. Photopatch test series used in Düsseldorf, Germany [25]

Tolbutamide	0.5% sal.
Hydrochlorothiazide	0.5% sal.
Frusemide	0.5% sal.
Thiourea	0.01% aq.
Chlorpromazine	0.5% pet.
Surgam	1% pet.
Quinidine sulphate	3.6% sal.
Cyclamate	1.25% aq.
Saccharine	0.4% pet.
Hexachlorophene	1% pet.
Bithionol	1% pet.
Buclosamide	1% pet.
Tetrabromosalicylanilide	1% pet.
Tetrachlorosalicylanilide	0.1% pet.
Salicylanilide mix	4% pet.
3,5-Dibromosalicylanilide	1% pet.
4',5-Dibromosalicylanilide	1% pet.
Monobromosalicylanilide	1% pet.
Tribromosalicylanilide	1% pet.
p-Aminobenzoic acid	5% 70% eth.
Benzophenone	1% pet.
Eugenol	1% pet.
6-Methylcoumarin	1% 70% eth.
Musk ambrette	1% 96% eth.
Balsam of Peru	25% pet.
Chrysanthemum oleoresin	70% eth.

Table 10.5.3. A photopatch test series used in the United States [26]

Bithionol	1% pet.
3,5-Dibromosalicylanilide	1% pet.
4',5-Dibromosalicylanilide	1% pet.
Dowicide-32	1% pet.
Hexachlorophene	1% pet.
6-Methylcoumarin	1% pet.
Musk ambrette	5% pet.
p-Aminobenzoic acid	10% pet.
Sandalwood oil	1% pet.
Tetrachlorocarbanilide	1% pet.
Tribromosalicylanilide	1% pet.

Table 10.5.4. St John's Dermatology Centre scheme of allergens for photopatch testing, 1991

Not for irradiation
Extended European standard series of contact allergens
a series of 'facial' and 'cosmetic' contact allergens
(Sect. 14.1), including:

   Sesquiterpene-lactone mix [20]
   Phosphorus sesquisulphide 0.5% pet.
   'Light series'

Drugs, as appropriate: suitable dilution
Other contact substances, as appropriate: suitable dilution

For irradiation ('light series')
Benzocaine	5% pet.
Chlorpromazine	0.1% pet.
Musk ambrette	5% pet.
Promethazine	1% pet.
Benzophenone-3 (Oxybenzone)	2% pet.
Benzophenone-10 (Mexenone)	2% pet.
Butyl methoxy dibenzoylmethane (Parsol 1789)	2% pet.
2-Ethoxyethyl *p*-methoxycinnamate (Cinoxate)	2% pet.
4-Isopropyldibenzoylmethane (Eusolex 8020)	2% pet.
3-(4-Methylbenzylidene) camphor (Eusolex 6300)	2% pet.
Octyl dimethyl PABA (Escalol 507)	2% pet.
Octyl methoxycinnamate (Parsol MCX)	2% pet.
p-Aminobenzoic acid (PABA)	2% pet.

Drugs, as appropriate: suitable dilution
Other contact substances, as appropriate: suitable dilution

10.5.4.2 UV-A Dose

As a rule, photoallergens are active in UV-A light (315–400 nm), but there are rare exceptions to this, and sulphanilamide and diphenhydramine are examples of compounds with action spectra involving UV-B. For normal investigations UV-A is used for photopatch testing. There are significant differences in the amount (dose, measured in J/cm^2) of UV-A light which is considered appropriate to use during photopatch testing to elicit allergic photocontact reactions.

In Scandinavia the recommendation is 5 J/cm^2 UV-A or 50% MED UV-A, whichever is smaller, for routine irradiation of patch tests during photopatch testing. In Düsseldorf, Germany, 10 J/cm^2 is used. In the United States a range of 5–15 J/cm^2 has been suggested, but 10 J/cm^2 is usual. At St John's Dermatology Centre 5 J/cm^2 is now used for routine photopatch testing, but this may be reduced for individuals with a low MED or increased for dark-skinned subjects.

The dermatologist undertaking photopatch testing generally does not know the MED of his patients, and this is usually not important. However, exposure to 5 J/cm^2 of UV-A can give a very severe sunburn-type reaction on the exposed skin of very light-sensitive individuals. If required, the MED can be determined by irradiating defined, small areas of the skin on the back in sequence, with increasing doses of UV-A from the same source of light as to be used for photopatch testing.

In the series reported by Cronin [5] the photoallergic contact reactions to musk ambrette were elicited by 1 J/cm^2 UV-A. The photoallergic contact reaction to 2-ethoxyethyl-p-methoxycinnamate [10] in a Guyanese man was elicited by 2 J/cm^2 UV-A. The threshold dose of UV-A to produce a photoallergic contact reaction to isopropyldibenzoylmethane was 2 J/cm^2 UV-A, determined by incremental exposures from 0.5 to 5 J/cm^2 [27].

Wennersten et al. [28] have commented that many of the reactions obtained to phenothiazines, during photopatch testing in their clinics using 5 J/cm^2 UV-A, may be phototoxic rather than photoallergic.

There is some evidence that irradiation with more than 5 J/cm^2 does not increase the rate of detection of photoallergic responses (C.T. Jansen, personal communication).

Recommended UV-A Dose. Although there needs to be a thorough evaluation of the optimum dose of UV-A exposure to elicit photoallergic patch test responses reliably in sensitized individuals, it seems appropriate to suggest that 5 J/cm^2 is normally suitable. 50% MED UV-A should be given when photosensitivity is exquisite.

Source of UV-A. Any artificial source of light with a good broad spectral output of UV-A (315–400 nm) is suitable for photopatch testing. A small unit used for giving hand and foot PUVA is an example. If significant amounts of UV-B are present, this needs to be filtered with window glass, as it is significantly more erythemogenic than UV-A. The energy output of the light source needs to be known and monitored at intervals as there may be fluctuation. The Waldmann Lichttechnik UV meter may serve as a standard monitoring device. At St John's Dermatology Centre the light source is a bank of Philips TL 44D 25/09 fluorescent tubes. There is now available the Philips TLK 40W/09N fluorescent tube, which is free from UV-B contamination.

10.5.4.3 Allergen Application and Readings

Individuals undergoing photopatch testing normally should also be patch tested with a standard series of contact allergens, allergens which cause contact reactions on the face, and cosmetics if appropriate. Patch testing to these allergens may take place at the same time as photopatch testing. Substances for photopatch testing are applied in duplicate as parallel series on either side of the back. Additional substances for photopatch testing may include drugs such as thiazide diuretics [29] or benzydamine [30], and occupational contactants such as thiourea, used as an antioxidant in photocopy paper [31].

After 2 days, the sites are examined for reactions, which are recorded in the accepted fashion. The photoallergens which are not for irradiation are masked with opaque material. The second series of photoallergens are irradiated with the UV-A and then covered with opaque material. After a further 2 days the opaque covers are removed, and any reactions are again recorded. In temperate climates it may not be necessary, in practical terms, to recover the allergens for this second 2-day period.

Some variations on this scheme are used. Sites for irradiation may be occluded with the allergen for 1 day only, and readings may be taken at a different time [25]. There is no evidence that this decreased time of occlusion affects the detection of photoallergens. It does, however, permit readings 1 day after irradiation, which may show early photoreactions, and a 3-day post-irradiation reading, at which time photoallergic reactions may be more obvious (E. Hölzle, personal communication).

In order to produce positive photopatch test reactions to methylcoumarin, the substance must be applied shortly before irradiation.

Photoscarification Test. If penetration of photopatch test substances through the stratum corneum is poor, increased penetration may be obtained by scarifying the skin or tape-stripping it [25].

10.5.4.4 Interpretation of Results

No reaction at the unirradiated site, but a reaction at the irradiated site, signifies a photoallergic response. Equal reaction at both sites is interpreted as simple contact allergy alone. Reactions at both sites, but with the irradiated site showing a significantly greater reaction, indicates that both contact and photocontact allergy may exist, but this should be interpreted with caution.

Although positive photoallergic contact reactions are usually quite clear, as with ordinary patch testing, it may sometimes be necessary to differentiate between a phototoxic and a photoallergic reaction. One method is to conduct a serial dilution series of the suspected photoallergen and also to vary the dose of irradiation. This technique has been called photopatch test mapping [32]. A positive response at a very low concentration and/or a very low light dose points to photoallergy rather than phototoxicity.

10.5.5 References

1. Norris PG, Hawk JLM (1990) Chronic actinic dermatitis: a unifying concept. Arch Dermatol 126: 376–378
2. Nater JP, De Groot AC (1985) Unwanted effects of cosmetics and drugs used in dermatology, 2 nd edn. Elsevier, Amsterdam, pp 109–118

304   Ian R. White

3. Wilkinson DS (1962) Patch test reactions to certain halogenated salicylanilides. Br J Dermatol 74: 302–306
4. Larsen W (1978) Photoallergy to musk ambrette found in aftershave lotion. Presented at the American Academy of Dermatology meeting, San Francisco
5. Cronin E (1984) Photosensitivity to musk ambrette. Contact Dermatitis 11: 88–92
6. LeRoy D, Dompmartin A (1989) Connubial photosensitivity to musk ambrette. Photodermatology 6: 137–139
7. Lindberg L, Larkö O, Roupe G (1986) Successful PUVA treatment for musk ambrette induced persistent light reaction. Photodermatology 3: 111–112
8. Cirne de Castro JL, Pereira MA, Prates Nunes F, Pereira dos Santos A (1986) Successful treatment of a musk ambrette sensitive persistent light reactor with azathiaprine. Photodermatology 3: 241–242
9. Thune P (1984) Contact and photocontact allergy to sunscreens. Photodermatology 1: 5–9
10. English JSC, White IR, Cronin E (1987) Sensitivity to sunscreens. Contact Dermatitis 17: 159–162
11. English JSC, White IR (1986) Allergic contact dermatitis from isopropyl dibenzoylmethane. Contact Dermatitis 15: 94
12. Schauder S, Ippen H (1986) Photoallergic and allergic contact dermatitis from dibenzoylmethanes. Photodermatology 3: 140–147
13. Schauder S, Ippen H (1988) Lichtschutzfilterhaltige Präparate in der Bundesrepublik Deutschland 1988. Z Hautkr 63: 707–763
14. Murphy GM, White IR (1987) Photoallergic contact dermatitis to 2-ethoxyethyl-p-methoxy cinnamate. Contact Dermatitis 16: 296
15. Bruze M, Gruvberger B, Thune P (1988) Contact and photocontact allergy to glyceryl para-aminobenzoate. Photodermatology 5: 162–165
16. Hjorth N, Roed-Petersen J, Thomsen K (1976) Airborne contact dermatitis from Compositae oleoresins stimulates photodermatitis. Br J Dermatol 95: 613–620
17. English JSC, Norris P, White I, Cronin E (1989) Variability in the clinical patterns of Compositae dermatitis. Br J Dermatol 121 [Suppl 34]: 27
18. Frain-Bell W, Johnson BE (1979) Contact sensitivity to chrysanthemum and the photosensitivity dermatitis and actinic reticuloid syndrome. Br J Dermatol 101: 491–501
19. Murphy GM, White IR, Hawk JLM (1990) Allergic airborne contact dermatitis to Compositae with photosensitivity–chronic actinic dermatitis in evolution. Photodermatol Photoimmunol Photomed 7: 38–39
20. Ducombs G, Benezra C, Talaga P et al. (1990) Patch testing with the "sesquiterpene lactone mix": a marker for contact allergy to Compositae and other sesquiterpene-lactone-containing plants. Contact Dermatitis to be published
21. Wrangsjö K, Ros AM, Wahlberg JE (1990) Contact allergy to Compositae plants in patients with summer exacerbating dermatitis. Contact Dermatitis 22: 148–154
22. Norris P, Hawk JLM, White IR (1988) Photoallergic contact dermatitis from fentichlor. Contact Dermatitis 18: 318–320
23. Jansen CJ, Wennersten G, Rystedt I, Thune P, Brodthagen H (1982) The Scandinavian standard photopatch test procedure. Contact Dermatitis 8: 155–158
24. Thune P, Jansen C, Wennersten G, Rystedt I, Brodthagen H, McFadden N (1988) The Scandinavian multicenter photopatch study (1980–85)–final report. Photobiology 5: 261–269
25. Hölzle E, Plewig G, Lehmann P (1987) Photodermatoses–diagnostic procedures and their interpretation. Photodermatol 4: 109–114
26. De Leo VA, Harber LC (1986) Contact photodermatitis. In: Fisher AA (ed) Contact dermatitis, 3rd edn. Lea and Febiger, Philadelphia, p. 465
27. Murphy GM, White IR, Cronin E (1990) Immediate and delayed photocontact dermatitis to isopropyl dibenzoylmethane. Contact Dermatitis 22: 129–131

28. Wennersten G, Thune P, Jansen CT, Brodthagen H (1986) Photocontact dermatitis: current status with emphasis on allergic contact photosensitivity (CPS) occurrence, allergens, and practical phototesting. Semin Dermatol 5: 277–289
29. White IR (1983) A positive photopatch test with hydrochlorothiazide. Contact Dermatitis 9: 237
30. Frosch PJ, Weickel R (1989) Photokontaktallergie durch Benzydamin (Tantum). Hautarzt 40: 771–773
31. Dooms-Goossens A, Chrispels MT, De Veylden H, Roelandts R, Willems L, Degreif H (1987) Contact and photocontact sensitivity problems associated with thiourea and its derivatives: a review of the literature and case reports. Br J Dermatol 116: 573–579
32. Takashima A, Yamatoto K et al. (1991) Allergic contact and photocontact dermatitis due to psoralens in patients with psoriasis treated with topical PUVA. Br J Dermatol 124: 37–42

10.6 In Vitro Testing in Contact Hypersensitivity

CLIFFORD MCMILLAN and DESMOND BURROWS

Contents

10.6.1 Introduction

The development of testing procedures to aid in the diagnosis of allergic contact dermatitis began with the introduction of the concept of patch testing by Jadassohn [1]. This involved reproducing allergic eczema, following application of antigen to a small area of unbroken skin in a sensitized individual. Almost a century later the technique, despite its empirical basis, has with refining and standardization developed into a useful tool in the investigation of contact dermatitis. Patch testing, however, gives rise to a number of problems. Interpretation is subjective and relies on observer experience. False-positive and false-negative reactions can occur [2–4]. In addition, the procedure is not without possible risks. In particular, patch testing may cause active sensitization of previously nonallergic patients.

Much of our current knowledge and increased understanding of the pathogenic mechanisms in contact allergy derives from the development of in vitro test systems. Such procedures, therefore, have provided useful investigative tools for use in research, but have not gained widespread acceptance in the clinical field. This is explained, at least in part, by the fact that these techniques all lack simplicity, are time-consuming and are not readily reproducible. While patch testing would continue to provide a useful screening technique, a simple reliable in vitro procedure would have the advantages of safety, could be carried out irrespective of the level of the patients' eczema ('angry back syndrome') [5] and could be used to investigate false-positive and false-negative results. There is, therefore, a requirement for a rapid, reproducible, in vitro test.

10.6.2 Immunology

Acute contact dermatitis is well established as a delayed cell-mediated hypersensitivity [6]. Most allergens are of low molecular weight and penetrate the skin, where they act as haptens by covalently binding to carrier proteins in the skin to become immunogenic. This antigenic complex is believed to be processed by Langerhans cells. These are dendritic cells found both in the skin and also in lymph nodes. They possess the ability to move from the epidermis to the dermis and, via the lymphatics, to regional lymph nodes. They act as antigen-presenting cells and their significance was first demonstrated by Silberberg et al. [7] showing apposition of Langerhans cells and lymphocytes at the site of positive patch test reactions. The Langerhans cell possesses similar surface markers to the macrophage, such as Ia antigen, complement and the FC fragment of immunoglobulin G (IgG). Antigenic information is transferred to adjacent T lymphocytes, which are complementary to the contact antigen, and receptors for the HLA-DR antigen on the membrane of the Langerhans cell. The small number of T cells thus activated are retained in the paracortical area of the draining lymph node where they differentiate into specific memory and effector cells.

Following epicutaneous challenge of hypersensitive patients, specific effector cells, present at or attracted to the site of application, are stimulated by the antigenic complex formed in the skin to release lymphokines [8]. These are soluble nonantibody products of lymphocytic activation by specific antigen; they modulate the inflammatory reaction, recruiting nonspecific cells and enabling amplification of the inflammation-inducing effect of a relatively small number of T effector cells. Langerhans cells release interleukin 1, which triggers activated T lymphocytes to release interleukin 2, which in turn promotes activated T-cell proliferation and release of immune interferon. The latter promotes expression of HLA-DR antigens on the Langerhans cell membrane and T-cell cytotoxic activity.

Lymphokines with a variety of biological activities have been demonstrated in contact sensitivity. Mitogenic factor [9] induces mitotic division of lymphocytes. Migration inhibitor factor (MIF) [10, 11] causes macrophages to remain in the reaction area. Others include cytotoxic factor [12], chemotactic factor [13] and angiogenic factor [14]. Many lymphokine activities have now been described, but as these substances become fully characterized it is possible that different activities may be ascribed to the same molecule. The detection of lymphokines provides a means of assessing cell-mediated immunity. Techniques which are of use in the in vitro investigation of contact allergy include migration inhibition, lymphocyte transformation, procoagulant activity and viral plaque inhibition. However, most attention has been directed to measurement of lymphocyte proliferative response (transformation) and cell migration inhibition.

10.6.3 In Vitro Tests

10.6.3.1 Migration Inhibition

Rich and Lewis [15] initiated in vitro studies on delayed hypersensitivity, by demonstrating that antigen inhibited the migration of cells from tissue explants taken from sensitized animals. George and Vaughan [16] demonstrated that exposure to the specific antigen inhibited the outward circular migrations from capillary tubes of peritoneal exudate cells from sensitized guinea pigs. Using this method, Bloom and Bennett [17] and David [18] showed that the inhibition was due to a soluble factor released by sensitized lymphocytes following stimulation. This factor was called 'migration inhibition factor'. A migration assay demonstrating the presence of this factor is a useful test in the evaluation of delayed hypersensitivity in man [19]. Two major lymphokines influencing cell migration have been described. Leucocyte inhibition factor [20] (LIF) inhibits the migration of polymorphonuclear leucocytes but not monocytes or macrophages. Migration inhibition factor (MIF) inhibits the migration of monocytes and macrophages but not polymorphonuclear leucocytes.

In order to measure cell migration inhibition, two different types of assay, namely the direct and indirect methods, are used (Fig. 10.6.1). In the direct migration system, leucocytes from hypersensitive patients are filled into capillaries. After centrifugation, the capillaries are cut at the liquid cell interface and the part containing cells placed in chambers filled with medium, with or without specific antigen. In positive tests, the migration of cells is inhibited by antigen-containing media compared to controls, and is expressed as the migration index (MI):

$$\text{MI} = \frac{\text{Average of migration areas with antigen}}{\text{Average of migration areas without antigen}} \times 100$$

Direct tests are quick and simple to perform but negative results fail to differentiate between lack of target cell response and lack of lymphokine production. It has also been suggested that inhibition may be mediated by mechanisms other than lymphokine release [21].

In the indirect test, lymphocytes from hypersensitive patients are incubated in the presence or absence of specific antigen, and the supernatants from these cultures are placed in chambers where capillaries filled with cells from nonsensitized guinea pigs are placed. Only media containing LIF or MIF inhibit the migration of the appropriate normal cells. This method, though more time consuming, provides stronger evidence that substances produced by the lymphocytes are indeed the source of inhibition.

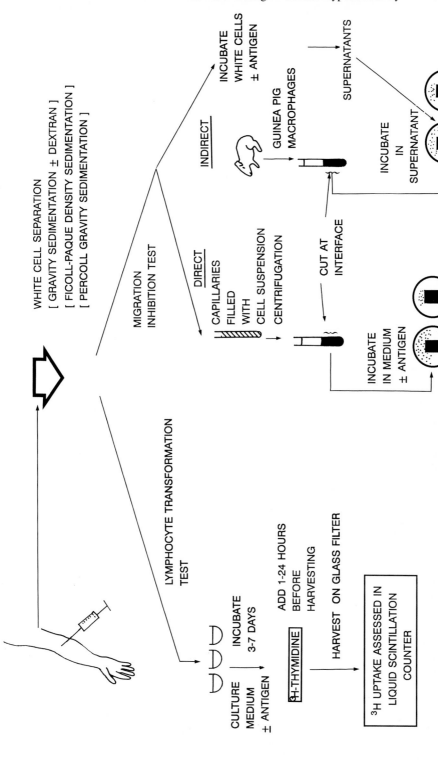

Fig. 10.6.1. Assessment of allergic contact dermatitis by means of lymphocyte transformation and migration inhibition.

Investigations of nickel-sensitive patients using these assays initially failed to show significant cell migration inhibition. Grosfeld et al. [22], using skin explants from patients allergic to nickel, did not find any differences in outgrowths compared to controls. Following improvements in methodology, Thulin and Zachariae [23] demonstrated specific leucocyte migration inhibition in chromate-sensitive patients. Shortly afterwards, Mirza [24, 25] found significant inhibition in patients with contact allergy to nickel. This was followed by similar reports from Thulin [26] and Jordan et al. [27]. Using the direct assay technique, these various investigators demonstrated significant differences in LIF production in affected patients compared to controls. Although toxic concentrations of allergens caused migration inhibition in both controls and hypersensitive patients, lower concentrations demonstrated a dose-dependent relationship, with optimum inhibition at just-below-toxic levels.

A modified technique, in which inhibition is assessed by measuring the linear migration of leucocytes along sealed capillaries, was described by Jones [28]. Results with purified protein derivative-(PPD)-induced migration inhibition of tuberculin-sensitive leucocytes suggested a good correlation with results using cut capillaries [28]. This sealed capillary method offfers the advantages of being simpler, more rapid and requiring less antigen [29]. Investigation of nickel-allergic subjects by Nordlind and Sandberg using this technique, however, failed to discriminate hypersensitive subjects from controls [29].

Nickel, because of the excellent solubility of its salts and its low cytotoxicity, has been one of the most frequently investigated antigens. In spite of this, in the absence of a standardized method, the various investigators have used different nickel salts as antigen and found differing optimal antigenic concentrations. The need to complex the nickel salt to a carrier protein was confirmed by some workers [25, 26] but found unnecessary by others [27]. Overlap of the migration indices between controls and hypersensitive patients [25, 26] led Thulin et al. to conclude that, while being a useful test to investigate groups of patients, migration indices taken in isolation could not be used to discriminate whether or not an individual was hypersensitive to nickel. In contrast, Jordan et al. [27] showed the two populations to be significantly different and without overlap between the groups. Interestingly, LIF responses were found in some patch-test-negative patients who had a past history suggestive of nickel contact allergy. This could be interpreted as increased sensitivity of the LIF method compared to patch testing but awaits further investigation.

10.6.3.2 Lymphocyte Transformation Test

In 1960 Nowell [30] first reported that lymphocytes, cultured in the presence of phytohaemagglutinin (PHA), enlarge and change into blast cells. This process, known as transformation, can be defined as the reversible rediffer-entiation of small lymphocytes to larger lymphoblasts, culminating in mitosis [31]. Such changes are associated with increased synthesis of phospholipids [32], lymphokines [17, 33], RNA [34] and DNA [35]. Blast transformation may be assessed morphologically, using various techniques to stain for RNA, DNA and nucleoli, or by evaluation of relative DNA content in the microden-sitometric assay [36]. The finding that uptake of radiolabelled thymidine by lymphocyte nucleic acids in culture correlates well with transformation [37], however, has led to this being used as a more objective and accurate method of assessment (Fig. 10.6.1). PHA causes nonspecific lymphocyte transformation. Pokeweed [38] and concanavalin A [39] also cause similar changes.

In addition to these nonspecific mitogens, antigens also possess the capability of transforming lymphocytes [40, 41]. Mills [42] demonstrated that this transformation was specific for the antigen to which the organism had become sensitized and that it correlated strongly with delayed hypersensitivity. In the mixed lymphocyte response (MLR) [43], specific transformation also occurs when two genetically different T-cell populations are mixed and react to each other's histocompatibility antigens.

Aspegren and Rorsman [44], following the report by Nowell [30], investigated the ability of nickel to transform lymphocytes from nickel-allergic subjects. At high nickel concentrations they found suppression of mitosis, while at lower concentrations they were unable to demonstrate any differences in transformation compared to controls. Pappas et al. [45] also found nonspecific transformation in response to nickel acetate, similar to previous reports of the nonspecific mitogenic effects of mercury salts [46, 47]. In contrast, Macleod et al. [48] found no significant thymidine uptake in controls, but significant uptake occurred in 7 out of 12 nickel-sensitive patients. The same authors, using nickel sulphate and nickel acetate as antigens, further reported specific transformation in nickel-sensitive patients, with neither salt acting in a nonspecific capacity [49]. Following this, there have been reports of similar findings [50, 51] but several authors [52–56], in addition to demonstrating transformation in response to nickel challenge of lymphocytes from nickel-allergic subjects, found a weak nonspecific mitogenic effect in control patients. Furthermore, cord blood lymphocytes showed the capacity to transform following incubation with nickel [55], being more pronounced at higher nickel concentrations.

Comparison of results by the various investigators using the lymphocyte transformation test as an in vitro means of assessing hypersensitivity to a particular contact allergen, such as nickel, is difficult because of numerous technical difficulties encountered in the test and the many different techniques used [57]. Methods of white cell separation vary among authors, even though the techniques used may affect the overall levels of transformation. These methods include gravity sedimentation with or without dextran, and density sedimentation using Ficoll-Paque or Percoll. Gravity sedimentation results in less pure lymphocyte cultures, but may lead to higher transformational values following stimulation with nickel [58] and PHA [49]. In contrast, Nordlind et al. [56] compared separation techniques in the in vitro study of nickel dermatitis using the lymphocyte transformation test and found highest lymphocyte thymidine uptake in Percoll-separated cells, with less uptake in those separated using Ficoll-Paque and the lowest in gravity sedimented lymphocytes.

In the case of the allergen nickel, while there is universal agreement among investigators that the concentration used to stimulate lymphocytes is critical, the optimum stimulatory concentration varies from laboratory to laboratory. Too high a concentration causes toxic effects, while too low a concentration fails to exhibit a mitogenic effect. Amounts of antigen vary from 23 770 μg with positive results, down to 0.01 μg with negative results [50]. Certain authors [51] suggest testing at more than one concentration because of 'high dilution responders' and 'low dilution responders'. Nickel sulphate is the most commonly used source of nickel and corresponds with that used in patch testing, but nickel acetate and chloride are also reported. Radiolabelled thymidine uptake, despite being the most widely used method of assessing lymphocyte transformation, is not standardized. Different radiolabelled isotopes may be added to cell culture from 1–24 h prior to assessment of uptake. Duration of cell culture varies from 3 to 7 days, with maximum response usually reported from 5 to 7 days. Following culture, the preparation of cells prior to measurement of thymidine uptake also varies.

The timing of the lymphocyte transformation test in relation to epicutaneous testing might be important. Powell et al. [59] noted increased transformation following epicutaneous challenge of human volunteers with experimentally induced contact allergy to dinitrochlorobenzene. This problem was considered by Veien et al. [60] in the context of nickel hypersensitivity. They found no difference in transformation before and after epicutaneous challenge, although they did report increased transformation following oral challenge.

Again taking nickel as one of the most frequently investigated allergens, in spite of the inability to compare results between different laboratories, several groups of investigators [53–56, 60] report significant differences between lymphocyte transformation in nickel-sensitive patients and controls. Unfortunately, however, there is often a degree of overlap between affected subjects and controls [53, 54, 56], which makes it unreliable to diagnose nickel allergy on the basis of the lymphocyte transformation test alone. Interestingly, the test was reported as positive in a nickel-sensitive patient whose patch testing had reverted to negative [52]. Similar findings were reported when testing in vitro using the migration inhibition assay [25]. It would, however, be premature to draw the conclusion that in vitro testing may, in certain circumstances, be more sensitive than testing in vivo.

Further points of interest resulting from in vitro investigation of contact allergy to nickel, using the lymphocyte transformation test, include the finding of significant lymphocyte transformation in an atopic who developed a pustular patch test reaction to nickel [52], suggesting that such a reaction is not necessarily nonspecific. Also reported is the case of a nickel-sensitive patient who was tested while taking 40-mg prednisone orally [50]. The lymphocyte transformation test was positive to nickel challenge but PHA stimulation, used as a control, was depressed. On repeat testing after discontinuation of steroid, the nickel transformation remained unchanged but the PHA stimulation reverted to normal.

10.6.3.3 Leucocyte Procoagulant Activity

Blood clotting mechanisms play an important role in cell-mediated hypersensitivity [61–63]. The cutaneous manifestation of delayed hypersensitivity in experimental animals is modified by anticoagulant therapy [62, 63]. In man, fibrin deposition is a consistent feature of allergic contact dermatitis [61]. Normal leucocytes can be stimulated in vitro to generate a procoagulant that activates the extrinsic cascade of blood clotting and is identified as tissue factor [64]. Human mononuclear cells produce significant levels of procoagulant activity following antigenic stimulation [65] and it is suggested that lymphokine-induced macrophage procoagulant activity may explain the inhibition of macrophage migration due to the cross-linking of fibrinogen on the cell surface [66]. Geczy and Meyer [67] assessed procoagulant activity in man, using mumps antigen and tuberculin (PPD) as antigenic stimuli, and found it to be in vitro correlate of delayed hypersensitivity. Comparison with blast transformation and migration inhibition suggested it to be a more sensitive assay.

In brief, this method involves leucocyte separation (Ficoll) followed by incubation in the presence or absence of antigen for 20 h. Procoagulant activity is assessed (in minutes) using a recalcification assay. This may be carried out visually or by automatic coagulocytometer. The activity is calculated from the clotting time of plasma incubated with cells in the absence of antigen (t^1) and clotting time of plasma incubated with cells in the presence of antigen (t^2)

$$\text{Activity} = \frac{t^1 - t^2}{t^1} \times 100$$

Investigation of nickel hypersensitivity using this method was carried out by Aldridge et al. [68]. These authors noted a marked increase in procoagulant activity in nickel-allergic subjects with increasing stimulatory concentrations of nickel. At concentrations of 5 and 10 μg/ml there was a statistically significant difference ($p < 0.01$) from controls. This method appears to have the advantages of sensitivity and rapid determination of results over other established in vitro techniques, but awaits confirmation by other laboratories.

10.6.3.4 Interferon

The ability of interferon (IFN) to inhibit viruses led to its discovery by Isaacs and Lindermann [69] in 1957. More recently, however, attention has focused on the role of IFN as an immune modulator. Three types of human IFN are recognized at present:
1. IFN-α or leucocyte interferon (type 1)
2. IFN-β or fibroblast interferon (type 1)
3. IFN-γ or immune interferon (type 2)

IFN-γ acts primarily as an immune modulator with some antiviral potential. In contrast, IFN-α and IFN-β are primarily antiviral with some potential for immune modulation [70]. Modulatory effects on immune function include activation of macrophages, promotion of antibody formation and natural killer cell function and increased expression of HLA-DR antigen, important in transfer of antigenic information to T lymphocytes. The ability of T lymphocytes to produce IFN-γ was first demonstrated by Wheelock et al. [33] using PHA mitogen. Green et al. [71] showed that sensitized T lymphocytes, following exposure to specific antigen, released a lymphokine which activated macrophages. Originally known as macrophage activity factor, this is now known to be IFN.

McKimm-Breschkin et al. [72] investigated the ability of antigen to induce IFN production in two continuous mouse T-cell lines which were shown to exhibit contact hypersensitivity to the sensitizing agent oxazalone. IFN was measured by means of its ability to inhibit growth of viral plaques, expressing titres as the reciprocal of the dilution causing a 50% reduction in the number of plaques compared to controls. These authors demonstrated antiviral activity, which they characterized as IFN-γ because it was species specific stable at 50°C for 30 min and inactivated by treatment at pH 2 (IFN-α and IFN-β are acid stable). Using an inhibitor of protein synthesis, they also demonstrated inhibition of IFN only when T lymphocytes were treated.

Using a similar viral plaque inhibition technique, McMillan et al. [73] investigated IFN production in nickel contact hypersensitivity (Figs. 10.6.2 and 10.6.3). Following incubation of leucocytes with nickel sulphate these investigators demonstrated significant ($p=0.002$) antiviral activity produced by cells taken from nickel-sensitive subjects compared to controls. This activity was found to be heat stable and acid labile, similar to the findings of McKimm-Breschkin et al., suggesting that this was caused by IFNγ. In addition, Sinigaglia et al. [74] demonstrated the production of IFN-γ by nickel-specific T-cell clones following their isolation and characterization in patients suffering from nickel allergy. In contrast, however, Karttunen et al. [75] were unable to demonstrate any measurable IFN-γ secretion in peripheral blood mononuclear cell cultures in nickel-sensitive subjects.

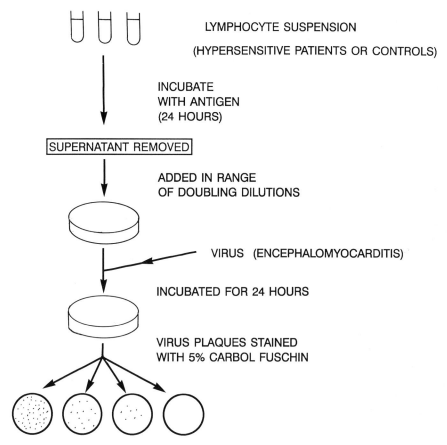

LYMPHOCYTE SUSPENSION

(HYPERSENSITIVE PATIENTS OR CONTROLS)

INCUBATE
WITH ANTIGEN
(24 HOURS)

SUPERNATANT REMOVED

ADDED IN RANGE
OF DOUBLING DILUTIONS

VIRUS (ENCEPHALOMYOCARDITIS)

INCUBATED FOR 24 HOURS

VIRUS PLAQUES STAINED
WITH 5% CARBOL FUSCHIN

Fig. 10.6.2. Interferon assay using viral plaque inhibition. Plaques are counted and antiviral activity is calculated against an interferon standard.

Tjernlund and coworkers [76] reported the expression of class II antigens on keratinocytes as a different approach to in vitro investigation of delayed-type cell-mediated hypersensitivity. These authors demonstrated that in nickel-sensitized patients, in contrast to healthy controls, expression of HLA-DR antigens in keratinocytes could be induced in vitro by coculture of normal skin biopsies with nickel-sulphate-stimulated autologous peripheral blood mononuclear cells. IFN-γ is known to induce HLA-DR expression on cultured keratinocytes, but while this may represent another alternative indirect method of assessing IFN-γ release, it is possible that a mediator other than IFN-γ may be responsible for the MHC class II antigen expression [77]. Irrespective of this, the suitability of this particular approach as an in vitro correlate of contact allergy may be limited by the finding that keratinocyte expression of MHC class II antigens can occur in irritant contact dermatitis as well as allergic contact dermatitis [78].

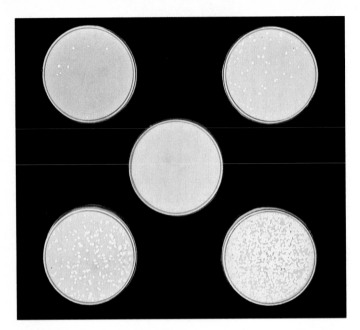

Fig. 10.6.3. Plates demonstrate increasing viral plaque inhibition as a measure of interferon activity

10.6.4 Discussion

In the investigation of contact allergy, several in vitro tests are capable of distinguishing sensitized subjects from controls. Indeed, in a review of the literature by Von Blomberg et al. [79] on those studies in which in vitro tests were used as a diagnostic test, positive reports were noted since 1962. Although these cover a broad range of antigens, most of the allergens currently used in the standard series have not been tested. Results from these studies, however, often reveal overlap between affected individuals and those who are nonallergic. These tests, therefore, while providing a useful means of looking at specific groups of individuals, cannot be relied upon to make the diagnosis of allergy when looking at an individual result taken in isolation.

Almost a century after its introduction, patch testing has, by refinement and standardization, become the single most important test in assessing contact allergy. In contrast, even in the more established in vitro tests such as the MIF and lymphocyte transformation assays, there is complete lack of standardization between laboratories.

In the case of nickel, despite it being the most frequently investigated allergen in vitro, no attempt has been made to reach agreement even on fundamental questions of which nickel salt to use and what the optimal concentration of nickel for antigenic challenge is. This lack of standardization makes difficult the comparison of data from different laboratories using the same test, and meaningful comparison of data from different laboratories using different tests is almost impossible.

In almost 40% of studies aimed at using in vitro procedures as diagnostic tests of contact allergy, nickel is the test allergen used. This is more a reflection of its in vitro suitability in terms of its solubility and low cytotoxicity than of its frequency as an allergen in clinical practice. Von Blomberg et al. [80] evaluated and compared the lymphocyte transformation and MIF tests as in vitro correlates of nickel allergy. They found the MIF test to be less sensitive (26% versus 7% false negatives), but more specific (13% versus 39% false positives) than the lymphocyte transformation test for predicting skin reactivity to nickel. These authors also found that although lymphocyte transformation and MIF data appeared to be only weakly correlated in the individuals tested, using a dual parameter analysis there was excellent correlation between skin test and in vitro reactivity for individuals with *matching* in vitro results (60% of all individuals tested). Silvennoinen-Kassinen [54], using the lymphocyte transformation test to assess in vitro response to nickel, reported a positive reaction in approximately 90% of patients with clinical allergy and a positive patch test. False-positive in vitro responses occurred in 10% of clinically healthy subjects. Al-Tawil et al. [81], also using the lymphocyte transformation test, investigated the correlation between quantitative in vivo and in vitro response in nickel-allergic patients. By testing in vivo, with a range of dilutions of nickel sulphate in water, they determined the lowest concentration eliciting a cutaneous response. This was then compared with the in vitro lymphocyte response. The best correlation coefficients obtained were 0.42 (linear) and 0.46 (logarithmic). In addition, there were several patients who showed a weak response in vivo, but had high lymphocyte reactivity in vitro and vice versa. Hutchinson et al. [49], comparing the clinical state of nickel-allergic subjects with their lymphocyte transformation responses, were unable to find any correlation. Gilboa and colleagues [82] noted that in subjects giving a history of earlobe dermatitis caused by wearing metal earrings containing nickel, in vivo testing was positive in less than 50%, while the in vitro response was negative in most of the subjects. This could be interpreted as suggesting that metallic nickel can elicit a nonimmunogical inflammatory response.

The series of events involving cellular interactions and release of many immunopharmacological mediators in contact dermatitis is extremely complex. Patch testing, through its production of a 'mini' patch of eczema, encompasses the entire reaction. It is almost certainly simplistic to consider that one single in vitro assay, such as measurement of a lymphokine, will provide a definitive test which is a direct correlate of the entire in vivo response. A single lymphokine may exert several different effects and may be released in inflammatory responses other than allergic contact hypersensitivity. Nevertheless, current investigative techniques enable differentiation of groups of allergic individuals from normal controls.

Refinement and standardization of procedures may enable in vitro assessment of an individual's susceptibility to a particular contact allergen such as nickel. Such a technique must be simple, quick and reproducible. Up to now the techniques used to assess lymphokines have tended to be indirect. Rather than measure the effects of these mediators, advances using developments in fields of monoclonal antibodies, radioimmunoassays and enzyme-linked immunosorbent assay (ELISA) [83] should enable direct measurement of specific lymphokines.

Positive reports on in vitro investigations in the diagnosis of contact allergy over the past 20 years have been based on measurement of the products of T-cell activation. More recently, however, attention has focused on direct identification of allergen-specific cells. The specificity for contact allergic hypersensitivity appears to reside within the T helper subset [74, 84, 85] and it has been possible to clone antigen-specific T cells for certain contact allergens (cobalt [85], nickel [74, 86]). The development of a method which could detect the presence of specific T cells within the circulation would have considerable advantages over current testing procedures. Such a test, however, will not only have to take into account the large number of allergen-specific T-cell receptors, but also the different MHC class II restriction patterns [79].

The diagnosis of contact allergy will continue to rely on the skills of the clinician, combined with in vivo testing [87]. The development of a suitable in vitro test, using a standardized technique, could provide complementary information to enable the correct diagnosis to be established, particularly in cases where patch testing is contraindicated or the results inconclusive. In vitro tests are likely to continue to be difficult to perform for substances of low solubility, such as colophony, wool alcohols or fragrances.

10.6.5 References

1. Jadassohn J (1895) Zur Kenntnis der medicamentosen Dermatosen. In: Verhandlungen der deutschen dermatologischen Gesellshaft, fünfter Congress. Jarish and Neisser, pp 103–129
2. Burrows D, Creswell SN, Merrett JD (1981) Nickel, hands and hip prostheses. Br J Dermatol 105: 437–444
3. Moller H, Svensson A (1986) Metal sensitivity: positive history but negative test indicates atopy. Contact Dermatitis 14: 57–60
4. Fisher AA (1982) Problems attending patch testing for nickel sensitivity. Cutis 29: 148–152
5. Mitchell JC (1981) Angry back syndrome. Contact Dermatitis 7: 359–361
6. Chase MW (1967) Hypersensitivity to simple chemicals. Harvey Lectures 61: 169–203
7. Silberberg I, Baer RL, Rosenthal SA (1974) The role of Langerhans cells in contact allergy. Acta Derm Venereol (Stockh) 54: 321–31.
8. Dumonde DC, Wolstencroft RA, Panayi GS, Matthew M, Morley J, Howsen WJ (1969) Lymphokines: non-antibody mediators of cellular immunity generated by lymphocyte activation. Nature 224: 38–42.
9. Maini RN, Bryceson ADM, Wolstencroft RA, Dumonde DC (1969) Lymphocyte mitogenic factor in man. Nature 224: 43–44

10. Nishioka K, Amos HE (1973) Contact sensitivity in vitro: the production of macrophage inhibition factors from DNCB sensitized lymphocytes by subcellular organelles obtained from DNCB epidermal tissue. Immunology 25: 423–432
11. Nishioka KL (1976) Detection of human contact sensitivity to dinitrochlorobenzene by the migration inhibition test. J Invest Dermatol 66: 351–354
12. Delescluse J, Turk JC (1970) Lymphocyte cytotoxocity: a possible in vitro test for contact dermatitis. Lancet I: 75–77
13. Cohen S, Ward PA, Yoshida T et al. (1973) Biologic activity of extracts of delayed hypersensitivity skin reaction sites. Cell Immunol 9: 363–376
14. Nishioka K, Katayama I (1978) Angiogenic activity in culture supernatant of antigen-stimulated lymph node cells. J Pathol 126: 63–69
15. Rich AR, Lewis MR (1932) The nature of allergy in tuberculosis as revealed by tissue culture studies. Bull Johns Hopkins Hospital 50: 115–131
16. George M, Vaughan JH (1962) In vitro cell migration as a model for delayed hypersensitivity. Proc Soc Exp Biol Med 111: 514–521
17. Bloom BR, Bennett B (1966) Mechanism of a reaction in vitro associated with delayed hypersensitivity. Science 153: 80–82
18. David JR (1966) Delayed hypersensitivity in vitro: its mediation by cell-free substances formed by lymphoid cell-antigen interaction. Proc Natl Acad Sci USA 56: 72–77
19. David JR (1973) Lymphocyte mediators and cellular hypersensitivity. N Engl J Med 288: 143–149
20. Rocklin RE (1974) Products of activated lymphocytes; leukocyte inhibitory factor (LIF) distinct from migration inhibitory factor (MIF). J Immunol 122: 1461–1466
21. Hamblin AS, Maini RN (1980) An evaluation of lymphokine measurement in man. In: Thompson RA (ed) Recent advances in clinical immunology, 2nd edn. Churchill Livingstone, Edinburgh pp 243–273
22. Grosfeld JCM, Penders AJM, de Grood R, Verwilghen L (1966) In vitro investigations of chromium- and nickel-hypersensitivity with culture of skin and peripheral lymphocytes. Dermatologica 132: 189–198
23. Thulin H, Zachariae H (1972) The leucocyte migration test in chromium hypersensitivity. J Invest Dermatol 58: 55–58
24. Mirza AM, Perera MG, Bernstein IL (1974) Leukocyte migration inhibition in nickel dermatitis. Fed Proc 33: 728
25. Mirza AM, Perera MG, Maccia CA, Dziubynskyj OG, Bernstein IL (1975) Leukocyte migration inhibition in nickel dermatitis. Int Arch Allergy Appl Immunol 49: 782–788
26. Thulin H (1976) The leukocyte migration test in nickel contact dermatitis. Acta Derm Venereol (Stockholm) 56: 377–380
27. Jordan WP, Dvorak (1976) Leukocyte migration inhibition assay (LIF) in nickel contact dermatitis. Arch Dermatol 122: 1741–1744
28. Jones BM (1973) Sealed capillary leucocyte migration test. Med Lab Tech 30: 245–249
29. Nordlind K, Sandberg G (1983) Leukocytes from patients allergic to chromium and nickel examined by the sealed capillary migration technique. Int Arch Allergy Appl Immunol 70: 30–3
30. Nowell PC (1960) Phytohemagglutinin, an initiator of mitosis in cultures of normal human leucocytes. Cancer Res 20: 462–466
31. Oppenheim JJ (1969) Immunological relevance of antigen and antigen antibody complex induced lymphocyte transformation. Ann Allergy 27: 305–315
32. Fisher DB, Mueller GC (1968) An early alteration in the phospholipid metabolism of lymphocytes by phytohemagglutinin. Proc Natl Acad Sci USA 60: 1396–1402
33. Wheelock EF (1965) Interferon-like virus inhibitor induced in human leukocytes by phytohemagglutinin. Science 149: 310–311

34. Cooper HL, Rubin AD (1965) RNA metabolism in lymphocytes stimulated by phytohemagglutinin: initial responses to phytohemagglutinin. Blood 25: 1014–1027
35. Mackinney AA, Stohlman F, Brecher G (1962) The kinetics of cell proliferation in cultures of human peripheral blood. Blood 19: 349–358
36. Cooper EH, Barkhan P, Hale AJ (1963) Observations on the proliferation of human leucocytes cultured with phytohaemagglutinin. Br J Haematol 9: 101–111
37. Caron GA, Sarkany I, Williams HS, Todd AP (1965) Radioactive method for the measurement of lymphocyte transformation in vitro. Lancet II: 1266–1268
38. Farnes P, Barker BE, Brownhill LE, Fanger H (1964) Mitogenic activity in *Phytolacca americana* (pokeweed). Lancet II: 1100–1101
39. Powell AE, Leon MA (1970) Reversible interaction of human lymphocytes with the mitogen concanavalin A. Exp Cell Res 62: 315–325
40. Marshall WH, Roberts KB (1963) Tuberculin-induced mitosis in peripheral blood leucocytes. Lancet I: 773
41. Pearmain G, Lycette RR, Fitzgerald PH (1963) Tuberculin-induced mitosis in peripheral blood leucocytes. Lancet I: 637–638
42. Mills JA (1966) The immunologic significance of antigen induced lymphocyte transformation in vitro. J Immunol 97: 239–247
43. Bach F, Hirschhorn K (1964) Lymphocyte interaction: a potential histocompatibility test in vitro. Science 143: 813–814
44. Aspegren N, Rorsman H (1962) Short-term culture of leucocytes in nickel hypersensitivty. Acta Derm Venereol (Stockh) 42: 412–417
45. Pappas A, Orfanos CE, Bertram (1970) Non-specific lymphocyte transformation in vitro by nickel acetate. A possible source of errors in lymphocyte transformation test (LTT). J Invest Dermatol 55: 198–200
46. Schopf E, Schulz KH, Isensee I (1969) Untersuchungen über den Lymphocyten-transformations-Test bei Quecksilber-Allergie, unspezifische Transformation durch Hg-Verbindungen. Arch Klin Exp Derm 234: 420–433
47. Schopf E, Schulz KH, Gromm M (1967) Transformation and Mitosen von Lympho-cyten in vitro durch Quecksilber II-Chlorid. Naturwissenschaften 5: 568–569
48. Macleod TM, Hutchinson F, Raffle EJ (1970) The uptake of labelled thymidine by leucocytes of nickel sensitive patients. Br J Dermatol 82: 487–492
49. Hutchinson F, Raffle EJ, Macleod TM (1972) The specificity of lymphocyte trans-formation in vitro by nickel salts in nickel sensitive subjects. J Invest Dermatol 58: 362–365
50. Millikan LE, Conway F, Foote JE (1973) In vitro studies of contact hypersensitivity: lymphocyte transformation in nickel sensitivity. J Invest Dermatol 60: 88–90
51. Gimenez-Camarasa JM, Garcia-Calderon P, Asensio J, De Maragas JM (1975) Lym-phocyte transformation test in allergic contact nickel dermatitis. Br J Dermatol 92: 9–15
52. Kim CW, Schopf E (1976) A comparative study of nickel hypersensitivity by the lymphocyte transformation test in atopic and non-atopic dermatitis. Arch Dermatol Res 257: 57–65
53. Svejgaard E, Morling N, Svejgaard A, Veien NK (1978) Lymphocyte transformation induced by nickel sulphate: an in vitro study of subjects with and without a positive nickel patch test. Acta Derm Venereol (Stockh) 58: 245–250
54. Silvennoinen-Kassinen S (1981) The specificity of a nickel sulphate reaction in vitro: a familial study and a study of chromium-allergic subjects. Scand J Imunol 13: 231–235
55. Al-Tawil NG, Marcusson JA, Moller E (1981) Lymphocyte transformation test in patients with nickel sensitivity: an aid to diagnosis. Acta Derm Venereol (Stockh.) 61: 511–515
56. Nordlind K (1984) Lymphocyte transformation test in diagnosis of nickel allergy. Int Arch Allergy Appl Immunol 73: 151–154

57. Hutchinson F, Macleod TM, Raffle EJ (1971) Lymphocyte transformation. Br J Dermatol 85: 300–301
58. Macleod TM, Hutchinson F, Raffle EJ (1982) In vitro studies on blastogenic lymphokine activity in nickel allergy. Acta Derm Venereol (Stockh) 62: 249–250
59. Powell JA, Whalen JJ, Levis WR (1975) Studies on the contact sensitization of man with simple chemicals (IV). Timing of skin reactivity, lymphokine production and blastogenesis following rechallenge with dinitrochlorobenzene using an automated microassay. J Invest Dermatol 64: 357–363
60. Veien NK, Svejgaard E, Menne T (1979) In vitro lymphocyte transformation to nickel: a study of nickel-sensitive patients before and after epicutaneous and oral challenge with nickel. Acta Derm Venereol (Stockh) 59: 447–451
61. Colvin RB, Johnson RA, Mihm MC Jr, Dvorak HF (1973) Role of the clotting system in cell-mediated hypersensitivity. I. Fibrin deposition in delayed skin reactions in man. J Exp Med 138: 686–698
62. Nelson DS (1965) The effects of anticoagulants and other drugs on cellular and cutaneous reactions to antigen in guinea-pigs with delayed-type hypersensitivity. Immunology 9: 219–234
63. Feinman L, Cohen S, Becker EL (1970) The effect of fumaropimaric acid on delayed hypersensitivity and cutaneous Forssman reactions in the guinea pig. J Immunol 104: 1401–1405
64. Rickles FR, Hardin JA, Pitlick FA, Hoyer LW, Conrad ME (1973) Tissue factor activity in lymphocyte cultures from normal individuals and patients with hemophilia A. J Clin Invest 52: 1427–1434
65. Edwards RL, Rickles FR, Bobrove AM (1979) Mononuclear cell tissue factor: cell of origin and requirements for activation. Blood 54: 359–370
66. Geczy CL, Hopper KE (1981) A mechanism of migration inhibition in delayed-type hypersensitivity reactions. II. Lymphokines promote procoagulant activity of macrophages in vitro. J Immunol 126: 1059–1065
67. Geczy CL, Meyer PA (1982) Leukocyte procoagulant activity in man: an in vitro correlate of delayed-type hypersensitivity. J Imunol 128: 331–336
68. Aldridge RD, Milton JI, Thompson AW (1985) Leukocyte procoagulant activity as an in vitro index of nickel contact hypersensitivity. Int Arch Allergy Appl Immunol 76: 350–353
69. Isaacs A, Lindenmann J (1957) Virus interference 1. The interferon. Proc R Soc Lond [Biol] 147: 258–267
70. Wardle EN (1987) Interferon-gamma: actions and importance. Br J Hosp Med 37: 446–448
71. Green JA, Cooperband SA, Kibrick S (1969) Immune specific induction of interferon production in cultures of human blood lymphocytes. Science 164: 1415–1417
72. McKimm-Breschkin JL, Mottram PL, Thomas WR, Miller JF (1982) Antigen-specific production of immune interferon by T cell lines. J Exp Med 155: 1204–1209
73. McMillan C, Adamson H, Burrows D, McNeill T (1986) Lymphokine antiviral activity in contact dermatitis. Presented at 8th international symposium on contact dermatitis, Cambridge
74. Sinigaglia F, Scheidegger D, Garotta G, Sheper R, Pletscher M, Lanzavecchia A (1985) Isolation and characterisation of Ni-specific T cell clones from patients with Ni-contact dermatitis. J Immuno 135: 3929–3932
75. Karttunen R, Silvennoinen-Kassinen S, Juutinen K, Andersson G, Ekre H-PT, Karvonen J (1988) Nickel antigen induces IL-2 secretion and IL-2 receptor expression on $CD4^+$ T cells, but no measurable gamma interferon secretion in peripheral blood mononuclear cell cultures in delayed type hypersensitivity to nickel. Clin Exp Immunol 74: 387–391
76. Tjernlund U, Scheynius A, Strand A (1987) In vitro testing of contact sensitivity. Acta Derm Venereol (Stockh) 67: 417–421

77. Groenewegen G, De Ley M, Jeunhomme GMAA, Buurman WA (1986) Supernatants of human leukocytes contain mediator, different from interferon, which induces expression of MHC class II antigens. J Exp Med 164: 131–143
78. Gawkrodger DJ, Carr MM, McVittie E, Guy K, Hunter JAA (1987) Keratinocyte expression of MHC class II antigens in allergic sensitization and challenge reactions and in irritant contact dermatitis. J Invest Dermatol 88: 11–16
79. Von Blomberg-van der Flier BME, Bruynzeel DP, Scheper RJ. Impact of 25 years of in vitro testing in allergic contact dermatitis. In: Frosch PJ, Dooms-Goossens A, Lachapelle J-M, et al (eds) Current topics in contact dermatitis. Springer, Berlin Heidelberg New York, pp 569–577
80. Von Blomberg BME, Bruynzeel DP, Scheper RJ (1987) In vitro diagnosis of allergic contact dermatitis. Presented at 17th world congress of dermatology, Berlin
81. Al-Tawil NG, Berggren G, Emtestam L, Fransson J, Jernselius R, Marcusson JA (1985) Correlation between quantitative in vivo and in vitro responses in nickel-allergic patients, Acta Derm Venereol (Stockh) 65: 385–389
82. Gilboa R, Al-Tawil NG, Marcusson JA (1988) Metal allergy in cashiers. Acta Derm Venereol (Stockh) 68: 317–324
83. Boerrigter GH, Vos A, Scheper RJ (1983) Direct measurement of in vitro antibody production using an enzyme-linked immunosorbent assay. J Immunol Methods 61: 377–384
84. Silvennoinen-Kassinen S, Jakkula H, Karvonen J (1986) Helper cells (Leu-3a$^+$) carry the specifity of nickel sensitivity reaction in vitro in humans. J Invest Dermatol 86: 18–20
85. Lofstrom A, Wigzell H (1986) Antigen specific human T cell lines specific for cobalt chloride. Acta Derm Venereol (Stockh) 66: 200–206
86. Kapsenberg ML, Res P, Bos JD, Schootemijer A, Teunissen MBM, Van Schooten W (1987) Nickel-specific T lymphocyte clones derived from allergic nickel-contact dermatitis lesions in man: heterogeneity based on requirement of dendritic antigenpresenting cell subsets. Eur J Immunol 17: 861–865
87. Milner JE (1986) In vitro tests for delayed skin hypersensitivity: lymphokine production in allergic contact dermatitis. In: Marzulli FN, Maibach HI (eds) Dermatotoxicology, 3rd edn. Hemisphere, New York, p 217

10.7 Noninvasive Techniques for Quantification of Contact Dermatitis

JØRGEN SERUP

Contents

10.7.1 Introduction

History and clinical examination are the main tools of clinical dermatologists. Inspection of the skin is rapid, and the lateral extension and severity of a dermatitis is easily assessed. The disadvantage is that this method is essentially subjective. As a research tool it is open to bias and thus difficult to use. With punch biopsy and microscopy, detailed information about the layers of the skin and their involvement with dermatitis is obtained; however, a punch usually represents only a very small fraction of diseased skin, and processing and staining are a kind of desirable artefact. The result still has a subjective element, related to the pathologist's examination.

Information and knowledge are not simply a matter of high magnification and fine detail. In the dermatological armamentarium there is an area between clinical evaluation and sophisticated technique where noninvasive bioengineering techniques may be relevant. Bioengineering techniques offer (a) noninvasiveness and in vivo information, with instant results; (b) objective assessment (quantitation or imaging as a basis for computerized analysis); (c) choice of body region and site of examination, with only few limitations depending on technique; and (d) the same site can be studied by different techniques, and follow-up examinations performed to study the spontaneous course and effect of treatment, without interfering with the subject being studied.

10.7.2 Prerequisites and Planning of Study by Noninvasive Techniques

Various devices for noninvasive evaluation of the skin have become available. It is straightforward to put a probe on the skin and to get a reading on a digital display. Generally, variation and inconclusiveness are more likely to be attributable to the way in which devices are used, rather than to inaccuracy of the equipment. Before a study based on bioengineering methods is conducted, the essentials of the method need be known, and a number of questions asked. These include the following:
– What information is expected?
– What is the most relevant variable to be measured, and which variables serve for description, comparison, support or exclusion?
– What is the expected time course of variables, and when should measurements be performed?
– Are variables expected to develop linearly, or not?
– What are the ranges of variables in relation to the expected phenomenon or structure being studied, including inter- and intraindividual variation and dependence of anatomical site, sex and age?
– What function or structure is actually being tested?
– What is the measuring area, and, if small, should more recordings be taken and averaged to overcome local site variation?
– Are recordings with the equipment reproducible, and is the accuracy acceptable relative to variables being measured and their expected range?
– What are the measuring standards and calibration procedures?
– Are there environmental standards and calibration procedures?
– Are there environmental influences, including season, and a need for special laboratory room facilities?
– Is preconditioning of the individual necessary before testing?
– What excludes measurements from being performed?
– Has the researcher or technician both the training and sufficient practical experience to conduct the study?

As in any other research field, the results depend essentially on the ratio between signal and noise, where noise means sources of variation, some predictable, others unknown. At the moment the success of studies based on noninvasive techniques depends mainly on the training of the researcher and appropriate planning, with an emphasis on proper control of predictable sources of variaton.

10.7.3 Review of Noninvasive Techniques Relevant to the Study of Contact Dermatitis

Essentials of skin structure and function as a basis for bioengineering studies were reviewed in the past by Rothman [1] and more recently by Goldsmith [2]. Various monographs about bioengineering methods and their technical principles and applications have appeared [3–7]. Recently, bioengineering and the patch test have been summarized [8].

Several noninvasive techniques were used in the past to study contact dermatitis, often prototypes or laboratory equipment. Some techniques such as polysulphide rubber replica are simple and can be used directly, while others are complicated, and validation, multiplication and commercialization are needed before they can attract general interest. This introduction deals mainly with techniques that are available and can be practiced in a variety of laboratories.

10.7.3.1 Changes in the Skin Surface

Change of colour and the skin surface are central to the visual assessment of contact dermatitis.

The colour of the skin, including erythema, can be measured by two different principles: (a) spectrophotometric scanning, using wavelengths of 400–800 nm and measurement of absorbance and reflectance, and (b) tristimulus analysis of reflected flash light. Spectrophotometric scanning has proven of little practical use because the broad melanin absorption band overlaps with the haemoglobin band, and because nonspecific optical phenomena of the skin, related to scaling and scattering, influence recordings significantly. However, devices that measure the haemoglobin band specifically and express erythema as an index of haemoglobin relative to melanin have appeared; if technically of high precision, these may prove useful [9].

The perception of colour by the human eye and brain is in the range of 400–800 nm, with a maximum of sensitivity between 500 and 600 nm, corresponding to the colour of blood and therefore redness. Equipment based on tristimulus analysis of reflected light and the Commission International d'Eclairage (CIE) takes this alinearity of the eye into account and expresses any colour in a three-dimensional system (Fig. 10.7.1) with green-red (a*), yellow-blue (b*) and L* axes, where L* expresses brightness [10]. In erythema, a* increases, L* decreases, and b* is unaltered [11]. Tristimulus devices are convenient and rapid to operate.

The contour of the skin surface, with scales, papules, vesicles, etc., can be studied by clinical photography and by various replica techniques. The main difficulty of close-up photography is that the flashgun light, after scattering within the skin, is reflected back to the camera lens from different layers of the skin with different microstructure and under different angles from the same

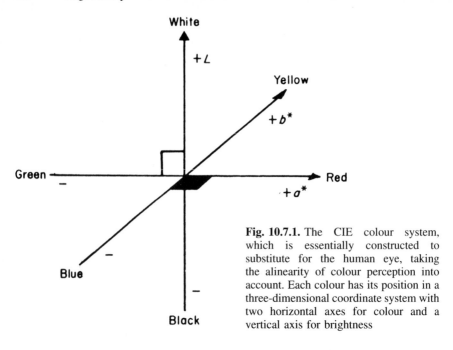

Fig. 10.7.1. The CIE colour system, which is essentially constructed to substitute for the human eye, taking the alinearity of colour perception into account. Each colour has its position in a three-dimensional coordinate system with two horizontal axes for colour and a vertical axis for brightness

structure. Skin surface pictures become much sharper if the surface is coated and transmission and scattering eliminated. If immersion oil is applied and optical effects of the surface thus eliminated, dermal structures such as blood vessels may be seen. In clinical photography the film and copy process is also subject to variation between batches, with significant influences on the photograph [12]. Using polysulphide rubber imprint material, 30° incident light and a stereomicroscope surface, details are clearly illustrated since the flexible rubber material is not transparent. Replica can be stored and evaluated blind and in batches under laboratory conditions. Replica can also be used as a basis for advanced quantification by stylus method and by computerized image analysis [13]. Recently a tape method was introduced, representing a development of the sticky slide technique for harvesting stratum corneum material. This may be useful for qualitative and quantitative evaluation of scaling and hyperkeratosis of dermatitis [14].

10.7.3.2 Epidermal Hydration and Water Barrier Function

Although invisibly, the water barrier of the skin is very often damaged in dermatitis, with consequences for the biology of the epidermis and the clinical manifestations.

Hydration of the skin surface can be measured by electrical methods [15, 16]. The construction of the detector and the technical specifications determine the layer of the epidermis that is measured. The contour of the skin and the size and shape of the detector determine the electrical contact and influence results. If the detector is small, more measurements need be taken and averaged to minimize local site variation. The conductance measurer described by Tagami [16] measures very superficially, and the Corneometer CM 420 based on electrical capacitance more deeply in the epidermis [17, 18]. Recent studies show that the compartment of the epidermis that is able to bind water is only small, and diffusional equilibrium between stratum corneum and ambient air takes place quickly, i.e. within 10 min [19]. Following occlusion, the biology of the epidermis changes, and equilibrium with ambient air takes a longer time, i.e. after 24 h of occlusion, 30 min or longer. Thus, when measuring skin surface hydration the skin needs be uncovered for a period before recordings. The temperature and humidity of the laboratory also need be kept within certain limits.

The parameter of transepidermal water loss (TEWL) expresses diffusional water loss through the skin and is of major importance in irritant reactions to detergents. Various closed chamber methods have been used in the past; however, these were cumbersome and interfered with the spontaneous TEWL. The method of open chamber, water vapour evaporation, and gradient estimation as described by Nilsson is widely used [20, 21]. The water vapour pressure gradient is measured with sensors (Fig. 10.7.2) at two different levels above the skin, and the TEWL is calculated [20, 21]. Proper preconditioning and good control of measuring conditions is essential for accurate recordings. Sources of variation were recently reviewed, and guidelines were given by the standardization group of the European Society of Contact Dermatitis [22]. The water barrier of the skin does not resemble a filter or membrane within the skin but a gradient across the skin, including a 10-mm layer of ambient air. Thus, the environment is part of the water barrier, and changes of temperature and humidity influence the passage of water out of the skin, and also the skin surface hydration. Eccrine sweating is, in most body regions, less important except after physical activity, when it has the capacity to increase by many times. Environmental changes related to season also need to be considered [23].

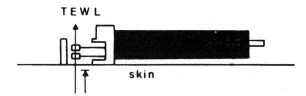

Fig. 10.7.2. Open chamber probe for measurement of TEWL. Pairs of sensors (hygrosensors coupled with thermistors) mounted in the chamber at different levels above the skin for determination of the humidity gradient in the chamber, representing the flux of water out of the skin, or the TEWL.

10.7.3.3 Parameters of Inflammation

Vasodilatation and oedema formation are the essential features of inflammation. Blood flow has been extensively studied while oedema formation has been comparatively overlooked.

The use of skin surface temperature as a measure of inflammatory activity is more or less obsolete in contact dermatitis. In normal skin the temperature varies within narrow limits. In dermatitis vasodilatation tends to increase the temperature towards the core temperature, but evaporation, crusting and scaling tend to decrease the temperature. Skin surface temperature can be measured by contact methods, including cholesteric crystal sheets, and by infrared nontouch methods. The main field of contact thermography in contact dermatitis is to image lateral temperature gradients, which may give detailed information about inflammation and crusting of patch test reactions [7, 24, 25].

The *vasodilatation* of inflammation and the increase in blood flow is often measured by laser Doppler flowmetry [6]. A variety of equipment is available. The tone of the cutaneous vasculature is normally in a relatively contracted condition, and it may be difficult to monitor vasoconstriction such as blanching due to corticosteroids. A 30-fold increase in flow may be seen in dermatitis; however, in advanced inflammation the oedema may compress vessels, and the degree of inflammatory activity may be underestimated. As compared to other methods, laser Doppler flowmetry is both sensitive and discriminative. The vasculature and its tone is in a state of dynamic balance, and factors such as mental stress and noise instantly influence the flow. Thus, both preconditioning and measuring conditions need be considered.

Measurement of the *oedema* of inflammatory reactions may be carried out by skin fold calipers and by high-frequency ultrasound (Fig. 10.7.3). Calipers inevitably compress the oedema, and it is unclear what layer of the skin is being included in the fold and measured. With ultrasound, high frequency and broad bandwidth are needed. Transducers of 20 MHz have provided a good compromise between the needs of resolution and depth of viewing field. With A-mode scanners the thickness of dermatitis skin can be measured and the increase in thickness representing oedema formation calculated [26]. With B-mode and C-mode scanners cross-sectional imaging of the skin is possible [27]. In vivo distances, areas, volume and structure analysis are possible by the use of computerized analysis. Ultrasound shows that inflammatory oedema

---

Fig. 10.7.3a,b. High-frequency B-mode scanning of a 1 + allergic reaction (**A**) and a 2 + allergic reaction (**B**) to nickel, obtained with Dermascan C.® A plastic membrane from the probe chamber is seen over the skin. Underneath the epidermis an echolucent band of oedema formation appears, with projections along the hair follicles and sebaceous glands. *White* and *blue* represent strong ultrasound reflections, *yellow* and *red* moderate, and *green* weak reflections. Subcutaneous fat is minimally echogenic and is seen *black*, as is the coupling medium between the ultrasound transducer and the skin surface with the plastic membrane

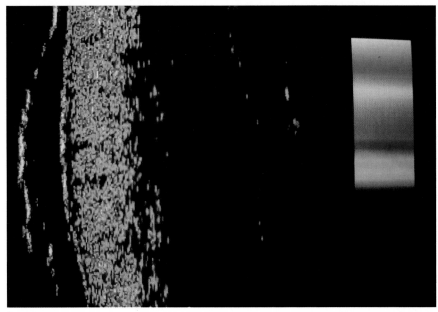

a

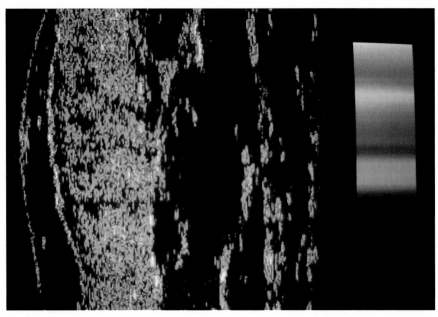

b

develops mainly in the papillary dermis, where it propagates and results in an echolucent band which can be measured and followed during the different stages of the inflammatory process (Fig. 10.7.3). Education and training is needed to perform ultrasound examination, as in any other specialty.

Generally, methods assessing static features such as structure and dimension are less vulnerable to measuring conditions and easier to standardize, compared to methods based on functions.

10.7.4 Allergic Contact Dermatitis

Erythema, oedema, papules, and vesicles are the well-known manifestations of acute allergic contact dermatitis that are read in diagnostic patch testing. Using noninvasive techniques, the same manifestations can be quantified. In strong reactions, bullae, erosions and crusts may appear. Once elicited, it is held that the cascade of events essentially follows the same course. In the chronic stage hyperkeratosis and scaling is often prominent. Unlike the situation in irritant contact dermatitis, allergic reactions have been relatively little studied by noninvasive techniques in the past.

Study of the skin surface contour by polysulphide rubber replica shows that counts of papules and vesicles correlate with clinical readings, and doubtful reactions may be divided into those with sporadic papules and those without but with an impression from the margin of the test chamber instead [28].

Studies of skin colour and allergic contact dermatitis have not appeared. It is likely that weak and moderate reactions can be ranked, but in strong reactions changes of the physical character of the skin surface are likely to influence the optical properties and create variation.

Epidermal hydration and TEWL depend very much on the clinical state of the dermatitis. In chronic dermatitis with scaling the conductance is decreased, due to a reduced water binding capacity, in contrast to TEWL, which is increased [29]. The value of conductance measurements seems not to lie in grading of early stage dermatitis but in assessment of chronic stages and documentation of healing. Decreased conductance and increased TEWL is very common in long-lasting dermatitis, irrespective of its origin. Nevertheless, increased TEWL is not a primary event in allergic reactions, but the water barrier becomes progressively damaged during the first few days as inflammation develops [30].

The surface temperature of acute allergic reactions is increased; however, if vesicles and bullae leaving crusts appear the temperature pattern of the surface may be irregular, with decreased temperature corresponding to the crusts [24, 25, 31]. Increased temperature may persist for a period after visible changes have disappeared [7].

Allergic reactions to nickel show increased blood flow as measured by laser Doppler flowmetry, and positive, doubtful and negative reactions can be distinguished [32]. However, the positive reactions may be difficult to rank. Probably the inflammatory response has an initial stage dominated by vasodilation and a more advanced stage dominated by oedema formation which compresses the vasculature. Allergic patch test reactions and irritant reactions to sodium lauryl sulphate (SLS) show increase of blood flow at the same level [33].

Ultrasound measurement of skin thickness and the oedema of allergic patch test reactions shows progressive thickening of the skin as the clinical reaction increases [26, 27, 34]. With ultrasound strong reactions can also be graded. The oedema formation of allergic reactions is more severe as compared to irritant reactions after SLS, matched with respect to strength of the reactions clinically [26]. With ultrasound B-mode scanning an echolucent band is seen in the papillary dermis immediately underneath the epidermis, representing more advanced oedema and swelling of the outer dermis (Fig. 10.7.3) [27]. It is a general feature that the inflammation of contact dermatitis mainly involves the papillary dermis, which is more easily distended under the influence of the pressure of oedema than the reticular dermis. Such changes cannot be evaluated by routine histology since histological processing is highly intrusive to tissue water, which is extracted and replaced by lipophilic media before embedding in paraffin.

10.7.5 Irritant Contact Dermatitis

Irritant contact dermatitis is not a uniform entity of disease, but each irritant exerts its particular noxious effects on the skin, and each occupation has its special set of risk substances and mode of physical contact [35]. Obviously, this creates diversity in the manifestations of irritancy and the way in which it is best assessed. Moreover, reactions are dependent on age, body region, menstrual phase, skin complexion and skin type, including sensitivity to sunlight etc. Thus, control of a great number of variables is needed as a prerequisite.

A number of substances and test procedures were evaluated in the past by Björnberg [36] and more recently by Frosch [37]. Monographs on irritant contact dermatitis and TEWL have been published by van der Valk [38], Pinnagoda [39] and Tupker [40]. Irritancy and laser Doppler flowmetry was studied by de Boer [41], and Agner has studied irritancy by various methods, including replica, thermography, TEWL, laser Doppler flowmetry, colorimetry, high-frequency ultrasound and conductance [42].

The change in colour in the direction of redness as elicited by the irritant SLS is characterized by an increase in a*, a minor decrease in L*, and unchanged b*, as measured according to the CIE system [11]. Colorimeters based on the CIE system and tristimulus colour analysis are especially suited to a busy routine and for situations in which preconditioning is difficult. Colorimetry appears accurate for the distinction of positive reactions from

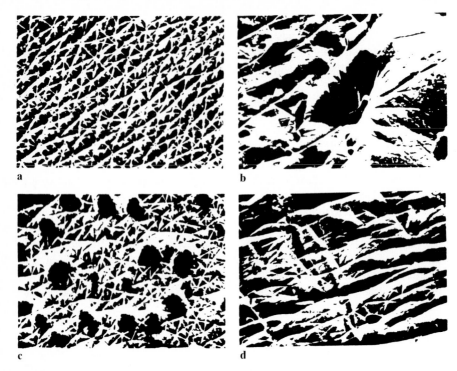

Fig. 10.7.4a–d. Replica from normal skin (*a*), allergic reaction with papules and bullae (*b*), irritant reaction to croton oil (*c*), and irritant reaction to sodium lauryl sulphate (*d*)

negative reactions; however, colorimetry is less precise for a more differentiated ranking of redness, depending on the irritant being studied [42, 43]. A major reason why grading of redness can be difficult is that the vasodilatation of inflammation, as mentioned, does not run linearly but fades out as the oedema progresses. Moreover, microanatomical changes in the skin surface of strong reactions influence the optical properties of the skin nonspecifically, with consequences for the measurement of colour. In chronic dermatitis, hyperkeratosis and scaling may influence colorimeter measurements.

The skin surface contour changes depending on the irritant and the time of examination, which studies with polysulphide rupper replica demonstrate [44]. Some irritants induce a papular pattern, others a nonpapular pattern (Fig. 10.7.4). Propanol, which is used as a vehicle for nonanoic acid, is itself irritant and changes the skin relief.

The skin surface hydration of irritant contact dermatitis is the result of damage to the cutaneous water barrier induced by the irritant on one side, resulting in increased water vapour pressure in and over the stratum corneum, and the formation of crusts, hyperkeratosis and scales on the other side, resulting in reduced water binding capacity and decreased stratum corneum hydration. Already in the acute stage of dermatitis, most irritants exert a noxious effect, with a decrease of electrical conductance and capacitance, depending on the specific irritant and its ability to coagulate the skin surface, while increased hydration is found only in some individuals and mainly from the detergent SLS [18]. In chronic-stage contact dermatitis the electrical measurements are almost without exception decreased [29]. Due to the variable structure and pathophysiology of acute irritant reactions, electrical methods have not been found very useful for the grading of irritancy [43].

Measurement of TEWL and damage of the water barrier has proven important for the characterization of irritant effects on skin elicited by detergents [38–40, 42]. Studies using mainly SLS as a model detergent have demonstrated that TEWL measurement is more accurate than other methods, such as laser Doppler flowmetry, colorimetry and ultrasound, for the grading of this irritant [39, 40, 42, 43, 45]. Impairment of the water barrier and increase of TEWL is not found only in the acute stage of dermatitis but also in chronic stages, with hyperkeratosis and scaling [29]. The difficulty with TEWL is that a number of prerequisites with respect to preconditioning and laboratory conditions need be fulfilled for measurements to be accurate, as described by the standardization group [21]. It must be stressed again that different irritants act differently on the skin, and experiences obtained with detergents cannot be uncritically extended to any other substance [35, 44, 45]. The use of TEWL to detect sensitive skin and predict the occupational risk of irritant contact dermatitis is described below.

Measurement of skin surface temperature, as mentioned above, is not an accurate measure of the inflammatory activity of irritant contact dermatitis. However, thermographic imaging of skin surface temperature gradients demonstrates that some reactions to irritants are cold due to the formation of a temperature-insulating crusting, while others are warm [24, 25, 31]. Different skin surface temperature patterns appear during the course of irritant reactions, and such patterns may be followed using thermographic methods and compared with allergic reactions.

Laser Doppler flowmetry has been used extensively for the evaluation of irritant contact dermatitis [41, 42, 46]. Experiments with SLS and laser Doppler flowmetry have demonstrated a dose-response relationship [41–43, 45, 46], and the method has proven valuable for the quantification of irritant reactions and their inflammatory component. In the evaluation of reactions elicited by SLS, laser Doppler flowmetry is, however, less acurate than TEWL and ultrasound measurements [43, 45]. As noted above, the oedema of strong reactions may compress the vasculature and influence the flow. Also changes in the skin surface, such as vesicles, bullae, crusts, hyperkeratosis and scaling, may influence the optics of the skin and the laser signal. Using probes covering a small surface area only, averaging of three or more recordings is necessary to overcome local site variation in the cutaneous blood supply. The laser Doppler method registers the total blood flow, and recordings are easily influenced by measuring conditions such as talking, breathing, noise and mental stress. Thus, preconditioning and laboratory conditions need to be carefully controlled.

High-frequency (20-MHz) ultrasound measurement of skin thickening and oedema formation has been used in numerous studies of SLS irritant reactions [26, 27, 42, 43, 45], and a dose-response relationship has been demonstrated. For the evaluation of SLS reactions in which damage of the water barrier is prominent ultrasound has an accuracy in between TEWL and laser Doppler flowmetry [43, 45]. In types of reactions with less-pronounced damage to the water barrier, ultrasound is probably more accurate. Hitherto, the cross-sectional ultrasound image of contact dermatitis has been relatively little studied. However, inflammatory oedema of the skin does not expand it in a uniform way. Oedema extends mainly in the more soft and pliable papillary dermis, and an echolucent band is seen by ultrasound [27]. Ultrasound has the advantage that structure is studied, and preconditioning and laboratory conditions are therefore not critical. Its disadvantage is that training in this special technique is necessary.

Sensitive Skin and Hyperirritable Skin. During his or her lifetime, almost every person on some occasion experiences a dermatitis, and skin sensitivity represents a spectrum of reactivity. Frosch and Kligman defined a group, on the basis of reactivity to SLS, who suffered more constantly from irritant contact dermatitis [47]. Recent studies show that a skin type with high basal TEWL reacts more strongly to SLS, and this may be used to predict occupational risk [39, 40, 42, 48], although prognostic and epidemiological studies are not yet available. Sensitive skin was also found to be more sensitive to light; more fair, with a higher L^* and lower b^* according to colorimetry; and thinner according to ultrasound. These findings may indicate a more profound structural and functional inferiority of sensitive skin, including deviations in both the epidermis and the dermis [42, 49]. However, skin sensitivity is not simply a constant but also changes with age, menstrual cycle, season of the year, etc.- factors which interfere and overlap, and which may occasionally create the preconditions for an irritant contact dermatitis to appear [23, 50]. All these variables need be taken into account whenever skin sensitivity is evaluated by noninvasive techniques, and determination of risk factors or dynamic testing by provocation with a standard noxious agent such as SLS is performed.

Patients with active hand dermatitis and young patients with atopic dermatitis have hyperirritable skin and react more strongly to SLS, while reactivity in chronic or healed eczema and in adult atopy and hand dermatitis is normal [51–53]. Thus, whenever groups of patients are studied by noninvasive techniques, they need to be clearly defined clinically.

10.7.6 Urticarial Wheals

Wheals or hives are very dynamic lesions with rapid changes during the initial 30 min when a triple response develops (Fig. 10.7.5). Thus, in the measurement of wheals the timing of recordings needs to be precise and relevant.

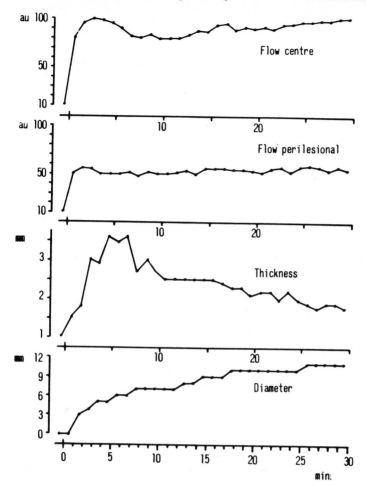

Fig. 10.7.5. Histamine wheal followed for 30 min with laser Doppler flowmetry (centre and perilesional flare), ultrasound measurement of wheal thickness, and measurement of mean diameter

Wheals have been only sporadically studied by noninvasive techniques. Laser Doppler flowmetry shows increase of blood flow in both the centre and the flare of the weal. The oedema formation interferes with the vasculature, and measurements in the flare are more suitable for distinction of the strength of reaction after different concentrations of histamine [54, 55].

Ultrasound examination of histamine wheals shows that the wheal is initially globoid, and at a diameter of about 5 mm it extends laterally in the skin and becomes more flat [27, 56]. With ultrasound the thickness and volume of wheals can be measured. Ultrasound cross-sectional imaging shows that the oedema of wheal reactions propagates mainly laterally in the skin in the papillary dermis, which is more easily distended [27]. At the same time this explains the formation of pseudopodia.

Wheal reactions to dimethyl sulphoxide have been studied by TEWL, conductance, ultrasound skin thickness and laser Doppler measurements, and all the methods were concluded to be suitable for quantification of responses except for laser Doppler flowmetry, this being due to the influence of oedema on the vasculature [57].

10.7.7 References

1. Rothman S (ed) (1954) Physiology and biochemistry of the skin. University of Chicago Press, Chicago
2. Goldsmith LA (ed) (1983) Biochemistry and physiology of the skin. Oxford University Press, New York
3. Leveque JL (ed) (1989) Cutaneous investigation in health and disease. Noninvasive methods and instrumentation. Dekker, New York
4. Rietschel RL, Spencer TS (eds) (1990) Methods for cutaneous investigation. Dekker, New York (Cosmetic science and technology series)
5. Marks R, Payne PA (eds) (1981) Bioengineering and the skin. MTP Press, Lancaster
6. Shepherd AP, Öberg PÅ(eds) (1990) Laser-Doppler blood flowmetry. Kluwer, Boston
7. Stüttgen G, Flesch U (1985) Dermatological thermography. In: Engel JM et al. (eds) Thermologic methods. VCH Weinheim
8. Berardesca E, Maibach HI (1988) Bioengineering and the patch test. Contact Dermatitis 18: 3–9
9. Diffey BL, Oliver RJ, Farr PM (1984) A portable instrument for quantifying erythema induced by ultraviolet radiation. Br J Dermatol 111: 663–672
10. Robertson AR (1977) The CIE 1976 color difference formulas. Color Res Appl 2: 7–11
11. Serup J, Agner T (1990) Colorimetric quantification of erythema - comparison of two colorimeters (Lange Micro Color and Minolta Chroma Meter CR-200) with a clinical scoring scheme and laser-Doppler flowmetry. Clin Exp Dermatol 15: 267–272
12. Slue WE (1989) Photographic cures for dermatologic disorders. Arch Dermatol 125: 960–962
13. Grove GL, Grove MJ (1989) Objective methods for assessing skin surface topography noninvasively. In: Leveque J-L (ed) Cutaneous investigation in health and disease Dekker, New York
14. Serup J, Winther A, Blichmann C (1989) A simple method for the study of scale pattern and effects of a moisturizer qualitative and quantitative evaluation by D-Squame tape compared with parameters of epidermal hydration. Clin Exp Dermatol 14: 277–282
15. Leveque J-L, deRigal J (1983) Impedance methods for studying skin moisturisation. J Soc Cosmet Chem 34: 419–426
16. Tagami H (1989) Impedance measurement for evaluation of the hydration state of the skin surface. In: Leveque J-L (ed) Cutaneous investigation in health and disease. Dekker, New York pp 79–111
17. Blichmann C, Serup J (1988) Assessment of skin moisture. Measurement of electrical conductance, capacitance and transepidermal water loss. Acta Derm Venereol (Stockh) 68: 284–290.
18. Agner T, Serup J (1988) Comparison of two electrical methods for measurement of skin hydration. An experimental study on irritant patch test reactions. Bioeng Skin 4: 263–269
19. Stender IM, Blichmann C, Serup J (1990) Effects of oil and water baths on the hydration state of the epidermis. Clin Exp Dermatol 15: 206–209

20. Nilsson GE (1977) Measurement of water exchange through skin. Med Biol Eng Comput 15: 209–218
21. Spencer TS (1990) Transepidermal water loss: methods and applications. In: Rietschel RL, Spencer TS (eds) Methods for cutaneous investigation. Dekker, New York, pp 191–217
22. Pinnagoda J, Tupker RA, Agner T, Serup J (1990) Guidelines for transepidermal water loss (TEWL) measurement. A report from the standardization group of the European Society of Contact Dermatitis. Contact Dermatitis 22: 164–178
23. Agner T, Serup J (1989) Seasonal variation of skin resistance to irritants. Br J Dermatol 121: 323–328
24. Agner T, Serup J (1988) Contact thermography for assessment of skin damage due to experimental irritants. Acta Derm Venereol (Stockh) 68: 192–195
25. Baillie AJ, Biagioni PA, Forsyth A, Garioch JJ, McPherson D (1990) Thermographic assessment of patch-test responses. Br J Dermatol 122: 351–360
26. Serup J, Staberg B (1987) Ultrasound for assessment of allergic and irritant patch test reactions. Contact Dermatitis 17: 80–84
27. Serup J (1991) Ten years of experience with high-frequency ultrasound examination of the skin: development and refinement of technique and equipments. In: Altmeyer P et al. (eds) Ultrasound examination of skin. Karger, Basel (in press)
28. Peters K, Serup J (1987) Papulo-vesicular count for the rating of allergic patch test reactions. A simple technique based on polysulfide rubber replica. Acta Derm Venereol (Stockh) 67: 491–495
29. Blichmann C, Serup J (1987) Hydration studies on scaly hand eczema. Contact Dermatitis 16: 155–159
30. Serup J, Staberg B (1987) Differentiation of allergic and irritant reactions by transepidermal water loss. Contact Dermatitis 16: 129–132
31. Serup J (1987) Contact thermography - towards the Sherlock Holmes magnifying glass for solving allergic and irritant patch test reactions? Contact Dermatitis 17: 61–63
32. Staberg B, Serup J (1984) Patch test responses evaluated by cutaneous blood flow measurements. Arch Dermatol 120: 741–743
33. Staberg B, Serup J (1988) Allergic and irritant skin reactions evaluated by laser Doppler flowmetry. Contact Dermatitis 18: 40–45
34. Serup J, Staberg B, Klemp P (1984) Quantification of cutaneous oedema in patch test reactions by measurement of skin thickness with high-frequency pulsed ultrasound. Contact Dermatitis 10: 88–93
35. Willis CM, Stephens CJM, Wilkinson JD (1989) Epidermal damage induced by irritants in man: a light and electron microscopy study. J Invest Dermatol 93: 695–699
36. Björnberg A (1968) Skin reactions to primary irritants in patients with hand eczema. An investigation with matched controls. Isacson, Göteborg
37. Frosch P (1985) Hautirritation und empfindliche Haut. Grosse, Berlin
38. van der Valk PGM (1983) Water vapour loss measurements on human skin. Thesis, State University Hospital, Gröningen
39. Pinnagoda J (1990) Transepidermal water loss. Its role in the assessment of susceptibility to the development of irritant contact dermatitis. Thesis, State University Hospital, Gröningen
40. Tupker Ra (1990) The influence of dertergents on the human skin. A study on factors determining the individual susceptibility assessed by transepidermal water loss. Thesis, State University Hospital, Gröningen
41. de Boer EM (1989) Occupational dermatitis by metalworking fluids. An epidemiological study and an investigation on skin irritation using laser Doppler flowmetry. Thesis, Vrije University, Amsterdam
42. Agner T (1991) Noninvasive measuring methods for the investigation of irritant contact dermatitis. Thesis, University of Copenhagen

43. Agner T, Serup J (1990) Sodium lauryl sulphate for irritant patch testing. A dose-response study using bioengineering methods for determination of skin irritation. J Invest Dermatol 95: 543–547

44. Agner T, Serup J (1987) Skin reactions to irritants assessed by polysulfide rubber replica. Contact Dermatitis 17: 205–211

45. Agner T, Serup J (1990) Individual and instrumental variations in irritant patch-test reactions - clinical evaluation and quantification by bioengineering methods. Clin Exp Dermatol 15: 29–33

46. Bircher AJ, Guy RH, Maibach HI (1990) Laser-Doppler blood flowmetry. Skin pharmacology and dermatology. In: Shepherd AP, Öberg PÅ (eds) Laser-Doppler blood flowmetry. Kluwer, Boston, pp 141–174

47. Frosch PJ, Kligman AM (1982) Recognition of chemically vulnerable and delicate skin. In: Frost PH, Horwitz SN (eds) Principles of cosmetics for the dermatologist. Mosby, St Luis, pp 287–296

48. Murahata RI, Crowe DM, Roheim JR (1986) The use of transepidermal water loss to measure and predict the irritation response to surfactants. Int J Cosmet Sci 8: 225–231

49. Frosch P, Wissing C (1982) Cutaneous sensitivity to ultraviolet light and chemical irritants. Arch Dermatol Res 272: 269–278

50. Agner T, Damm P, Skouby SO (1991) Menstrual cycle and skin rectivity. J Am Acad Dermatol 24: 566–570

51. Werner Y, Lindberg M (1985) Transepidermal water loss in dry and clinically normal skin in patients with atopic dermatitis. Arch Dermatol Res 65: 102–105

52. Agner T (1991) Skin susceptibility in uninvolved skin of hand eczema patients and healthy controls. Br J Dermatol 125: 140–146

53. Agner T (1990) Susceptibility to sodium lauryl sulphate in patients with atopic dermatitis and controls. Acta Derm Venerol (Stockh) 71: 296–300

54. Serup J, Staberg B (1985) Quantification of weal reactions with laser Doppler flowmetry. Comparative blood flow measurements of the oedematous centre and the perilesional flare of skin-prick histamine weals. Allergy 40: 233–237

55. van Neste D (1991) Skin response to histamine: reproducibility study of the dry skin prick test method and of the evaluation of microvascular changes with laser Doppler flowmetry. Acta Derm Venereol (Stockh) 71: 25–28

56. Serup J (1984) Diameter, thickness, area, and volume of skin-prick histamine weals. Allergy 39: 359–364

57. Agner T, Serup J (1989) Quantification of the DMSO-response, a test for assessment of sensitive skin. Clin Exp Dermatol 14: 214–217

Chapter 11
Occupational Contact Dermatitis

11 Occupational Contact Dermatitis

RICHARD J.G. RYCROFT

Contents

11.1 Introduction

Contact dermatitis caused by patients' work has an unrivalled claim to our attention within the field of contact dermatitis: first, it is simply so common; second, work is such a vital psychological part of most human lives [1,2]; and third, work matters financially to almost all individuals and to absolutely all their countries. Occupational contact dermatitis can therefore destroy the psychosocial and economic stability of patients as well as that of their skin [3]. It also overlaps with investigative, preventive, rehabilitative and medicolegal aspects of occupational medicine that are not immediately familiar to most clinicians. For all these reasons, it is an area of the subject not without its difficulties, but also one with a particular appeal.

11.2 Definition and Setting

There is no universally accepted definition of occupational contact dermatitis. Definitions vary according to the use to which they are to be put. A broad definition is contact dermatitis due wholly or partially to the patient's occupation. Being somewhat stricter, occupational exposure should be a major factor [4]. A stricter definition still is contact dermatitis that would not have occurred if the patient had not been doing the work of that occupation [5]. A broader definition tends to be more suitable for everyday clinical practice, a narrower definition when deciding medicolegal questions of causation.

Occupational contact dermatitis is the major part, 90%–95% [6], of the broader spectrum of occupational dermatoses. Occupational dermatoses that are not contact dermatitis include [7] contact urticaria, oil folliculitis (oil acne), chloracne, leukoderma, scleroderma-like disease, ulceration (Fig. 11.1) and epidermal carcinoma. In their turn, occupational dermatoses are part of occupational disease generally, which includes conditions such as occupational asthma that may be caused by the same agents as occupational dermatoses [8]: colophony (rosin), for example, causes both asthma and allergic contact dermatitis in the electronics industry [9,10]. Some chemicals that cause occupational dermatoses are also capable of causing ocular and neurobehavioural disorders, notably formaldehyde and ammonia (eye irritation), hexavalent chromium (anosmia), methyl methacrylate and synthetic pyrethroid insecticides [11] (paraesthesia) and organotin compounds (psychiatric symptoms) [12].

11.3 History

There are three classic texts that embody the work involved in establishing occupational dermatology as a subspecialty in its own right (Table 11.1). The preeminent British exponent of the subject, Charles Calnan [13], has charted its beginnings from the first approaches of the enthusiastic English physician

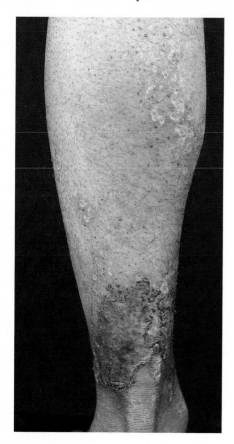

Fig. 11.1. Cement ulceration (cement burns) from acute occlusion of wet cement. (Courtesy of The St John's Institute of Dermatology)

Table 11.1. The three classic texts of occupational dermatology

Author	Country	Date[a]	Title
R. Prosser White	UK	1915	The Dermatergoses or Occupational Affections of the Skin [14]
Poul Bonnevie	Denmark	1939	Aetiologie und Pathogenese der Eczemkrankheiten [15]
Louis Schwartz, Louis Tulipan, Samuel M. Peck, and, later, Donald Birmingham	USA	1939	Occupational Diseases of the Skin [16]

[a]Of first edition, when applicable.

Table 11.2. Major modern texts of occupational dermatology

Author	Country	Date[a]	Title
Robert M. Adams	USA	1990	Occupational Skin Disease [7]
Jean Foussereau, Claude Benezra	France	1970	Les Eczémas Allergiques Professionnels [17]
Jean Foussereau, Claude Benezra, Howard Maibach	France	1982	Occupational Contact Dermatitis [18][b]
Jean Foussereau	France	1991	Guide de Dermato-Allergologie Professionelle [352]
Eberhard Zschunke	Germany	1985	Grundrißder Arbeitsdermatologie [19]

[a]Of latest edition, when applicable.
[b]English updated version of [17].

Prosser White, through the scientific and scholarly interest of the Dane Poul Bonnevie and the public-health-oriented experience of the Americans Louis Schwartz, Louis Tulipan, Samuel Peck and, later, Donald Birmingham.

It was Professor Hageman at the University of Lund in southern Sweden who gave Sigfrid Fregert the opportunity to make Europe the latest pioneer of occupational dermatology over the past 30 years [21]. This impetus was strongly supported by the International Contact Dermatitis Research Group, sustained over the past 25 years by Bonnevie's younger compatriot, Niels Hjorth, who died in 1990. Major modern texts in occupational dermatology are listed in Table 11.2

11.4 Frequency

Nowhere is the frequency of occupational contact dermatitis in the general population accurately known. Statistics generated by governmental compensation systems have to date been underestimates, due to underdiagnosis, underreporting and misclassification, though better statistics may be compiled in the future [22]. Changes in the regulations determining entitlement to compensation can drastically, though meaninglessly, alter the statistics [23].

Dermatological diseases accounted for approximately one-third of all cases of chronic occupational diseases recently identified in the United States Bureau of Labor Statistics Annual Survey [24]. The overall rate of new cases was around 1 per every 1000 full-time workers per annum, the greatest number of cases occurring in manufacturing, where the corresponding incidence rate was 2.85 per 1000 full-time workers. The true rates of occupational skin disease may be 10–50 times higher than those reflected in the Annual Survey [25]. In the United States, as many as 20%–25% of all reported occupational dermatological conditions resulted in an average of 10–12 days lost from work. Assuming an underreporting of 10–50 times, the estimated annual costs of occupational dermatological diseases in the United

Table 11.3. Important population prevalence studies of eczema reported over the last three decades

Authors	Site	Place	Prevalence of eczema (%)
Lomholt [26]	All sites	Faroe Islands	1.7
Agrup [4]	Hands	Southern Sweden	0.6
Rea et al. [27]	All sites	Inner London	6.1
Johnson [28]	All sites	USA	2.1/4.7[a]
	Hands		0.5
Coenraads et al. [29]	Hands and arms	Netherlands	6.2
Meding and Swanbeck [30]	Hands	Gothenburg, Sweden	11.8

[a]Active/remission.

States due to lost productivity, medical care and disability payments, may range between $222 and $1000 million [31].

A different approach to estimating how much occupational contact dermatitis there is in the working community is to look at population studies of the prevalence of eczema, particularly hand eczema. The essential findings of important examples of such studies are summarized in Table 11.3.

On direct examination of a sample of over 3000 adults from a mixture of urban and rural communities in the Netherlands [29], 4.6% of men and 8% of women had eczema on the hands and/or arms, totalling 6.2% over the whole sample. Without patch testing, it was considered that irritancy was a factor in the eczema of 3.6% of the whole sample, more than half: 53% of the men with eczema of the hands and forearms and 61% of the women. Most of the affected women were housewives (homemakers). The highest prevalence of hand and arm eczema (all forms combined) among men was observed in those working in the chemical industry (prevalence 14.5%) and the metal industry (prevalence 10.7%); age was not a factor. The figure for the chemical industry is surprisingly high and may reflect local industry.

From an initial questionnaire survey of 20 000 persons in a Swedish industrial city, 1238 were confirmed as having hand eczema [30]. Of these, 976 were patch tested, and a further 105 had been so tested within 2 years of the examination, making a total of 1081 with available patch test results. Allergy to colophony was found to be statistically more frequent among female office workers–it was thought from paper contact. The highest 1-year period prevalence of hand eczema was 21.3% in cleaners, compared to an overall figure of 11.8%. The most harmful reported contacts included dust and dry dirt as well as water and detergents. The prevalence of hand eczema in women was almost twice as high as in men.

Clinical experience strongly suggests that occupational contact dermatitis constitutes a sizable proportion of the total burden of contact dermatitis, particularly on the hands. These statistics, taken together, therefore provide some indication of how much occupational contact dermatitis there actually

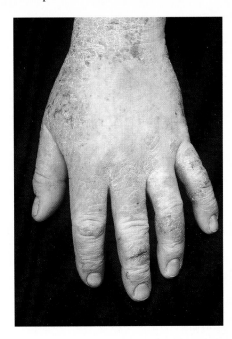

Fig. 11.2. Allergic contact dermatitis from chromate in cement. (Courtesy of The St John's Institute of Dermatology)

is in the general population. In a population the size of that in the United Kingdom, an estimate is that at least many tens of thousands must be affected at any one time, equivalent perhaps to the total population of one of its provincial cities (50 000–100 000).

The cost of occupational contact dermatitis to the community is a human as well as a financial one. Disablement from an occupational dermatosis can be as great as that from the loss of a limb, though financial compensation is likely to be much less. In the case of one particularly disabling form of the disease, allergic contact dermatitis from chromate (Fig. 11.2), the term 'chrome cripple' [32] is a graphic reminder of this.

11.5 Age

In Fregert's thought-provoking study [21], occupational contact dermatitis tended to begin under the age of 20 years in hairdressing and housework; under the age of 30 in the food industry, hospital cleaning and bakery; between the ages of 20 and 30 in other hospital work; at any age after 20 in the plastics industry, nonhospital cleaning, rubber industry, metal industry and cement casting; and over the age of 40 in the building industry and brick-laying. Most women's dermatitis started earlier in life than most men's, but only because they had jobs such as hairdressing more than men.

Griffiths, looking at skin disease keeping people away from work, concluded that the maximum impact of such skin disease was in those aged in their 20s and 30s [33]. This statistic probably does not give the whole picture, however, as Fregert's study showed, and a characteristic bimodal curve has been described [34, 35], in which the prevalence of an occupational dermatosis decreases progressively from the very youngest workers, who have a high prevalence, to rise again in those aged over 55, their prevalence being higher than that of those in the 35–55 age group. The peak age of onset of dermatitis in the pottery industry in the United Kingdom is the early 20s, with a second lower peak in the 40s [36]. Many authors state that the resistance to occupational contact dermatitis decreases with age [37] or find that the risk of occupational contact dermatitis increases progressively with age [38].

Peaks of prevalence at either end of working life are probably often realistic, since they reflect both the so-called 'green' (i.e. new) labour effect and the influence of ageing on the skin. Younger workers perhaps get dermatitis because their skins are in some way unaccustomed to contact with their working materials, older workers perhaps either because their skins have become progressively 'worn out' somehow by such contact, or because ageing changes in the skin render it more susceptible, or because of a combination of the two. There may also perhaps be other factors increasing the risk in younger workers, such as an initial lack of caution brought on by the healthy feeling in the young that they are just as immune to skin disease as to everything else.

11.6 Occupations

In Fregert's [21] study, occupations were ranked as to frequency of contact dermatitis in the following descending order for men: metalworking, cement casting, building, plastics, woodworking, rubber, food, service, agriculture, painting, baking and confectionery, pharmaceutical and chemical, horticulture and floristry, graphics, glass, tanning and catering. And for women: hospital, hospital cleaning, cleaning, hairdressing, food, catering, rubber, plastics, textiles, laboratory, horticulture and floristry, and housework.

In the United States, the highest rates of occupational skin disease are consistently found in three major industries: agriculture, manufacturing and construction [25, 39]. Crop and livestock production in agriculture, and leather products, food products, rubber and plastic products are specifically identifiable as being of high risk. Skin diseases account for almost two-thirds of all occupational illnesses within agriculture [25]. Coenraads et al. [29] found the highest prevalence of eczema of the hands and arms in men in the Netherlands to be among those in the chemical and metal industries. In the United Kingdom, the industries recently most at risk have been, for men, again in descending order, mining and quarrying, construction and vehicle manufacture, and, for women, professional and scientific services; food, drink and tobacco industries; and hotels, public houses, snack bars and other catering establishments [33].

Table 11.4. Prevalence of occupational contact dermatitis in studies of selected occupations reported over the past decade

Authors	Country	Occupation	Prevalence (%)[a]
Högberg and Wahlberg [40]	Sweden	Housepainters	3.9 (minimum)
Varigos and Dunt [41]	Australia	Tyre factory workers	3.7
		Cement factory workers	6.8
Lammintausta [42]	Finland	Hospital workers (cleaners)	8 (10)
Hansen [43]	Denmark	Hospital cleaners	15.3
Peltonen et al. [44]	Finland	Shipyard cleaners	11
Coenraads et al. [45]	Netherlands	Construction workers	6.2
Van Putten et al. [46]	Netherlands	Construction workers exposed to epoxy resins	17
Kavli et al. [47]	Norway	Shrimp peelers	6
Coenraads et al. [38]	Singapore	Metalworkers	4.5
Peltonen et al. [48]	Finland	Food industry workers	8.5
Hogan et al. [49]	Canada	Grain elevator workers	13.1
Singgih et al. [50]	Netherlands	Hospital cleaners	12
Goh et al. [51]	Singapore	Prefabricated concrete workers	14
Wahlberg and Högberg [52]	Sweden	Flooring installers	13
Bruze and Almgren [53]	Sweden	Phenol-formaldehyde resin workers	12.6
Avnstorp [54]	Denmark	Prefabricated concrete workers	10.5 (1981)
		Cr allergy	2.6 (1987)
De Boer et al. [55]	Netherlands	Metalworkers	14

[a]The different figures are not directly comparable because of multiple differences in methods of arriving at prevalence rates.

Some recent studies of the prevalence of occupational contact dermatitis in selected occupations are listed in Table 11.4. Although the various figures are not directly comparable because of differences in the methods used to determine prevalence, it can be seen that rates between 4% and 17% have commonly been found in these high-risk groups; that the rate tends to rise as the high-risk group is increasingly accurately defined; and that concrete workers, metalworkers and hospital cleaners feature prominently in studies with prevalence rates of over 10%.

11.7 Period of Exposure

How soon workers develop dermatitis after the onset of exposure varies considerably from one occupation to another. There may be more than one peak of prevalence, as discussed in Sect. 11.5. In Fregert's study

[21], among women 40% of allergic contact dermatitis and 53% of irritant contact dermatitis started within the 1st year in the occupation; in men the corresponding figures were 23% and 34%. This difference arose because of differences in occupational choice between the sexes. Hairdressers, for example, generally develop their dermatitis early in their career [56], whereas bricklayers and hod carriers commonly develop theirs after more than 10 years of exposure [57].

Recent reports have shown that the true picture may be still more variable and complex. The risk of developing chromate allergy or hand eczema in wet-cement workers was not influenced by age or exposure time as much as by exposure to particular work processes [54]. The exposure time for 28 patients with occupational contact dermatitis from epoxy resins (Fig. 11.3) was less than 1 month for 14.3%, between 1 month and 1 year for 32.1% and more than 1 year for 53.6%, the mean being just less than 3 years. The mean exposure time for patients with allergic contact dermatitis from epoxy reactive diluents was much less (just under 1 year), and it was less still (6 months) for those with irritant contact dermatitis from epoxy resin systems [58].

Thus the influence of length of exposure on the onset of occupational contact dermatitis depends upon the precise type and degree of that exposure and cannot necessarily be predicted simply from the occupation.

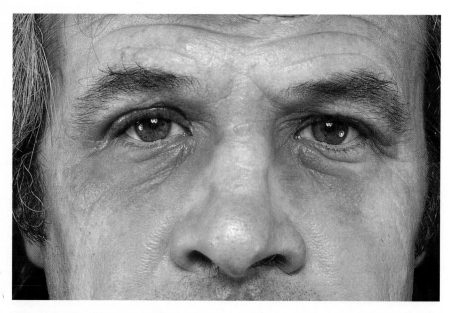

Fig. 11.3. Allergic contact dermatitis from epoxy resin in a spray paint. (Courtesy of The St John's Institute of Dermatology)

11.8 Aetiology

The relative proportions of irritant contact dermatitis and allergic contact dermatitis in reported studies of occupational contact dermatitis vary widely and they depend on three main variables: the thoroughness of patch testing, whether the study is clinic-based or workplace-based, and what criteria are used to define dermatitis.

The more thoroughly that patch testing is carried out on a clinic-based population, where minor degrees of dermatitis, for example irritant reactions (see Chap. 8), are less likely to be included, the higher the proportion of allergic contact dermatitis becomes, until it may achieve parity or even the ascendance [21]. Workplace-based studies, where patch testing may not be quite as thorough, and where degrees of skin change that might be regarded only as dry skin or fissuring may be included in the total figure for skin disease, tend to show irritant contact dermatitis as predominant, sometimes overwhelmingly so. This contrast is illustrated by comparing the studies of Grattan et al. [59] and de Boer et al. [60] on machine operatives exposed to metalworking fluids, the first of which was clinic-based and the second workplace-based; allergy was detected in 43% of the first study population and in 2.8% of the second.

With a substance that can cause both irritant and allergic contact dermatitis, such as phenol-formaldehyde resin [53], cases of irritancy often greatly outnumber those of allergy.

In general, irritant contact dermatitis probably still remains the commoner condition, though the proportion of occupational contact dermatitis that is either primarily or secondarily allergic is much higher than many yet accept. A major monograph on the aetiology and clinical patterns of eczema has been published by Bäurle [61].

11.8.1 Irritants

Acute irritant contact dermatitis may take from 1 h to 1 day to appear [62, 63] and is usually traceable to a single contact factor. Chronic irritant contact dermatitis may take months or years and is often multifactorial [64].

Mechanical irritancy should not be overlooked, though chemical irritancy is the commoner cause of dermatitis [65]. Irritants can cause contact urticaria as well as contact dermatitis [66].

Susceptibility to one irritant does not necessarily imply susceptibility to another [67], though Frosch [68] has found a reasonably good correlation and identified a susceptible group (14%) within the human population [69]. Blacks in general are less easily irritated than whites of Celtic extraction [70], and susceptibility to sunburn and chemical irritants tends to go together [71].

The influence of atopy on susceptibility to chronic irritant contact dermatitis has recently been studied in detail in four investigations, all in Scandinavia, three of which were completed by the time of Rystedt's 1986 review [72]. Lammintausta and Kalimo [73], in Finland, found a greatly increased risk of hand dermatitis among those engaged in hospital wet work in persons with previous or current atopic dermatitis, atopic mucosal symptoms associated with atopic skin diathesis ("an obviously dry skin with an abnormally low threshold of pruritus for two or three ... non-specific irritants"), or atopic skin diathesis combined with a family history of eczema, asthma or hay fever.

A subsequent study by Rystedt [74] in Sweden demonstrated that the risk of hand eczema in adult atopics was particularly increased by having more severe eczema in childhood, and especially by having eczema on the hands in childhood. The importance of a previous history of childhood hand eczema in predicting the risk of hand dermatitis in hospital wet work has since been confirmed in Sweden by Nilsson and Bäck [75].

Most recently of the four, Meding and Swanbeck [76], again in Sweden, concur with previous reports that for individuals with only mucous membrane symptoms of atopy only a minor increase in hand eczema risk is contracted in adulthood, whereas a history of childhood eczema was the most important predictive factor for adult hand eczema that they identified, followed in order of importance by female sex and a history of occupational exposure to solvents, oils, paints, glues, unspecified chemicals, cement (Fig. 11.4), water and detergents, foodstuffs, plants and soil, dust and dry dirt, or coins [73].

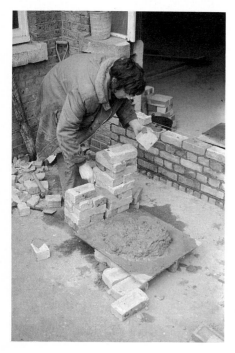

Fig. 11.4. A bricklayer's apprentice meeting the irritant and allergic risks from cement

A significantly increased risk of occupational irritant contact dermatitis therefore appears at present to be limited to those with severe, rather than mild, childhood eczema and in particular to those who had eczema on their hands as children. As to the reason for such susceptibility, Gehring [77] has proposed that it is connected with a diminished resistance within the epidermis as a whole, rather than being confined to a reduced barrier function.

Occupational irritants have recently been reviewed by Bruze and Emmett [78] and by Andersen et al. [79], and irritant contact dermatitis in general by Frosch [70], Mathias [80] and Griffiths and Wilkinson [81] (see also Sect. 2.2). Common high-risk occupations for irritant contact dermatitis [64, 78] are listed in Table 11.5; the principal occupational irritants [82, 83] are listed in Table 11.6.

The occurrence of occupational irritant contact dermatitis is not as widely reported in the literature as it should be. One of the main reasons for this is simply that it is harder to write a convincing report about it than about allergic

Table 11.5. Common high-risk occupations for irritant contact dermatitis

Housewives
Bakers
Butchers
Caterers
Cleaners
Construction workers
Food processors
Hairdressers
Horticulturalists
Masseurs
Metalworkers
Motor mechanics
Nurses
Painters
Printers

Table 11.6. The principal occupational irritants

Water
Soaps and detergents
Alkalis
Acids
Metalworking fluids
Organic solvents
Other petroleum products
Oxidizing agents
Reducing agents
Animal products
Physical factors

Table 11.7. Some instances of irritant contact dermatitis in the workplace reported over the past 5 years

Authors	Occupation	Irritant
Gan et al. [84]	Furniture sanders	Hardwoods
Rycroft et al. [85]	Horticultural workers	Chicory sap
Lovell et al. [86]	Plastic lens makers	Diallylglycol carbonate monomer
Vale and Rycroft [87]	Furniture makers	Urea-formaldehyde resin
Bruynzeel et al. [88]	Electronics assemblers	Chrome-passivated metal
Halkier-Sørensen and Thestrup-Pedersen [89]	Fish processors	Raw fish
Bruze and Almgren [53]	Laminate makers	Phenol-formaldehyde resin
Thestrup-Pedersen et al. [90]	Plastics workers	Heated polyethylene
Goh and Ho [91]	Electrodischarge machinists	Dielectric fluids

contact dermatitis. Some recent reports of specific instances of occupational irritant contact dermatitis are listed in Table 11.7.

11.8.2 Allergens

Common high-risk occupations for allergic contact dermatitis [21] are listed in Table 11.8, and the principal occupational allergens in Table 11.9. When evaluating certain rates of patch test positivity in occupational groups it is sometimes useful to remember that the rates of patch test reactivity in adults without dermatitis range from 3.5% to 12.5% [92]. Atopics do not incur a generally increased risk of allergic contact dermatitis along with their increased risk of irritant contact dermatitis (but see Sect. 5.1.6).

Table 11.8. Common high-risk occupations for allergic contact dermatitis

Adhesives/sealants/resins/plastics workers
Agriculturalists
Cement casters
Construction workers
Glass workers
Graphics workers
Horticulturalists
Leather tanners
Painters
Pharmaceutical/chemical workers
Rubber workers
Textile workers
Tilers
Woodworkers

Table 11.9. The principal occupational allergens

Biocides (including isothiazolinones)
Chromate (cobalt)
Dyes
Epoxy resin systems
Essences and fragrances
Formaldehyde
Formaldehyde resins
(Meth)acrylates
Nickel (primary sensitization usually nonoccupational)
Plants
Rubber-processing chemicals

11.9 Pathology

The mechanisms underlying irritant contact dermatitis have recently been reviewed by Frosch [70] and Mathias [80], and the immunology of allergic contact dermatitis by Thestrup-Pedersen et al. [93] and Scheper and von Blomberg [94] (see Chap. 2).

11.10 Clinical Features

The hands are involved in 80%–90% of all cases of occupational contact dermatitis [83]. Dermatitis starting on the trunk is rarely occupational [95]. Exclusive localization of contact dermatitis to the hands is commoner in women than in men [21]. Among 59 women with occupational hand eczema there was no single predominant distribution pattern [96]. In the larger group of 263 women with hand eczema that Cronin studied [96], allergic contact dermatitis could present equally with any of the four patterns that she delineated (palmar, dorsal, fingers only, whole hand), whereas irritant contact dermatitis less often presented with a palmar pattern (see Chap. 8).

Many cases of occupational irritant contact dermatitis start as erythema and scaling over the backs of the metacarpophalangeal joints and adjacent parts of the backs of the fingers, and in the web spaces between the fingers [56]. A generalized, rather shiny, superficially fissured, scaly fingertip dermatitis is also characteristic of certain forms of irritant contact dermatitis, perhaps particularly when combined with endogenous factors.

Exclusive or more severe involvement of the thumb, index finger and/or middle finger of the dominant hand (or of their nails) is an indication of possible occupational causation [97].

Patterns of dermatitis suggesting endogenous eczema (atopic, discoid, seborrhoeic and stasis) are seen in an appreciable percentage of cases of chromate sensitivity [98]. Discs of dermatitis on the backs of the hands and forearms are also seen in contact dermatitis from water-based metalworking

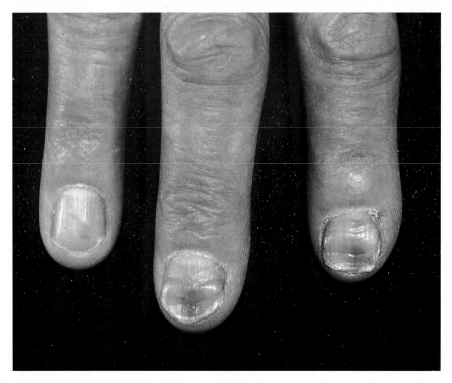

Fig. 11.5. Koilonychia from dipping a (gloved) hand into organic solvent (Carbitol). (Courtesy of The St John's Institute of Dermatology)

fluids (soluble oils) [99]. Hand eczema that is palmar and vesicular and can therefore look like dyshidrotic eczema may be caused by occupational allergens such as N-isopropyl-N' − p-phenylenediamine [100] and even sometimes by occupational irritants [101].

Involvement of the fingernails in occupational contact dermatitis is ignored at the risk of missing some diagnoses altogether, since occupational cases can present exclusively with nail, subungual or paronychial involvement [102, 103]. Some occupational contactants, such as organic solvents, may cause nail changes, such as koilonychia [104], with little or no associated eczema (Fig. 11.5). Others, such as (di)methacrylate-containing screw sealants [105], may focus their contact dermatitis on the fingertips, but with encroachment under the nail in the form of subungual hyperkeratosis and onycholysis. The nail changes being slower to recover, the clinician may later be presented with a patient who appears to have nail changes only.

Psoriasis and tinea of the hands are commonly confused with occupational contact dermatitis in the workplace. Psoriasis may be aggravated on the hands by irritant or mechanical occupational contact [106, 107]. Scabies, lichen planus and keratolysis exfoliativa (dermatitis lamellosa sicca) can also cause confusion on the hands.

Facial contact dermatitis can arise occupationally from both irritants and allergens [95, 108, 109], and this is often from airborne contact [110].

The aggravating effect of stress on occupational contact dermatitis may require assessment, and the assistance of a medical social worker enlisted in relieving it. The stress may have emotional, financial or medicolegal origins. psychoneuroses may present in many ways to dermatologists and occupational physicians [111, 112] and sometimes as suspected occupational contact dermatitis. Dermatitis artefacta [113] rarely presents as suspected occupational contact dermatitis. What is more common in an occupational group is an employee with a clearly visible nonoccupational skin disease becoming the focus of widespread anxiety about possible contact dermatitis [114].

The clinical management of hand dermatitis has been reviewed by Epstein [115] and the management of contact dermatitis generally in Chap. 16.

11.11 Prognosis

In a Swedish questionnaire study with a 65% response rate, Fregert [21] found that, 2–3 years after diagnosis, only one-quarter of 555 patients diagnosed as having occupational contact dermatitis over a 10-year period had completely healed; one-half still had periodic symptoms, and one-quarter permanent symptoms. Among the 40% who had changed their occupation, the change had not improved their overall prognosis.

Wall and Gebauer [116] in Western Australia built on this study by attempting to follow up 993 cases of occupational skin disease documented over an 8-year period, 95% of whom had contact dermatitis. In all, 954 patients (96%) were reviewed, over 60% more than 2 years after diagnosis. 522 (55%) were still suffering from their original occupational skin disease or from its consequences. 387 (41%) had changed their job, but of these more than one-quarter had chosen new jobs in which the work environment further aggravated their skin. 550 (57%) were still in the same job or the same type of occupation, and 68% were still symptomatic. 404 had changed to an entirely different work environment, from the dermatological point of view, and 37% were still symptomatic. 110 patients (11.5% overall) had an ongoing skin disease for which there was no obvious present cause; this was termed persistent postoccupational dermatitis.

Rosen and Freeman [117] in New South Wales refined such studies still further by documenting improvement as well as complete healing, obtaining overall improvement figures of 76% among those who changed industry, 82% among those who changed duties within the same industry, and 61% among those who remained with the same duties in the same industry.

The main findings of these three studies can be summarized as follows. The prognosis for occupational contact dermatitis severe enough to be referred to a dermatologist (known to have a special interest in occupational contact dermatitis) is one of persistence in over half, though with improvement in around half of these. Appropriate occupational changes improve the prognosis for most, but around 10% of patients overall develop persistent postoccupational dermatitis.

In more detail, all studies found chromate to be the major allergen in persistent occupational contact dermatitis, though a wide range of other allergens were also found to be causal. Allergic contact dermatitis from plastics, including epoxy resin, had the best prognosis [21]. Of nine cases reported by Wall and Gebauer [116] as having more than 50% disability (according to the guidelines of the American Medical Association) seven were related to chromate allergy. Burry and Kirk [32] coined the phrase 'chrome cripples' when describing five cases of manual workers sensitized to chromate who became disabled, and in some cases virtually unemployable, from recurrent or continuous dermatitis, though Burrows [98] did detect some improvement in prognosis among younger chromate-sensitive patients. Breit and Turk [118] have reviewed this topic further.

Recent follow-up studies of cutting fluid dermatitis (predominantly irritant) have shown varying results. In a small study in Birmingham, United Kingdom, clearance was found in 45% of the 40 patients surveyed for up to 2.5 years after diagnosis: only one patient had had to change his occupation as a direct result of the dermatitis [119].

In a larger questionnaire study in London, United Kingdom, comprising 100 patients with soluble oil dermatitis, a generally poor prognosis was found whether or not patients continued in their work [120]. Of those who continued to work with soluble oils 78% had not healed 2 years after diagnosis; of those who stopped working with soluble oils 70% had not healed 2 years after discontinuing contact. Patients who discontinued contact with soluble oils fell into two groups. those who healed rapidly and those who developed a chronic dermatitis. Of the 15 patients who had healed after 2 years 11 had done so within the first 3 months following cessation of contact. Numbers were not large enough to determine whether prognosis was influenced by whether or not the patient was sensitized.

The prognosis for catering workers studied by Cronin [121] was also poor. Of 32 followed up, the majority for at least 2 years, 12 had to give up their work because of their contact dermatitis (and one was made redundant). Of the 19 who remained in catering only 4 healed completely; of the 13 who left only 4 healed.

The reasons for this generally poor prognosis, in both irritant and allergic contact dermatitis, are hard to be sure of [69]. Patch test positivity certainly tends to persist [122], but dermatitis seems often to persist even in the apparent absence of continuing contact. The three main contending explanations are that inapparent sources of contact with the original cause of the contact dermatitis continue, that contacts with other causes of contact dermatitis (to which the patient's skin is rendered more susceptible by the original dermatitis) maintain the dermatitis, or that there is some inherent chronicity to contact dermatitis. The truth, when discovered, will probably incorporate all three explanations.

A nihilistic interpretation [123] of the comparatively poor prognosis in cases of occupational contact dermatitis severe enough to see a dermatologist specializing in such cases – suggesting that their patch test results are therefore invalidated – can legitimately be resisted. Many less severe cases can be seen to be making much better progress during factory surveys [124], and even severe cases often become less severe and hence more manageable at work, even if persistent, after adequate investigation and treatment [117].

The prognosis of contact dermatitis (mainly occupational) has recently been reviewed by Hogan et al. [125, 126].

11.12 Diagnosis

The criteria for establishing occupational causation of contact dermatitis have recently been reviewed by Rietschel [127] and Mathias [128].

11.12.1 Clinical

More than simply ascertaining the patient's occupation (though even that is still too often omitted from the patient's records [129]) the dermatologist must strive to acquire a mental picture of precisely how the patient carries out his or her work, exactly what comes into contact with the skin as a result, and to what extent such contact occurs. While it is certainly worth studying the types of question that are useful in this enterprise [130], the taking of the history is a clinical skill needing adaptation to the individual patient. The essential facts that from the basis of every history in cases of suspected occupational contact dermatitis are reviewed below.

The Time of Onset of the Earliest Signs. This is frequently initially underestimated because we tend to remember the exacerbation that finally led us to seek medical advice more readily than the original onset. In general, short histories are more suggestive of occupational causation than long, but many patients do not seek medical advice until they have had milder degrees of contact dermatitis for extensive periods. In Fregert's [21] study, 22% of cases of occupational contact dermatitis had a history of less than 1 month, but 29% a history of more than 1 year.

The Primary Site of Onset. In occupational contact dermatitis this is usually the hands [83]. In a minority of cases the wrists, forearms, lower legs or face is the primary site. Initial involvement of the covered areas of the trunk and feet is rare [83].

The Route (and Timing) of any Secondary Spread. Local spread from one hand to the other and from the hands to the forearms commonly occurs, often quite rapidly, in occupational contact dermatitis [95]. Distant spread from the hands to the feet is commoner when the patient is sensitized [95] but can sometimes also occur in severe irritant contact dermatitis. Distant spread from the hands to the face is also commoner in allergic contact dermatitis [95] or photodermatitis, but again can sometimes also occur in irritant contact dermatitis [108]. Facial involvement may be becoming less common [95].

Occupation. The essential questions that need to be asked about occupation are its title, length of time in it, and what precisely it involves the patient in doing. A reply of "machine operator", for example, should prompt further questions as to what kind of machine(s), the mode of operation, and what substance(s) and how much, gets onto the skin as a result. Visiting the workplace (see Sect. 11.12.4) enormously increases the dermatologist's subsequent capacity to gain a meaningful picture of a job from such questioning of the patient, not least because of the 'inside' knowledge that it imparts concerning the terms used to describe different machines, processes and materials.

Particularly useful additional questions in suspected occupational contact dermatitis are reviewed below.

Whether the Dermatitis Improves away from Work and Worsens on Return to Work. This question can usefully be refined further by attempting to determine how much improvement or deterioration occurs, and how quickly. Primarily nonoccupational eczemas may also show some improvement on holidays but occupational contact dermatitis usually shows greater and more consistent improvement (and deterioration on return to work). Occupational allergic contact dermatitis tends to deteriorate more rapidly on return to work than irritant contact dermatitis; it may also sometimes be slower to improve away from work. As an occupational contact dermatitis of either type becomes more chronic, the work-relatedness of its pattern of improvement and worsening often becomes progressively obscured.

Whether any Attempt Has Been Made to Prevent or Remove Skin Contamination with any Product or Clothing, and if so, with What. Occupational contact dermatitis may have been prevented, at least in certain skin areas, by such precautions or, alternatively, exacerbated, particularly if allergy has been contracted secondarily to gloves or skin care products. The risk of such allergies arising primarily in noneczematous skins, however, has sometimes been exaggereated by dermatologists [131].

Whether Fellow Workers Have Experienced Similar Symptoms. The involvement of a sizable proportion of working colleagues is more indicative of irritant than allergic contact dermatitis, though sometimes heavy exposure to a potent allergen may also sensitize as many as one-third or more of small workforces. Patients' own assessments of the similarity of their workmates' dermatoses are, understandably, often unreliable.

11.12.2 Patch Tests

Patch testing in suspected occupational contact dermatitis is widely acknowledged to be essential [132] but difficult [133]. Discussion of particularly occupational aspects of patch testing is to be found in several recent publications [83, 127, 132–135].

A standard series is rarely sufficient in occupational cases, and its supplementation with additional series [133, 136, 137] and the patient's own samples is frequently required [133, 138]. Useful additional series that are commercially available are listed in Table 11.10.

Table 11.10. Commercially available additional series useful in suspected occupational cases

Series	Supplier
Dental	C, H
Hairdressing	C, H
Isocyanates	C
Metal compounds	H
Meth(acrylate)	C
Oil and cooling fluid	C
Photographic chemicals	C, H
Plastics and glues	C, H
Textile colours and finishes	C

C, Chemotechnique Diagnostics AB, Tisdagsgatan 11, 216 19 Malmo, Sweden H, Hermal Kurt Herrmann, PO Box 12 28, 2057 Reinbek/Hamburg, FRG

The dermatologist is between Scylla and Charybdis, as it were, when patch testing an occupational patient; by trying to steer clear of the whirlpool of the false positive, he or she may be eaten alive by the monster of the false negative. While trying to navigate this narrow strait, it is encouraging to remind ourselves that the greatest abuse of patch testing is failure to use it [134].

The most crucial part of patch testing is interpreting the results and especially determining when they are false positive or false negative [133, 134]. Repetition, serial dilution and control testing are the keys to avoiding the false positive. The false negative can only be avoided by constant vigilance, including mental disciplines such as batch consciousness [139].

A major difficulty is the patch testing of unfamiliar substances. An approach to this problem has recently been outlined [133]. Serial dilutions of 1.0%, 0.1% and 0.01% (or, when severe irritancy is to be expected, 0.1%, 0.01% and 0.001%) can be useful to apply under such circumstances, but for many products, such as metalworking fluids, these would be overdilutions.

The most accessible current source of known patch test dilutions is de Groot's systematic handbook [140].

11.12.3 Other Tests

Besides bacteriological culture and mycological examination and culture [115], there are certain other tests of diagnostic use in cases of suspected occupational contact dermatitis. These are discussed below.

Tests for Immediate Hypersensitivity. These are described in Sect. 10.4.

Simple Chemical Tests for Identification of Specific Allergens. These are described in Sect. 10.3 and by Fregert [141].

More Advanced Chemical Methods. Analytical methods such as gel permeation and high-performance liquid chromatography have become more widely employed to identify and prepare fractions of allergenic mixtures, since Fregert and coworkers put them to such good use in the elucidation of the allergenic fraction of epoxy resin [142]. Notable examples in the occupational field are the studies of phenol-formaldehyde resin [143] and colophony [144].

Measurement of Degree of Skin Contamination. Several methods of quantifying the degree of skin contamination by occupational contact factors have been devised and are listed in Table 11.11. More use could be made of them than at present.

Table 11.11. Methods of quantifying degree of skin contamination

Method	References
Skin wiping	[145]
Skin rinsing	[146]
Exposure pads	[147, 148]
Natural fluorescence (oils, tars)	[145, 149]
Fluorescent tracer	[150, 151]

11.12.4 Workplace Visits

Fregert and his colleagues in Lund, Sweden, "soon found that the opportunity of visiting working-places and factories was a requisite for adequate solving of problems of occupational dermatology" [152]. In their specialized unit, 200–300 patients were seen per year, and as many as 50 workplaces were visited as a result. A dermatologist who can regularly find one half-day per week for workplace visiting, as well as adequate time for patch testing, has the opportunity to become reasonably proficient in clinical occupational dermatology within a few years; additional time for laboratory investigations allows greater proficiency.

Table 11.12. Information useful to acquire and record from workplace visits

Type of information	Details
Organizational	Name, address (including postcode) and telephone number of workplace
	Names and status of all medical, nursing, employer and employee representatives met
Demographic	Numbers employed overall and in relevant work area(s)
	Current expansion, contraction, turnover of workforce
	Shift system and pay scheme
Technological	Broad concept of production as a whole
	Detailed understanding of work in relevant area(s)
	Names and addresses of suppliers of materials meeding further identification
Preventive	Broad impression of working conditions (space, lighting, ventilation)
	Detailed review of protective installations, protective clothing, skin care products and education
	Assessment of actual uptake and effectiveness of above
Miscellaneous	Industrial relations, psychological, sociological and economic factors; comparison with sister factory; etc.
Clinical	Assessment (often provisional) of skin complaints in employees other than index case
Epidemiological	Prevalence of skin complaints as a proportion of the total exposed
	Estimate of prevalence of occupational dermatoses
Aetiological	Opinions of others (with attributions)
	Own opinion, with grounds (may be inconclusive)
Operational	Summary of findings
	Recommendations for prevention and/or further investigation
	Follow-up

The types of information worth acquiring and recording from such workplace visits are listed in Table 11.12. The benefits associated with making such visits are listed in Table 11.13. An alternative to visiting the workplace, and one to which similar principles apply, is to communicate with medical, nursing, employer or employee representatives by letter or telephone. But the dermatologist should remain aware that the answer obtained to a question depends upon who is asked, whereas direct observation, once trained, should generally provide the right answer (Fig. 11.6).

11.12.5 Epidemiological Surveys

Sometimes the clinical assessment of individual patients may be inadequate to identify or characterize clearly enough an occupational dermatosis [153]. An epidemiological survey of dermatoses within a work area may then be needed, for example, when skin complaints arise that are particularly widespread or

Table 11.13. Benefits of workplace visiting

Benefits	References
Finding the relevance of initially unexplained positive patch test reactions to the standard series	
Finding missed allergens	[154]
Confirmation of diagnosis of irritant contact dermatitis	
Diagnosis of mild or unfamiliar occupational dermatoses by their occurrence together in more than one member of a workforce, e.g. low-humidity occupational dermatoses, sick building syndrome	[154–156]
Confirmation that various nonoccupational dermatoses grouped together as a pseudo-occupational dermatosis, and why	[83, 157]
Recognition of a visible dermatosis, occupational or nonoccupational, causing imitative anxiety symptoms in fellow employees (psychic possession)	[114]
Opportunity for the dermatologist to test concepts derived from the literature and clinically against reality	
Initiation of research into new occupational dermatoses	
Incidental effects, including improved dermatologist-occupational-physician and dermatologist-patient relationships	[158]
Progressive increase in dermatologist's overall knowledge of the working contactants of his/her patients	

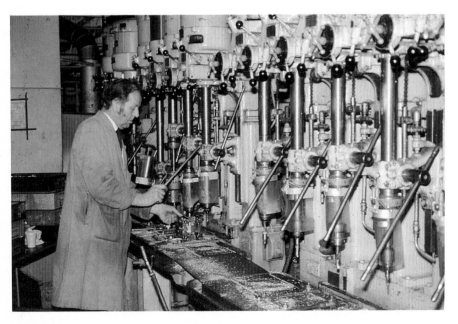

Fig. 11.6. Direct observation of machine operators may be needed to explain their dermatitis

without any identifiable cause. Such surveys should always be planned with epidemiological and statistical advice from the very beginning, since this may affect the essential design of the study. Coenraads and Nater [159] have published an introduction to problems such as those of determining true prevalence, bias, confounding variables and sample size, and Coenraads and Smit have written further on this in Chap. 6 of the present volume.

Exposed and control groups may need to be identified and checked for matching. Particular care should be taken regarding what is required of control groups; the slight risk of inducing sensitization by patch testing control subjects, for example, should be considered. Problems of observer variation, grading of clinical signs, and the design of questionnaires [160] frequently arise. Successful communication with the group(s) being studied is vital before, during and after a survey. The ethics of taking part in such a study, and also of leaving it, should be clearly explained.

11.13 Treatment

The treatment of occupational contact dermatitis rests on the foundation of accurate diagnosis and, depending on that, partial or complete separation of the patient from the cause. General aspects of treatment are to be found in the major dermatology textbooks [161–163] and specific aspects relevant to contact dermatitis in Chap. 16.

11.13.1 Acute

It may sometimes be necessary to advise that a patient stay away from work during an acute phase of an occupational contact dermatitis. The primary objective in preventing disability in the long-term, however, is to enable the patient to remain at work [5], and therefore everything possible should be done to limit this period of work absence to the minimum; every week that passes increases the disability. The cooperation of the patient's employer may need actively to be enlisted in providing the patient with temporary alternative work, so as to allow an early but safe return to work.

Many reasons other than the dermatological can delay patients' return to work [125, 126], including a lack of insight into the adverse effects of being off work on the part of the patients' medical advisers [5]. Being off work for as long as 3 months, which could occur, for example, between two dermatological outpatient appointments, can produce a demoralization so profound that a patient may never again feel capable of regular employment.

11.13.2 Chronic

With certain exceptions, indicated below, the primary aim in the management of the chronic case of occupational contact dermatitis is to return the patient to his or her original work. The basis for this view has previously been presented in this chapter (see Sect. 11.11). There are two main classes of exception to this general rule [5]. The first is isolated uncomplicated allergic contact dermatitis from substances such as epoxy resin, biocides, other specific chemicals or plant allergens. A permanent change of occupation in such cases usually results in complete clearance and no change of occupation in almost certain chronicity.

The second exception is in certain types of wet work in which there is evidence of an enhanced susceptibility to irritation in individuals with sensitive skins (see Sect. 11.8.1). The prognosis for such individuals tends to be bad even after a change of occupation, but it is made so much worse by continuation in the job, for example, metalworking, hairdressing and catering, that the only advice that can realistically be given is to change occupation.

11.14 Prevention

Because of the poor prognosis associated with many forms of occupational contact dermatitis (see Sect. 11.11), its prevention is of extreme importance. There are several recent relevant reviews [164–167].

11.4.1 Preemployment Examination

Guidelines have been published for the preemployment screening of prospective employees with skin disease [168, 169]. Those with a history of severe childhood eczema, especially if with hand involvement, should be advised against the types of occupation listed in Table 11.5, though sometimes there may be specific areas of work, even within such generally high-risk occupations that may present much less of a risk. Each individual case should be assessed on its own merits. There is one additional occupational risk for those with active eczema of the exposed skin in nursing, the transmission of hepatitis B or HIV infection; precautions nowadays in place to prevent such transmission in all nurses should minimize this, however.

There are two ways in which skin conditions may pose a threat to the job being done, rather than vice versa. The first is the health hazard that arises from staphylococcal colonization of chronic dermatoses involving the exposed skin of the hands, forearms or scalp, mainly eczema and psoriasis. The resulting increased risks of food poisoning in catering staff [170] and cross-infection in hospital staff constitute a contraindication to the employment of persons with such conditions, especially if currently active, in foodhandling or in the 'hands-on' care of patients, particularly if some of these patients are likely to be immunologically compromised. Sustained clearance

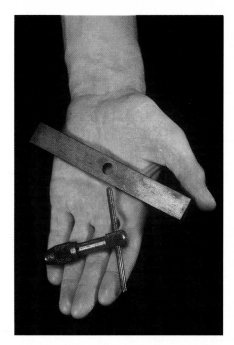

Fig. 11.7. The hyperhidrotic hand of a 'ruster' and ferrous metal handled by him. (Courtesy of The St John's Institute of Dermatology)

of such conditions from exposed skin might be held to remove the contraindication under certain circumstances, though the tendency to recurrence of the dermatosis might still remain a contraindication under others.

The second way in which a skin condition may pose a threat to the job is via the phenomenon known as the 'ruster' [171, 172]. Rusters are those whose touch is capable of rusting ferrous metals (Fig. 11.7), with a delay dependent upon the ambient relative humidity. They were once thought to have some special quality of sweat, but palmar hyperhidrosis now appears to be the reason. Their employment in engineering may result in the rusting of finished metal products while in transit to the customer. Successful control of the hyperhidrosis by methods such as tapwater iontophoresis, difficult though this may be to achieve, can therefore legitimately be held to remove the contraindication [173].

11.14.2 Alkali Tests

The role of alkali and other tests as predictors of susceptibility to occupational irritants [174] remains controversial. None is in practice as simple and reliable as it would need to be to gain widespread clinical use [70, 175]. The diagnostic value of older tests such as the alkali resistance test of Burckhardt has been overestimated. Frosch [68, 70] has used more sophisticated tests with panels of irritants as a research procedure to identify the 14% among the general population with hyperirritable skin. One may not, however, be able to predict the susceptibility to one irritant from the susceptibility to another [67, 71]. Preemployment patch testing with potential sensitizers should not be performed [83].

11.14.3 Industrial Hygiene

The design of systems of work, handling procedures, segregation of a process in a confined area, local exhaust ventilation, and partial or 'total' enclosure of a process are all aspects of industrial hygiene that influence the amount of skin contact and hence the risk of dermatitis [83, 165–167]. Other important aspects include allergen replacement [176] and the fact that even processes described as 'totally enclosed' or 'fully automated' in practice provide multiple opportunities for skin contact [177]. Maintenance fitters (service engineers) are particularly at risk in this respect [178]. Wearing gloves may be considered unsafe in the operation of rapidly rotating machinery [179].

11.14.4 Personal Hygiene

The issues of protective clothing, skin care products and skin cleansers are complex but becoming clearer [164].

Protective Gloves and Clothing. There is now an extensive literature on the penetration of protective gloves and clothing by substances such as organic solvents (Fig. 11.5), making the choice of material crucial to effective protection against specific occupational contacts [180]. Useful practical information on this choice is provided by Wilkinson [181], Wahlberg [165], Mellström et al. [182], Mellström and Carlsson [183], and Estlander and Jolanki [184], as well as in a highly detailed handbook [180]. Some general guidance as to the suitability of various glove materials is given in Table 11.14.

Thickness remains one of the most important criteria to consider when selecting a glove [185], and this may vary considerably from one part of the glove to another [186]. The presence of one chemical may reduce the 'breakthrough time' [180] of another [187]. Gloves consisting of ethylene vinyl alcohol copolymer sandwiched between polyethylene have been shown to be highly effective in protecting against epoxy resin [188], methyl methacrylate [189] and many other organic compounds.

As methods of measuring permeation of materials have become increasingly sophisticated and standardized [190], a data base (DAISY) on protective gloves has been developed in Sweden to centralize all such information [183, 191], and the detailed handbook mentioned above is also available electronically with an expert computer system (GlovES+) [180]. Publications in specialized areas, such as the handling of cytotoxic drugs [192], are also appearing.

Table 11.14. General guidance as to the suitability of various glove materials[a]

Material	Chemical basis	Protective against	Notes
Natural rubber	cis-Isoprene	Soaps and detergents (preferably heavyweight), water-soluble irritants, dilute acids and alkalis	Not good for organic solvents, strong acids and alkalis, many other organic compounds
Butyl rubber	Isobutene, isoprene	Aldehydes, amines (except butylamine and triethylamine), amides, ketones, formaldehyde resins, epoxy resins, acrylates (except butyl acrylate), isocyanates	
Chloroprene	Chloroprene (Neoprene)	Soaps and detergents, dilute acids and alkalis, certain amines and esters, most alcohols, vegetable oils	Not good for aldehydes, ketones, nitro- and halogenated compounds
Fluorocarbon	Vinylidene fluoride, hexafluoropropene	Organic solvents, particularly halogenated and aromatic hydrocarbons	Cost 30–40 × as much as natural rubber
Nitrile rubber	Acrylonitrile, butadiene	Organic acids, certain alcohols, amines, ethers, peroxides, inorganic alkalis, vegetable oils	Also protect against organophosphorus compounds to some extent
Styrene-butadiene rubber	Styrene, butadiene		Hypoallergenic surgical gloves only
Polyethylene	Ethylene	Mainly intended for food-handlers and medical personnel	Chemical resistance depends on seams
Polyvinyl alcohol	Vinyl alcohol	Several organic solvents, esters (except di-n-octyl-phthalate)	Not resistant to water or aqueous solutions
Polyvinyl chloride	Vinyl chloride	Soaps and detergents, oils, metalworking fluids, dilute acids and alkalis, vegetable oils	Not good for most organic solvents

[a]Actual protection depends on manufacturing quality, glove thickness, chemical concentration, duration of contact, environmental temperature and humidity, etc.

Apart from the well-known ability of rubber gloves to sensitize, causing either contact dermatitis or contact urticaria [183], protective clothing has also been incriminated as a cause of outbreaks of occupational contact dermatitis from residues of perchloroethylene remaining in dry-cleaned garments [183, 193]. Dermatitis from other protective equipment has recently been reviewed by Foussereau et al. [194].

Barrier Creams. 'Barrier' creams, better skin care or skin protection creams, have been reviewed by Orchard [195] and Cronin [196]. These authors are agreed that their effectiveness in practice still remains to be scientifically established. In the laboratory, in contrast, data demonstrating beneficial effects have been generated, for example, by Lachapelle and colleagues with a histological method in the guinea pig [197–200]. A guinea pig skin absorption model [201], however, showed only poor skin protection by barrier cream against the organic solvents that they studied, and glove material, if properly selected, was demonstrably much more effective [202]. A repetitive patch test model in man [203], an excised human skin model [200] and, more recently, a repetitive irritation test in the guinea pig and man [305] have, like Lachapelle's method, shown good discriminatory ability between different protective applications and different irritants.

Results in practice can fall so far below those in the laboratory that the sole use of barrier cream is banned in Denmark [206]. One was successfully applied, however, underneath polyethylene disposable gloves by car painters and generally preferred to wearing cotton inner gloves. Skin care creams may also be of some use in allowing easier cleansing of the skin. Clinical experience suggests that the application of emollient creams after washing or at the end of the working day may be beneficial in prevention [164], though this has not been scientifically established [207, 208]. Products marketed for protection against glass fibre were found to be of only limited value [209], though methacrylate spray coatings and barrier creams may provide some protection against epoxy resins [210]. Perhaps the most effective 'barrier' creams are the sunscreens [167], which may have the potential to prevent phototoxic reactions to plants [211] as well as sun-induced neoplasia.

Barrier creams may give weak irritant reactions on patch testing. True sensitization is rare [196].

Skin Cleansers. The scientific basis of the relative merits in practice of different types of industrial skin cleanser remains extremely insecure. There is a frequent tendency for greater effectiveness of skin cleansing to be associated with greater irritant potential [212]. Laboratory studies associate such irritancy particularly with components such as aromatic organic solvents, anionic surfactants and abrasive particles. Yet the results of such studies are highly dependent upon the experimental conditions and evaluation techniques employed [213]; the real-life situation may be far more complex, with interaction between the effects of more than one skin cleanser [214] and of skin care creams.

11.14.5 Dermatitic Potential

The development of methods for assessing the irritant and the sensitization potential of chemicals proceeds apace [165, 215]; the methods now available are reviewed in Chap. 18.

If formulated products are to be properly assessed for sensitization potential, it is their individual constituents that must be so tested, excepting those whose sensitization potential is already well-known, and it is not possible from such tests to determine any concentration limits that may be regarded as safe in use [216]. Applying tests for sensitization potential to the whole formulated product must not therefore be considered as indicating the 'actual' sensitization risk in use, as opposed to the 'theoretical' sensitization potential (or hazard) of its individual constituents.

Data on the results of tests for sensitization potential on whole formulated products cannot therefore be assessed without additional data on the results of tests for sensitization potential on the individual constituents of such products.

11.15 Medical Report

The preparation of a medical report for compensation purposes has been reviewed for British dermatologists by McMillan et al. [217] and North American dermatologists by Goldstein [218] (see Chap. 19). In general, the items listed in Table 11.15 should always be considered for inclusion. It is strongly recommended that such reports be prepared with much thought and care as to clarity and accuracy of presentation. Medical terms not of common currency should be explained as they occur.

The dermatologist should distinguish carefully between opinion as to causation (was the dermatosis occupational?) and opinion as to liability (whose responsibility was the dermatosis?). Most legal systems expect a medical report to confine itself to the question of causation (and associated questions such as prognosis and disability), and comments as to liability render such a report unusable for the purpose intended. If a dermatologist in the United Kingdom wishes to make comments on liability, or is asked for them, these are best included in a letter or additional report, separate from the main report.

At all times, the dermatologist should remember that he or she may eventually have to bear witness in court to anything written in a medical report. A comment made in too much haste may later be acutely embarrassing if challenged during cross-questioning.

11.16 Examples of Occupational Contact Dermatitis

11.16.1 Soluble Oil Dermatitis

'Soluble oil' is a term frequently given to water-based metalworking fluids based on oil-in-water emulsions, often extended to include synthetic metalworking fluids that consist essentially of wetting agents and corrosion inhibitors in water [219]. Soluble oils have become very widely used in the engineering industry as neat (or 'insoluble') oils have come to be used less [219]. Skin contact with soluble oils among machine tool operatives can still be heavy and prolonged on the hands and forearms (Fig. 11.8), even though computer-controlled technology is gradually reducing such exposure [124].

Table 11.15. Items of information to consider including in a medical report

Item	Notes
Sources of information other than the patient	Previous case notes, previous medical reports, workplace inspections.
Family history	Atopy, other allergies, other dermatoses.
Previous personal history	Atopy, other allergies, other dermatoses.
Previous occupations	Job titles, employers, types of contact, dates (patient may need to consult).
Present occupation	Job title, employer's name and address (including postcode), dates.
Time in contact with suspected causal factor(s)	May be shorter (or longer) than time in present occupation.
Description of the working process	In sufficient detail to give accurate assessment of degree of skin contact as well as range of contactants.
Details of working background	Skin care creams, skin cleansers, protective clothing. Other cases of dermatitis?
Time and site of initial skin complaint	Previous injury at initial site? Who reported to? What treatment given?
Progress, with approximate dates	Gradual/sudden aggravations/improvements, influence of weekends, holidays, sickness absences; early on, later on.
Degree of incapacity during course	Dates of absence from work (patient may need to consult); levels of earnings before and after dermatosis.
Changes in occupation	Job titles, dates, details of changes in contactants.
Treatment and its effectiveness	Patient may need to consult.
Clinical findings	Present state. Have lesions been suppressed by topical corticosteroids?
Special investigations	Patch tests, prick tests, open tests (positive and negative), reading times, vehicles, concentrations. Bacteriological/mycological examinations.
Intercurrent diseases	Mycotic infections, light eruptions, fevers.
Diagnosis	
Common knowledge of risk	Could the employer be expected to have foreseen the risk?
Conclusions in terms understandable to nonmedical readers	Probable connection between occupation and dermatosis: balanced against predisposing factors and leisure activities. Possibility of continuing in occupation: prospect of rehabilitation if change of occupation required. Probable medical prognosis (state of the dermatosis). Probable socioeconomic prognosis (capacity for work).

As many as one-third of those working occupationally with soluble oils can experience varying degrees of dermatitis in the course of a year [124]. 'Outbreaks' of soluble oil dermatitis, in reality usually increases in the severity and/or frequency of this endemic background level, occur from time to time in production machining [220], the cause(s) rarely being simple to identify.

Experimentally, soluble oils are only marginal irritants [124, 221]. Yet, in practice, their emulsifier or wetting agent fraction appears primarily

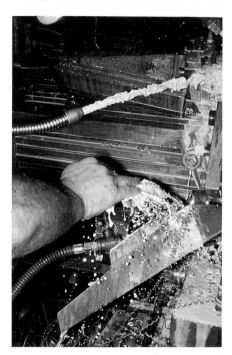

Fig. 11.8. A machine tool operative deflecting soluble oil to check the machine setting

responsible for chronic irritant contact dermatitis in a varying proportion of machine operatives and to a varying degree. In a study of 174 consecutive cases of suspected cutting fluid (mainly soluble oil) dermatitis in London and Birmingham, irritant contact dermatitis was diagnosed in 63% and was considered to be the sole diagnosis in 21% [59]. In the same study, allergic factors were thought to be relevant in 43% of patients and to be the sole cause in 20%.

Soluble oils, then, are capable of sensitizing as well as irritating the skin. The most frequent allergens are emulsifiers based on tall oil (allergenically overlapping with colophony) and the biocides, especially formaldehyde releasers, that they contain to control microbial contamination [59, 222–226]. Roles for amines, thiazoles, isothiazolinones, fragrances and leached metals have also been stressed [219, 227–230]. Much smaller percentages of allergy are found if unselected factory dermatitis populations, rather than selected outpatient dermatitis populations, are studied [55, 60, 124, 221, 231]. De Boer et al. [60] have recently established sensitization to alkanolamine-borate complexes in soluble oils not requiring conventional biocides.

The clinical presentation of soluble oil dermatitis is somewhat variable and does not allow reliable distinction between irritant and allergic types [232]. A characteristic pattern is a patchy eczema of the forearms, wrists (Fig. 11.9) and backs of the hands [233], but vesicular palmar eczema can also occur, and without the need for sensitization [101, 220, 227]. There is a commercially

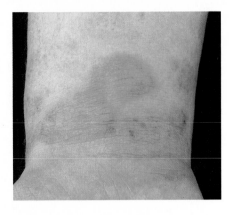

Fig. 11.9. Patches of soluble oil dermatitis on the flexor aspect of the wrist. (Courtesy of The St John's Institute of Dermatology)

available cutting oil series (Table 11.10), which greatly assists in detecting sensitization to soluble oils by patch testing.

The management of established cases of soluble oil dermatitis can usually be directed towards enabling the patient to continue in the same work [119, 232–234], though in severe cases occurring early in apprenticeships or in severe persistent cases later in working life, particularly when there is sensitization, the patient may be better advised to change occupation. In primary prevention, the degree of skin exposure [235] and maintenance of the correct dilution of the emulsion [232] are key factors, and a multifactorial approach to this multifactorial dermatitis is essential [236]. Recent reviews of this very frequent occupational contact dermatitis are [219, 232, 237]. The technology [238, 239] and health effects [240] of metalworking fluid additives have also been reviewed in recent years.

11.16.2 Hairdressers' Dermatitis

Some degree of dermatitis in hairdressers is almost universal at the early stage of their careers, mainly because of continual shampooing [56]. It seems, however, that few hairdressers have to give up the job as a result of what is usually a mild irritant contact dermatitis of the backs of the metacarpophalangeal joints and finger webs. The early development of finger eczema in junior hairdressers, often associated with atopy, has a worse prognosis than the more usual pattern just described [56]. In the United Kingdom at least, many hairdressers eventually give up the work anyway for better pay elsewhere [241]. Giving up hairdressing generally improves the prognosis for hairdressers' dermatitis, even in atopics.

When hairdressers become stylists, they no longer have to shampoo hair regularly, and irritant contact dermatitis from shampoo ceases to be a problem. Stylists who develop dermatitis are much more likely to become sensitized. A few junior hairdressers also become sensitized. *p*-Phenylene-diamine (PPD)

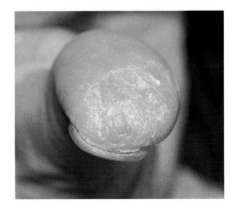

Fig. 11.10. Allergic contact dermatitis on pulps of hairdresser's hands from glyceryl monothioglycolate. (Courtesy of P.J. Frosch)

in hair dyes and glyceryl monothioglycolate (GMTG) in acid permanent wave solutions are currently the most frequent sensitizers among hairdressing chemicals [242–244], GMTG being reported with increasing frequency over the past decade [245, 246] (Fig. 11.10).

Ammonium persulphate allergy from bleaching agents is a complex phenomenon, involving an urticarial [247] as well as a dermatitic response [248]. Other common hairdressing allergens are *p*-toluylenediamine and *o*-nitro-*p*-phenylenediamine in hair dyes, and ammonium thioglycolate in alkaline permanent wave solutions [242]. Maceration of the nail ends, upward curving of the nails and subungual pseudomembranes have also been attributed to ammonium thioglycolate [249].

Allergies to nickel, formaldehyde, quaternium 15 and isothiazolinones may also be specifically relevant to hairdressing equipment or materials, as may allergies to thiurams or mercaptobenzothiazole in the rubber gloves that may be resorted to after the onset of iritant contact dermatitis from shampoo. Gloves can also be a source of contact urticaria from rubber latex.

In addition, hairdressers of both sexes may contract pilonidal sinuses between the fingers [250], and female hairdressers the same condition on the periareolar region of the breasts [251, 252]. (Pilonidal sinuses on the hands have also been reported in dog groomers, milkers and sheep shearers and on the breasts in female sheep shearers [251].)

The prognosis of hairdressers' dermatitis most probably depends on how many adverse factors are present, the worst prognosis accompanying a recent history of atopic dermatitis, current shampoo irritation and a relevant difficult-to-avoid allergen such as PPD or GMTG. The combination of even two such factors still often makes the dermatologist's best eventual advice to the patient be to seek an alternative occupation.

The Hairdressing Training Board in the United Kingdom has recently decided to make occupational health a mandatory item at all levels of their assessment of competence [253], largely in an attempt to improve the education of young hairdressers about risks to the skin.

Czarnecki [254] reviewed the German-language literature on hairdressers' dermatitis in 1977, and more recent reviews, though mainly of the English language literature, have also appeared [242, 243, 255].

11.16.3 Catering Workers' Dermatitis

After a tentative description by Seeberg in 1952 [256], Hjorth and Roed-Petersen [257] brought general attention to the phenomenon that they termed protein contact dermatitis in 1976: foods eliciting hand eczema via a type I rather than a type IV mechanism. The foods that they drew particular attention to were fish and shellfish. The importance of type I allergies to foods in the hand eczema of catering workers has since been confirmed by many authors [121, 258–261].

Cronin [121] found that hand eczema in catering workers was occupational in as many as 47/50 cases seen. Irritation was a commoner cause of dermatitis than sensitization (Fig. 11.11). There was an association between atopy and sensitization for type I but not for type IV allergy. The commonest type I sensitizer was fish, followed by tomato, melon, carrot, cucumber, lettuce, potato, watercress, orange, green pepper, onion and garlic. The commonest type IV allergen was garlic, followed by onion, herring, kidney bean, red cherry, carrot, red pepper and tomato skin. Garlic and onion needed to be diluted to 50% in olive oil to prevent patch test irritancy. The clinical pattern of hand eczema in catering workers provided little information as to its aetiology. Prognosis was not good, the hand eczema of some continuing even after a change of job.

Many workers in the food and catering industries experience irritant contact dermatitis (Fig. 11.11) from continual contact with detergents in washing-up and surface cleaning in kitchens, as well as with fruit, vegetable and meat juices [48, 121, 262]. Occasionally allergic contact dermatitis occurs from sanitizing chemicals [263].

Garlic and onion are widely regarded as the commonest causes of allergic contact dermatitis in cooks and chefs [121, 257, 264]. Type I allergy to onion and garlic also occurs [121, 257, 265]. Type I allergy to potato is particularly common in atopics [266]; potato can also be positive on patch testing [262, 267]. While there remains some disagreement as to how closely atopy is generally associated with type I sensitivities [121, 258], it seems likely that such allergies would be commoner in atopics.

The majority of food handlers with positive patch or prick tests to foods can eat the cooked foods without systemic symptoms, though this does not necessarily apply to spices [268] (see Sect. 16.13.17).

There is one further aspect to catering workers' dermatitis that should concern clinicians: the public health implications of staphylococcal colonization (Fig. 11.11) of food handlers' hand eczema (see Sect. 11.14.1.).

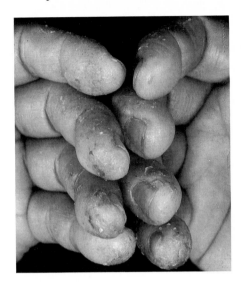

Fig. 11.11. Irritant catering workers' dermatitis, with heavy staphylococcal colonization. (Courtesy of The St John's Institute of Dermatology)

Food handlers' dermatitis has recently been reviewed by Hausen and Hjorth [269] and Cronin [270], the latter providing fully referenced tables of the foods reported as causing type I and type IV allergies.

11.17 Specific Occupational Harzards

The following is a checklist of the contact irritants and sensitizers, and causes of contact urticaria (CU) and/or protein contact dermatitis (PCD), in various occupations.

Agriculture

Irritants.   Artificial fertilizers, milking equipment cleansers, engine fuels [271].

Sensitizers.   Rubber (boots, gloves, milking machines), cement, plants, pesticides [272], wood preservatives, fertilizers (nickel, cobalt [273]), soil disinfectants [274], animal feed additives [275] (antibiotics [276], cobalt, vitamin K3 [277], ethoxyquin, quinoxaline and derivatives, dinitolmide, phenothiazines), veterinary medicaments [271].

CU/PCD.   Animal hair and dander [271].

Art

Irritants.   Organic solvents, clay, plaster.

Sensitizers.   Turpentine, pigments (nickel, cobalt, chromium), azo dyes, colophony, epoxy, (meth)acrylate, formaldehyde and polyurethane resins.

Automobile and Aircraft Manufacture and Maintenance

Irritants.   Organic solvents, hydraulic oils, engine fuels, metalworking fluids, fibreglass, skin cleansers.

Sensitizers.   Chromate [278] (primers, passivated metal, anticorrosives, welding fumes, metalworking fluids), nickel, cobalt, rubber (multiple sources other than tyres), epoxy [58], (meth)acrylate [279], polyurethane, polyester [280] and polysulfide [281] resins.

Baking and Pastry Making

Irritants.   Flour, washing-up liquids, hard-surface cleaners.

Sensitizers.   Flavourings and spices [268] (cinnamon [282], cardamom, nutmeg, clove, eugenol, vanilla), essential oils, citrus fruits, dyes, fat preservatives (lauryl gallate), flour improvers (benzoyl peroxide), sodium carboxymethyl cellulose [283].

CU/PCD.   Flour [260], flavourings and spices, essential oils, citrus fruits [270].

Bartending

Irritants.   Washing-up liquids, hard-surface cleaners, citrus fruits.

Sensitizers.   Flavourings, citrus fruits [284], antibacterials in sanitizing washing-up liquids [285].

Bookbinding

Irritants.   Organic solvents, glues, paper.

Sensitizers.   Glues [286], formaldehyde, size (colophony, meleopimaric acid [287]).

Butchering

Irritants.   Washing-up liquids, hard-surface cleaners, meat, entrails.

Sensitizers.   Nickel, softwood sawdust (colophony), hardwood knife handles [288], meat [289], antiseptics [290].

CU/PCD.   Meat [289], blood.

Cable Jointing and Pipe Repairing

Irritants.   Solvents, (meth)acrylate resins.

Sensitizers.   Epoxy and (meth)acrylate resins, fluxes.

Carpentry and Cabinetmaking

Irritants.   French polish, organic solvents, glues, woods [84], wood preservatives, fibreglass, skin cleansers.

Sensitizers.   Hardwoods [291–294] (mahogany, rosewood, teak, etc.), softwoods (colophony), glues, fillers and varnishes [epoxy, (meth)acrylate, formaldehyde and polyurethane resins], stains (chromate), turpentine.

CU/PCD.   Woods [295].

Catering and Food Processing Industries

Irritants.   Washing-up liquids, hard-surface cleaners, meat, fish, fruit and vegetable juices.

Sensitizers.   Fruit and vegetables [269, 270] (onion, garlic, carrot, lettuce, citrus fruits), hardwood knife handles, flavourings and spices [268], formaldehyde, rubber gloves.

CU/PCD.   Meat, fish, shellfish, fruit and vegetables [269, 270, 296].

Ceramics and Pottery Industries

Irritants.   Wet clays, lithographic solutions and glazes [36].

Sensitizers.   Cobalt (pigments) [297], 1,2-benzisothiazolin-3-one [36], epoxy resin, turpentine, formaldehyde (gum arabic).

Chemical and Pharmaceutical Industries

Irritants and sensitizers are many and varied according to the specific process. Halogenated chemical intermediates are frequent sensitizers [298, 299].

Cleaning

Irritants.   Washing-up liquids, hard-surface cleaners, descaling agents, organic solvents.

Sensitizers.   Rubber gloves, nickel, formaldehyde, fragrances [300].

CU/PCD.   Rubber gloves [301], fragrances, alcohols [300].

Coal Miners

Irritants.   Rock dust, coal dust, hydraulic fluids [302], greases, engine fuels, filling paste (calcium sulphate) [303].

Sensitizers.   Rubber boots, face masks, explosives, chromate and cobalt (cement), fragrances [304], coconut diethanolamide (hydraulic fluid) [305].

Construction Industry

Irritants.   Cement, chalk, fly ash [306], hydrochloric and hydrofluoric acids, fibreglass, rockwool, wood preservatives, organotin compounds, oil in brick-making.

Sensitizers.   Cement and fly ash [306] (chromate [54, 98], cobalt [307], epoxy resin [46], rubber and leather gloves, adhesive (phenol- or urea-formaldehyde resins), woods, wood preservatives, fibreglass impregnated with phenol-formaldehyde, epoxy and polyurethane resins, rubber weatherseals, jointing materials.

Dentistry

Irritants.   Soap, detergents, skin cleansers, plaster of Paris, acrylic monomer.

Sensitizers.   Rubber gloves, local anaesthetics (amethocaine, procaine), mercury [308], UV-curing acrylates, aromatic epoxy acrylates [309], aliphatic acrylates [310], disinfectants and sterilants (formaldehyde, glutaraldehyde [311], eugenol [308]), nickel, chromate [308], epoxy resin (filling), periodontal dressings (balsam of Peru, eugenol, colophony), catalysts in dental impression and sealant materials (methyl-*p*-toluenesulphonate, methyl-1,4-dichlorobenzenesulphonate).

CU/PCD.   Saliva, rubber gloves.

Electrics and Electronics Industry

Irritants.   Soldering flux [10], organic solvents, hydrofluoric acid, fibreglass, antistatic agents [312], chrome-passivated metal [88].

Sensitizers.   Soldering flux, insulating tape (rubber, colophony, tar), rubber, chromate [313], cobalt, nickel, phenol-formaldehyde, epoxy and polyurethane resins, anaerobic acrylic sealants.

CU/PCD.   Soldering flux [10], epoxy hardener [58].

Electroplating (and Electroforming)

Irritants.   Organic solvents, detergents, acids, alkalis, heat, metal dust.

Sensitizers.   Nickel, chromate [98, 314], cobalt, mercury, gold [315], rubber gloves.

Embalmers

Irritants.   Formaldehyde[316], glutaraldehyde [311].

Sensitizers.   Formaldehyde[316], glutaraldehyde [311], rubber gloves

CU/PCD.   Formaldehyde, rubber gloves.

Enamelling

Irritants.   Enamel powder.

Sensitizers.   Chromate, nickel, cobalt.

Fishing

Irritants.   Wet work, friction, engine fuels.

Sensitizers.   Tars, net dyes, rubber (boots, gloves), marine organisms (Dogger Bank itch) [317] and plants [318].

CU/PCD.   Fish, marine organisms and plants.

Floor Laying

Irritants.   Organic solvents, cement (including ulceration).

Sensitizers.   Chromate (cement), epoxy resin, glues (phenol-formaldehyde, *p-tert*-butylphenol-formaldehyde [52], urea-formaldehyde resins), varnish (urea-formaldehyde resin), (meth)acrylates, polyurethanes, hardwoods.

Floristry, Horticulture, Gardening

Irritants.   Plants [319] (daffodils, narcissi, jonquils, *Dieffenbachia*), manure, fertilizers, pesticides, wet work, friction (wire).

Sensitizers.   Plants [319, 320] [Asteraceae (Compositae) from chrysanthemums to weeds, daffodils, narcissi, jonquils, *Primula obconica,* tulips, *Alstroemeria*], lichens, pesticides, fertilizers, soil disinfectants (see "Agriculture"), rubber (gloves, boots).

Foundry Work

Irritants.   Oils, phenol-formaldehyde resins, skin cleansers.

Sensitizers.   Phenol- and urea-formaldehyde resins, furan and epoxy resins, chromate [98] (cement, bricks, leather gloves).

Hairdressing

Irritants.   Shampoos [56], permanent-waving and bleaching solutions.

Sensitizers.   Hair dyes [242], thioglycolates [242, 246], ammonium persulphate [248], nickel, formaldehyde, isothiazolinones, resorcinol, pyrogallol, fragrances, rubber gloves

CU/PCD.   Ammonium persulphate.

Hospital Work

Irritants.   Washing-up liquids, hard-surface cleaners, skin cleaners, disinfectants, formaldehyde, foods, organic solvents (histopathology), wet work [42, 300].

Sensitizers.   Rubber gloves, formaldehyde, glutaraldehyde [311], fragrances, antibiotics, phenothiazines, foods, epoxy resin and (meth)acrylates (histopathology).

CU/PCD.   Rubber gloves [301], formaldehyde [300].

Housework

Irritants.   Washing-up liquids, hard-surface cleaners, foods, wet work.

Sensitizers.   Foods [269, 270], flavourings and spices [268], chromate (bleaches), formaldehyde (household products), plants and flowers, hand creams and lotions, rubber gloves.

CU/PCD.   Meat, fish, shellfish, fruit and vegetables [269, 270], rubber gloves [301].

Jewellers

Irritants.   Organic solvents [321], fluxes.

Sensitizers.   Nickel, precious metals [322], epoxy resins (see also "Enamelling").

Metalworking

Irritants.   Metalworking fluids [219, 232, 237], organic solvents, skin cleansers.

Sensitizers.   Chromate (antirust agents, welding fumes), nickel, cobalt [323], metalworking fluids [219, 232, 237] (biocides, colophony, mercaptobenzothiazole, leached metals, ethylenediamine [324]).

Office Work

Irritants.   Indoor climate [155, 325], paper [326], fibreglass [327].

Sensitizers.   Rubber (finger stalls), nickel (paper clips, scissors), paper [326] (correction, copying, carbon), glues.

Sick Building Syndrome.   [156].

Painting

Irritants.   Thinners, organic solvents [328], emulsion paints, wallpaper adhesives, organotin compounds.

Sensitizers.   Turpentine, dipentene, cobalt (pigments, driers), chromate (pigments, antirust), nickel (pigment) [329], epoxy, acrylic [330] and polyurethane resins, glues (urea- and phenol-formaldehyde resins), varnish (urea-formaldehyde, colophony) preservatives in water-based paints and glues (chloroacetamide [40], methylol-chloroacetamide, chlorothalonil [331]), triglycidyl isocyanurate in polyester powder paints [332].

Photographic Processing

Irritants.   Reducing and oxidizing agents, alkalis, organic solvents.

Sensitizers.   Metol (*p*-aminophenol), hydroquinone, pyrogallol, amidol, phenidone, ethylenediamine, ethylenediaminetetraacetate (EDTA), resorcinol, pyrocatechol, phloroglucinol, salicylaldoxime, triazine, formaldehyde, glutaraldehyde, chromate, sodium metabisulphite, colour developers, persulphate bleach accelerator (PBA) 1 [333], rubber gloves.

Plastics Industry

Irritants.   Organic solvents, acids, oxidizing agents, styrene.

Sensitizers.   Monomers and low molecular weight oligomers [53, 334], hardeners, additives (organic cobalt salts, colophony), pigments, styrene [335].

Plumbing

Irritants.   Wet work, soldering fluxes, skin cleansers.

Sensitizers.   Rubber (gloves, hoses, packing), chromate (cement, antirust paint), epichlorohydrin (solvent cement) [336].

Printing

Irritants.   Organic solvents, multifunctional acrylates in UV-curing inks, lacqueres and printing plates [337].

Sensitizers.   Chromate [98], cobalt, paper (colophony, maleopimaric acid [287]), turpentine, rubber (offset printing roller blanket), formaldehyde and isothiazolinones [338] (gum arabic and fountain solutions), multifunctional acrylates in UV-curing inks, lacquers and printing plates [337, 339].

Road Construction and Repair

Irritants.   Sand-oil mix, asphalt (phototoxic), skin cleansers.

Sensitizers.   Cement (chromate, epoxy resin), epoxy resin, tars, chromate (antirust paint).

Rubber Manufacture

Irritants.   Friction, organic solvents, talc, zinc stearate [100].

Sensitizers.   Rubber chemicals [340, 341], colophony, chromate, cobalt, phenol-formaldehyde resin, dyes.

Shoe Making and Repairing

Irritants.   Organic solvents.

Sensitizers.   Glues (*p-tert*-butylphenol-formaldehyde resin [342]), leather (chromate, formaldehyde, chloroacetamide [343], dyes), rubber, colophony, turpentine, bisphenol A [344].

Swimming Bath Attendants

Irritants.   Free or combined chlorine/bromine [345].

Sensitizers.   Biocides, sodium hypochlorite [346], formaldehyde, essential oils.

Tanning

Irritants.   Alkalis, acids, reducing and oxidizing agents, hair removers.

Sensitizers.   Chromate [98], formaldehyde, glutaraldehyde, vegetable tans [347], finishes, biocides, dyes [348].

CU/PCD.   Formaldehyde [349].

Textile and Upholstery Trades

Irritants.   Organic solvents, oxidizing, reducing and bleaching agents, friction, fibre types, formaldehyde (from crease-resistant resins and fire retardants).

Sensitizers.   Formaldehyde (as above), dyes [348, 350–352], chromate [98] (mordant), dimethylthiourea [353] (paper cutting patterns).

CU/PCD.   Formaldehyde, reactive dyes [354].

Veterinary Medicine (and Slaughtering)

Irritants.   Disinfectants, wet work, animal fluids and entrails [355], rectal and vaginal examinations of livestock.

Sensitizers.   Rubber gloves, veterinary medicaments [356, 357] (penicillin, streptomycin, neomycin, tylosin tartrate, spiramycin, virginiamycin, mercaptobenzothiazole [7], 3-ethylamine-1,2-benzisothiazole hydrochloride [358]), glutaraldehyde [311], Bronopol (2-bromo-2-nitropropan-1,3-diol) (preservative in rectal lubricant) [359].

CU/PCD.   Animal tissues, obstetric fluids, hair and dander [360].

Woodworking

Irritants.   Woods [84, 361], fibreboard (urea-formaldehyde resin) [87], wood preservatives [361], organic solvents, skin cleansers.

Sensitizers.   Woods [291], wood preservatives, colophony, turpentine, balsams, tars, lacquers, glues (urea-, phenol- and *p*-tert-butylphenol-formaldehyde resins), lichens, *Frullania*

CU/PCD.   Woods [295].

Acknowledgements.   I thank Charles Calnan and Etain Cronin for introducing me to the ways of thinking in this chapter, Robert Adams for allowing me access to his reference resources, Pat Tharratt for her librarianship, and Claire Sinicka for her word-processing skills.

11.18 References

1. Warr P (1983) Work, jobs and unemployment. Bull Br Psychol Soc 36: 305–311
2. Sass B (1988) The centrality of work. Work Stress 2: 255–260
3. Meding B, Swanbeck G (1990) Consequences of having hand eczema. Contact Dermatitis 23: 6–14
4. Agrup G (1969) Hand eczema and other dermatoses in South Sweden. Acta Derm Venereol (Stockh) 49 Suppl 61
5. Calnan CD, Rycroft RJG (1981) Rehabilitation in occupational skin disease. Trans Coll Med S Afr 25 [Suppl Rehabil]: 136–142
6. Mathias CGT (1988) Occupational dermatoses. J Am Acad Dermatol 19: 1107–1114
7. Adams RM (1990) Occupational skin disease, 2nd edn. Saunders, Philadelphia
8. Parkes WR (1982) Occupational asthma (including byssinosis). In: Parkes WR (ed) Occupational lung disorders, 2nd edn. Butterworths, London, pp 415–453
9. Lam S, Chan-Yeung M (1987) Occupational asthma: natural history, evaluation and management. Occup Med: State Art Rev (Occup Pulm Dis) 2: 373–381
10. Koh D, Foulds IS, Aw TC (1990) Dermatological hazards in the electronics industry. Contact Dermatitis 22: 1–7
11. Flannigan SA, Tucker SB, Key MM, Ross CE, Fairchild EJ II, Grimes BA, Harrist RB (1985) Synthetic pyrethroid insecticides : a dermatological evaluation. Br J Ind Med 42 : 363–372.
12. Anger WK, Johnson BL (1985) Chemicals affecting behaviour. In: O'Donaghue JL (ed) Neurotoxicity of industrial and commercial chemicals, vol 1. CRC, Boca Raton, pp 51–148
13. Calnan CD (1977) Dermatology and industry (Prosser White Oration). Clin Exp Dermatol 3: 1–16
14. White RP (1928) The dermatergoses or occupational affections of the skin, 3rd edn. Lewis, London
15. Bonnevie P (1939) Aetiologie and Pathogenese der Ekzemkrankheiten. Busck, Copenhagen
16. Schwartz L, Tulipan L, Birmingham DJ (1957) Occupational diseases of the skin, 3rd edn. Kimpton, London
17. Foussereau J, Benezra C (1970) Les eczémas allergiques professionels. Masson, Paris
18. Foussereau J, Benezra C, Maibach HI (1982) Occupational contact dermatitis. Munksgaard, Copenhagen
19. Foussereau J (1991) Guide de dermato-allergologie professionnelle. Masson, Paris
20. Zschunke E (1985) Grundriss der Arbeitsdermatologie. VEB Verlag Volk und Gesundheit, Berlin
21. Fregert S (1975) Occupational dermatitis in a 10-year material. Contact Dermatitis 1: 96–107
22. Taylor JS (1988) Occupational disease statistics in perspective. Arch Dermatol 124: 1557–1558 (editorial)
23. Health and Safety Commission (1991) Annual report 1989/90. HMSO, London, pp 79–85, 102
24. Association of Schools of Public Health (1988) Proposed national strategies for the prevention of leading work-related diseases and injuries, pt 2. Washington, pp 65–93
25. Mathias CGT, Morrison JH (1988) Occupational skin disease, United States: results from the Bureau of Labor Statistics Annual Survey of Occupational Injuries and Illnesses, 1973 through 1984. Arch Dermatol 124: 1519–1524
26. Lomholt G (1963) Psoriasis, prevalence, spontaneous course and genetics. A census study on the prevalence of skin diseases in the Faroe Islands. Gad, Copenhagen
27. Rea JN, Newhouse ML, Halil T (1976) Skin disease in Lambeth. A community study of prevalence and use of medical care. Br J Prev Soc Med 30: 107–114

28. Johnson MLT (1977) Skin conditions and related needs for medical care among persons 1–74 years, United States 1971–1974. US Department of Health, Education and Welfare, Washington DC (DHEW publications no (PHS) 79–1660, ser 11, no 212)

29. Coenraads PJ, Nater JP, van der Lende R (1983) Prevalence of eczema and other dermatoses of the hands and arms in the Netherlands. Association with age and occupation. Clin Exp Dermatol 8: 495–503

30. Meding B, Swanbeck G (1990) Occupational hand eczema in an industrial city. Contact Dermatitis 22: 13–23

31. Mathias CGT (1985) The cost of occupational skin disease. Arch Dermatol 121: 332–334

32. Burry JN, Kirk J (1975) Environmental dermatitis: chrome cripples. Med J Aust 2: 720–721

33. Griffiths WAD (1985) Industrial dermatitis – a national problem. In: Griffiths WAD, Wilkinson DS (eds) Essentials of industrial dermatology. Blackwell, Oxford, pp 1–11

34. Newhouse ML (1964) The epidemiology of noninfective skin diseases in an automobile factory. Dissertation, University of London, pp 262–264

35. Campion KM, Rycroft RJG (1993) A study of attenders at an occupational dermatology clinic. Contact Dermatitis 28: 307

36. Smith AG (1989) Skin disease in the poetry industry. Ann Occup Hyg 33: 365–368

37. Schmunes E (1988) Predisposing factors in occupational skin disease. Dermatol Clin 6: 7–13

38. Coenraads PJ, Foo SC, Lun KC (1985) Dermatitis in small-scale metal industries. Contact Dermatitis 12: 155–160

39. O'Malley M, Thun M, Morrison J, Mathias CGT, Halperin WE (1988) Surveillance of occupational skin disease using the supplementary data system. Am J Ind Med 13: 291–299

40. Högberg M, Wahlberg JE (1980) Health screening for occupational dermatoses in house painters. Contact Dermatitis 6: 100–106

41. Varigos GA, Dunt DR (1981) Occupational dermatitis. An epidemiological study in the rubber and cement industries. Contact Dermatitis 7: 105–110

42. Lammintausta K (1983) Hand dermatitis in different hospital workers who perform wet work. Dermatosen 31: 14–19

43. Hansen KS (1983) Occupational dermatoses in hospital cleaning women. Contact Dermatitis 9: 343–351

44. Peltonen L, Wickström G, Selonen R (1983) Occupational skin diseases in shipyard workers. Dermatosen 31: 87–91

45. Coenraads PJ, Nater JP, Hansen JA, Lantinga H (1984) Prevalence of eczema and other dermatoses of the hands and forearms in construction workers in the Netherlands. Clin Exp Dermatol 9: 149–158

46. Van Putten PB, Coenraads PJ, Nater JP (1984) Hand dermatoses and contact allergic reactions in construction workers exposed to epoxy resins. Contact Dermatitis 10: 146–150

47. Kavli G, Gram IT, Moseng D, Ørpen G (1985) Occupational dermatitis in shrimp peelers. Contact Dermatitis 13: 69–71

48. Peltonen L, Wickström G, Vaahtoranta M (1985) Occupational dermatoses in the food industry. Dermatosen 33: 166–169

49. Hogan DJ, Dosman JA, Li KYR, Graham B, Johnson D, Walker R, Lane PR (1986) Questionnaire survey of pruritus and rash in grain elevator workers. Contact Dermatitis 14: 170–175

50. Singgih SIR, Lantinga H, Nater JP, Woest TE, Kruyt-Gasperz JA (1986) Occupational hand dermatoses in hospital cleaning personnel. Contact Dermatitis 14: 14–19

51. Goh CL, Gan SL, Ngui SJ (1986) Occupational dermatitis in a prefabrication construction factory. Contact Dermatitis 15: 235–240

52. Wahlberg JE, Högberg M (1987) Health screening for occupational dermatoses in flooring installers. Boll Dermatol Allergol Prof 2: 95–102
53. Bruze M, Almgren G (1988) Occupational dermatoses in workers exposed to resins based on phenol and formaldehyde. Contact Dermatitis 19: 272–277
54. Avnstorp C (1989) Prevalence of cement eczema in Denmark before and since addition of ferrous sulphate to Danish cement. Acta Derm Venereol (Stockh) 69: 151–155
55. De Boer EM, van Ketel WG, Bruynzeel DP (1989) Dermatitis in metalworkers. I. Irritant contact dermatitis. Contact Dermatitis 20: 212–218
56. Cronin E, Kullavanijaya P (1979) Hand dermatitis in hair-dressers. Acta Derm Venereol (Stockh) 59 [Suppl 85]: 47–50
57. Høvding G (1970) Cement eczema and chromium allergy. An epidemiological investigation. Dissertation, University of Bergen
58. Jolanki R, Kanerva L, Estlander T, Tarvainen K, Keskinen H, Henriks-Eckerman M-L (1990) Occupational dermatoses from epoxy resin compounds. Contact Dermatitis 23: 172–173
59. Grattan CEH, English JSC, Foulds IS, Rycroft RJG (1989) Cutting fluid dermatitis. Contact Dermatitis 20: 372–376
60. De Boer EM, van Ketel WG, Bruynzeel DP (1989) Dermatoses in metalworkers. II. Allergic contact dermatitis. Contact Dermatitis 20: 280–286
61. Bäurle G (1986) Handekzeme. Studie zum Einfluß von konstitutionellen and Umweltfaktoren auf die Genese. Schattauer, Stuttgart
62. Deschamps D, Garner R, Savoye J, Chabaux C, Efthymiou M-L, Fournier E (1988) Allergic and irritant contact dermatitis from diethyl-β-chloroethylamine. Contact Dermatitis 18: 103–105
63. Warshaw TG (1988) Primary irritant effect of 3,4,5-trichloropyridazine. Contact Dermatitis 18: 257–258
64. Malten KE (1981) Thoughts on irritant contact dermatitis. Contact Dermatitis 7: 238–247
65. Kligman AM, Klemme JC, Susten AS (eds) (1985) The chronic effects of repeated mechanical trauma to the skin. Am J Ind Med 8: 253–513
66. Lahti A (1980) Non-immunologic contact urticaria. Dissertation, University of Oulu
67. Bjornberg A (1968) Skin reactions to primary irritants in patients with hand eczema. An investigation with matched controls. Isacsons, Göteborg
68. Frosch PJ (1985) Hautirritation und empfindliche Haut. Grosse, Berlin
69. Maibach HI, Lamminstausta K, Berardesca E, Freeman S (1989) Tendency to irritation: sensitive skin. J Am Acad Dermatol 21: 833–835
70. Frosch PJ (1989) Irritant contact dermatitis. In: Frosch PJ, Dooms-Goossens A, Lachapelle J-M, Rycroft RJG, Scheper RJ (eds) Current topics in contact dermatitis. Springer, Berlin Heidelberg New York, pp 385–398
71. Frosch PJ, Wissing C (1982) Cutaneous sensitivity to ultraviolet light and chemical irritants. Arch Dermatol Res 272: 269–278
72. Rystedt I (1986) Atopy, hand eczema and contact dermatitis: summary of recent large scale studies. Semin Dermatol 5: 290–300
73. Lammintausta K, Kalimo K (1981) Atopy and hand dermatitis in hospital wet workers. Contact Dermatitis 7: 301–308
74. Rystedt I (1985) Factors influencing the occurrence of hand eczema in adults with a history of atopic dermatitis in childhood. Contact Dermatitis 12: 185–191
75. Nilsson E, Bäck O (1986) The importance of anamnestic information of atopy, metal dermatitis and earlier hand eczema for the development of hand dermatitis in women in wet hospital work. Acta Derm Venereol (Stockh) 66: 45–50
76. Meding B, Swanbeck G (1990) Predictive factors for hand eczema. Contact Dermatitis 23: 154–161

77. Gehring W (1990) Effects of irritants in atopic dermatitis. Contact Dermatitis 22: 292–293
78. Bruze M, Emmett EA (1990) Occupational exposures to irritants. In: Jackson EM, Goldner R (eds) Irritant contact dermatitis. Dekker, New York, pp 81–106
79. Andersen KE, Benezra C, Burrows D, Camarasa J, Dooms-Goossens A, Ducombs G, Frosch P, Lachapelle J-M, Lahti A, Menné T, Rycroft R, Scheper R, White I, Wilkinson J (1987) Contact dermatitis. A review. Contact Dermatitis 16: 55–78
80. Mathias CGT (1987) Clinical and experimental aspects of cutaneous irritation. In: Marzulli FN, Maibach HI (eds) Dermatotoxicology, 3rd edn. Hemisphere, Washington, pp 173–189
81. Griffiths WAD, Wilkinson DS (1985) Primary irritants and solvents. In: Griffiths WAD, Wilkinson DS, (eds) Essentials of industrial dermatology. Blackwell, Oxford, pp 58–72
82. Rycroft RJG, Wilkinson JD (1986) The principal irritants and sensitizers. In: Rook A, Wilkinson DS, Ebling FJG, Champion RH, Burton JL (eds) Textbook of dermatology, 4th edn. Blackwell Oxford, pp 533–535
83. Fregert S (1981) Manual of contact dermatitis, 2nd edn. Munksgaard, Copenhagen
84. Gan SL, Goh CL, Lee CS, Hui KH (1987) Occupational dermatosis among sanders in the furniture industry. Contact Dermatitis 17: 237–240
85. Rycroft RJG, Lovell CR, Harries PG, Winter P, Mallet AI (1987) Occupational irritant contact dermatitis from chicory. Boll Dermatol Allergol Prof 2: 77–82
86. Lovell CR, Rycroft RJG, Vale PT (1988) Irritant contact dermatitis from diallyglycol carbonate monomer and its prevention. Contact Dermatitis 18: 284–286
87. Vale PT, Rycroft RJG (1988) Occupational irritant contact dermatitis from fibreboard contining urea-formaldehyde resin. Contact Dermatitis 19: 62
88. Bruynzeel DP, Hennipman G, van Ketel WG (1988) Irritant contact dermatitis and chrome-passivated metal. Contact Dermatitis 19: 175–179
89. Halkier-Sørensen L, Thestrup-Pedersen K (1988) Skin temperature and skin symptoms among workers in the fish processing industry. Contact Dermatitis 19: 206–209
90. Thestrup-Pedersen K, Madsen JB, Rasmussen K (1989) Cumulative skin irritancy from heat-decomposed polyethylene plastic. In: Frosch PJ, Dooms-Goossens A, Lachapelle J-M, Rycroft RJG, Scheper RJ (eds) Current topics in contact dermatitis. Springer, Berlin Heidelberg New York, pp 412–415
91. Goh CL, Ho SF (1993) Contact dermatitis from dielectric fluids in electrodischarge machining. Contact Dermatitis 28: 134-138
92. Seidenari S, Manzini BM, Danese P, Motolese A (1990) Patch and prick test study of 593 healthy subjects. Contact Dermatitis 23: 162–167
93. Thestrup-Pedersen K, Larsen CG, Rønnevig J (1989) The immunology of contact dermatitis. A review with special reference to the pathophysiology of eczema. Contact Dermatitis 20: 81–92
94. Scheper RJ, von Blomberg BME (1989) Allergic contact dermatitis: T-cell receptors and migration. In: Frosch PJ, Dooms-Goossens A, Lachapelle J-M, Rycroft RJG, Scheper RJ (eds) Current topics in contact dermatitis. Springer, Berlin Heidelberg New York, 412–415
95. Meneghini CL, Angelini G (1984) Primary and secondary sites of occupational contact dermatitis. Dermatosen 32: 205–207
96. Cronin E (1985) Clinical patterns of hand eczema in women. Contact Dermatitis 13: 153–161
97. English JSC, White IR, Rycroft RJG (1986) Sensitization to 1-methylquinoxalinium-p-toluene sulfonate. Contact Dermatitis 14: 261–262
98. Burrows D (1983) Adverse chromate reactions on the skin. In: Burrows D (ed) Chromium: metabolism and toxicity. CRC, Boca Raton, pp 137–163
99. Rycroft RJG (1981) Soluble oil dermatitis. Clin Exp Dermatol 6: 229–234

100. White IR (1988) Dermatitis in rubber manufacturing industries. Dermatol Clin 6: 53–59

101. De Boer EM, Bruynzeel DP, van Ketel WG (1988) Dyshidrotic eczema as an occupational dermatitis in metal workers. Contact Dermatitis 19: 184–188

102. Baran R (1990) Occupational nail disorders. In: Adams RM (ed) Occupational skin disease. Saunders, Philadelphia, pp 160–171

103. Rycroft RJG, Baran R (1984) Occupational abnormalities and contact dermatitis. In: Baran R, Dawber RPR (eds) Diseases of the nails and their management. Blackwell, Oxford, pp 267–287

104. Ancona-Alayón A (1975) Occupational koilonychia from organic solvents. Contact Dermatitis 1: 367–369

105. Mathias CGT, Maibach HI (1984) Allergic contact dermatitis from anaerobic acrylic sealants. Arch Dermatol 120: 1202–1205

106. Fisher AA (1979) Occupational palmar psoriasis due to safety prescription container caps. Contact Dermatitis 5: 56

107. Moroni P, Cazzaniga R, Pierini F, Panella V, Zerboni R (1988) Occupational contact psoriasis. Dermatosen 36: 163–164

108. Dooms-Goossens AE, Debusschere KM, Gevers DM, Dupré KM, Degreef HJ, Loncke JP, Snauwaert JE (1986) Contact dermatitis caused by airborne agents. A review and case reports. J Am Acad Dermatol 15: 1–10

109. Lachapelle J-M (1987) The concept of industrial airborne irritant or allergic contact dermatitis. In: Maibach HI (ed) Occupational and industrial dermatology, 2nd edn. Year Book, Chicago, pp 179–189

110. Dahlquist I, Fregert S (1979) Allergic contact dermatitis from volatile epoxy hardeners and reactive diluents. Contact Dermatitis 5: 406–407

111. Sneddon IB (1979) The presentation of psychiatric illness to the dermatologist. Acta Derm Venereol (Stockh) 59 [Suppl 85]: 177–179

112. Rosenberg SJ, Freedman MR, Schmaling KB, Rose C (1990) Personality styles of patients asserting environmental illness. J Occup Med 32: 678–681

113. Sneddon IB (1983) Simulated disease: problems in diagnosis and management (Parkes Weber lecture 1982). J R Coll Physicians Lond 17: 199–205

114. Maguire A (1978) Psychic possession among industrial workers. Lancet i: 376–378

115. Epstein E (1984) Hand dermatitis: practical management and current concepts. J Am Acad Dermatol 10: 395–424

116. Wall LM, Gebauer KA (1991) A follow-up study of occupational skin disease in Western Australia. Contact Dermatitis 24: 241–243

117. Rosen RH, Freeman S (1993) Prognosis of occupational contact dermatitis in New South Wales, Australia. Contact Dermatitis 29 : 88–93

118. Breit LR, Turk RBM (1976) The medical and social fate of the dichromate allergic patient. Br J Dermatol 94: 349–351

119. Grattan CEH, Foulds IS (1989) Outcome of investigation of cutting fluid dermatitis. Contact Dermatitis 20: 377–378

120. Pryce DW, Irvine D, English JSC, Rycroft RJG (1989) Soluble oil dermatitis: a follow-up study. Contact Dermatitis 21: 28–35

121. Cronin E (1987) Dermatitis of the hands in caterers. Contact Dermatitis 17: 265–269

122. Keczkes K (1984) Does contact sensitivity last? Int J Dermatol 23: 108–109

123. Comaish JS (1976) Validity of patch test results. Contact Dermatitis 2: 285–286 (letter)

124. Rycroft RJG (1982) Soluble oil as a major cause of occupational dermatitis. Dissertation, Cambridge University

125. Hogan DJ, Dannaker CJ, Maibach HI (1990) The prognosis of contact dermatitis. J Am Acad Dermatol 23: 300–307

126. Hogan DJ, Dannaker CJ, Maibach HI (1990) Contact dermatitis: prognosis, risk factors, and rehabilitation. Semin Dermatol 9: 233–246

127. Rietschel RL (1988) Patch testing in occupational hand dermatitis. Dermatol Clin 6: 43–46
128. Mathias CGT (1989) Contact dermatitis and workers compensation: criteria for establishing occupational causation and aggravation. J Am Acad Dermatol 20: 842–848
129. Cowles S (1982) Inadequate occupational histories in case records. N Engl J Med 307: 1713–1714 (letter)
130. The Occupational and Environmental Health Committee of the American Lung Association of San Diego and Imperial Counties (1983) Taking the occupational history. Ann Intern Med 99: 641–651
131. Kligman AM (1983) Lanolin allergy: crisis or comedy? Contact Dermatitis 9: 99–107
132. Rycroft RJG (1990) Is patch testing necessary? In: Champion RH, Pye RJ (eds) Recent advances in dermatology, no 8. Churchill Livingstone, Edinburgh, pp 101–111
133. Rycroft RJG (1986) False reactions to nonstandard patch tests. Semin Dermatol 5: 225–230
134. Calnan CD (1987) The use and abuse of patch tests. In: Maibach HI (ed) Occupational and industrial dermatology, 2nd edn. Year Book, Chicago, pp 28–31
135. Fregert S (1989) Patch testing with isolated and identified substances in products: basis for prevention. J Am Acad Dermatol 21: 857–860
136. Cronin E (1986) Some practical supplementary trays for special occupations. Semin Dermatol 5: 243–248
137. Adams RM (1989) Panels of allergens for specific occupations. J Am Acad Dermatol 21: 869–874
138. Rycroft RJG (1982) Contact sensitization to 2-monomethylol phenol in phenol formaldehyde resin as an example of the recognition and prevention of industrial dermatoses. Clin Exp Dermatol 7: 285–290
139. Fregert S (1979) Batch consciousness in dermatological management. Acta Derm Venereol (Stockh) 59 [Suppl 85]: 63–65
140. De Groot AC (1986) Patch testing. Test concentrations and vehicles for 2800 allergens. Elsevier, Amsterdam
141. Fregert S (1988) Physicochemical methods for detection of contact allergens. Dermatol Clin 6: 97–104
142. Thorgeirsson A, Fregert S, Ramnäs A (1978) Sensitization capacity of epoxy resin oligomers in the guinea pig. Acta Derm Venereol (Stockh) 58: 17–21
143. Bruze M, Fregert S, Zimerson E (1985) Contact allergy to phenol-formaldehyde resins. Contact Dermatitis 12: 81–86
144. Karlberg A-T, Bohlinder K, Boman A, Hacksell U, Hermannson J, Jacobsson S, Nilsson JLG (1988) Identification of 15-hydroperoxyabietic acid as a contact allergen in Portuguese colophony. J Pharm Pharmacol 40: 42–47
145. Hill RH (1984) Ultraviolet detection of synthetic oil contamination of skin. Am Ind Hyg Assoc J 45: 474–484
146. Keenan RR, Cole SB (1982) A sampling and analytical procedure for skin contamination evaluation. Am Ind Hyg Assoc J 43: 473–476
147. Jongeneelen FJ, Scheepers PTJ, Groenendijk A, van Aerts LAGJM, Anzion RBM, Bos RP, Veestra SJ (1988) Airborne concentrations, skin contamination, and urinary metabolite excretion of polycyclic aromatic hydrocarbons among paving workers exposed to coal tar derived road tars. Am Ind Hyg Assoc 49: 600–607
148. Cohen B-SM, Popendorf W (1989) A method for monitoring dermal exposure to volatile chemicals. Am Ind Hyg Assoc J 50: 216–223
149. Vo-Dinh T, Gammaga RB (1981) The lightpipe luminoscope for monitoring occupational skin contamination. Am Ind Hyg Assoc J 42: 112–120

150. Fenske RA, Leffingwell JT, Spear RC (1986) A video imaging technique for assessing dermal exposure I. Instrument design and testing. Am Ind Hyg Assoc J 47: 764–770

151. Fenske RA, Wong SM, Leffingwell JT, Spear RC (1986) A video imaging technique for assessing dermal exposure. II. Fluorescent tracer testing. Am Ind Hyg Assoc J 771–775

152. Fregert S (1963) The organization of occupational dermatology in Lund. Acta Derm Venereol (Stockh) 43: 203–205

153. Emmett EA (1984) The skin and occupational disease. Arch Environ Health 39: 144–149

154. Rycroft RJG (1988) Looking at work dermatologically. Dermatol Clin 6: 1–5

155. Rycroft RJG (1987) Low-humidity occupational dermatoses. In: Gardner AW (ed) Current approaches to occupational health 3. Wright, Bristol, pp 1–13

156. Skov P, Valbjørn O, Pedersen BV (1989) Influence of personal characteristics, job-related factors and psychosocial factors on the sick building syndrome. Scand J Work Environ Health 15: 286–295

157. Rycroft RJG (1980) Occupational dermatoses in perspective. Lancet ii: 24–26

158. Valsecchi R, Cassina G, Leghissa P, Migliori M, Cainelli T, Seghizzi P (1987) Cooperation between departments of dermatology and occupational disease: an eighteen months' experience results. Boll Dermatol Allergol Prof 2: 192–198

159. Coenraads PJ, Nater JP (1987) Some general epidemiological and statistical considerations in the design of studies on dermatitis in selected occupational populations. Boll Dermatol Allergol Prof 2: 105–116

160. Berg M, Axelson O (1990) Evaluation of a questionnaire for facial skin complaints related to work at visual display units. Contact Dermatitis 22: 71–77

161. Wilkinson DS, Champion RH. General aspects of treatment (1986) In: Rook A, Wilkinson DS, Ebling FJG, Champion RH, Burton JL (eds) Textbook of dermatology, 4th edn. Blackwell, Oxford, pp 2479–2499

162. Pye RJ, Roberts SOB, Champion RH (1986) Systemic therapy. In: Rook A, Wilkinson DS, Ebling FJG Champion RH, Burton JL (eds) Textbook of dermatology, 4th edn. Blackwell, Oxford, pp 2501–2527

163. Griffiths WAD, Ive FA, Wilkinson JD (1986) Topical therapy. In: Rook A, Wilkinson DS, Ebling FJG, Champion RH, Burton JL (eds) Textbook of dermatology, 4th edn. Blackwell, Oxford, pp 2529–2573

164. Burrows D (1985) Industrial dermatitis today and its prevention. In: Griffiths WAD, Wilkinson DS (eds) Essentials of industrial dermatology. Blackwell, Oxford, pp 12–23

165. Wahlberg JE (1986) Prophylaxis of contact dermatitis. Semin Dermatol 5: 255–262

166. Burrows D, Beck MH (1986) Prevention of industrial dermatitis. In: Recent advances in dermatology no 7. Churchill Livingstone, Edinburgh, pp 75–76

167. Tucker SB (1988) Prevention of occupational skin disease. Dermatol Clin 6: 87–96

168. Engel HO, Rycroft RJG (1988) Dermatology. In: Edwards FC, McCallum RI, Taylor PJ (eds) Fitness for work. The medical aspects. Oxford University Press, Oxford, pp 114–125

169. Lammintausta K, Maibach HI (1988) Dermatologic considerations in worker fitness evaluation. Occup Med State Art Rev 3: 341–350

170. Tranter HS (1990) Foodborne staphylococcal illness. Lancet 336: 1044–1046

171. Jensen O (1979) 'Rusters'. The corrosive action of palmar sweat. I. Sodium chloride in sweat. Acta Derm Venereol (Stockh) 59: 135–138

172. Jensen O (1979) 'Rusters'. The corrosive action of palmar sweat. II. Physical and chemical factors in palmar hyperhidrosis. Acta Derm Venereol (Stockh) 59: 139–143

173. Zschunke E (1978) Metallkorrosion (Rost) durch Hyperhidrose. Dermatol Monatsschr 164: 727–728

174. Ummenhofer B (1980) Zur Methodik der Alkaliresistenzprüfung. Dermatosen 28: 104–109
175. Foussereau J, Benezra C, Maibach HI (1982) Occupational contact dermatitis. Munksgaard, Copenhagen, pp 76–77
176. Calnan CD (1970) Studies in contact dermatitis XXIII. Allergen replacement. Trans St John's Hosp Dermatol Soc 56: 131–138
177. Fregert S (1980) Possibilities of skin contact in automatic processes. Contact Dermatitis 6: 23
178. Zschunke E (1980) Management of industrial dermatitis. Contact Dermatitis 6: 18–19
179. Church RE (1981) Prevention of dermatitis and its medicolegal aspects. Br J Dermatol 105 [Suppl 21]: 85–90
180. Forsberg K, Keith LH (1989) Chemical protective clothing performance index book. Wiley, New York
181. Wilkinson DS (1985) Protective gloves. In: Griffiths WAD, Wilkinson DS (eds) Essentials of industrial dermatology. Blackwell. Oxford, pp 101–105
182. Mellström GA, Boman AS, Wahlberg JE (1986) Protective gloves. Reduction of skin exposure to chemicals. In: Maibach HI (ed) Occupational and industrial dermatology, 2nd edn. Year Book, Chicago, pp 126–133
183. Mellström G, Carlsson B (1987) 2nd Scandinavian symposium on protective clothing against chemicals and other health risks. Arbete och Hälsa. Vetenskaplig skriftserie, Vol 12
184. Estlander T, Jolanki R (1988) How to protect the hands. Dermatol Clin 6: 105–113
185. Jensen DA, Hardy JK (1989) Effect of glove material thickness on permeation characteristics. Am Ind Hyg Assoc J 50: 623–626
186. Berardinelli SP, Hall R (1985) Site-specific whole glove chemical penetration. Am Ind Hyg Assoc J 46: 60–64
187. Michelsen RL, Roder MM, Berardinelli SP (1986) Permeation of chemical protective clothing by three binary solvent mixtures. Am Ind Hyg Assoc J 47: 236–240
188. Henriksen H (1982) Selection of materials for protective gloves. Polymer membranes for protection against contact with epoxy preparations. Report no 8/1982. Danish Directorate of Labour Inspection Services, Copenhagen
189. Darre E, Vedel P, Jensen JS (1987) Skin protection against methyl methacrylate. Acta Orthop Scand 58: 236–238
190. Moody RP, Ritter L (1990) Pesticide glove permeation analysis: comparison of the ASTM F739 test method with an automated flow-through reverse-phase liquid chromatography procedure. Am Ind Hyg Assoc J 51: 79–83
191. Mellström G (1985) Protective effect of gloves – compiled in a data base. Contact Dermatitis 13: 162–165
192. Thomas PH, Fenton-May V (1987) Protection offered by various gloves to carmustine exposure. Pharm J 20: 775–777
193. Redmond SF, Schapper KR (1987) Occupational dermatitis associated with garments. J Occup Med 29: 243–244
194. Foussereau J, Tomb R, Cavelier C (1990) Allergic contact dermatitis from safety clothes and individual protective devices. Dermatol Clin 8: 127–132
195. Orchard S (1984) Barrier creams. Dermatol Clin 2: 619–629
196. Cronin E (1985) Barrier creams. In: Griffiths WAD, Wilkinson DS (eds) Essentials of industrial dermatology. Blackwell, Oxford, pp 106–110
197. Mahmoud G, Lachapelle J-M, van Neste D (1984) Histological assessment of skin damage by irritants: its possible use in the evaluation of a 'barrier cream'. Contact Dermatitis 11: 179–185
198. Mahmoud G, Lachapelle J-M (1985) Evaluation expérimentale de l'efficacité de crèmes-barrière et de gels antisolvants dans la prévention de l'irritation cutanée provoquée par des solvants organiques. Cah Méd Travail 22: 163–168

199. Nouaigui H, Antoine JL, Lachapelle J-M (1988) An experimental study of the protective value of a silicone cream versus its vehicle against skin irritation provoked by sodium hydroxide. Arch Mal Prof 49: 383–387
200. Lachapelle J-M, Nouaigui H, Marot L (1990) Experimental study of the effects of a new protective cream against skin irritation provoked by the organic solvents *n*-hexane, trichlorethylene and toluene. Dermatosen 38: 19–23
201. Boman A, Mellström G (1989) Percutaneous absorption of three organic solvents in the guinea pig. III. Effect of barrier creams. Contact Dermatitis 21: 134–140
202. Boman A, Mellström G (1989) Percutaneous absorption of three organic solvents in the guinea pig. IV. Effect of protective gloves. Contact Dermatitis 21: 260–266
203. Komp B (1985) Skin protection creams. Their importance in the prophylaxis of occupational dermatoses. Dermatosen 33: 20–26
204. Lodén M (1986) The effect of 4 barrier creams on the absorption of water, benzene, and formaldehyde into excised human skin. Contact Dermatitis 14: 292–296
205. Frosch PJ, Kurte A, Pilz B (1993) Efficacy of skin barrier creams. III. The repetitive irritation test (RIT) in humans. Contact Dermatitis 29 : 113–118
206. Jepsen JR, Jørgensen AS, Kyst A (1985) Hand protection for car-painters. Contact Dermatitis 13: 317–320
207. Blanken R, van der Valk PGM, Nater JP, Dijkstra H (1987) Afterwork emollient creams: effects on irritant skin reactions. Dermatosen 35: 95–98
208. Serup J, Winther A, Blickmann CW (1989) Effects of repeated application of a moisturizer. Acta Derm Venereol (Stockh) 69: 457–459
209. Bendsoë N, Björnberg A, Löwhagen G-B, Tengberg J-E (1987) Glass fibre irritation and protective creams. Contact Dermatitis 17: 69–72
210. Blanken R, Nater JP, Veenhoff E (1987) Protective effect of barrier creams and spray coatings against epoxy resins. Contact Dermatitis 17: 79–83
211. Vale PT (1993) Prevention of phytophotodermatitis from celery. Contact Dermatitis 29 : 108
212. Dobson RL (1979) Evaluation of hand cleansers. Contact Dermatitis 5: 305–307
213. De Boer EM, Scholten RJPM, van Ketel WG, Bruynzeel DP (1990) Quantitation of mild irritant reactions due to repeated patch test application of liquid cleaners. A laser Doppler flowmetry study. Int J Cosmet Sci 12: 43–52
214. Malten KE, den Arend JACJ (1985) Irritant contact dermatitis. Traumiterative and cumulative impairment by cosmetics, climate and other daily loads. Dermatosen 33: 125–132
215. Kimber I (1989) Aspects of the immune response to contact allergens: opportunities for the development and modification of predictive test methods. Food Chem Toxicol 27: 755–762
216. Magnusson B, Fregert S, Wahlberg J (1979) Determination of skin sensitization potential of chemicals. Predictive testing in guinea pigs. Arbete och Hälsa. Vetenskaplig skriftserie, vol 26
217. McMillan EM, McKenna WB, Milne CM (1982) Guidelines on preparing a medical report for compensation purposes. Br J Dermatol 106: 489–494
218. Goldstein A (1984) Writing report letters for patients with skin disease resulting from on-the-job exposures. Dermatol Clin 2: 631–641
219. Rycroft RJG (1990) Petroleum and petroleum derivatives. In: Adams RM (ed) Occupational skin disease, 2nd edn. Saunders, Philadelphia, pp 486–502
220. Weidenbach T, Takoski J (1985) Gehäuftes Auftreten von dyshidrosiformen Handekzem durch eine Öl-in-Wasser-Emulsion bei Metallarbeiten. Dermatosen 33: 121–124
221. De Boer EM (1989) Occupational dermatitis by metalworking fluids. An epidemiological study and an investigation on skin irritation using laser Doppler flowmetry. Dissertation, Free University, Amsterdam

222. Robertson MH, Storrs FJ (1982) Allergic contact dermatitis in two machinists. Arch Dermatol 118: 997–1002

223. Van Ketel WG, Kisch LS (1983) The problem of the sensitizing capacity of some Grotans used as bacteriocides in cooling oils. Dermatosen 31: 118–121

224. Ernst B, Schmidt O (1983) Bestrahlung von Kühlschmierstoffen mit harter Gamma-Strahlung: ein Weg zur Reduktion von Hautschäden. Arbeitsmed Sozialmed Präventivmed 18: 79–82

225. Dahlquist I (1984) Contact allergy to the cutting oil preservatives Bioban CS-1246 and P-1487. Contact Dermatitis 10: 46

226. Wrangsjö K, Mårtensson A, Widström L, Sundberg K (1986) Contact dermatitis from Bioban P 1487. Contact Dermatitis 14: 182–183

227. Alomar A, Conde Salazar L, Romaguera C (1985) Occupational dermatoses from cutting oils. Contact Dermatitis 12: 129–138

228. Shrank AB (1985) Allergy to cutting oil. Contact Dermatitis 12: 229

229. Mitchell DM, Beck MH (1988) Contact allergy to benzyl alcohol in a cutting oil reodorant. Contact Dermatitis 18: 301–302

230. Lachapelle J-M (1990) A European overview of occupational dermatology. Occup Health Rev Oct/Nov: 21–24

231. Wolfram H (1987) Gesundheitsgefahren durch Kühl-und Schmiermittel. Arbeitsmed Sozialmed Präventivmed 22: 135–139

232. Pryce DW, White J, English JSC, Rycroft RJG (1989) Soluble oil dermatitis: a review. J Soc Occup Med 39: 93–98

233. Rycroft RJG (1980) Soluble oil dermatitis. Tijdschr Soc Geneeskd 58: 765–767

234. Gross J, Wolfram H (1990) Hautgefährdung durch Kühlschmierstoffe. Arbeitsmed Sozialmed Präventivmed 25: 36–38

235. Rietschel E (1982) Kombinierte Belastung der Haut am Beispiel des Schleifens und Honens als Folge von Rationalisierungsmaßnahmen. Arbeitsmed Sozialmed Präventivmed 17: 272–273

236. Geretzki P (1983) Diseases caused by soluble oil emulsions in the metal processing industry. Suggestions for solving this problem of multifactorial action. Dermatosen 31: 10–14

237. Foulds IS, Koh D (1990) Dermatitis from metalworking fluids. Clin Exp Dermatol 15: 157–162

238. Kajdas C (1988) Additives for metalworking lubricants – a review. Proceedings of the 6th International colloquium on industrial lubricants, properties, application, disposal. Technical Academy, Esslingen, sect 11.2-1–11.2-14

239. Shennan JL (1983) Selection and evaluation of biocides for aqueous metal-working fluids. Tribol Int 16: 317–330

240. Hausser M, Dicke F, Ippen H (1985) Kühlschmiermittelbestandteile und ihre gesundheitliche Wirkung. Zentralbl Arbeitsmed 35: 176–181

241. Rivett J, Merrick C (1990) Prevalence of occupational contact dermatitis in hairdressers. Contact Dermatitis 22: 304–305

242. Holness DL, Nethercott JR (1990) Dermatitis in hairdressers. Dermatol Clin 8: 119–126

243. Nethercott JR, MacPherson M, Choi BCK, Nixon P (1986) Contact dermatitis in hairdressers. Contact Dermatitis 14: 73–79

244. Lynde CW, Mitchell JC (1982) Patch test results in 66 hairdressers 1973–81. Contact Dermatitis 8: 302–307

245. Warshawki L, Mitchell JC, Storrs FJ (1981) Allergic contact dermatitis from glyceryl monothioglycolate in hairdressers. Contact Dermatitis 7: 351–352

246. Storrs FJ (1984) Permanent wave contact dermatitis: contact allergy to glyceryl monothioglycolate. J Am Acad Dermatol 11: 74–85

247. Calnan CD, Shuster S (1963) Reactions to ammonium persulphate. Arch Dermatol 88: 812–815

248. Kellett JK, Beck MH (1985) Ammonium persulphate sensitivity in hairdressers. Contact Dermatitis 13: 26–28
249. Hannuksela M, Hassi J (1980) Hairdresser's hand. Dermatosen 28: 149–151
250. Grobe J-W (1978) Pilonidal-sinus bei einem Friseur. Dermatosen 26: 190–191
251. Bowers PW (1982) Roustabouts' and barbers' breasts. Clin Exp Dermatol 7: 445–447
252. Gannon MX, Crowson MC, Fielding JWL (1988) Periareolar pilonidal abscesses in a hairdresser. Br Med J 297: 1641–1642
253. Hairdressing Training Board Bulletin (1990) Feb 1990; Issue 6: 8
254. Czarnecki N (1977) Zur Klinik und Pathogenese des Friseurekzems. Z Hautkr 52: 1–10
255. Heacock HJ, Rivers JK (1986) Occupational diseases of hairdressers. Can J Public Health 77: 109–113
256. Seeberg G (1952) Eczematous dermatoses from contact with, or ingestion of beef, pork and mutton (4 case reports). Acta Derm Venereol (Stockh) 32 [Suppl 29]: 320–322
257. Hjorth N, Roed-Petersen J (1976) Occupational protein contact dermatitis in food handlers. Contact Dermatitis 2: 28–42
258. Tosti A, Guerra L (1988) Protein contact dermatitis in food handlers. Contact Dermatitis 19: 149
259. Niinimaki A (1987) Scratch-chamber tests in food handler dermatitis. Contact Dermatitis 16: 11–20
260. Veien NK, Hattel T, Justesen O, Nørholm A (1983) Causes of eczema in the food industry. Dermatosen 31: 84–86
261. Tosti A, Fanti PA, Guerra L, Piancastelli E, Poggi S, Pilleri S (1990) Morphological and immunohistochemical study of immediate contact dermatitis of the hands due to foods. Contact Dermatitis 22: 81–85
262. Greig D (1983) Dermatitis in catering workers. Dissertation, University of Auckland
263. Sinclair S, Hindson C (1988) Allergic contact dermatitis from dodecyldiaminoethyl glycine. Contact Dermatitis 18: 320
264. Lautier R, Wendt V (1985) Contact allergy to Alliaceae. Case-report and literature-survey. Dermatosen 33: 213–215
265. Campolmi P, Lombardi P, Lotti T, Sertoli A (1982) Immediate and delayed sensitization to garlic. Contact Dermatitis 8: 352–353
266. Cronin E (1980) Contact dermatitis. Churchill Livingstone, Edinburgh, p 183
267. Carmichael AJ, Foulds IS, Tan CY (1988) Allergic contact dermatitis from potato flesh. Contact Dermatitis 20: 64–65
268. Dooms-Goossens A, Dubelloy R, Degreef H (1990) Contact and systemic contact-type dermatitis to spices. Dermatol Clin 8: 89–93
269. Hausen BM, Hjorth N (1984) Skin reactions to topical food exposure. Dermatol Clin 2: 567–578
270. Cronin E (1989) Dermatitis in food handlers. In: Callen JP, Dahl MV, Golitz LE, Schachner LA, Stegman SJ (eds) Advances in dermatology 4. Year Book, Chicago, pp 113–123
271. Veien N (1987) Occupational dermatoses in farmers. In: Maibach HI (ed) Occupational and industrial dermatology, 2nd edn. Year Book, Chicago, pp 436–446
272. Jung H-D, Rothe A, Heise H (1987) Zur Epikutantestung mit Pflanzenschutz- und Schädlingsbekämpfungsmitteln (Pestiziden). Dermatosen 35: 43–51
273. Pecegueiro M (1990) Contact dermatitis due to nickel in fertilizers. Contact Dermatitis 22: 114–115
274. Bousema MT, Wiemer GR, van Joost T (1991) A classic case of sensitization to DD-95. Contact Dermatitis 24: 132–133
275. Mancuso G, Staffa M, Errani A, Berdondini RM, Fabbri P (1990) Occupational dermatitis in animal field mill workers. Contact Dermatitis 22: 37–41

276. De Groot AC, Conemans JMH (1990) Contact allergy to furazolidone. Contact Dermatitis 22: 202–205

277. Dinis A, Brandão M, Faria A (1988) Occupational contact dermatitis from vitamin K3 sodium bisulphite. Contact Dermatitis 18: 170–171

278. Hjerpe L (1986) Chromate dermatitis at an engine assembly department. Contact Dermatitis 14: 66–67

279. Condé-Salazar L, Guimaraens D, Romero LV (1988) Occupational allergic contact dermatitis from anaerobic acrylic sealants. Contact Dermatitis 18: 129–132

280. Dooms-Goossens A, de Jonge G (1985) Letter to the editor. Contact Dermatitis 12: 238

281. Wilkinson SM, Beck MH (1993) Allergic contact dermatitis from sealants containing polysulphide polymers (Thiokol). Contact Dermatitis 29 : 273–274

282. Nethercott JR, Holness DL (1989) Occupational dermatitis in food handlers and bakers. J Am Acad Dermatol 21: 485–490

283. Hamada T, Horiguchi S (1978) A case of allergic contact dermatitis due to sodium carboxymethyl cellulose. Jpn J Ind Health 20: 207–211

284. Cardullo AC, Ruszkowski AM, De Leo VA (1989) Allergic contact dermatitis resulting from sensitivity to citrus peel, geraniol, and citral. J Am Acad Dermatol 21: 395–397

285. Sonnex TS, Rycroft RJG (1986) Allergic contact dermatitis from orthobenzyl parachlorophenol in a drinking glass cleaner. Contact Dermatitis 14: 247–248

286. English JSC, Lovell CR, Rycroft RJG (1985) Contact dermatitis from dibutyl maleate. Contact Dermatitis 13: 337–338

287. Karlberg A-T, Gäfvert E, Hagelthorn G, Nilsson JLG (1990) Maelopimaric acid – a potent sensitizer in modified rosin. Contact Dermatitis 22: 193–201

288. Fancalanci S, Giorgini S, Gola M, Sertoli A (1984) Occupational dermatitis in a butcher. Contact Dermatitis 11: 320–321

289. Beck H-I, Nissen BK (1982) Type I and type IV allergy to specific chicken organs. Contact Dermatitis 8: 217–218

290. Lachapelle J-M (1984) Occupational allergic contact dermatitis to povidone-iodine. Contact Dermatitis 11: 189–190

291. Beck MH, Hausen BM, Dave VK (1984) Allergic contact dermatitis from *Machaerium scleroxylum* Tul. (Pao ferro) in a joinery shop. Clin Exp Dermatol 9: 159–166

292. Irvine C, Reynolds A, Finlay AY (1988) Erythema multiforme-like reaction to "rosewood". Contact Dermatitis 19: 224–225

293. Goh CL (1987) Occupational allergic contact dermatitis from rengas wood. Contact Dermatitis 18: 300

294. Tilsley DA (1990) Australian blackwood dermatitis. Contact Dermatitis 23: 40–41

295. Schmidt H (1978) Contact urticaria to teak with systemic effects. Contact Dermatitis 4: 176–177

296. Halkier-Sørensen L, Thestrup-Pedersen K (1989) The relevance of low skin temperature inhibiting histamine-induced itch to the location of contact urticarial symptoms in the fish processing industry. Contact Dermatitis 21: 179–183

297. Seidenari S, Danese P, Di Nardo A, Manzini BM, Motolese BM (1990) Contact sensitization among ceramics workers. Contact Dermatitis 22: 45–49

298. Pedersen NB, Thormann J, Senning A (1980) Occupational contact allergy to bis-(4-chlorophenyl)-methyl chloride. Contact Dermatitis 6: 56

299. Niklasson B, Björkner B, Hansen L (1990). Occupational contact dermatitis from antitumor agent intermediates. Contact Dermatitis 22: 233–235

300. Nilsson E (1985) Contact sensitivity and urticaria in "wet" work. Contact Dermatitis 13: 321–328

301. Turjanmaa K, Reunala T (1988) Contact urticaria from rubber gloves. Dermatol Clin 6: 47–51

302. Puttick LM (1989) Skin disorders in the coal mining industry. Dissertation, University of London

303. Lachapelle J-M, Mahmoud G, Vanherle R (1984) Anhydrite dermatitis in coal mines. An airborne irritant reaction assessed by laser Doppler flowmetry. Contact Dermatitis 11: 188–189

304. Maurice PDL, Saihan EM (1984) Fragrance mix sensitivity in coal miners. Contact Dermatitis 10: 50–51

305. Hindson C, Lawlor F (1983) Cocount diethanolamide in a hydraulic mining oil. Contact Dermatitis 9: 168

306. Kiec-Swierczynska M (1990) Occupational dermatoses and allergy to metals in Polish construction workers manufacturing prefabricated building units. Contact Dermatitis 23: 27–32

307. Garcia J, Armisen A (1985) Cement dermatitis with isolated cobalt sensitivity. Contact Dermatitis 12: 52

308. Rudzki E, Rebandel P, Grzywa Z (1989) Patch tests with occupational contactants in nurses, doctors and dentists. Contact Dermatitis 20: 247–250

309. Kanerva L, Estlander T, Jolanki R (1989) Allergic contact dermatitis from dental composite resins due to aromatic epoxy acrylates and aliphatic acrylates. Contact Dermatitis 20: 201–211

310. Farli M, Gasperini M, Francalanci S, Gola M, Sertoli A (1990) Occupational contact dermatitis in 2 dental technicians. Contact Dermatitis 22: 282–287

311. Nethercott JR, Holness DL, Page E (1988) Occupational contact dermatitis due to glutaraldehyde in health care workers. Contact Dermatitis 18: 193–196

312. Bennett DE, Mathias CGT, Susten AS, Fannick NL, Smith AB (1988) Dermatitis from plastic tote boxes impregnated with an antistatic agent. J Occup Med 30: 252–255

313. Stevenson CJ, Morgan PR (1983) Investigation and prevention of chromate dermatitis in colour television manufacture. J Soc Occup Med 33: 19–20

314. Lee HS, Goh CL (1988) Occupational dermatoses among chrome platers. Contact Dermatitis 18: 89–93

315. Goh CL (1988) Occupational dermatitis from gold plating. Contact Dermatitis 18: 122–123

316. Holness CL, Nethercott JR (1989) Health status of funeral service workers exposed to formaldehyde. Arch Environ Health 44: 222–228

317. Ashworth J, Curry FM, White IR, Rycroft RJG (1990) Occupational allergic contact dermatitis in east coast of England fisherman: newly described hypersensitivities to marine organisms. Contact Dermatitis 22: 185–186

318. Van der Willigen AH, Habets JMW, van Joost T, Stolz E, Nienhuis PH (1988) Contact allergy to iodine in Japanese sargassum. Contact Dermatitis 18: 250–252

319. Schmidt R (1990) Plants. In: Adams RM (ed) Occupational skin disease, 2nd edn. Saunders, Philadelphia, pp 503–524

320. Hausen BM, Oestmann G (1988) Untersuchungen über die Häufigkeit berufsbedingter allergischer Hauterkrankungen auf einem Blumengroßmarkt. Dermatosen 36: 117–124

321. McCunney RJ (1988) Diverse manifestations of trichloroethylene. Br J Ind Med 45: 122–126

322. Bedello PG, Goitre M, Roncarolo G, Bundino S, Cane D (1987) Contact dermatitis to rhodium. Contact Dermatitis 17: 111–112

323. Gawkrodger DJ, Lewis FM (1993) Isolated cobalt sensitivity in an etcher, Contact Dermatitis 29 : 46

324. Matthieu L, Weyler J, Deckers I, Van Sprundel M, Van Andel A, Dockx P (1993) Occupational contact sensitization to ethylenediamine in a wire–drawing factory. Contact Dermatitis 29 : 39

325. Thestrup-Pedersen K, Bach B, Petersen R (1990) Allergic investigations in patients with the sick building syndrome. Contact Dermatitis 23: 53–55

326. Marks JG (1988) Dermatologic problems of office workers. Dermatol Clin 6: 75–79

327. Verbeck SJA, Buise-van Unnik EMM, Malten KE (1981) Itching in office workers from glass fibres. Contact Dermatitis 7: 354

328. Mathias CGT (1984) Dermatitis from paints and coatings. Dermatol Clin 2: 585–602

329. Banner-Martin BR, Rycroft RJG (1990) Nickel dermatitis from a powder paint. Contact Dermatitis 22: 50

330. Cofield BG, Storrs FJ, Strawn CB (1985) Contact allergy to azaridine paint hardener. Arch Dermatol 121: 373–376

331. Lidén C (1990) Facial dermatitis caused by chlorothalonil in a paint. Contact Dermatitis 22: 206–211

332. Dooms-Goossens A, Bedert R, Vandaele M, Degreef H (1989) Airborne contact dermatitis due to triglycidylisocyanurate. Contact Dermatitis 21: 202–203

333. Lidén C (1990) Persulfate bleach accelerator – a potent contact allergen in film laboratories. chemical identification, purity studies, and patch testing. Am J Contact Dermatitis 1: 21–24

334. Malten KE (1987) Old and new, mainly occupational dermatological problems in the production and processing of plastics. In: Maibach HI (ed) Occupational and industrial dermatology, 2nd edn. Year Book, Chicago, pp 290–340

335. Sjöborg S, Dahlquist I, Fregert S, Trulson L (1982) Contact allergy to styrene with cross reaction to vinyltoluene. Contact Dermatitis 8: 207–208

336. Beck MH, King CM (1983) Allergic contact dermatitis to epichlorohydrin in a solvent cement. Contact Dermatitis 9: 315

337. Andrews LS, Clary JJ (1986) Review of the toxicity of multifunctional acrylates. J Toxicol Environ Health 19: 149–164

338. Reid CM, Rycroft RJG (1993) Allergic contact dermatitis from multiple sources of MCI/MI biocide and formaldehyde in a printer. Contact Dermatitis 28 : 252–253

339. Malten KE (1987) Printing plate manufacturing processes. In: Maibach HI (ed) Occupational and industrial dermatology, 2nd edn. Year Book, Chicago, pp 351–366

340. Kilpikari I (1982) Occupational contact dermatitis among rubber workers. Contact Dermatitis 8: 359–362

341. Menezes Brandão F (1990) Rubber. In: Adams RM (ed) Occupational skin disease, 2nd edn. Saunders, Philadephia, pp 462–485

342. Foussereau J, Cavelier C, Selig D (1976) Occupational eczema from para-tertiary-butylphenol formaldehyde resins; a review of the sensitizing resins. Contact Dermatitis 2: 254–258

343. Jelen G, Cavelier C, Protois JP, Foussereau J (1989) A new allergen responsible for shoe allergy: chloroacetamide. Contact Dermatitis 21: 110–111

344. Srinivas CR, Devadiga R, Aroor AR (1989) Footwear dermatitis due to bisphenol A. Contact Dermatitis 20: 150–151

345. Rycroft RJG, Penny PT (1983) Dermatoses associated with brominated swimming pools. Br Med J 286: 462

346. Hostynek JJ, Patrick E, Younger B, Maibach HI (1989) Hypochlorite sensitivity in man. Contact Dermatitis 20: 32–37

347. Calnan CD, Cronin E (1978) Vegetable tans in leather. Contact Dermatitis 4: 295–296

348. Estlander T, Kanerva L, Jolanki R (1990) Occupational allergic dermatoses from textile, leather and fur dyes. Am J Contact Dermatitis 1: 13–20

349. Helander I (1977) Contact urticaria from leather containing formaldehyde. Arch Dermatol 113: 1443

350. Kiec-Swierczynska M (1982) Occupational contact dermatitis in the workers employed in production of texas textiles. Dermatosen 30: 41–43

351. Fujimoto K, Hashimoto S, Kozuka T, Tashiro M, Sano S (1985) Occupational pigmented contact dermatitis from azo-dyes. Contact Dermatitis 12: 15–17
352. Sadhra S, Duhra P, Foulds IS (1989) Occupational dermatitis from Synacril Red 3B liquid (CI Basic Red 22). Contact Dermatitis 21: 316–320
353. Dooms-Goossens A, Chrispeels MT, de Veylder H, Roelandts R, Willems L, Degreef H (1987) Contact and photocontact sensitivity problems associated with thiourea and its derivatives: a review of the literature and case reports. Br J Dermatol 116: 573–579
354. Estlander T (1988) Allergic dermatoses and respiratory diseases from reactive dyes. Contact Dermatitis 18: 290–297
355. Hjorth N (1978) Gut eczema in slaughterhouse workers. Contact Dermatitis 4: 49–52
356. Hjorth N, Roed-Petersen J (1980) Allergic contact dermatitis in veterinary surgeons. Contact Dermatitis 6: 27–29
357. Falk ES, Hektoen H, Thune PO (1986) Skin and respiratory tract symptoms in veterinary surgeons. Contact Dermatitis 12: 274–278
358. Dahlquist I (1977) Contact allergy to 3-ethylamino-1,2-benzisothiazoal-hydrochloride, a veterinary fungicide. Contact Dermatitis 3: 277–286
359. Wilson CL, Powell SM (1990) An unusual case of allergic contact dermatitis in a veterinary surgeon. Contact Dermatitis 23: 42–43
360. Prahl P, Roed-Petersen J (1979) Type I allergy from cows in veterinary surgeons. Contact Dermatitis 5: 33–38
361. Jagels R (1985) Health hazards of natural and introduced chemical components of boatbuilding woods. Am J Ind Med 8: 241–251

Chapter 12
Contact Dermatitis in Children

Contact Dermatitis in Children

CARLO LUIGI MENEGHINI

Contents

12.1 Introduction

In spite of its apparent fragility, children's skin deals very effectively with the various stimuli or insults arising in the environment. Nevertheless, the skin of the newborn, babies and youngsters shows evidence of irritation more frequently than in either older children or adults; at the same time, the incidence of contact allergy seems lower in the younger age groups. These differences in the behaviour of the skin in children, compared to adults, cease to be apparent in older children, more specifically towards 8–10 years of age. Children can thus present with either irritant contact dermatitis (ICD), or allergic contact dermatitis (ACD).

12.2 Irritant Contact Dermatitis

From birth, children are exposed to a variety of chemical, physical or biological (microbial, animal or vegetable) irritants capable of inducing irritant contact reactions. The most common forms of this type of dermatitis are:
- Napkin dermatitis (synonyms: napkin area dermatitis or diaper dermatitis)
- Perioral contact dermatitis and contact cheilitis
- Contact urticaria

12.2.1 Napkin Dermatitis

Napkin dermatitis occurs in the first 2 years of life in approximately 20% of babies, and involves the area covered by absorbent nappies, i.e. genital, pubic and gluteoischial regions. Of 11061 children (5396 boys) under 12 years of age presenting for the first time in the Bari Dermatological Clinic over a period of 5 years, the condition was recorded in 527 patients (4.8%) [1]. This form of ICD is caused by multiple factors:
- Contact with urine and faeces
- Persistent moisture and maceration of the nappy-covered skin [2, 3]
- Growth of fungi, especially *Candida albicans,* and bacteria
- High acidity of faeces
- Release of ammonia from the operation of the faecal flora and, in particular, of *Bacillus ammoniagenes* and *B. proteus,* a factor supported by some authors [4] but held to be not clearly proved by others [5]
- Predisposition [6], health conditions [7].

The increase in pH resulting from the accumulation of ammoniacal compounds would seem to play a dominant role in the activation of faecal lipases and proteases, responsible for the high irritant potential of faeces mixed with urine [8]. Other possible contributory factors are:
- Detergent or soap residues in insufficiently rinsed napkins
- Deodorants and preservatives contained in commercially supplied absorbent nappies
- Cosmetic products applied several times a day as emollients or antiirritants (these are not always well tolerated, especially under occlusion)
- Mechanical irritation as from rubbing during napkin changes.

The clinical appearance of napkin dermatitis varies considerably. The condition may present as ICD with erythema, oedema, vesiculation, exudative abrasions, or dry but intensely erythematous, smooth, tense, shiny skin. In other cases papulopustular lesions and haemorrhagic erosions may be found. In still others blisters and nodules may also be present. The dermatitis may persist in the napkin area for weeks or months, or – encouraged by superficial infections or by inappropriate or poorly tolerated medication – it may extend onto the abdomen and trunk.

However, napkin dermatitis may also present clinically in a very different way i.e. that of psoriasiform dermatitis (Fig. 12.1). The rash, consisting of erythematous, scaly, pityriasiform or psoriasiform lesions, involves the genital and perigenital region, but in time it may spread in the form of scattered patches to involve the trunk or even the face. Under these circumstances the differential diagnosis from infantile psoriasis may present some difficulty, and the problem is usually resolved only after a variable period of observation. Contrary to what might be expected, the incidence of napkin dermatitis is not higher in children with atopic dermatitis. This conclusion has been arrived at

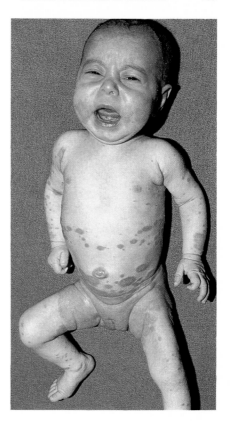

Fig. 12.1. Psoriasiform napkin
dermatitis with secondary spread

after perusal of the records of 2400 of our own cases of atopy and of 100
subjects with haemangioma taken as controls.

Prevention of irritant contact napkin dermatitis consists of minimizing the
operation of the various causative factors. The nappies should be changed
very frequently and the currently available superabsorbent disposable napkins
are preferable. Cleansing at every napkin change should avoid all irritation
and should be done with copious water, a not-too-strongly-degreasing soap
and a very simple emollient, such as a natural vegetable oil, liquid paraffin,
water-oil emulsion or bland ointment.

The treatment of napkin dermatitis is practically only topical. In the
presence of weeping lesions, at every napkin change the area involved
should be washed with 5% aluminium acetate solution diluted with water
1:10–1:40, or wet packs may be applied for a few minutes; alternatively a
blandly antiseptic 0.1% solution of potassium permanganate may be used.
Subsequently, Castellani's carbol-fuchsin paint (1:6 in water) is applied,
followed by one of the following pastes, as suggested by Fisher [9], or by
water-in-oil lotion, with a small amount of Tween 80 as the emulsifier.

Burow's solution	5.0 ml
Anhydrous lanolin	20.0 g
Plain Lassar's paste up to	60.0 g

or:

Zinc oxide	25 g
Mineral oil	10 g
White soft paraffin	40 g

with or without 1% clioquinol

In the absence of exudation or erosions, various creams or ointments may be used, with or without 1% clioquinol. In the napkin area topical corticosteroids are not required; moreover, in order to avoid atrophy and the development of granulomas, the long-term use of topical fluorinated corticosteroids is contraindicated.

12.2.2 Perioral Contact Dermatitis and Contact Cheilitis

These forms of dermatitis result from irritant contact with specific foods, such as citrus fruits, tomato, fish, fruit juices, and fermented cheeses. They occur relatively frequently, especially in the first 2–3 years of life, and not only in atopics but also in nonatopic subjects. The irritation may be induced by saliva, especially if the child bites or sucks the lips or adjoining tissues, or chews gum. Irritant contact dermatitis of the fingers, as well as lesions ot the nails and periungual tissues, can develop as a result of the mechanical irritation of sucking and of infection.

12.2.3 Contact Urticaria

Contact urticaria, in the form of circumscribed erythemato-oedematous reaction with wealing, also occurs in children. It usually develops within a few minutes, lasts up to 30–60 min and resolves without a trace in several hours. It can occur on intact as well as on altered skin in both atopic and nonatopic subjects, as a result of the topical action of physical, chemical and biological agents, including foods, cheeses, and other animal and vegetable products. Some act directly as irritants, while others involve an immunological mechanism of the immediate type. Less frequently a third type of action may observed, whose mechanism is still incompletely understood [10] (see Sect. 2.3).

12.3 Allergic Contact Dermatitis

Allergic contact dermatitis (ACD) can be observed, albeit rarely in the first few months of life, from rubber pants [11], epoxy resin in identification bracelets, nickel in earrings, neomycin, balsam of Peru, ethylenediamine [12], metals and *p*-phenylenediamine [13]. Experimental contact allergy has also been induced in very young babies to plants of the *Rhus* genus, which includes poison ivy [14].

Subsequently, acting on the assumption that young babies rarely develop poison ivy dermatitis, Epstein [15] demonstrated experimentally that, compared with children over 3 years of age, babies under 1 year old are less susceptible to the sensitizing action of the purified pentadecyl catechol which is the allergen of the *Rhus* genus. Further clinical research has shown that allergy to a potent sensitizer such as poison ivy is rare under the age of 5 years [16]. It is generally agreed that the incidence of ACD from other allergens is also less common in young children [9, 17–19], especially those under 3–4 years old, than in older children. This view has been tested in studies that were initiated in 1967 [20], continued thereafter [21] and that were recently productive of some discordant data [22]. The differences in question may result from the diversity of the parameters taken into consideration in the relevant clinicoepidemiological and allergological studies:

- The age, clinical type, presence or absence of atopy, habits and the area of origin of the patients.
- The size of the series.
- The patch test methods employed, the patch testing materials, the reading of results and interpretation (not always easy in small children), and the occurrence of doubtful reactions, especially with such substances as mercurial compounds, formaldehyde, balsam of Peru, and fragrances.
- The method of data analysis in relation to age groups etc.: some studies included children over 12 years up to 16 years of age or even more, in whom the sensitization process is the same as in adults.

In summary, the data in the literature reflect the diversity of the methodologies employed.

Levy et al. [23], in their 10-year research material in the allergy department of the Strasbourg dermatological clinic, recorded 87 cases of ACD in children, the main sensitizers being mercurial compounds, followed by drugs and then metals. Veien et al. [24], in a series of 3664 patients with a presumptive diagnosis of contact dermatitis collected over a period of 5 years, patch tested 168 children up to 14 years of age: 77 had positive reactions to one or more allergens, headed by nickel and followed by chromate and components of rubber. Members of the Spanish Contact Dermatitis Research Group [25] reported the results of allergological studies in a series of 1023 children up to the age of 14 years; they diagnosed ACD in 318 cases, including 143 patients with either a personal or family history of atopy showing one or more positive reactions, most frequently to nickel, mercurial compounds, cobalt and chromate. The proportion of allergic children proved higher among those over 7–8 years of age.

In their 10-year research material, other authors [26] patch tested 147 children aged 3–14 years and recorded positive reactions, most frequently to nickel, cobalt, para dyes and chromate, in 104 subjects. They concluded that (a) positive patch test results are relatively infrequent and (b) the high incidence of negative patch tests indicates that standard allergen concentrations used in adults can also be employed in patch testing children.

In their comprehensive paper, Weston and Weston [27] summarize their experience with ACD in children in the light of available knowledge. ACD accounts for up to 20% of all cases of dermatitis in children. The most common allergens responsible are nickel, other metals, rubber chemicals contained in shoe materials, preservatives and plants. Contact allergy to the latter is particularly common in certain parts of the United States, especially California.

In 1970–1986 a Polish research team [28] patch tested 200 children aged 3–18 years with eczematous lesions. The majority of the subjects were atopic. In the subgroup of 109 subjects aged 6–15 years who patch tested positively, the most common allergen responsible was nickel, followed by formaldehyde, neomycin, rubber chemicals, drugs and others. Of 361 children aged 6 months to 16 years, forming part of a series of 8994 subjects patch tested in three Belgian university clinics (Belgium Tri-Contact) over a period of 10 years, contact allergy was demonstrated in 156 cases, most frequently to nickel, followed by cobalt, p-phenylenediamine, mercurial compounds and fragrances. One-third of the patients suffered from atopic dermatitis [29].

Rademaker and Forsyth [30] carried out a 7-year follow-up of 5986 patients patch tested for contact dermatitis. The series included 125 children under 12 years of age, and 60 of these (48%) tested positively to one or more allergens, headed by nickel and followed by cobalt, chromate and fragrances. Using the European standard series of allergens, the researchers encountered no problems of irritancy, only a certain lack of space on the limited area of the children's backs.

The findings of a recent study [31] in a series of 585 children aged 4 months to 14 years suffering from various forms of dermatitis, mainly eczematous, and consecutively patch tested, were as follows. Positive results with at least one allergen were recorded in 85 subjects (36 boys and 49 girls), of whom a majority were aged 9 to 14 years: 60% showed foot lesions, with positive reactions to nickel, cobalt and chromate in cases of dorsal lesions and to rubber chemicals in cases of plantar lesions.

12.4 Personal Observations

From 1975 to June 1987, using the standard International Contact Dermatitis Research Group technique [32] (in children aged 4 months to 5 years, because of the limited space available on the back, we used small (Epitest) chamber tests) we patch tested consecutively four groups of children, as follows [33]:

1. 122 children aged 4 months to 2 years with napkin area dermatitis with (the majority) or without secondary rash

2. 422 nonatopic children aged 1–16 years with eczematous contact dermatitis
3. 282 children aged 1–16 years with atopic dermatitis
4. 40 children aged 4 months to 2 years with various dermatoses ('cradle cap', cheilitis, impetigo).

The group of 422 patch-tested nonatopic children (group 2) with eczematous contact dermatitis represented 3.7% of the total of 11440 patients with contact dermatitis investigated in the period 1975 to June 1987. These findings demonstrate the low incidence of contact dermatitis in paediatric patients, especially in the first few years of life. Of this group of 422 children, 94 (22.3%) were 1–12 years old and 328 (77.7%) were 13–16 years old.

The incidence of contact allergy in the group of children with eczematous nonatopic dermatitis (group 2) was significantly higher (57.8%) than that recorded in children with atopic eczema (group 3; 16.7%). In both sexes the incidence of sensitization in nonatopics increased with age, and similar results were observed in the group of atopics (Table 12.1, Figs. 12.2, 12.3).

Table 12.1. Contact allergy incidence according to patch test results in four groups of children with different dermatitis

Clinical pattern of dermatitis	No. of children tested		Incidence of Contact Allergy		
	Total	(male female)	Total	(male female)	%
1. Napkin dermatitis	122	(65 57)	0		
2. Eczematous contact dermatitis	422	(129 293)	244	(74 170)	57.8
3. Atopic dermatitis	282	(147 135)	47	(16 31)	16.7
4. Noneczematous dermatoses (controls)	40	(22 18)	0		

Published data on the incidence of contact allergy in children with cutaneous atopy vary from equal [34], to higher [35] or lower [36] than in the nonatopic population. The various series differ also in composition, patient selection criteria, the ages of the patients and the allergens employed in testing. Some of the results are also vitiated by the interpretation of positive reactions recorded to certain known irritants as allergic.

Clinical appearances of ACD in children are no different from those in adults. Signs develop at the site of allergenic contact. In addition to the various clinical pictures of contact dermatitis of the hands, or lesions in areas of contact with earrings or other metal objects, both younger and older children not infrequently present with vesicular or vesicobullous, pompholyx-like dermatitis of the feet, due to allergy to glues or additives in rubber, or to metals, especially chromate (Fig. 12.4). Another type of ACD in children to

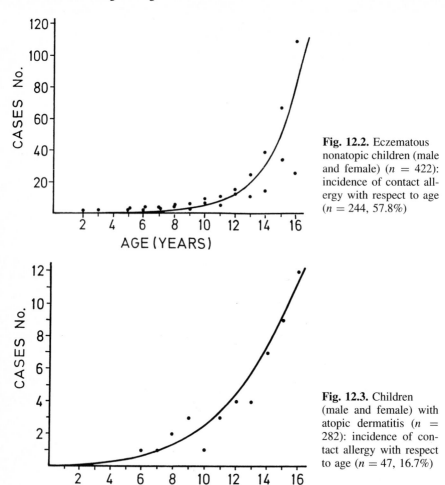

Fig. 12.2. Eczematous nonatopic children (male and female) ($n = 422$): incidence of contact allergy with respect to age ($n = 244$, 57.8%)

Fig. 12.3. Children (male and female) with atopic dermatitis ($n = 282$): incidence of contact allergy with respect to age ($n = 47$, 16.7%)

be kept in mind is allergic contact cheilitis due to constituents of toothpastes, cosmetics and medicaments [37].

Prevention and treatment of these conditions are based on the same principles as those of contact dermatitis in general (see Chap. 16).

12.5 Conclusions

Children are as susceptible to sensitization as adults, but sensitization is less common in the first 2–3 years of life. In those with napkin dermatitis the chances of sensitization are not increased, though the likelihood of exposure to such potential sensitizers as preservatives, cosmetic preparations, creams or ointments and essential oils is relatively high.

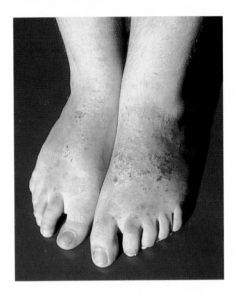

Fig. 12.4. Chromate dermatitis from leather children's shoes

Clinically diagnosable eczematous contact dermatitis is thus not being missed by alert clinicians in departments of dermatology and paediatrics, but is not common in the first 4–5 years of life. The incidence of contact allergy increases with age, especially in children aged 6–10 and over, when the chances of environmental exposure to sensitizers also increase.

The incidence of contact allergy in subjects with cutaneous atopy may be equal, slightly lower or even higher than in nonatopic children. The technique of patch testing used in adults also proves to be a valid diagnostic tool in children, in whom the same test compounds in the same standard concentrations may be used.

12.6 References

1. Bonifazi E, Garofalo L, Angelini G, Pisani V, Scardigno A (1981) Diaper rash with secondary eruptions. Ital Gen Rev Dermatol 18: 127–131
2. Aly R, Maibach HI (1982) Effects of prolonged skin occlusion. In: Maibach HI, Boisits EK (eds) Neonatal skin: structure and function. Dekker, New York
3. Jordan WE, Blaney TL (1982) Factors influencing infant diaper dermatitis. In: Maibach HI, Boisits EK (eds) Neonatal skin: structure and function. Dekker, New York
4. Brown CP, Wilson FH (1964) Diaper region irritations. Pertinent facts and methods of prevention. Clin Pediatr 3: 409–413
5. Leyden JJ, Katz S, Stewart R, Kligman AM (1977) Urinary ammonia and ammonia-producing microorganisms in infants with and without diaper dermatitis. Arch Dermatol 113: 1689–1690
6. Boisits EK, McCormack JJ (1982) Diaper dermatitis and the role of predisposition. In: Maibach HI, Boisits EK (eds) Neonatal skin: structure and function. Dekker, New York
7. Berg RW, Buckingham KW, Stewart RL (1986) Etiologic factors in diaper dermatitis: the role of urine. Pediatr Dermatol 3: 102–106
8. Longhi F, Carlucci G, Bellucci R et al. (1992) Diaper dermatitis: a study of contributing factors. Contact Dermatitis 26: 248–252

9. Fisher AA (1986) Contact dermatitis, 3rd edn. Lea and Febiger, Philadelphia
10. von Grogh G, Maibach HI (1981) The contact urticaria syndrome – and update review. J Am Acad Dermatol 5: 328–342
11. Reiffers J, Hunziker N, Brun R, Vidmar B (1974) Sensibilizations cutanées allergiques peu communes. Dermatologica 148: 285–291
12. Fisher AA (1985) Allergic contact dermatitis in early infancy. Cutis 35: 315–316
13. Seidenari S, Manzini BM, Motolese A (1992) Contact sensitization in infants: report of 3 cases. Contact Dermatitis 27: 319
14. Strauss HW (1931) Artificial sensitization of infants to poison ivy. J Allergy 2: 137–144
15. Epstein WL (1961) Contact-type delayed hypersensitivity in infants and children: induction of *Rhus* sensitivity. Pediatrics 27: 51–53
16. Mobley SL, Mansmann HC (1974) Current status of skin-testing in children with contact dermatitis. Cutis 13: 995–1000
17. Desmons F (1974) L'eczéma de contact de l'enfant. Bull Actual Thér 19: 1499–1510
18. Cronin E (1980) Contact dermatitis. Churchill Livingstone, Edinburgh
19. Hjorth N (1981) Contact dermatitis in children. Acta Derm Venereol (Stockh) [Suppl] 95: 36–39
20. Meneghini CL, Rantuccio F (1967) Eczematous contact hypersensitivity in children. Newsletter 2: 5
21. Angelini G, Meneghini CL (1977) Contact and bacterial allergy in children with atopic dermatitis. Contact Dermatitis 3: 163–174
22. Gonçalo S, Gonçalo M, Azenha A, Barros MA et al. (1992) Allergic contact dermatitis in children. Contact Dermatitis 26: 112–115
23. Levy A, Hanau D, Foussereau J (1980) Contact dermatitis in children. Contact Dermatitis 6: 260–262
24. Veien NK, Hattel T, Justesen O, Nørholm A (1982) Contact dermatitis in children. Contact Dermatitis 8: 373–375
25. Romaguera C, Alomar A, Camarasa JNG, Garcia Bravo B et al. (1985) Contact dermatitis in children. Contact Dermatitis 12: 283–284
26. Pevny I, Brennenstuhl M, Razinskas G (1984) Patch testing in children. Contact Dermatitis 11: 201–206, 302–310
27. Weston WL, Weston JA (1984) Allergic contact dermatitis in children. Am J Dis Child 138: 932–936
28. Rudzki E, Grzywa Z, Rebandel P (1987) Patch testing in children. Contact Dermatitis 17: 117–118
29. Degreef H, Dooms-Goossens A (1987) Allergic contact dermatitis in children in Belgium. Pediatr Dermatol News 6: 209–211
30. Rademaker M, Forsyth A (1989) Contact dermatitis in children. Contact Dermatitis 20: 104–107
31. Balato N, Lembo G, Patruno C, Ayala F (1989) Patch testing in children. Contact Dermatitis 20: 305–307
32. Fregert S, Hjorth N, Magnusson B et al. (1969) Epidemiology of contact dermatitis. Trans St John's Hosp Dermatol Soc 55: 17–34
33. Angelini G, Meneghini CL (1987) Contact allergy in children. Pediatr Dermatol News 6: 195–204
34. Seidenari S, Mosca M, Motolese A, Manzini BM et al. (1989) La sensibilizzazione per contatto nei bambini affetti da dermatite atopica. G Int Dermatol Pediatr 1: 39–45
35. Epstein S, Mohajerin AH (1964) Incidence of contact sensitivity in atopic dermatitis. Arch Dermatol 90: 284–287
36. Palacios J, Fuller EW, Blaylock WK (1966) Immunological capabilities of patients with atopic dermatitis. J Invest Dermatol 47: 490–494
37. Tosti A, De Padova MP, Manuzzi P, Bardazzi F (1987) Contact cheilitis in children. Pediatr Dermatol News 6: 212–215

Chapter 13
Allergens from
the Standard Series

Allergens from the Standard Series

KLAUS E. ANDERSEN, DESMOND BURROWS and IAN R. WHITE

Contents

13.1 Introduction

The distinction between allergic and irritant contact dermatitis is usually made by patch testing. This test procedure is indicated in the investigation of long-standing cases of contact dermatitis and should also be used to exclude contact allergy as a complicating factor in stubborn cases of other eczematous diseases such as atopic dermatitis, stasis eczema, seborrhoeic dermatitis and vesicular hand eczema. A patch test is the cutaneous application of a small amount of the suspected allergen in a suitable concentration and vehicle. The test site, usually the back, is covered with an occlusive dressing for 2 days. The skin condition, vehicle and concentration and volume of the test substance, test site, application time, and the number of readings influence the result, and frequent errors are possible [1–3] (see Sect. 10.1). The proper performance and interpretation of this bioassay require considerable training and experience.

Patch testing is routinely performed by applying a standard series of the most frequently occurring contact allergens. The choice of test concentration is based on patch test experience to the level where there are a minimum of irritant reactions and a maximum of clinically explainable allergic positive reactions. Test concentrations are generally expressed in percentages. This can be misleading as the molecular weight of allergens can be very different. A better way of expressing concentration would be both the percentage and molality, (m = number of moles per 1000 g solvent or vehicle) [14].

An experienced contact dermatologist is able to guess correctly the clinically relevant contact allergen in some patients, based on the history and the clinical appearance of the eczema. The guess is more prone to be correct for common allergens as nickel (50%–80%) and less so for less common allergens (<10%) [5, 6]. This failure to guess correctly explains the general acceptance of the use of a standard series in the evaluation of all patients suspected of having a contact dermatitis.

Table 13.1. The current standard patch test series of 24 allergens

Potassium dichromate	0.5%pet.
Neomycin sulphate	20% pet.
Thiuram mix	1% pet.
p-Phenylenediamine free base	1% pet.
Cobalt chloride	1% pet.
Benzocaine	5% pet.
Formaldehyde	1% aq.
Colophony	20% pet.
Clioquinol	5% pet.
Balsam of Peru	25% pet.
IPPD	0.1% pet.
Wool alcohols (lanolin)	30% pet.
Mercapto mix	2% pet.
Epoxy resin	1% pet.
Paraben mix	15% pet.
p-tert-Butylphenol-formaldehyde resin	1% pet.
Fragrance mix	8% pet.
Ethylenediamine dihydrochloride*	1% pet.
Quaternium 15	1% pet.
Nickel sulphate	5% pet.
Cl- + Me-Isothiazolinone	0.01% aq.
Mercaptobenzothiazole	2% pet.
Primin	0.01% pet.
Sesquiterpene lactone mix	0.1% pet.

* No longer included

Supplementary tests with working materials properly diluted, and extra allergens selected on the basis of patient history and known exposures, are often required in order to determine the nature of the patient's suspected contact dermatitis.

The standard series is dynamic and subject to continual modification rather than an enshrined and permanent truth. It is regularly updated jointly by the International Contact Dermatitis Research Group (ICDRG) and the European Environmental and Contact Dermatitis Research Group (Table 13.1). The standard series can be extended to include allergens of local importance to specific departments. The frequency of allergic contact sensitization to the allergens of the standard series varies from study to study depending on the composition of the study population. Comparison of the frequencies in different populations is valid only when the results are standardized with respect to such confounding factors as age, sex, presence of atopy, presence of diseased skin, and occupational exposure – the MOAHL index, indicating the frequency of occurrence of males, occupational dermatitis, atopy, hand dermatitis and leg ulcers or stasis dermatitis [7, 8].

13.1.1 References

1. Adams RM (1981) Patch testing – a recapitulation. J Am Acad Dermatol 5: 629–643
2. Fisher AA (1986) Contact dermatitis, 3rd edn. Lea and Febiger, Philadelphia
3. Cronin E (1980) Contact dermatitis. Churchill Livingstone, Edinburgh
4. Benezra C et al. (1978) Concentrations of patch test allergens: are we comparing the same things? Contact Dermatitis 4: 103–105
5. Cronin E (1972) Clinical prediction of patch test results. Trans St Johns Hosp Dermatol Soc 58: 153–162
6. Podmore P, Burrows D, Bingham EA (1984) Prediction of patch test results. Contact Dermatitis 11: 283–284
7. Christophersen J et al. (1989) Clinical patch test data evaluated by multivariate analysis. Contact Dermatitis 21: 291–299
8. Wilkinson JD, Hambly EM, Wilkinson DS (1980) Comparison of patch test results in two adjacent areas of England. II. Medicaments. Acta Derm Venereol (Stockh) 60: 245–249

13.2 Nickel

Nickel is a metal which is used in a large number of alloys and chemical compounds. Only iron, chromium and lead are produced in larger amounts. Nickel is ubiquitous in the environment and constitutes about 0.008% of the earth's crust. Humans are constantly exposed, although in variable amounts [1]. Metallic nickel as well as nickel salts give rise to contact allergy, metallic nickel only after corrosion. The corrosiveness of sweat, saliva and other body fluids to nickel and nickel alloys is of primary importance [2].

Nickel is the commonest allergen in the standard series. The incidence of nickel allergy in women has been doubling every 10 years and is now around 30% [3, 4]. The commonest cause of sensitization is ear piercing [5], particularly if there is a history of irritation at the time of piercing. The clinical pattern of nickel dermatitis is described in the classic paper of Calnan and Wells [6]. The primary sites of dermatitis develop as a result of direct contact. The secondary sites are unrelated to direct contact. The eruption is symmetrical and often includes the neck and face, eyelids, elbow flexures and forearms, hands, inner thighs and anogenital region, and it may be generalized.

The mechanism behind the spread is controversial. It is sometimes called autosensitization, haematogenous spread following percutaneous absorption, and several experimental studies in humans point to the importance of oral provocation [7]. It is argued that some of the experimental studies have utilized unrealistically high amounts of inorganic nickel for the oral provocation. Can oral nickel produce exacerbation of dermatitis on the hands or elsewhere, and, if it can, are the amounts required to do this likely to be met with in the everyday diet? This is doubtful and remain to be proved [8]. However, nickel-sensitive patients with vesicular hand eczema worsened after an oral challenge with a diet naturally high in nickel [9].

The relationship between nickel allergy and hand eczema is controversial. It is evident that allergic contact dermatitis of the hands occurs as a result of contact with solubilized nickel and more rapidly if the patient has preexisting irritant hand dermatitis [10]. Menné et al. [11] found that nickel allergy in women predisposes to the development of hand eczema, and that hand eczema predisposes to the development of nickel allergy.

Other problems about nickel allergy remain unsolved: for instance, does nickel allergy render a person, even with normal skin, more vulnerable to irritant contact dermatitis? It would appear that it can [12].

The incidence of allergy in men, even in those with earrings, is lower than in women, the reason not being clear. Some experimental studies claim that women are more easily sensitized than men [13]. More likely explanations for the fewer nickel-allergic men may be ear piercing at a later age, the use of less nickel-containing jewelry, or piercing only one ear.

Certainly in nickel allergy one can see patterns of dermatitis which are unusual for contact dermatitis, for instance, the palmar aspects of the fingers and adjacent palm. This can sometimes be explained by local contact. It is to be expected that a solid such as metal produces a different distribution from liquids and detergents.

There is no method of desensitization, but it is possible to produce immune tolerance in animals fed nickel prior to attempted sensitization [12], and this has been confirmed in humans in a study of young girls with dental prostheses (assuming ingestion of nickel) prior to ear piercing [14]. This is clearly not a practical method of solving this big problem. Oral administration of nickel sulphate 5.0 mg once a week for 6 weeks in nickel-allergic patients lowered the degree of contact allergy significantly, as measured by the patch test reactions before and after nickel administration [15].

There is little doubt that metal plates on bones can initiate a dermatitis which occurs particularly over the areas of the plate [16, 17], but it is now well accepted that nickel allergy is not a contraindication to a metal hip of stainless steel or vitallium type. There is no evidence that these sensitize or exacerbate a preexisting dermatitis or lead to rejection of the hip.

Nickel allergy does not seem to increase the chance of developing other allergies [18, 19], with the exception of cobalt, copper and palladium. This may be due simply to the fact that these metals are commonly associated. It is difficult to obtain pure compounds and most of these metals are contaminated with the others. However, Moss et al. [20] suggested that the acquisition of sensitivity to one allergen might predispose to the acquisition of another unrelated sensitivity – based on a statistical analysis of patch test data from 2200 consecutive patients and experimental sensitization using dinitrochlorobenzene. Further, guinea pigs sensitized to nickel were found to be more easily sensitized to cobalt [21], and it has been shown that lymphocytes with monoclonal sensitivity to nickel react to palladium and copper but not to cobalt (Scheper, personal communication).

The dimethylglyoxime test is accurate to about 10 ppm (0.001% = 2.1 µg Ni/g) and is a good routine test to eliminate metals as a source of nickel which may be causing allergy.

However, metals containing lower amounts can still produce an exacerbation of nickel dermatitis [22, 23], and therefore the dimethylglyoxime test cannot be relied upon absolutely to rule out a piece of metal as the cause of a patient's dermatitis. Emmett et al. [24] examined the bioavailability of nickel from consumer products and found the provocation threshold in sensitive patients to vary from 5.2 mg to 0.47 µg – the lowest amount of nickel producing a reaction. A reduction of nickel in jewelry could considerably reduce the amount of nickel allergy, and governmental regulation is in effect in Denmark to achieve this [25]. An equivalent proposal is under consideration in the European Union.

Nickel sulphate 5% pet. is the standard patch test concentration and produces a few irritant reactions. A follicular reaction can occur. A problem in patch testing is that 15%–50% of those who give a clear history of reaction to metal jewelry, strongly suggesting clinically a nickel allergy, produce a negative patch test [8, 26], depending on the questioning procedure. The reason for this is not clear. It does not appear to be due to a fault in the test reagent or method of testing, as other salts, for instance, nickel chloride or intradermal testing, increase the positive yield very little [27]. Some consider that these cases indicate an atopic tendency and that the metal in such cases is an irritant [27, 28].

13.2.1 References

1. Grandjean P, Nielsen GD, Andersen O (1989) Human nickel exposure and chemobiokinetics. In: Maibach HI, Menné T (eds) Nickel and the skin: immunology and toxicology. CRC, Boca Raton, pp 9–34
2. Morgan LG, Flint GN (1989) Nickel alloys and coatings: release of nickel. In: Maibach HI, Menné T (eds) Nickel and the skin: immunology and toxicology. CRC, Boca Raton, pp 45–54
3. Cronin E (1980) Contact dermatitis. Churchill Livingstone, Edinburgh
4. Romaguera C, Grimalt F, Vilaplana J (1988) Contact dermatitis from nickel: an investigation of its source. Contact Dermatitis 19: 52–57
5. Larsson-Stymne B, Widström L (1985) Ear piercing – a cause of nickel allergy in schoolgirls. Contact Dermatitis 13: 289–293
6. Calnan CD, Wells GC (1956) Suspender dermatitis and nickel sensitivity. Br Med J 2: 1265–1268
7. Veien N (1989) Systemically induced eczema in adults. Acta Derm Venereol [Suppl] (Stockh) 147
8. Burrows D (1989) Prosser White Oration. Mischievious metals – chromate, cobalt, nickel and mercury. Clin Exp Dermatol 14: 266–272
9. Nielsen GD et al. (1990) Nickel-sensitive patients with vesicular hand eczema: oral challenge with a diet naturally high in nickel. Br J Dermatol 122: 299–308
10. Wilkinson DS, Wilkinson JD (1989) Nickel allergy and hand eczema. In: Maibach HI, Menné T (eds) Nickel and the skin: immunology and toxicology. CRC, Boca Raton, pp 133–163

11. Menné T, Borgan O, Green A (1982) Nickel allergy and hand dermatitis in a stratified sample of the Danish female population: an epidemiological study including statistic appendix. Acta Derm Venereol (Stockh) 62: 35–41

12. Van der Burg CKH, Bruynzeel DP, Vreeburg KJJ et al. (1986) Hand eczema in hairdressers and nurses: a prospective study. Contact Dermatitis 14: 275–279

13. Rees JL, Friedmann PS, Matthews JN (1989) Sex differences in susceptibility to development of contact hypersensitivity to dinitrochlorobenzene (DNCB). Br J Dermatol 120: 371–374

14. Hoogstraten IMW, Andersen KE, von Blomberg BME et al. (1991) Reduced frequency of nickel allergy upon oral nickel contact at an early age. Clin Exp Immunol 85: 441–445

15. Sjövall P, Christensen OB, Möller H (1987) Oral hyposensitization in nickel allergy. J Am Acad Dermatol 17: 774–778

16. Thomas RHM, Rademaker M, Goddard NJ, Munro D (1987) Severe eczema of the hands due to an orthopedic plate made of vitallium. Br Med J 294: 106–107

17. Wilkinson JD (1989) Nickel allergy and orthopedic prostheses. In: Maibach HI, Menné T (eds) Nickel and the skin: immunology and toxicology. CRC, Boca Raton, pp 187–193

18. Lammintausta K, Kalimo K (1987) Do positive nickel reactions increase nonspecific patch test reactivity? Contact Dermatitis 16: 160–163

19. Paramsothy Y, Collins M, Smith AG (1988) Contact dermatitis in patients with leg ulcers: the prevalence of late positive reactions and evidence against systemic ampliative allergy. Contact Dermatitis 18: 30–36

20. Moss C et al. (1985) Susceptibility and amplification of sensitivity in contact dermatitis. Clin Exp Immunol 61: 232–241

21. Lammintausta K, Pitkanen OP, Kalimo K et al. (1985) Interrelationship of nickel and cobalt contact sensitization. Contact Dermatitis 13: 148–152

22. Menné T, Andersen KE, Kaaber K et al. (1987) Evaluation of dimethylglyoxine stick tests for detection of nickel. Derm Beruf Umwelt 35: 128–130

23. Menné T, Brandrup F, Thestrup-Pedersen K et al. (1987) Patch test reactivity to nickel alloys. Contact Dermatitis 16: 255–259

24. Emmett EA et al. (1988) Allergic contact dermatitis to nickel: bioavailability from consumer products and provocation threshold. J Am Acad Dermatol 19: 314–322

25. Menné T, Rasmussen K (1990) Regulation of nickel exposure in Denmark. Contact Dermatitis 23: 57–58

26. Kieffer M (1979) Nickel sensitivity: relationship between history and patch test reaction. Contact Dermatitis 5: 398–401

27. Möller H, Svensson A (1986) Metal sensitivity: positive history but negative test indicates atopy. Contact Dermatitis 14: 57–60

28. Gilboa R, Al-Tawil NG, Marcusson JA (1988) Metal allergy in cashiers: an in vitro and in vivo study for the presence of metal allergy. Acta Derm Venereol (Stockh) 68: 317–324

13.3 Chromium

It is probably more accurate to use the term chromate, because chromium is unique in that the metal itself does not sensitize, but rather its salts. There is a question as to which valence causes the allergy, hexavalent ($Cr_2O_7^{2-}$) or trivalent (Cr^{3+}). Trivalent chromium penetrates the skin very poorly, binding with proteins on the surface skin, whilst hexavalent penetrates easily but binds poorly with proteins. It is though that hexavalent chromium penetrates the skin and is then reduced enzymatically to trivalent chromium, which combines with protein as the hapten. Using standard patch test techniques, Fregert and Rorsman [1] showed that if the concentration of trivalent chromium is high enough and the exposure time sufficiently prolonged, positive patch tests will also result. However, the evidence would suggest that, at a cellular level, the body develops an allergy to both hexavalent and trivalent chromium [2].

The true frequency of patch test positives to chromate on routine patch testing is probably 2%–4%. Where higher rates are reported, some irritant reactions may be included. Patch test studies investigating the trend in chromate sensitivity over the years give conflicting results [3–6]. It is difficult to compare these results unless the patient materials are examined for such confounding factors as age, sex, atopy, occupational dermatitis, site of dermatitis, etc.

The commonest cause of chromate allergy by far remains cement [7]. Some consider that cement dermatitis is decreasing in prevalence, and it has been suggested that this may be due to the addition of ferrous sulphate [8, 9]. However, this was occurring before its addition [5, 6], and the decline is also occurring in countries where ferrous sulphate has not been added. Adding ferrous sulphate to cement increases the cost by 1%, and it is still debatable whether addition of ferrous sulphate or better mechanization in the building industry is the most likely reason for the reduction in prevalence of cement dermatitis.

There are many causes of chromate allergy other than cement, including chrome-tanned leather, anti-rust paint, timber preservatives, the wood pulp industry, ash either from burnt wood in general or matches with chromate in the match head, coolants and machine oils, galvanizing, defatting solvents, brine added to yeast residues, welding, the dye industry (due to either a dye, a reducing agent or a mordant), printing, glues, foundry sand, boiler linings, television work (ammonium bichromate to produce cross-linking of light-sensitive polyvinyl alcohol), magnetic tapes (chromium dioxide), solutions used to facilitate tyre fittings, chromium plating, hardeners and resins in the aircraft industry, preservative used in milk testing, bleaches and detergents. An extensive list of possible sources of contact allergy is presented in Table 13.2. Of these many are rare, and one-off contacts. The commonest sources of chromate allergy by far still remain cement, followed by welding, chrome tanning, leather, pigments and chrome plating. More detailed information can be obtained in references [7] and [10].

Chromate dermatitis tends to have a bad prognosis. Fregert [11] found that only 7% of women and 10% of men with chromate allergy were healed after 5 years. Burrows [12] found that only 8% of his cases of cement dermatitis were cleared 10–14 years later. The cause for this is not clear. It may be due to chromate remaining in the skin for a long time, or it may only require minute quantities of chromate to induce a contact allergy reaction, and minute quantities of an amount similar to that in cement are found in many everyday objects, such as paper, soil, ash, etc. Purschel and Furst [13] found a large

Table 13.2. Occupational exposure to chromium is possible during contact with the following compounds or work procedures. (From [10])

Analytic standards reagents
Anticorrosion agents
Batteries
Catalysts (for hydrogenation, oxidation, polymerization)
Ceramics
Drilling muds
   Chromium lignosulphonates (from sodium dichromate using lignosulphate waste)
Electroplating and anodizing agents
Engraving
Explosives
Fire retardant
Hardeners and resins in the aircraft industry
Magnetic tapes
Metallic chromium
Milk preservatives
Paints and varnishes
Paper
   "Chrome cake" (containing sodium sulphate and small amounts
   of sodium dichromate)
Photography
Roofing
Sutures
Tanning leather
Textile mordants and dyes
Television screens
Wood preservatives

---

percentage of their cases were still in contact with chromate in spite of a change of occupation.

It has been suggested that dermatitis can be aggravated in those allergic to chromate by oral ingestion, but this remains unproven and has not received the attention that the same theory has received in nickel allergy [14].

Chromium is an essential element in the body, especially for glucose metabolism.

Potassium dischromate 0.5% pet. is the standard dilution for testing. However, this percentage can produce an irritant reaction, which may explain the wide difference in dichromate allergy reported through the world. It has been suggested that 0.25% would be more accurate, but while this produces fewer reactions, it does miss some true dichromate allergies [15]; the same applies to 0.375% [16]. This closeness of irritant concentration to that to detect contact allergy is a problem in assessing the true incidence of chromate allergy and in diagnosing individual patients. Patch testing with trivalent salts such as chromium trichloride and chromium sulphate produces a high percentage of false negatives [17]. The patch test activity of trivalent compounds compared with hexavalent chromium is of the order of 1/10 for oxalate, 1/100 for chloride, 1/1000 for the acetate [18].

13.3.1 References

1. Fregert S, Rorsman H (1964) Allergy to trivalent chromium. Arch Dermatol 90: 4–6
2. Burrows D (1984) The dichromate problem. Int J Dermatol 23: 215–220
3. Edman B, Möller H (1982) Trends and forecasts for standard allergens in a 12-year patch test material. Contact Dermatitis 8: 95–104
4. Kiec-Swierczynska M (1990) Allergy to chromate, cobalt and nickel in Lodz 1977–1988. Contact Dermatitis 22: 229–231
5. Färm G (1986) Changing patterns in chromate allergy. Contact Dermatitis 15: 298–310
6. Gailhofer G, Ludvan M (1987) Zur Änderung des Allergenspektrums bei Kontaktekzemen in den Jahren 1975–1984. Derm Beruf Umwelt 35: 12–16
7. Burrows D (1983) Chromium: metabolism and toxicity. CRC, Boca Raton
8. Avnstorp C (1992) Cement eczema. An epidemiological intervention study. Acta Derm Venereol (Stockh) 72 [Suppl 179]: 1–22
9. Avnstorp C (1989) Follow-up of workers from the prefabricated concret cement. Contact Dermatitis 20: 365–371
10. Burrows D, Adams RM (1990) Metals. In: Adams RM (ed) Occupational skin disease, 2nd edn. Saunders, Philadelphia, pp 349–386
11. Fregert S (1975) Occupational dermatitis in a 10-year material. Contact Dermatitis 1: 96–107
12. Burrows D (1972) Prognosis in industrial dermatitis. Br J Dermatol 87: 145–148
13. Purschel W, Furst G (1972) Berufsbedingtes Kontaktekzem – Katamnesen und Rehabilitation. Berufsdermatosen 20: 174
14. Kaaber K, Veien N (1977) The significance of chromate ingestion in patients allergic to chromate. Acta Derm Venereol (Stockh) 57: 321–323
15. Andersen KE, Burrows D, Cronin E et al. (1988) Recommended changes to standard series. Contact Dermatitis 19: 389–390
16. Burrows D, Andersen KE, Camarase JG et al. (1989) Trial of 0.5% versus 0.375% potassium dichromate. Contact Dermatitis 21: 351
17. Frosch P, Aberer W (1988) Chrom-Allergie. Dermatosen 36: 168–169
18. Fregert S, Rorsman H (1966) Allergic reactions to trivalent chromium compounds. Arch Dermatol 66: 711–714

13.4 Cobalt

A positive patch test to cobalt usually occurs in association with a positive test to nickel or chromate, more particularly nickel. This association is thought to be due to the metals being commonly associated with one another, so that considerable contact with nickel means a correspondingly high contact with cobalt, and hence a corresponding possibility of sensitization to both. This may not be completely true (see Sect. 13.2). Cobalt allergy is therefore usually synonymous with metal or nickel allergy. A positive test to cobalt occurs 20 times more frequently in those allergic to nickel than in those not allergic, and a person with a 3+ nickel-positive patch test is 50 times more likely to have a 3+ positive cobalt reaction [1]. Rystedt and Fischer [2] reported 7% positive patch tests in 4034 eczema patients; of these only 50 were isolated cobalt reactions.

Cases of allergy have been reported due to contact with nonmetal sources, such as cobalt naphthenate and oleate used as dryers for varnishes, paints and printing inks, or as a contact catalyst in polyester resin systems, an oxidizing agent in automobile exhaust controls, in electroplating, and in the rubber tyre industry. Exposure and allergy have also occurred to cobalt in wet alkaline clay in pottery and china plants: the latter may be due to porcelain dyes. Cobalt is often added to animal feeds, and dermatitis has been described due to it. Some consider it important in cement dermatitis, like chromate but of less significance. This is controversial, as cements from some countries do not contain cobalt or only very little indeed. It is often difficult to identify the source of isolated positive cobalt patch test, that is, one with negative nickel and chromate tests. However, most of these patients are probably allergic to jewelry, as with nickel. Cobalt chloride 1% pet. is the standard dilution for patch testing.

13.4.1 References

1. Van Joost T, van Everdingen JJ (1982) Sensitization to cobalt associated with nickel allergy: clinical and statistical studies. Acta Derm Venereol (Stockh) 62: 525–529
2. Rystedt T, Fischer T (1983) Relationship between nickel and cobalt sensitization in hard metal workers. Contact Dermatitis 9: 195–210

13.5 Fragrance Mix

Fragrance and flavour substances are strong-smelling organic compounds with characteristic, usually pleasant odors [1]. Fragrances are ubiquitous and used in perfumes and perfumed products. They are found not only in cosmetics but also in detergents, fabric softeners and other household products. Flavours are used for the flavouring of toothpastes, foods and beverages.

Perfume allergy evaluation may be difficult. A complete perfume compound consists of from 10 to more than 300 basic components selected from over 5000 raw materials, which can be divided into the following [1, 2]: (a) 500 natural products isolated from various parts of plants, e.g. blossoms, buds, fruit, peel, seeds, leaves, bark, wood, roots or resinous exudates; (b) 5 animal products and their extracts (ambergris from the sperm whale, musk tonkin from the testes of musk deer, castoreum from beaver glands, beeswax absolute from beeswax, and civet from glands of the civet cat); (c) over 4000 synthetic fragrances.

In a recent European study comprising 2455 consecutive patients, the overall incidence of allergy to fragrance materials as measured by fragrance mix was 7.8% [3]. The most common reaction to fragrance materials is allergic contact dermatitis, but contact urticaria, photodermatitis, irritation and depigmentation may occur.

Perfume allergy evaluation is made more difficult by the fact that labelling of perfumes with their ingredients is not required by law and by the secrecy

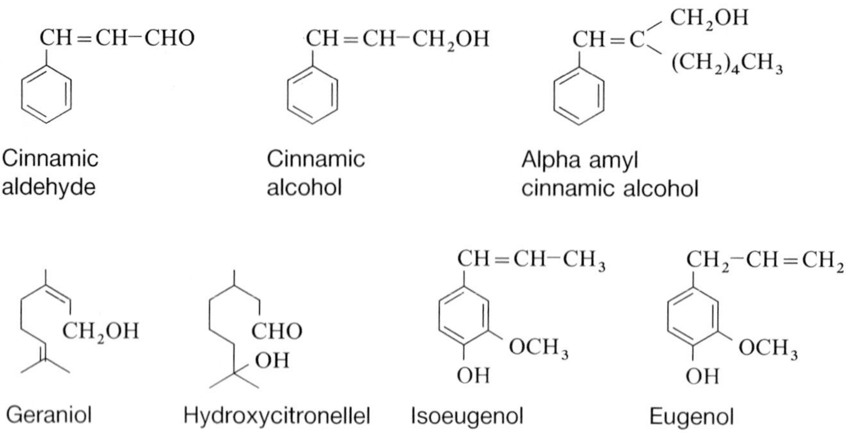

Fig. 13.1. Components of the fragrance mix

policy of perfume manufacturers. That certain perfumes are sensitizers and photosensitizers (others are solely photosensitizers) adds to the investigator's frustration. The composition of a perfume may change depending on the product that it is meant for. To avoid false-negative reactions, ingredient testing is necessary.

Screening with individual fragrances is impractical and time consuming and may give rise to multiple positive reactions and the excited-skin syndrome. Therefore, a perfume screening mix for patch testing has been developed to increase the ability to detect perfume allergy [4]. It is not a perfect detector of fragrance allergy, and constant work is necessary to improve the quality, reproducibility and relevance of the mix [3]. The current fragrance mix consists of eight ingredients, each at a concentration of 1%: cinnamaldehyde, cinnamyl alcohol, eugenol, alpha amyl cinnamaldehyde, hydroxycitronnellal, geraniol, isoeugenol and oak moss absolute, with sorbitan sesquioleate as emulsifier (Fig. 13.1). It has been shown to be a valuable screening agent for perfume dermatitis [5]. It is estimated that fragrance mix currently detects about 75% of all cases of fragrance sensitivity [6]. However, both false-positive and false-negative reactions are quite common [3]. Marginal reactions may in some cases be regarded as being irritant, while in other cases retesting of the patient with the ingredients of the mix may reveal positive patch tests to one or more of them.

Some patients with definite reactions to the mix may prove negative when tested with the ingredients. However, the choice of patch test concentration when testing the components separately is important. The ICDRG recently lowered the fragrance mix concentration from 8 × 2% to 8 × 1% due to the frequent occurrence of weak positive irritant patch test reactions, but when tested separately, at least some of the components can be applied in higher concentrations, for example 2%–5% [7].

13.5.1 References

1. Bauer K et al. (1988) Flavors and fragrances. In: von Arpe HJ et al. (eds) Ullmann's encyclopedia of industrial chemistry, vol A11. VCH, Weinheim, pp 144–246
2. Larsen WG (1986) Perfume dermatitis. In: Fisher AA (ed) Contact dermatitis, 3rd edn. Lea and Febiger, Philadelphia, pp 394–404
3. Wilkinson JD, Andersen K, Camarasa J et al. (1989) Preliminary results on the effectiveness of two forms of fragrance mix as screening agents for fragrance sensitivity. In: Frosch PJ, Dooms-Goossens A, Lachapelle J-M, Rycroft EJ, Scheper EJ (eds) Current topics in contact dermatitis. Springer, Berlin Heidelberg New York, pp 127–131
4. Larsen WG (1977) Perfume dermatitis. A study of 20 patients. Arch Dermatol 113: 623–627
5. De Groot AC (1988) Adverse reactions to cosmetics. Thesis, State University of Groningen
6. Larsen WG, Maibach HI (1982) Fragrance contact allergy. Semin Dermatol 1: 85–90
7. De Groot AC, van der Kley AMJ, Bruynzeel DP, Meinardi MMHM, Smeenk G, van Joost T, Pavel S (1993) Frequency of false-negative reactions to the fragrance mix. Contact Dermatitis 28: 139–140

13.6 Balsam of Peru

Balsam of Peru is the natural resinous balsam which exudes from the trunk of the Central American tree *Myroxylon pereirae* after scarification of the bark. It consists of essential oil and resin, and is thus of the oleoresin type. The composition varies, and standardization is based on physical characteristics and the identification of some major chemical constituents. Balsam of Peru contains 30%–40% of resins of unknown composition, while the remaining 60%–70% consists of well-known chemicals: benzyl benzoate, benzyl cinnamate, cinnamic acid, benzoic acid, vanillin, farnesol and nerolidol.

Many perfumes and flavourings contain components either identical with, or cross-reacting with, materials contained in balsam of Peru and other natural resins. Positive patch tests with one or more of these substances are often an indication of perfume allergy. In medicinal preparations balsam of Peru is still sometimes used for its dermatological effects.

The early epidemiology of perfume allergy is based on Hjorth's [1] classic monograph on balsam of Peru. It gave positive reactions in 4.0% of men and 4.0% of women in a Danish epidemiological study comprising 2166 eczema patients [2]. Immediate reactions to patch tests with balsam of Peru occur. The high incidence of perfume allergy is attributed to the widespread use of perfumes in cosmetics, topical preparations, and household products. Generally, the fragrance concentration is about 0.1% but may be many times higher. Systemic reactions following ingestion of balsams in eczema patients may result in flare-ups of their dermatitis [3].

Regarding the safety of perfume and fragrance ingredients, the Research Institute of Fragrance Materials evaluates and publishes regularly in the journal *Food and Chemical Toxicology*. Opdyke [4] has reviewed the subject, and *Ullmann's Encyclopedia of Industrial Chemistry* [5] is a major source of information. The International Fragrance Association recommends that balsam of Peru should not be used as a fragrance ingredient due to its sensitizing properties.

Fisher and Dooms-Goossens [6] suggest that sensitizing ingredients in a perfume may become hypoallergenic by interacting with other ingredients during the aging process of the perfume. Another interesting phenomenon regarding perfume allergy is the quenching phenomenon described by Opdyke [7]. The sensitizing properties of cinnamaldehyde, citral and phenylacetaldehyde were inhibited by eugenol, (+) limonene and phenylethyl alcohol, respectively. The mechanism behind quenching of sensitization is not known. The quenching effect seems to operate at two levels: induction and elicitation. It may exert its effect through blockade of antigen-presenting cells or by physicochemical mechanisms [8, 9]. Though the clinical implications of quenching are uncertain, from a research point of view it remains interesting.

A product use test is important in the evaluation of a patient with suspected perfume allergy because of false-positive patch test reactions. Generally, the composition of perfumes is complex, and the ingredients are not known to the investigator. The patient may tolerate some and not other perfumed products. Balsam of Peru 25% pet. is the standard dilution for patch testing.

13.6.1 References

1. Hjorth N (1961) Allergy to balsams, allied perfumes and flavouring agents. Munksgaard, Copenhagen
2. Christophersen J et al. (1989) Clinical patch test data evaluated by multivariate analysis. Contact Dermatitis 21: 291–297
3. Veien N (1989) Systemically induced eczema in adults. Acta Derm Venereol [Suppl] (Stockh) 147
4. Opdyke DL (1975) The safety of fragrance materials. Br J Dermatol 93: 351
5. Bauer K et al. (1988) Flavors and fragrances. In: von Arpe HJ et al. (eds) Ullmann's encyclopedia of industrial chemistry, vol A11. VCH, Weinheim, pp 144–246
6. Fisher AA, Dooms-Goossens A (1976) The effect of perfume "ageing" on the allergenicity of individual perfume ingredients. Contact Dermatitis 2: 155–159
7. Opdyke DLK (1976) Inhibition of sensitization reactions induced by certain aldehydes. Food Cosmet Toxicol 14: 197–198
8. Hanau D et al. (1983) The influence of limonene on induced delayed hypersensitivity to citral in guinea pigs. I. Histological study. Acta Derm Venereol (Stockh) 63: 1–7
9. Barbier P, Benezra C (1983) The influence of limonene on induced delayed hypersensitivity to citral in guinea pigs. II. Label distribution in the skin of ^{14}C-labelled citral. Acta Derm Venereol (Stockh) 63: 93–96

13.7 Colophony

Colophony (rosin) is a widespread, naturally occurring material, which is the residue left after distilling off the volatile oil from the oleoresin obtained from trees of the family *Pinaceae*. The chemical composition is complex and variable, depending on the manufacturing process, geographical area and storage conditions [1, 2]. Three kinds of colophony may be identified: (a) gum rosin comes from the trunks of living trees (the resin is distilled to yield turpentine oil and the gum resin residue); (b) wood rosin is a distillate from dead pine tree stumps; and (c) tall oil rosin is a byproduct from pine wood pulp [3].

Colophony is composed of about 90% resin acids and 10% neutral substances. The principal allergens in colophony are not yet determined. Oxidation products of abietic acid (Fig. 13.2) and dehydroabietic acid have been identified as allergens [4]. Synthetically prepared derivatives and the neutral fraction also contain allergenic compounds [5–7]. In a Danish study, comprising 2166 consecutive eczema patients, 3.7% were colophony sensitive [8].

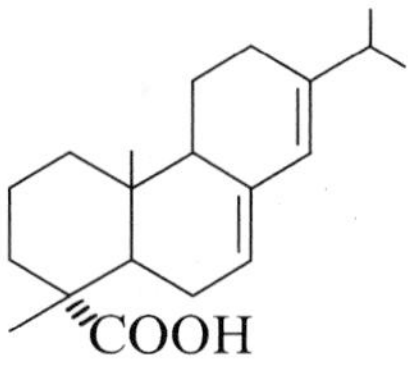

Fig. 13.2. Abietic acid   ''''COOH

Cross-reactions between rosin, balsam of Peru, oil of turpentine, wood tar, pine resin, and spruce resin may occur [3, 9].

The possible exposure to colophony is widespread both at work and in leisure time (Table 13.3). In cosmetics, colophony occurs in depilatories, tonics, dressing and hair grooming aids, make-up products, mascara and hair products. Colophony allergy from adhesives has been known for 70

Table 13.3. Products commonly containing colophony

Paper	Polishes
Printing inks	Wood wool
Soldering flux	Ostomy appliances
Cutting fluids	Violinists' rosin
Glues	Dentistry products
Adhesives	Cosmetics
Ulcer bandages	Brown soaps
Surface coatings	Chewing gums
Insulating tapes	Varnishes
Cleansing agents	

years, but the use of adhesives based on acrylate polymers has reduced the incidence of contact dermatitis from this source. However, when strong adhesive effects are wanted, colophony is still needed as an ingredient. In the modern electronics industry the use of colophony as a fluxing agent in assembly work produces a significant number of contact allergies, appearing as allergic hand dermatitis and airborne facial dermatitis.

The occurrence of contact allergy to colophony has been increasing over the past few decades [10]. The allergenicity of colophony can be reduced by chemical modification, i.e. by hydrogenation of the nonaromatic double bonds in the resin, which minimizes the content of easily oxidized acids of the abietic type [11]. Unmodified Chinese colophony is used in the standard series at a concentration of 20% pet. Further studies are necessary to improve our understanding of colophony contact allergy and the optimal choice of patch test material.

13.7.1 References

1. Hausen BM, Kuhlwein A, Schultz KH (1982) Kolophonium-Allergie. Derm Beruf Umwelt 30: 145–152
2. Karlberg A-T (1988) Contact allergy to colophony. Thesis, University of Stockholm
3. Fisher AA (1986) Contact dermatitis, 3rd edn. Lea and Febiger, Philadelphia, pp 665–674
4. Karlberg A-T, Bohlinder K, Boman A, Hacksell U, Hermansson J, Jacobsson S, Nilsson JLG (1988) Identification of 15-hydroxyperoxyabietic acid as a contact allergen in Portuguese colophony. J Pharm Pharmacol 40: 42–47
5. Hausen BM, Krueger JM, Mohnert J, Hahn H, König WA (1989) Contact allergy due to colophony. III. Sensitizing potency of resin acids and some related products. Contact Dermatitis 20: 41–50
6. Hausen BM, Jensen S, Mohnert J (1989) Contact allergy to colophony. IV. The sensitizing potency of commercial products. An investigation of French and American modified colophony derivatives. Contact Dermatitis 20: 133–143
7. Hausen BM, Mohnert J (1989) Contact allergy to colophony. V. Patch test results with different types of colophony and modified-colophony products. Contact Dermatitis 20: 295–301
8. Christoffersen J et al. (1989) Clinical patch test data evaluated by multivariate analysis. Contact Dermatitis 21: 291–299
9. Hjorth N (1961) Allergy to balsams, allied perfumes and flavouring agents. Munksgaard, Copenhagen
10. Edman B (1988) Computerized patch test data in contact allergy. Thesis, University of Lund
11. Karlberg A-T, Boman A, Nilsson JLG (1988) Hydrogenation reduces the allergenicity of colophony. Contact Dermatitis 19: 22–29

13.8 Neomycin

Neomycin is a widely used antibiotic (Fig. 13.3). The frequency of neomycin sensitivity in the general population in San Francisco was 1.1% [1], while 5%–8% of patients with eczema have been sensitive to it in earlier studies.

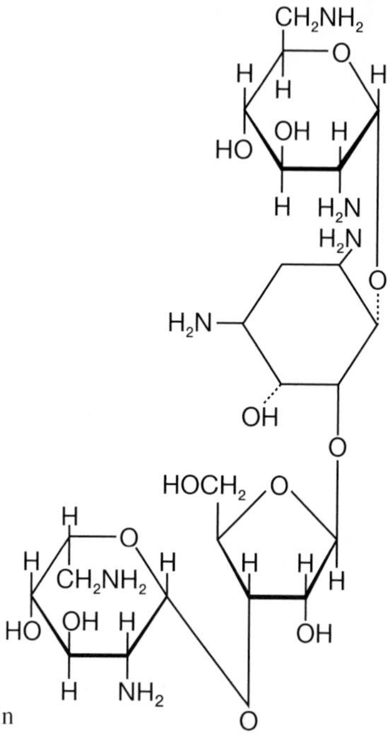

Fig. 13.3. Neomycin

In a Danish study comprising 2 166 consecutive patients, the frequency of neomycin sensitivity was 2.9%. Several patch test studies agree that the trend in the occurrence of neomycin sensitivity is upward over the years, probably due to increased use of topical drugs containing this antibiotic [2, 3]. The patients particularly at risk of neomycin sensitivity appear to be those with stasis dermatitis, external otitis and perianal eczema.

The diagnosis of neomycin allergy may be difficult because the dermatitis is not vesicular or bullous but often appears instead as an aggravation or continuation of a preexisting dermatitis. It is instructive to note that the therapeutic concentration of neomycin is often 0.5%, while the patch test concentration is 20%. Even at this concentration some positive may be missed and Frosch et al. [4] recommend stripping half the thickness of the epidermis off the patch test site before application. The positive neomycin patch test appears late, after 3–4 days in many cases.

The cross-sensitization pattern of neomycin is complex. Regular cross-sensitivity occurs between neomycin, framycetin, and paromomycin, which all contain a neosamine group [5]. Among neomycin-positive patients in Helsinki, 48% had reactions to kanamycin, 36% to gentamycin, 21% to sisomycin and 25% to tobramycin [6].

13.8.1 References

1. Prystowsky SD, Nonomura JH, Smith RW, Allen AM (1979) Allergic hypersensitivity to neomycin. Arch Dermatol 115: 713–715
2. Edman B, Möller H (1982) Trends and forecasts for standard allergens in a 12-year patch test material. Contact Dermatitis 8: 95–104
3. Gollhausen R, et al. (1988) Trends in allergic contact sensitization. Contact Dermatitis 18: 147–154
4. Frosch PJ, Weickel R, Schmitt T, Krastel H (1987) Nebenwirkungen von ophthalmologischen Externa. Z Hautkr 63: 126–136
5. Pirilä V, Förström L, Rouhunkoski S (1967) Twelve years of sensitization to neomycin in Finland: report of 1760 cases of sensitivity to neomycin and/or bacitracin. Acta Derm Venereol (Stockh) 47: 419–425
6. Förström L, Pirilä V (1978) Cross sensitivity within the neomycin group of antibiotics. Contact Dermatitis 4: 312

13.9 Benzocaine

Benzocaine is a *p*-aminobenzoic acid derivative used as a local anaesthetic (Fig. 13.4). It is a fairly weak sensitizer [1]. The incidence of contact sensitivity reported varies widely from country to country, probably dependent entirely on the level of use of benzocaine in the community. The incidence of positive reactions to topical anaesthetics is in the range of 0.8%–1.5%. In some countries, such as the United States, it is widely used in over-the-counter preparations, whereas in others, such as the United Kingdom, its use is much less frequent. While it does not have a high sensitizing potential, it is usually applied in the orifices of the body and to raw intertriginous areas, which renders sensitization easier.

It can cross-react with other compounds; 25% of benzocaine-sensitive patients react to para-phenylenediamine and para-aminobenzoic acid esters used in sunscreening agents [2]. It also cross-reacts with procaine, sulphonamides and certain dyes [3, 4]. However benzocaine-sensitive individuals do not react with xylocaine (lidocaine). In order to detect more patients sensitive to topical anaesthetics it is necessary to test with other "caine" anaesthetics [5, 6]. The standard patch test dilution of benzocaine is 5% pet.

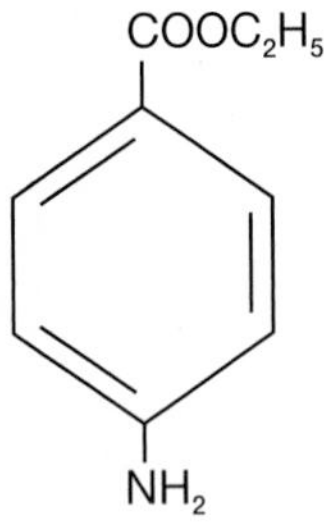

COOC$_2$H$_5$

NH$_2$ **Fig. 13.4.** Benzocaine

13.9.1 References

1. Kligman AM (1966) The identification of contact allergens by human assay. III. The mazimization test: a procedure for screening and rating contact sensitizers. J Invest Dermatol 47: 393–409
2. Hjorth N, Wilkinson D, Magnusson B et al. (1978) Glyceryl-p-aminobenzoate patch testing in benzocaine sensitive subjects. Contact Dermatitis 4: 46–48
3. Adriani J, Dalili H (1971) Penetration of local anesthetics through epithelia barriers. Anesth Analg 50: 834–841
4. Fisher AA (1986) Local anaesthetics in contact dermatitis, 3rd edn. Lea and Febiger, Philadelphia, pp 220–227
5. Wilkinson JD et al. (1990) Preliminary patch testing with 25% and 15% "caine" mixes. Contact Dermatitis 22: 244–245
6. Beck MH, Holden A (1988) Benzocaine – an unsatisfactory indicator of topical local anaesthetic sensitization for the U.K. Br J Dermatol 118: 91–94

13.10 Clioquinol

Due to stability problems, clioquinol 5% pet. has replaced the quinoline mix in the standard series. The mix contained a mixture of clioquinol and chlorquinaldol (Fig. 13.5). These substances have both antibacterial and antifungal activity and are commonly used in creams and ointments to treat skin conditions in which an anti-infective agent is required. A concentration of 3% in such preparations is usual, and they may be combined with a topical steroid. Clioquinol has been used in medicines for oral administration. Synonyms for clioquinol are: chinoform, chloroiodoquine, cliochinolum, iodochlorhydroxyquin, iodochlorhydroxyquinoline, and 5-chloro-7-iodoquinolin-8-ol (Vioform). Chlorquinaldol is 5,6-dichloro-2-methylquinol-8-ol (Sterosan, Steroxin).

These quinolines are not strong allergens. The acquisition of allergic sensitivity to them does not generally cause a marked worsening of an eczema, and when combined with a topical steroid, the steroid causes some suppression of the inflammatory response.

Cronin [1] found that no particular pattern of eczema predisposed to clioquinol sensitivity, although geographical variation in incidence depends on the types of products locally available and the type of patient being investigated. In London the incidence of sensitivity to clioquinol was 1.6% in the period 1971–1976, but in a similar period a decade later it was 0.8%.

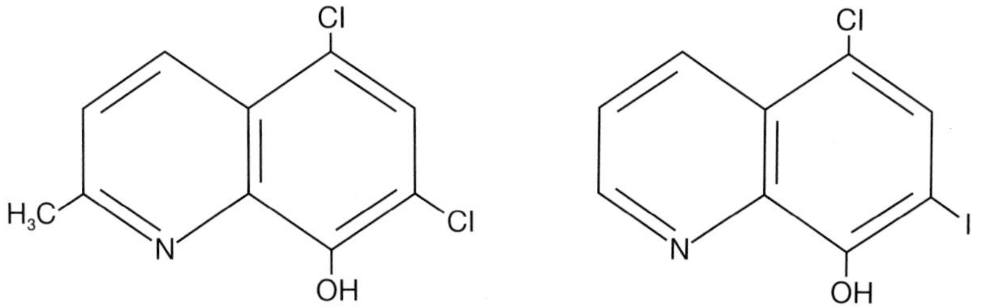

Fig. 13.5. Clioquinol (*right*) and chlorquinaldol (*left*)

The oral administration of either clioquinol or chlorquinaldol has resulted in a generalized eruption in individuals allergic to these compounds [2, 3]. An immediate-type reaction occurred in a woman intolerant of oral quinine when clioquinol was applied topically [4]; a quinoline ring is common to both.

Cross-reactions between clioquinol and chlorquinaldol are not common, and clioquinol is the more important of the two allergens. Testing with clioquinol alone may cause a loss of reactions compared to the mix [5]. However, in three patients believed to have been sensitized previously to clioquinol, a spectrum of reactions was recorded to other halogenated hydroxyquinolines [6].

A cream containing 3% clioquinol was reported as causing scrotal and inguinal irritant contact dermatitis in some men [7].

13.10.1 References

1. Cronin E (1980) Contact dermatitis. Churchill Livingstone, Edinburgh
2. Ekelund A, Möller H (1969) Oral provocation in eczematous contact allergy to neomycin and hydroxyquinolines. Acta Derm Verereol (Stockh) 49: 422–426
3. Skog E (1975) Systemic eczematous contact-type dermatitis induced by iodochlorhydroxyquin and chloroquine phosphate. Contact Dermatitis 1: 187
4. Simpson JR (1974) Reversed cross-sensitisation between quinine and iodochlorhydroxyquinoline. Contact Dermatitis Newslett 15: 431
5. Agner T, Menné T (1993) Sensitivity to clioquinol and chlorquinaldol in the quinoline mix. Contact Dermatitis 29 : 163
6. Allenby CF (1965) Skin sensitisation to Remiderm and cross-sensitisation to hydroxyquinoline compounds. Br Med J: 208–209
7. Kero M, Hannuksela M, Sothman A (1979) Primary irritant dermatitis from topical clioquinol. Contact Dermatitis 5: 115–117

13.11 Wool Alcohols

Lanolin is a natural product from sheep fleece and consists of a complex mixture of esters and polyesters of high molecular weight alcohols and fatty acids. The composition varies from time to time and from place to place. Wool alcohols (lanolin alcohols) are a complex mixture of alcohols derived from hydrolysis of the oily, wavy fraction of sheep fleece. The general incidence of lanolin allergy is low [1]. Lanolin and wool alcohols are weak allergens and experimental sensitization is difficult to achieve in man and animals [2]. Wool alcohols are included in the European standard series because of the high incidence of lanolin allergy among eczema patients. Lanolin allergy is most common among leg ulcer patients.

The use of lanolin extends from topical preparations to polishes, anticorrosives, printing inks, and paper constituents. The literature on contact allergy to lanolin is extensive and has been reviewed up to 1973 by Breit and Bandmann [3]. Hjorth and Trolle Lassen [4] described the clinical picture of lanolin allergy, emphasizing the frequent occurrence of lanolin allergy in elderly women with a long history of eczema. Spread of eczema to secondary sites was common. The majority of positive patch test reactions were rather weak, with only few strong reactions.

In epidemiological studies of patients, the frequency of sensitization ranges form 1.1% [5] to 6.0% [6], depending on group selection and prescription habits. The detection of weak lanolin allergy was improved by testing with wool alcohols in a concentration of 30% pet. However, this concentration may give false-positive patch tests [2]. Mortensen [7], testing with wool alcohols 30% pet., found 2.7% positive patch tests in 1230 patients, while supplementary testing of 899 other eczema patients with lanolin derivatives, including hydrogenated lanolin (90% lanolin alcohols) and Amerchol L 101 (lanolin sterols and alcohols), yielded 6.6% positive reactions.

The true frequency of lanolin allergy requires definition. We believe that lanolin allergy is uncommon on normal skin and with cosmetic usage, in contrast to the significant rate when applied to leg ulcers and other diseased skin. Because of the rarity of lanolin sensitization when applied to normal skin, we carefully verify every positive patch test to wool alcohols and lanolin to ensure that it represents allergy and not the excited-skin syndrome.

The allergens in lanolin are unknown but are probably present in its alcoholic fraction. Their allergenicity is increased by the simultaneous presence of detergent. Removal of the free fatty alcohols and detergent from lanolin reduced the hypersensitivity by 99% in selected lanolin-sensitive patients [8].

Several modifications of lanolin have been tested to produce one with less sensitizing capacity. Acetylated lanolin (Modulan) was less of a sensitizer than plain lanolin [9]. De-waxed lanolin (Lantrol) has also been claimed to cause less sensitization than lanolin. Hydrogenated lanolin, used frequently because of its hydrophilic, colourless and odourless properties, caused a higher incidence of hypersensitivity than anhydrous lanolin in Japan [10]. A patient hypersensitive to one brand of lanolin may tolerate another. The patch test concentration in the standard series is wool alcohols 30% pet.

13.11.1 References

1. Clark EW (1975) Estimation of the general incidence of specific lanolin allergy. J Soc Cosmet Chem 26: 323–335
2. Kligman AM (1983) Lanolin allergy: crisis or comedy. Contact Dermatitis 9: 99–107
3. Breit R, Bandmann HJ (1973) Dermatitis from lanolin. Br J Dermatol 88: 414–416
4. Hjorth N, Trolle Lassen C (1963) Skin reactions to ointment bases. Trans St Johns Hosp Dermatol Soc 49: 127–140
5. Iden DL, Schroeter AL (1977) The vehicle tray revisited: the use of the vehicle tray in assessing allergic contact dermatitis by a 24-hours application method. Contact Dermatitis 3: 122–126
6. Fisher AA et al. (1971) Allergic contact dermatitis due to ingredients of vehicles. Arch Dermatol 104: 286–290
7. Mortensen T (1979) Allergy to lanolin. Contact Dermatitis 5: 137–139
8. Clark EW, Blondeel A, Cronin E, Oleffe JA, Wilkinson DS (1981) Lanolin of reduced sensitizing potential. Contact Dermatitis 7 : 80–83
9. Cronin E (1966) Lanolin dermatitis. Br J Dermatol 78: 167–174
10. Sugai T, Higashi J (1975) Hypersensitivity to hydrogenated lanolin. Contact Dermatitis 1: 146–157

13.12 Ethylenediamine Dihydrochloride[*]

For patch testing, 1% pet. is the standard concentration of ethylenediamine dihydrochloride (Fig. 13.6). Allergy to this compound is commonest by far in the United States, where Mycolog cream, a preparation containing neomycin, nystatin and triamcinolone, is widely used. A similar preparation is used in the United Kingdom (Tri-Adcortyl cream) and is by far the commonest cause of sensitization there. In these preparations it is used as a stabilizer; the corresponding ointment does not contain it.

$$H_2N-CH_2-CH_2-NH_2, 2\,HCl$$

Fig. 13.6. Ethylenediamine dihydrochloride

Ethylenediamine has other uses, and dermatitis has been described due to it from the following sources: floor polish remover [1], epoxy hardener [2] and coolant oil [3]. Its use has also been described in a number of other industries, rubber, dyes, insecticides, and synthetic waxes.

There is a potential problem with systemic administration in those sensitized, either with drugs which contain ethylenediamine, for instance aminophylline, or with drugs chemically related to it, including various antihistamines, among which are hydroxyzine hydrochloride, piperazine and cyclizine. Cases have been described with generalized erythroderma in patients who have become allergic to piperazine in local applications, who received piperazine phosphate for threadworms [4].

Patients seldom, if ever, become sensitized through systemic administration, and problems arise only in those already sensitized who receive the drugs, and it is surprising how few reactions occur considering the number of patients sensitized. Few patients become sensitized through contact in industry, and ethylenediamine is a rare sensitizer outside the local application which contains it. For this reason, it was recently recommended that ethylenediamine be removed from the standard series and included in a medicament series.

13.12.1 References

1. English JSC, Rycroft RJG (1989) Occupational sensitization to ethylenediamine in a floor polish remover. Contact Dermatitis 20: 220–221
2. Crow KD, Peachey RDG, Adams JE (1978) Coolant oil dermatitis due to ethylenediamine. Contact Dermatitis 4: 359–361
3. Angelini G, Meneghini CL (1977) Dermatitis in engineers due to synthetic coolants. Contact Dermatitis 3: 219–220
4. Price ML, Hall-Smith SP (1984) Allergy to piperazine in a patient sensitive to ethylenediamine. Contact Dermatitis 10: 120

[*] No longer included in standard series.

13.13 Parabens

The most widely used preservatives in foods, drugs, and cosmetics are the parabens (esters of *p*-hydroxbenzoic acid). About one-third of the cosmetics registered at the United States Food and Drug Administration contain parabens. Used in combination, parabens have a synergistic effect. Cross-reactions between the four paraben esters methyl, ethyl, propyl and butyl paraben (Fig. 13.7) are common, but exceptions occur. The paraben mix used to contain these four esters plus benzyl paraben. Benzyl paraben has recently been removed because it is suspected to be a carcinogen.

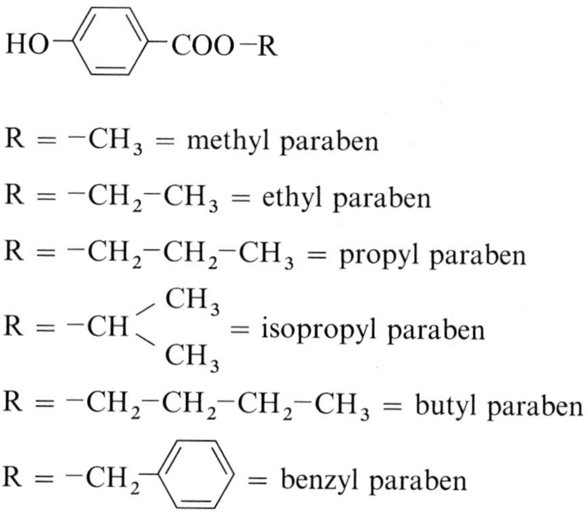

$$HO-\langle\bigcirc\rangle-COO-R$$

$$R = -CH_3 = \text{methyl paraben}$$

$$R = -CH_2-CH_3 = \text{ethyl paraben}$$

$$R = -CH_2-CH_2-CH_3 = \text{propyl paraben}$$

$$R = -CH\begin{smallmatrix}\nearrow CH_3 \\ \searrow CH_3\end{smallmatrix} = \text{isopropyl paraben}$$

Fig. 13.7. Esters of *p*-hydroxybenzoic acid: methyl, ethyl, propyl, isopropyl and butyl parabens

$$R = -CH_2-CH_2-CH_2-CH_3 = \text{butyl paraben}$$

$$R = -CH_2-\langle\bigcirc\rangle = \text{benzyl paraben}$$

In diagnostic patch testing Menné and Hjorth [1] found that approximately 1.0% of more than 8000 eczema patients tested were sensitized. The frequency of positive reactions was remarkably constant over a 15-year period. Clinical experience suggests that the incidence of paraben sensitization in healthy persons is likely to be small, and agrees with the impression that occasional cases of paraben sensitivity occur and are important to the particular patient's welfare, but sensitization is low when the extensive use of the material is considered [2]. Patients with stasis dermatitis and leg ulcers are at increased risk.

Fisher et al. [2] and Schorr [3] assumed that repeated topical application of low concentrations of parabens in medicaments or cosmetics could cause sensitization, while Hjorth and Trolle Lassen [4] stated that higher concentrations were necessary for the majority of cases. They reported a 1% incidence of paraben sensitivity, suggesting that this was due to the frequent use in Denmark of topical anti-fungal agents containing up to 5% paraben (Amycen). Cross-reactions may occur to other para compounds such as benzocaine, para-phenylenediamine and sulphonamides [5]. Note that paraben-sensitive leg ulcer patients can often use paraben-preserved consmetics on normal skin without adverse effect [6].

In the European standard series, the parabens are now tested as a mix of 3% of methyl, ethyl, propyl and butyl p-hydroxybenzoates, a total of 12% pet. The previous mix, which contained the same ingredients plys benzyl paraben, a total of 15% pet., could be irritant and enhance the occurrence of multiple false-positive patch tests (angry back) [7]. In Menné and Hjorth's study [1] two-thirds of the patients reacting to the mix showed positive reactions to one or more of the individual esters. Multiple patch test reactivity is probably due to cross-sensitization, but concomitant sensitization to individual esters is a possibility because the esters are often used in combination.

The final details of the paraben story remain to be elucidated. Certainly many patients labelled as paraben allergic have instead irritant responses to the marginally irritating 15% mix; others have excited skin syndrome with nonspecific false positives. It is our impression that, except for high concentration (i.e. ¿ 1%) drug use and application to leg ulcers, the parabens are rare sensitizers. Combined with the extensive chronic toxicity data available on their systemic effects, these compounds set a standard for relative safety that new preservatives have difficulty in matching. Technical and microbiological considerations sometimes make alternative preservatives necessary. However, the paraben mix is important in the standard series because paraben allergy is difficult to diagnose from the history or clinical appearance.

13.13.1 References

1. Menné T, Hjorth N (1988) Routine patch testing with paraben esters. Contact Dermatitis 19: 189–191
2. Fisher AA et al. (1971) Allergic contact dermatitis due to ingredients of vehicles. Arch Dermatol 104: 286–290
3. Schorr WF (1968) Paraben allergy: a cause of intractable dermatitis. JAMA 204: 859–862
4. Hjorth N, Trolle Lassen C (1963) Skin reactions to ointment bases. Trans St Johns Hosp Dermatol Soc 49: 127–140
5. Maucher OM (1974) Beitrag zur Kreuz-oder Kopplingsallergie zur Parahydroxybenzoe-Säure-Ester. Berufsdermatosen 22: 183–187
6. Fisher AA (1973) The paraben paradox. Cuits 12: 830–832
7. Mitchell JC (1977) Multiple concomitant positive patch test reactons. Contact Dermatitis 3: 315–320

13.14 Formaldehyde

Formaldehyde is a ubiquitous and potent sensitizer, industrially, domestically, and medically. Formaldehyde exposure is difficult to estimate because the chemical – besides being manufactured, imported and used as such – is incorporated into a large variety of products and reactants in many chemical processes, including formaldehyde releasers, polymerized plastics, metal-working fluids, medicaments, fabrics, cosmetics and detergents (Table 13.4) [1, 2].

Table 13.4. Formaldehyde uses and exposure

Clothing, wash and wear, crease-resistant clothing
Medications: wart remedies, anhidrotics
Antiperspirants
Preservative in cosmetics
Photographic paper and solutions
Paper industry
Disinfectants and deodorizers
Cleaning products
Polishes
Paints and coatings
Printing and etching materials
Tanning agents
Dry-cleaning materials
Chipboard production
Mineral wool production
Glues
Phenolic resins and urea plastics in adhesives and footwear
Fish meal industry
Smoke from wood, coal and tobacco (relevance controversial)

Shampoos may contain formaldehyde. Because they are quickly diluted and washed off, only exquisitely formaldehyde-sensitive consumers develop dermatitis on the scalp and face from such formaldehyde-containing wash-off products. However, hairdressers may develop hand dermatitis from similar products due to their more intense exposure.

Formaldehyde dermatitis from textiles is rare today because manufacturers have improved the fibric finish treatment and reduced the amount of formaldehyde residues in new clothing. Garments made from 100% acrylic, polyester, linen, silk, nylon and cotton are generally considered to be formaldehyde-free [3]. Formaldehyde sensitivity is not necessarily accompanied by simultaneous sensitivity to formaldehyde resins and formaldehyde releasers, and vice versa [4–6]. It depends on the exposure conditions and the actual release of formaldehyde. The frequency of formaldehyde-positive patch tests in eczema patients is around 3%–4% [7].

Inexplicable positive patch test reactions frequently occur, where no clinical relevance is found. A harder search, however, might often reveal it. Hidden sources of formaldehyde about the home may be a cause of hand eczema in some women with formaldehyde allergy [8]. In certain cases a positive patch test should be confirmed by a repeated test and by a use test. The threshold level of formaldehyde required to elicit an eczematous reaction in the axilla of formaldehyde-sensitive volunteers was 30 ppm [9]. Formaldehyde releasers used as preservatives in cosmetics and technical products are often concealed by trade names or synonyms (Table 13.5) [10]. The epidemiology of formaldehyde sensitization requires reevaluation. Most early studies utilized irritant patch test concentrations. The current recommended patch test concentration is 1% aq.

Table 13.5. Formaldehyde releasers. (From [10])

Bakzid P (mixture of cyclic aminoacetals and organic amine salts)
Biocide DS 5249 (1,2-benzisothiazolin-3-one and a formaldehyde releaser)
Bronopol (2-bromo-2-nitropropane-1,3-diol)
Dantoin MDMH (methyladimethyoxymethan formal)
DMDM hydantoin (dimethylodimethyl hydantoin)
Dowicil 200 (quaternium 15)
Germall 115 (imidazolidinyl urea)
Germall II (diazolidinyl urea)
Grotan BK [1,3,5-tris(hydroxyethyl)hexyhydrotriazine]
Hexamethylenetetramine, methenamine [1,3,5,7-tetraazaadamantan-1,3,5,7-tetraazatri-cyclo(3,3,1,1^{3,7}decan]
KM 103 (substituted triazine)
Paraformaldehyde (polyoxymethylene)
Parmetol K50 (N-methylochloracetamide, O-formal of benzyl alcohols)
Polynoxylin (polyoxymethylene urea)
Preventol D1 [1-(3-chlorallyl)-3,5,7-triaza-1-azoniaadamantanchloride benzyl formal]
Preventol D2 (benzylhemiformal)
Preventol D3 (chlormethylacylamino methanol)

13.14.1 References

1. Feinman SE (1988) Formaldehyde sensitivity and toxicity. CRC, Boca Raton
2. Flyvholm M-A, Andersen P (1993) Identification of formaldehyde releasers and occurrence of formaldehyde and formaldehyde releasers in registered chemical products. Am J Ind Med 24: 533–552
3. Adams RM, Fisher AA (1986) Contact allergen alternatives: 1986. J Am Acad Dermatol 14: 951–969
4. Ford GP, Beck MH (1986) Reactions to Quaternium 15, Bronopol and Germall 115 in a standard series. Contact Dermatitis 14: 271–274
5. De Groot AC, et al. (1988) Patch test reactivity to DMDM hydantoin. Relationship to formaldehyde allergy. Contact Dermatitis 18: 197–201
6. Storrs F (1983) Allergic contact dermatitis to 2-bromo-2-nitro-propane-1,3-diol in a hydrophilic ointment. J Am Acad Dermatol 2: 157–170
7. Christoffersen J, et al. (1989) Clinical patch test data evaluated by multivariate analysis. Contact Dermatitis 21: 291–299
8. Cronin E (1991) Formaldehyde is a significant allergen in women with hand eczema. Contact Dermatitis 25: 276–282
9. Jordan W, Sherman W, King S (1979) Threshold responses in formaldehyde-sensitive subjects. J Am Acad Dermatol 1: 44–48
10. Fiedler HP (1983) Formaldehydabaspalter. Derm Beruf Umwelt 31: 187–189

13.15 Quaternium 15

Quaternium 15 is a formaldehyde releaser used chiefly as a cosmetic preservative (Fig. 13.8). Formaldehyde releasers are in widespread usage in industry, household products and cosmetics [1]. They are marketed under a multitude of trade names. Chemically they are linear or cyclic reversible polymers of formaldehyde, and formaldehyde is formed in different amounts depending mainly on temperature and pH.

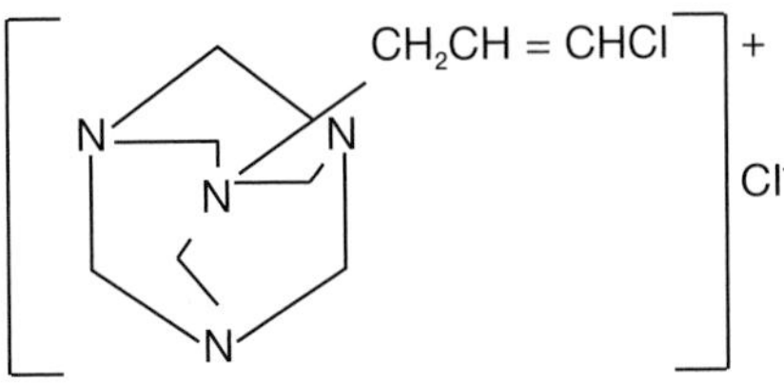

Fig. 13.8. Quaternium 15

Quaternium 15 has several synonyms: Dowicil 200, −100 and −75, N-(3-chlorallyl)-hexaminium chloride, chlorallyl methenamine chloride, 1-(3-chlorallyl)-3,5,7-triaza-1-azonioadamantane chloride. Formaldehyde is released in small amounts, and formaldehyde-sensitive patients may react simultaneously to this preservative. However, quaternium 15 sensitivity may also be directed against the entire molecule. Allergic contact dermatitis from a formaldehyde-releasing agent may thus be due to the entire molecule, to formaldehyde, or to both [2, 3]. The usual preservative concentration of 0.1% releases about 100 ppm free formaldehyde, and this concentration can elicit dermatitis in formaldehyde-sensitive patients [4].

The repeated use of lotions and creams with this preservative may provoke dermatitis by mild irritation from the vehicles and subsequent sensitivity to the preservative. Sensitive patients should request cosmetics without formaldehyde releasers, even though some alternative formaldehyde releasers might be tolerated due to reduced formaldehyde production. In the United States, mandatory cosmetic labelling makes it easy to avoid specific ingredients, while this is difficult in the European Community where cosmetic labelling is not yet required.

The frequency of positive reactions varies from country to country, possibly due to variations in the frequency of use. A recent Danish study comprising 2166 consecutive patients showed the frequency of quaternium 15 positives to be 1.2% [5], while none of 501 patients in Holland were positive [6]. The patch test concentration is 2% pet.

13.15.1 References

1. Flyvholm M-A, Andersen P (1993) Identification of formaldehyde releasers and occurrence of formaldehyde and formaldehyde releasers in registered chemical products. Am J Ind Med 24: 533–552
2. Storrs F (1983) Allergic contact dermatitis to 2-bromo-2-nitro-propane-1,3-diol in a hydrophilic ointment. J Am Acad Dermatol 2: 157–170
3. De Groot AC et al. (1988) Patch test reactivity to DMDM hydantoin. Relationship to formaldehyde allergy. Contact Dermatitis 18: 197–201
4. Jordan WP, Sherman WT, King SE (1979) Threshold responses in formaldehyde-sensitive subjects. J Am Acad Dermatol 1: 44–48
5. Christoffersen J et al. (1989) Clinical patch test data evaluated by multivariate analysis. Contact Dermatitis 21: 291–299
6. De Groot AC et al. (1986) Contact allergy to preservatives. II. Contact Dermatitis 15: 218–222

13.16 Cl- + Me-Isothiazolinone

Isothiazolinones (5-chloro-2-methyl-4-isothiazolin-3-one and 2-methyl-4-isothiazolin-3-one, 3:1 ratio by weight; Fig. 13.9) are the active ingredients in Kathon CG (Rohm & Haas, Philadelphia), a cosmetic preservative. The CTFA-adopted names for the active chemicals are methylchloroisothiazolinone and methylisothiazolinone. Cl- + Me-Isothiazolinone has currently been chosen as a shorter name for the patch test preparation. Isothiazolinones are used extensively as effective biocides to preserve the water content of cosmetics, toiletries, household and industrial products such as metal-working fluids, cooling-tower water, latex emulsions, and for slime control in paper mills.

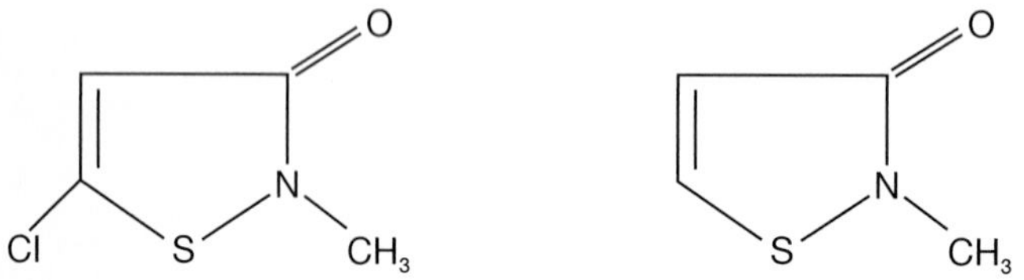

Fig. 13.9. Isothiazolinones: 5-chloro-2-methyl-4-isothiazolin-3-one (*left*) and 2-methyl-4-isothiazolin-3-one (*right*)

Isothiazolinones are marketed under many brand names [1], which makes it easy to overlook the presence of these chemicals in formulations (Table 13.6). Approximately 25% of all cosmetic products and toiletries – in particular wash-off products – in the Netherlands contain Kathon CG or synonymous preservatives [2]. A Danish study examined the content of Kathon CG in 156 of the most commonly used cosmetic products in Denmark. Kathon CG was present in 48% of wash-off and 31% of leave-on cosmetic products [3]. In a

Table 13.6. Biocides containing Cl- + Me-isothiazolinone (some also contain other ingredients)

Kathon CG	Metatin GT
Kathon 886 MW	Mitco CC 31 L
Kathon LX	Mitco CC 32 L
Kathon WT	Special Mx 323
Acticide	Parmetol DF 35
Algucid CH 50	Parmetol DF 12
Amerstat 250	Parmetol A 23
Euxyl K 100	Parmetol K 50
Fennosan IT 21	Parmetol K 40
GR 856 Izolin	Parmetol DF 18
Grotan TK 2	P 3 Multan D
Mergal K 7	Piror P 109

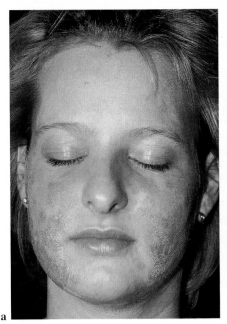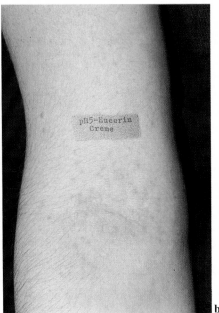

a   b

Fig. 13.10. a Allergic contact dermatitis from Cl-Me-isothiazolinone in a popular moisturizing cream. **b** Positive repeated open application test in same patient. (Courtesy of P.J. Frosch)

few years Kathon CG has reached the rank of the 13th most frequently used preservative for cosmetics in the United States [4]. However, this ranking list is 5–6 years old and may have changed considerably.

Methylchloroisothiazolinone and methylisothiazolinone are strong sensitizers in guinea pig sensitization tests [5, 6], and a number of reports have documented a varying and, in some countries, an increasing incidence of allergic contact dermatitis from these chemicals [2, 7-9]. Kathon CG is an important allergen for the hands and for the face (Fig. 13.10.a). A use test may be helpful in cases of doubtful relevance (Fig. 13.10.b), although it may be negative even in patients with true allergic patch test reactions.

Cl- + Me-Isothiazolinone was recently included in the standard series. Patch test reactions may show unusually sharp borders and can still be true allergic reactions. The patch test concentration is 100 ppm aq. This is the best compromise, as higher concentrations (200–300 ppm) may produce irritation and patch test sensitization [1, 10]. On the other hand, 100 ppm may in some cases perhaps give false-negative test results on normal back skin in patients with an isothiazolinone-induced aggravation of a hand dermatitis.

Due to the activity of isothiazolinones on the skin it is imperative that exact dosing be used when isothiazolinones are used for patch testing. The correct dose for a standard Finn Chamber is 20 µl.

13.16.1 References

1. Björkner B, Bruze M, Dahlquist I, Fregert S, Gruvberger B, Persson K (1986) Contact allergy to the preservative Kathon CG. Contact Dermatitis 14: 85–90
2. De Groot AC, Weyland JW (1988) Kathon CG: a review. J Am Acad Dermatol 18: 350–358
3. Rastogi SC (1990) Kathon CG and cosmetic products. Contact Dermatitis 22: 155–160
4. Decker RL Jr (1985) Frequency of preservative use in cosmetic formulas as disclosed to FDA – 1984. Cosmet Toilet 100: 65–68
5. Chan PK, Baldwin RC, Parsons RD, et al. (1983) Kathon biocide: manifestation of delayed contact dermatitis in guinea pigs is dependent on the concentration for induction and challenge. J Invest Dermatol 81: 409–411
6. Bruze M, Dahlquist I, Fregert S, Gruvberger B, Persson K (1987) Contact allergy to the active ingredients of Kathon CG. Contact Dermatitis 16: 183–188
7. Cronin E, Hannuksela M, Lachapelle J-M, Maibach HI, Malten KE, Meneghini CL (1988) Frequency of sensitization to the preservative Kathon CG. Contact Dermatitis 18: 274–279
8. Frosch PJ, Schulze-Dirks A (1987) Kontaktallergie auf Kathon CG. Hautarzt 38: 422–425
9. Menné T, Frosch PJ, Veien NK et al. (1991) Contact sensitization to 5-chloro-2-methyl-4-isothiazolin-3-one and 2-methyl-4-isothiazolin-3-one (MCI/MI). Contact Dermatitis 24: 334–341
10. Maibach HI (1985) Diagnostic patch test concentration for Kathon CG. Contact Dermatitis 13: 242–245

13.17 p-Phenylenediamine

p-Phenylenediamine (PPD) is a colourless compound that acts as a primary intermediate in hair dyes (Fig. 13.11). It is oxidized by hydrogen peroxide and then polymerized to a colour within the hair by a coupler. Most cases of contact allergy to PPD occur due to contact with hair dyes, in either the client or the hairdresser. In the 1930s, cases were very common and occurred in the clients, but severe dermatitis from PPD in the hairdressing client has become much rarer (1). Many cases of PPD allergy are seen in men from the Indian subcontinent who are resident in the UK, but most cases now probably occur in hairdressers. Sensitization seems to be facilitated by irritation of their hands from detergents, wetness and perming lotions. Once the hair is dyed and polymerized, it has been said to be nonallergic; however, cases are occasionally

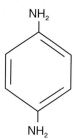

Fig. 13.11. p-Phenylenediamine

seen in which people react to other persons' dyed hair. This may be due to the dyeing not being carried out properly, leaving unpolymerized hair dye. Cases can occur in which the hair appears to be dyed properly, and yet the dyed hair produces a reaction in the patient and others in contact with it.

Patients with PPD allergy may cross-react with benzocaine, procaine, sulphonamides and PABA sunscreens, azo- and aniline dyes, anthraquinone, antihistamines and the rubber antioxidant 4-isopropylaminodiphenylamine [2–4]. However, Cronin did not find that any of 47 hairdressers positive to PPD reacted to the PPD-rubber mix [5]. Similarly, in a Swedish study in which there were 25 patients positive to PPD and 16 positive to PPD-rubber mix, there were no cross-reactions between the two test substances (Lidén, personal communication). The cross-reaction pattern may explain the difficulty in finding the relevance of many PPD positives. Cross-reactions occur to other related hair dyes, such as p-toluenediamine, p-aminodiphenylamine, 2,4-diaminoanisole and o-aminophenol.

Immediate-type hypersensitivity to PPD, with extensive urticarial reactions, has been reported [6].

PPD 1% pet. is the standard dilution for patch tests. PPD base 1% pet. was replaced by PPD dihydrochloride 0.5% pet. in the standard series in 1984. There was a general impression that this had lead to fewer positives. A multi-centre trial confirmed that the dihydrochloride missed some true positives, and so it was replaced in 1988 by PPD free base 1% pet. [7].

13.17.1 References

1. Corbett JF, Menkart J (1973) Hair colouring. Cutis 12: 190
2. Herve-Bazin B et al. (1977) Occupational eczema from n-isopropyl-n'-phenyl-paraphenylenediamine (IPPD) and n-dimethyl-1,3-butyl-n'-phenylparaphenylenedi-amine (DMPPD) in tyres. Contact Dermatitis 3: 1–15
3. MacKie BS, Mackie LE (1964) Cross sensitization in dermatitis due to hair dyes. Aust J Dermatol 7: 189
4. Schønning L, Hjorth N (1969) Cross sensitization between hair dyes and rubber chemicals. Berufsdermatosen 17: 100
5. Cronin E (1980) Contact Dermatitis. Churchill Livingstone, Edinburgh, p 137
6. Calnan CD (1967) Reaction to artificial colouring materials. J Soc Cosm et Chem 18: 215
7. Dooms-Goosens A, Scheper RS, Andersen KE et al. (1988) Comparative patch testing with PPD base and PPD dihydrochloride: human and animal data compiled by the European Contact Dermatitis Group. In: Frosch P et al. (eds) Current topics in contact dermatitis. Springer, Berlin Heidelberg New York, pp 281–285

13.18 Thiuram Mix

The thiuram mix used in the standard series contains the following four compounds, each at a dilution of 0.25% (Fig. 13.12):
– Tetraethylthiuram disulphide (TETD; disulfiram)
– Tetramethylthiuram disulphide (TMTD)

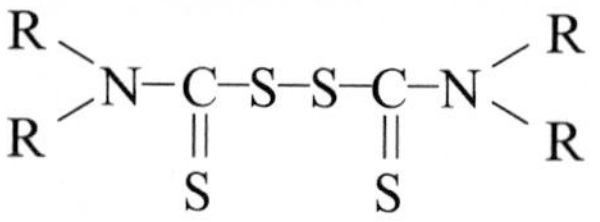

$$
\begin{array}{c}
R \\ \diagdown \\[-4pt] N-C-S-S-C-N \\[-2pt] R \diagup \quad \| \qquad \| \quad \diagdown R \\[-2pt] S \qquad S
\end{array}
\quad
\begin{array}{c} R \\ R \end{array}
$$

R = CH$_3$ TMTD
R = C$_2$H$_5$ TETD
R = –(CH$_2$)$_5$–   PTD

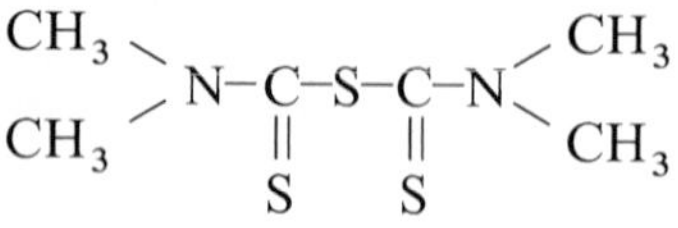

$$
\begin{array}{c}
CH_3 \\ \diagdown \\[-4pt] N-C-S-C-N \\[-2pt] CH_3 \diagup \quad \| \quad \| \quad \diagdown \\[-2pt] S \quad S
\end{array}
\quad
\begin{array}{c} CH_3 \\ CH_3 \end{array}
$$

TMTM

Fig. 13.12. Components of thiuram mix: tetramethylthiuram disulphide (TMTD), tetraethylthiuram disulphide (TETD), dipentamethylenethiuram disulphide (PTD), tetramethylthiuram monosulphide (TMTM)

- Tetramethylthiuram monosulphide (TMTM)
- Dipentamethylenethiuram disulphide (PTD)

These chemicals are used in the vulcanization of rubber as accelerating agents. They increase the rate of cross-linking by sulphur between the hydrocarbon chains of the uncured rubber and may also donate some sulphur to the reaction. In the fully cured product, unreacted accelerators remain. Some of these may migrate over time onto the surface of the finished article, together with other rubber chemicals. By thorough washing with hot water of thin rubber items, such as latex-dipped gloves or condoms, it is possible to leach out most of these thiuram residues. Some hypoallergenic rubber articles are accelerated by thiurams but have been treated by washing as described.

The use of thiurams is ubiquitous in the rubber industry. The compounds are encountered in rubbers for both industrial and domestic use. Different manufacturers have preferences for particular thiurams which they use for particular applications. This fact probably explains geographical variations in the incidence of sensitivity to components of the mix [1]. Gloves are the commonest cause of rubber dermatitis, and the allergen is usually a thiuram. Release of thiuram from rubber gloves into synthetic sweat may vary between brands [2]. Thiuram sensitivity is more common in women than in men.

An allergic contact dermatitis from a thiuram in rubber often has no clear clinical pattern, and in a glove dermatitis the classical distribution of the eczematous reaction is usually not present. This classical pattern consists of a diffuse eczema over the back of the hands and a band of eczema to the mid-forearm at the level of the cuff of the glove. Rubber sensitivity is often clinically significant for an eczema.

In individuals who are sensitive to thiurams the use of polyvinyl chloride plastic gloves, shoes with leather or polyurethane soles, and clothing elasticated with Lycra (a polyurethane elastomer) may be required where indicated to reduce personal exposure to the allergens. A list of suppliers of hypoaller-genic latex and polyurethane gloves is available [3].

Thiurams have found wide use as fungicides, particularly for agricultural purposes but also for such applications as wallpaper adhesives and paints. They have also been used in animal repellents. TETD has been used in a scabicidal soap. TETD, when administered systemically, causes inhibition of the enzyme aldehyde dehydrogenase. On taking an alcoholic drink there is a buildup of acetaldehyde, which causes skin irritation, erythema and urticaria. In the form of Antabuse, TETD is used to treat alcoholism. Topical exposure to TETM and systemic taking of alcohol has caused a similar toxic reaction [4], as has also the taking of Antabuse and topical exposure to alcohol in toiletries [5]. TETD has been used to treat vesicular hand eczema in nickel-sensitive individuals [6].

A widespread eczematous reaction may develop after the systemic admin-istration of TETD to previously sensitized individuals [7]. The carbamates are no longer included in the standard series of contact allergens [8]. It has been shown that the majority of individuals who give an allergic reaction to carbamix also react to thiuram mix [9]. Thiuram mix is, therefore, a good detector of rubber sensitivity to this group of rubber chemicals, to which they are chemically similar. The carba mix produced false-positive irritant reactions which were frequently misinterpreted.

13.18.1 References

1. Cronin E (1980) Contact dermatitis. Churchill Livingstone, Edinburgh, p 729
2. Knudsen BB, Larsen E, Egsgaard H, Menné T (1993) Release of thiurams and carbamates from rubber gloves. Contact Dermatitis 28: 63–69
3. Frosch PJ, Born CM, Schütz R (1987) Kontaktallergien auf Gummi-, Operations- und Vinylhandschuhe. Hautarzt 38: 210–217
4. Gold S (1966) A skinful of alcohol. Lancet 2: 1417
5. Stole D, King LE (1980) Disulfiram-alcohol skin reaction to beer-containing shampoo. JAMA 244: 2045
6. Kaaber K, Menné T, Veien N, Hougaard P (1983) Treatment of dermatitis with Antabuse; a double blind study, Contact Dermatitis 9: 297–299
7. Van Hecke E, Vermander F (1984) Allergic contact dermatitis by oral disulfiram. Contact Dermatitis 10: 254
8. Andersen KE, Burrows D, Cronin E, Dooms-Goossens A, Rycroft RJG, White IR (1988) Recommended changes to the standard series. Contact Dermatitis 19: 389–390
9. Logan RA, White IR (1988) Carbamix is redundant in the patch test series. Contact Dermatitis 18: 303–304

13.19 Mercapto Mix

The mercapto mix contains the following four compounds, each at a concen-tration of 0.5% pet. (Fig. 13.13):
- 2-Mercaptobenzothiazole (MBT)
- N-Cyclohexyl-2-benzothiazole sulphenamide (CBS)
- 2,2'-Dibenzothiazyl disulphide (MBTS)

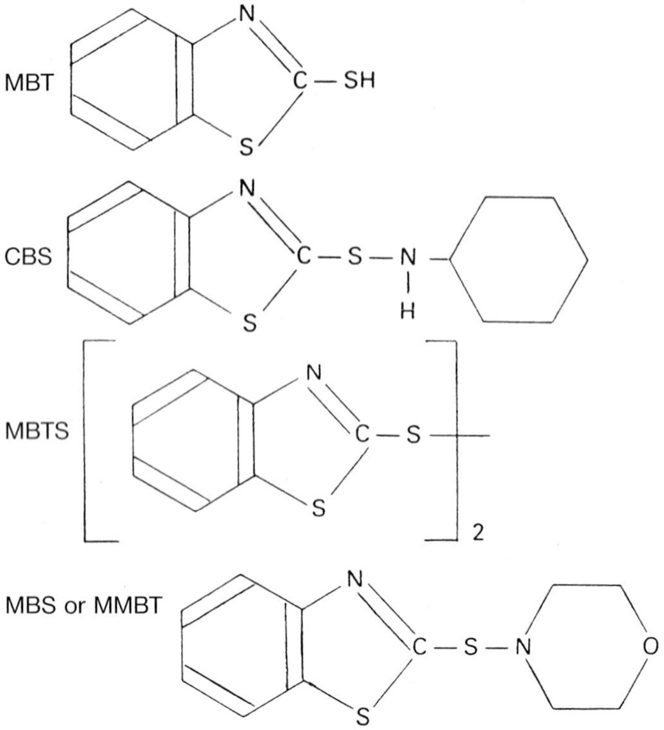

Fig. 13.13. Components of mercapto mix: 2-mercaptobenzothiazole (*MBT*), *N*-cyclohexyl-2-benzothiazole sulphenamide (*CBS*), 2,2'-dibenzothiazyl disulphide (*MBTS*) and morpholinyl mercaptobenzothiazole [2-(morpholinothio) benzothiazole, or *N*-oxydiethylene benzothiazole sulphenamide; *MBS, MMBT*]

– Morpholinyl mercaptobenzothiazole [2-(Morpholinothio) benzothiazole, *N*-oxydiethylene benzothiazole sulphenamide; MBS, MMBT]

These chemicals are present in many rubbers, to which they are added as accelerators before vulcanization takes place (see Sect. 13.18) and like thiurams are ubiquitous in rubber products. The majority of individuals who react to the mix react to MBT if tested to the individual components of the mix, and therefore it is not possible to determine the nature of the primary allergen. Fregert [1] observed that benzene with a thiazole ring and a thiol group in the 2 position were required for cross-sensitization to occur.

According to Cronin [2], women who react to MBT have probably been sensitized by gloves or shoes, but in men the sensitization is probably by footwear. Among numerous other sources of contact with rubbers containing MBT are rubber handles, masks, elastic bands, tubing, elasticated garments and artificial limbs [3]. MBT may be present in a variety of nonrubber products, including cutting oils, greases, coolants, anti-freezes, fungicides, adhesives and veterinary medicaments [4].

As well as in the mercapto mix, MBT is included in the standard series on its own at 2% pet. The mix failed to detect 30% of patients who were MBT allergic when compared to simultaneous testing with 1% MBT, and 12 of 24 individuals who reacted to 2% MBT did not react to the mix [5]. The mercapto mix used in North America does not contain MBT, which is tested separately at 1% pet., the concentration of the remaining three allergens being 0.33%. Recent analysis of the stability of the mercaptobenzothiazole compounds has shown that the so-called cross-sensitivity reported for this group is the result of chemical interaction resulting in one main hapten [6].

13.19.1 References

1. Fregert S (1969) Cross-sensitivity pattern of 2-mercaptobenzothiazole (MBT). Acta Derm Venereol (Stockh) 49: 45–48
2. Cronin E (1980) Contact dermatitis. Churchill Livingstone, Edinburgh, pp 734–735
3. Condé-Salazar L, LLinas Volpe MG, Guimaraens D, Romero L (1988) Allergic contact dermatitis from a suction socket prosthesis. Contact Dermatitis 19: 305–306
4. Taylor JS (1986) Rubber. In: Fisher AA (ed) Contact dermatitis. Lea and Febiger, Philadelphia, p 623
5. Andersen KE, Burrows D, Cronin E, Dooms-Goossens A, Rycroft RJG, White IR (1988) Recommended changes to the standard series. Contact Dermatitis 5: 389–390
6. Hansson C, Agrup G (1993) Stability of the mercaptobenzothiazole compounds. Contact Dermatitis 28: 29–34

13.20 N -Isopropyl-N ′-phenyl-p -phenylenediamine (IPPD)

Due to difficulties in supply of the other two components, IPPD 0.1% pet. has replaced, in the standard series, the PPD-black-rubber mix, which contains the following three compounds in pet. [1] (Fig. 13.14):

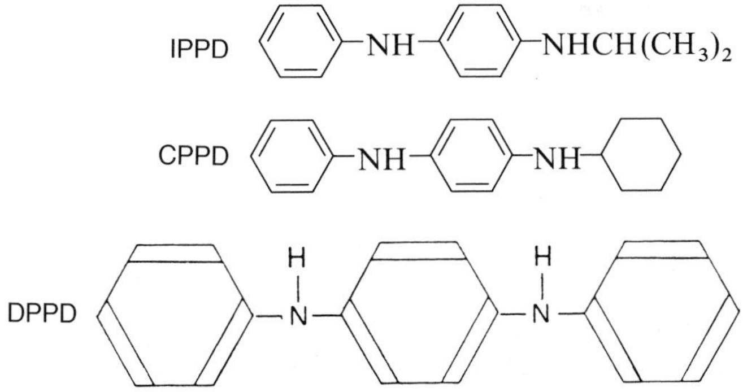

Fig. 13.14. Components of PPD – black-rubber mix: *N*-isopropyl-*N′*-phenyl-*p*-phenylenediamine (4-isopropylamino-diphenylamine; *IPPD*), *N*-phenyl-*N′*-cyclohexyl-*p*-phenylenediamine (*CPPD*) and *N*, *N′*-diphenyl-*p*-phenylenediamine (*DPPD*)

- *N*-Isopropyl-*N'*-phenyl-*p*-phenylenediamine   (phenylisopropyl-*p*-pheny-lenediamine, 4-isopropylamino-diphenylamine; IPPD) 0.1%
- *N*-Phenyl-*N'*-cyclohexyl-*p*-phenylenediamine (CPPD) 0.25%
- *N*, *N'*-Diphenyl-*p*-phenylenediamine (DPPD) 0.25%

With time, vulcanized rubber gradually reacts with atmospheric oxygen and ozone to crack and crumble, a process known as weathering or perishing. In order to reduce this effect, antioxidants and antiozonants may be added before vulcanization, particularly to those rubbers intended for heavy and stressful uses such as tyres and industrial applications. A number of antiozonant types are available, but those based on derivatives of *p*-phenylenediamine (PPD derivatives, staining antidegradents) are in common use.

The chemicals within the PPD-black-rubber mix are not related in use to *p*-phenylenediamine, which is a hair dye.

IPPD has been established as a contact allergen in heavy-duty rubber goods since Bieber and Foussereau [2] reported nine cases, including four men who had occupational contact with tyres. Manufacturers of rubber chemicals have attempted to produce an antiozonant with the desired technical properties of IPPD but having a reduced potential for inducing sensitization.

A substitute that has been promoted for IPPD is *N*-(1,3-dimethylbutyl)-*N'*-phenyl-*p*-phenylenediamine (DMPPD; Fig. 13.15). Manufacturers of DMPPD have claimed for it a low potential for inducing cutaneous sensitization, and as a result it has replaced IPPD and some of its derivatives in many applications, particularly in the United States but not in Eastern Europe. However, in practice it has been noted that individuals who are allergic to IPPD usually react to DMPPD on patch testing. Herve-Bazin et al. [3] evaluated 42 tyre handlers who were IPPD sensitive and found that all 15 who were also tested to DMPPD reacted to it. Guinea pig maximization performed independently by this group showed DMPPD to be a more potent allergen than IPPD in this animal model. DMPPD is not present in the standard series mix.

In factories where IPPD continues to be used as an antiozonant there is no significant excess of allergic reactions to it [4]; this may be related to the considerably improved hygiene in rubber factories in recent years.

The hand dermatitis induced by hypersensitivity to PPD-derived antiozonants often has a palmar distribution, because this is the usual area of skin contact with rubbers most likely to contain these agents. Clinically, a PPD-derivative hand dermatitis can look endogenous. The prognosis of such a PPD-derivative hand dermatitis can be adversely affected by allowing chronic

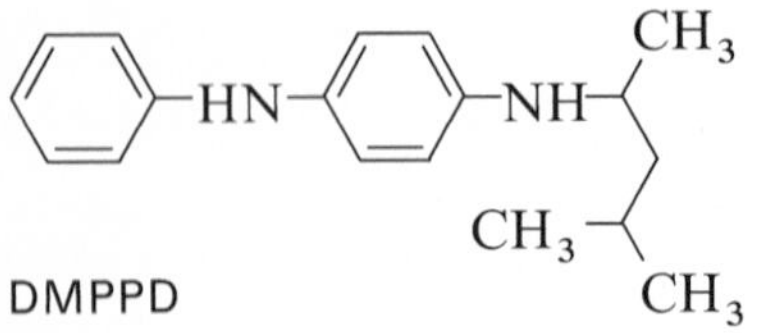

DMPPD

Fig. 13.15. *N*-1,3-Dimethylbutyl-*N'*-phenyl-*p*-phenylenediamine (DMPPD)

exposure to the offending allergen, and may cause the dermatitis to persist after avoidance of further contact.

Although PPD-derived antiozonants are commonly present in rubber for heavy-duty applications, they may also be present in other rubber. Examples include squash balls, scuba masks [5], motorcycle handles [6], boots [7], watch straps [8], spectacle chains [9] and orthopaedic bandages [10].

A purpuric contact dermatitis has been described in some individuals sensitive to IPPD. The dermatitis was summarized by Fisher [11] as being pruritic, petechial and purpuric. The reaction is usually localized to the area of skin contact but may be widespread. Purpuric patch tests to IPPD have been reported.

A lichenoid contact dermatitis from IPPD has been observed [12], although the histological features of the reaction were those of a lichenified dermatitis.

By testing with IPPD alone, approximately 10% of those sensitized to this group of industrial rubber chemicals may escape a correct diagnosis [1].

13.20.1 References

1. Menné T, White IR, Bruynzeel DP, Dooms-Goossens A (1992) Patch test reactivity to the PPD-black-rubber-mix (industrial rubber chemicals) and individual ingredients. Contact Dermatitis 26: 354
2. Bieber MP, Foussereau J (1968) Role de deux amines aromatiques dans l'allergie au caoutchouc; PBN et 4010 NA, amines anti-oxydantes dans l'industrie du pneu. Bull Soc Fr Dermatol Syphiligr 75: 63–67
3. Herve-Bazin B, Gradiski D, Marignac B, Foussereau J (1977) Occupational eczema from N-isopropyl-N'-phenylparaphenylenediamine (IPPD) and N-dimethyl-1,3-butyl-N-phenylparaphenylenediamine (DMPPD) in tyres. Contact Dermatitis 3: 1–15
4. White IR (1988) Dermatitis in rubber manufacturing industries. Dermatol Clin 6: 53–59
5. Tuyp E, Mitchell JC (1983) Scuba diver dermatitis. Contact Dermatitis 9: 334–335
6. Goh CL (1987) Hand dermatitis from a rubber motorcycle handle. Contact Dermatitis 16: 40–41
7. Ho VC, Mitchell JC (1985) Allergic contact dermatitis from rubber boots. Contact Dermatitis 12: 110–111
8. Romaguera C, Aquirre A, Diaz Perez JL, Grimalt F (1986) Watch strap dermatitis. Contact Dermatitis 14: 260–261
9. Conde-Salazar L, Guimaraens D, Romero LV, Gonzalez MA (1987) Unusual allergic contact dermatitis to aromatic amines. Contact Dermatitis 17: 42–44
10. Carlsen L, Andersen KE, Egsgaard H (1987) IPPD contact allergy from an orthopedic bandage. Contact Dermatitis 17: 119–121
11. Fisher AA (1984) Purpuric contact dermatitis. Cutis 33: 346
12. Ancona A, Monroy F, Fernandez-Diez J (1982) Occupational dermatitis from IPPD in tyres. Contact Dermatitis 8: 91–94

13.21 Epoxy Resin

Of all epoxy resins 95% consist of a glycidyl ether group formed by the reaction of bisphenol A with epichlorohydrin (Fig. 13.16). Theoretically there

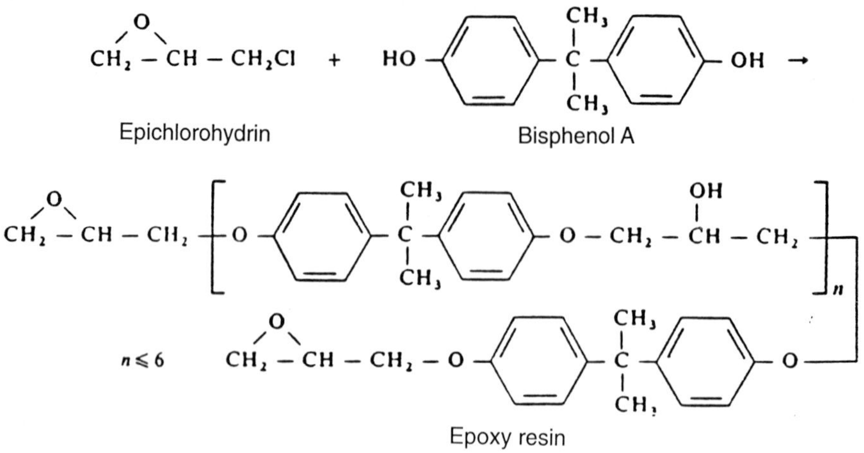

Epichlorohydrin   Bisphenol A

Epoxy resin

Fig. 13.16. Epichlorohydrin, bisphenol A and epoxy resin

are many different chemical compositions which can be used to make an epoxy resin. Until recently these have not been important, but they are fast becoming so as epoxy resins with different properties are required, for instance, with carbon fibre [1]. Epoxy resins are commonly used in everyday life as adhesives. As well as the resin itself in these compounds, there are fillers, pigments, plasticizers, reactive diluents and solvents, and these compounds are then mixed with a hardening agent which cures the resin.

Epichlorohydrin/bisphenol A epoxy resin can vary in molecular weight from 340 to much larger polymers, the larger polymers having a much lower sensitizing capacity [2]. Epoxy resin compounds therefore should contain little or no low molecular weight epoxy resin. The higher the molecular weight, the less sensitizing the compound is. Once epoxy resin becomes hardened, its sensitizing capacity becomes markedly reduced, but so-called cured resins can contain uncured molecules and so have been known to sensitize.

Epoxy resins are used as adhesives and in paints requiring great hardness and durability, for instance, in ships, in electrical insulation, as an additive to cement for quick bonding and strength. A negative patch test to epoxy resin does not necessarily mean that the patient is not allergic to the epoxy product which they have been using, for the following reasons: (a) there may be some other epoxy resin in the compound; (b) they may be allergic to some other compound in the resin, for instance, dyes, fillers, plasticizers, etc.; (c) they may be allergic to the hardener.

Hardeners are not contained in the routine series because, while 95% of epoxy resins are of one particular chemical, very many different hardeners are used. Both epoxy resins and hardeners can be irritant, as well as sensitizing, and if a patch test is applied at more than 1%, it may produce an irritant reaction. It is said [3] that epoxy resins are not volatile, so that a facial dermatitis suggests sensitization to the hardener, rather than the resin. This is not a reliable rule, however.

One of the commonest sources of sensitization in industry is the use of epoxy resin with fibreglass to make strong sheeting used for various purposes, such as hulls for boats. It is increasingly used in the impregnation of carbon fibre cloth, as this is used in situations of stress and heat, such as aeroplanes, and is acquiring an increasingly wide use. Different epoxy resins are used, as well as standard epoxy resin, for fibreglass which withstands high stress and bonds to carbon fibre.

Many patients give a positive patch test to epoxy resin without any obvious contact with uncured epoxy resin. It may be that the source of sensitization is contact with so-called cured epoxy which may contain pockets of uncured resin. Fregert and Trulsson [4] and Fregert [5] have suggested that chemical tests may be of value in demonstrating uncured resin. There are two tests for epoxy resin, one a simple colour reaction, which is not specific for uncured resin, the other thin layer chromatography, which is (see Chap. 10.3). In the standard series epoxy resin is tested at 1% pet.

13.21.1 References

1. Burrows D, Campbell H, Fregert S, Trulsson L (1984) Contact dermatitis from epoxy resins, tetraglycidyl-4, 4-methylene dianiline and O-diglycidyl phthalate in composite material. Contact Dermatitis 11: 80–83
2. Fregert S, Thorgeirsson A (1977) Patch testing with low molecular oligomers of epoxy resin in humans. Contact Dermatitis 3: 301–303
3. Dahlquist E, Fregert S (1979) Contact allergy to Cardura E, an epoxy reactive diluent of the ester type. Contact Dermatitis 5: 121–122
4. Fregert S, Trulsson L (1978) Simple methods for demonstration of epoxy resins in bisphenol A type. Contact Dermatitis 4: 69–72
5. Fregert S (1988) Physicochemical methods for detection of contact allergens. Dermatol Clin 6: 97–104

13.22 p -tert-Butylphenol-Formaldehyde Resin

p-tert-Butylphenol-formaldehyde resin (PTBP resin) is made by reacting the substituted phenol, p-tert-butylphenol, with formaldehyde (Fig. 13.17). It is a useful adhesive which sticks rapidly, is durable and pliable, and has good strength at raised temperatures. Because of its flexibility it is used in shoe construction and in leather goods. It is also used in other contact adhesives such as those used in laminating surfaces. These contact adhesives based on PTBP resin are often formulated with neoprene (a synthetic rubber), which causes initial bonding until the resin cures.

PTBP resins have commonly been reported as causing both occupational and nonoccupational allergic contact dermatitis. The first occupational cases were described in those making or repairing shoes [1, 2] who developed hand eczema. The cobblers reported by Malten reacted to both p-tert-butylphenol itself and also to PTBP resin. PTBP resins can also cause allergic contact dermatitis on the feet of those who wear shoes containing the adhesive [3].

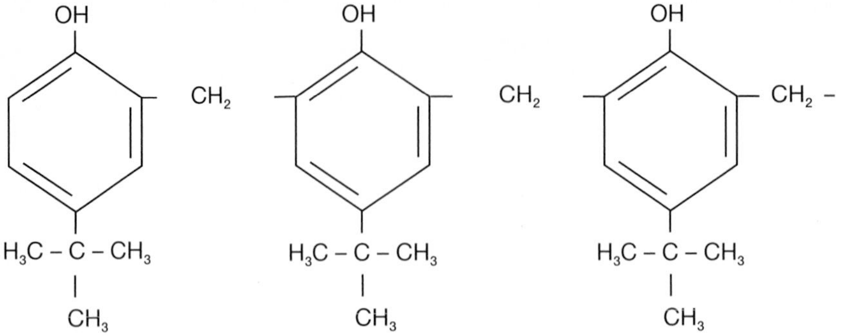

Fig. 13.17. *p-tert*-Butylphenol (*left*) and *p-tert*-butylphenol-formaldehyde resin (*above*)

Phenolic resin adhesives are used in the rubber industry for bonding rubber to rubber and to metal surfaces. Such a resin caused allergic contact dermatitis of the eyelids, chin, legs and popliteal fossae of a man in a rubber factory. The adhesive contained 8% phenol-formaldehyde polymers. On patch testing h reacted to the resin and the polymers at a dilution of 1% and also to the standard PTBP resin in the patch test series [4]. It has been pointed out, however, that patch testing with PTBP resin is not sufficient to detect allergy to phenol-formaldehyde resins based on phenols other than *p-tert*-butylphenol [5].

PTBP resin adhesives have been used in car assembly plants for fixing rubber weather strip car door seals in place. In one factory over a 3-year period, 50 men exposed to the adhesive developed a dermatitis. It was believed that toluene used as a tackifying agent contributed to the problem by causing irritation, but on patch testing 35 of the men produced a positive reaction to the PTBP resin adhesive. An improvement in working conditions and the discarding of toluene as tackifying agent resulted in resolution of the problem [6]. Nonoccupational causes of hypersensitivity to PTBP resin include the wearing of leather watch straps glued with the adhesive [7], the use of some brands of plastic fingernail adhesive [8], and also the use of PTBP resin adhesives for do-it-yourself purposes [9]. It may also be present on adhesive labels [10].

The incidence of PTBP resin sensitivity and the relevance of it has been tabulated by Cronin [11] from her own data. She found 28 men to be allergic to PTBP resin on routine patch testing and in 10 of these the relevance was occupational: shoe mender/maker [3], glues [6], lacquer in research chemist [1]. Of 33 women in her series only one reaction was of occupational relevance, and this occurred in a shoe mender. The remaining nonoccupational sources of contact were: own shoes [12], watch strap [7], glue [3], woodwork [1], or unknown [9]. There are probably a number of allergens in PTBP resin, but *p-tert*-butylphenol itself is a rare allergen. It has been shown [2] that in guinea pigs PTBP and PTBP resin sensitize independently. Malten recommended that PTBP resins should be made without any excess *p-tert*-butylphenol present, in order to eliminate one allergen [12]. In a polychloroprene/PTBP resin adhesive which caused an allergic contact dermatitis, the allergens were found to be 2-hydroxy-5-*tert*-butyl benzyl alcohol and a condensate of 4-*p-tert*-butylphenol molecules joined by methylene bridges [13]. Formaldehyde is not a main allergen in PTBP resin.

Depigmentation of the skin caused by *p-tert*-butylphenol and other substituted phenols has been reported as occurring in those workers manufacturing the chemical when exposure has been excessive. Such depigmentation has also occurred in those using PTBP resin adhesives in a car factory, where the problem was probably due to the excess *p-tert*-butylphenol present in the adhesive. It has been pointed out that this depigmentation can occur without irritant damage occurring to the skin [14].

The patch test concentration is 1% pet.

13.22.1 References

1. Calnan CD, Harman RRM (1959) Studies in contact dermatitis X. Sensitivity to para-tertiary butylphenol. Trans St Johns Hosp Dermatol Soc 43: 27–32
2. Malten KE (1967) Contact sensitizations caused by p. tert. butylphenol and certain phenol-formaldehyd-containing glues. Dermatologica 135: 54–59
3. Van Ketel WG (1974) Plastics and glues. Contact Dermatitis Newslett 16: 470–471
4. Van der Willingen AH, Stolz E, van Joost T (1987) Sensitisation to phenol formaldehyde in rubber glue. Contact Dermatitis 16: 291–292
5. Bruze M (1987) Contact dermatitis from phenol-formaldehyde resins. In: Maibach HI (ed) Occupational and industrial dermatology, 2nd edn. Year Book Medical Publishers, Chicago, pp 430–435
6. Engel HO, Calnan CD (1966) Resin dermatitis in a car factory. Br J Ind Med 23: 62–66
7. Mobacken H, Hersle K (1976) Allergic contact dermatitis caused by para-tertiary butylphenol-formaldehyde resin in watch straps. Contact Dermatitis 2: 59
8. Rycroft RJG, Wilkinson JD, Holmes R, Hay RJ (1980) Contact sensitization to p-tertiary butylphenol (PTBP) resin plastic nail adhesive. Clin Exp Dermatol 5: 441–445
9. Moran M, Martin-Pascual A (1978) Contact dermatitis to para-tertiary-butylphenol formaldehyde. Contact Dermatitis 4: 372–373
10. Dahlquist I (1984) Contact allergy to paratertiary butylphenol formaldehyde resin in an adhesive label. Contact Dermatitis 10: 54
11. Cronin E (1980) Contact dermatitis. Churchill Livingstone, Edinburgh, pp 617–619
12. Malten KE (1973) Occupational dermatoses in the processing of plastics. Trans St Johns Hosp Dermatol Soc 59: 78–113
13. Schubert H, Agatha G (1979) Zur Allergennatur der para-tert. Butylphenolformaldehydharze. Derm Beruf Umwelt 27: 49–52
14. Malten KE, Rath R, Pastors PMH (1983) Para-tert-butylphenol formaldehyde and other causes of shoe dermatitis. Derm Beruf Umwelt 31: 149–153

13.23 Primin

Primin, or 2-methoxy-6-pentylbenzoquinone, is the major allergen in primula dermatitis (Fig. 13.18). Primin is included in the European standard series because it is an important allergen in certain countries, especially in Northern Europe. However, the current sensitization rate is so low in some countries, for example, Germany, that it is not incorporated into the local standard series. Primin allergy may be difficult to suspect because patients may be unaware of contact with the plant.

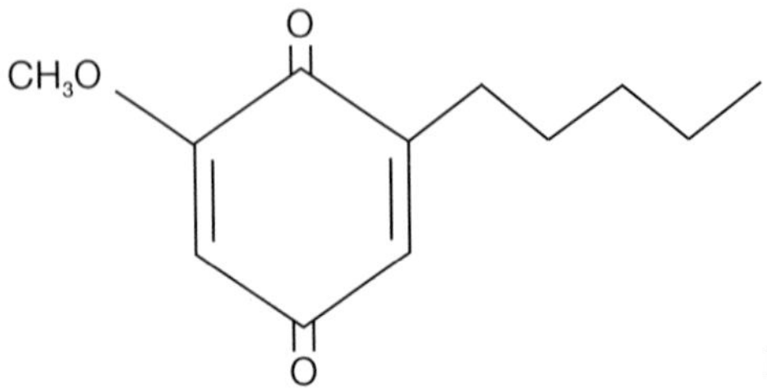

Fig. 13.18. Primin

Primula obconica, which has round leaves covered with visible fine hairs and microscopical trichomes, is the usual cause; other species of *Primula* rarely cause dermatitis. Primin is a powerful sensitizer contained in the fine hairs, and the content varies with the season, hours of sunshine, and care of the plant [1, 2]. Higher concentrations of the allergen are irritant and may sensitize the patient. Testing may invoke flare reactions. In primula dermatitis, lesions are often arranged in linear streaks and most often appear on exposed skin. The parts most often affected are the eyelids, cheeks, chin, neck, fingers, hands and arms. Other plants and woods containing quinones may show cross-reactivity with primin [3].

The patch test concentration is 0.01% pet.

13.23.1 References

1. Hjorth N (1967) Seasonal variations in contact dermatitis. Acta Derm Venereol (Stockh) 47: 409–418
2. Benezra C, Ducombs G, Sell Y, Foussereau J (1985) Plant contact dermatitis. Decker, Toronto, pp 200–201
3. Fregert S, Hjorth N, Schulz KH (1968) Patch testing with synthetic primin in persons sensitive to *Primula obconica.* Arch Dermatol 98: 144–147

13.24 Sesquiterpene Lactone Mix

The sesquiterpene lactone (SL) mix contains the following three sesquiterpene lactones in pet. (See Fig. 10.5.3): alantolactone 0.033%, dehydrocostus lactone 0.033%, and costunolide 0.033%. The SL mix was developed by Ducombs et al. [1]. These sesquiterpene lactones are contact allergens present in Compositae plants (syn. Asteraceae), which constitute one of the largest flowering plant families in the world. More than 200 of the about 25 000 known Compositae species have caused allergic contact dermatitis. The Compositae family includes many of the common weeds, milfoil (*Achillea millefolium*), tansy (*Tanacetum vulgare*), mugwort (*Artemisia vulgaris*), and wild camomile (*Chamomilla recutita* Rauschert) – and many cultivated garden flowers such as chrysanthemum (*Chrysanthemum indicum*), marguerite (*Laucanthemum vulgare*), marigold (*Calendula officinalis*), goldenrod (*Solidago virgaurea*), African marigold (*Tagetes*), feverfew (*Tanacetum parthenium* Schultz-Bip.) and sunflower (*Helianthus annuus*). The edible types of Compositae include ordinary lettuce, endive and artichoke [2]. Besides localized eczema caused by direct contact between skin and the plants, the Compositae may give rise to a more widespread dermatitis of light and air exposed skin areas causing suspicion of airborne contact dermatitis. Seasonal variation in the severity of the eczema with summer exacerbation is frequently seen [3, 4]. Many patients have had localized eczema for a number of years when it suddenly turns into a widespread dermatitis one summer [5]. This may reflect the fact that many Compositae-sensitive patients have multiple contact allergies, and/or that Compositae sensitivity may predispose to photosensitivity [6]. The allergens may be present in all parts of the plant and also in dried plant material. The SL mix does not reveal all cases of Compositae contact allergy and supplementary tests with ether extracts of Compositae plants under suspicion are recommended. However, these extracts are not commercially available and have to be manufactured on a local basis. Further, it is important to emphasize that the content of allergenic sesquiterpene lactones may vary from season to season and from one geographical area to another. The experience with routine testing with the SL mix in Northern Europe suggests a varying frequency (1%–4%) of sensitization among eczema patients. This is high enough to justify inclusion in the standard series in this area. The SL mix is safer to use for screening purposes than plant material, which may irritate or sensitize [2, 4].

13.24.1 References

1. Ducombs G, Benezra C, Talaga P et al. (1990) Patch testing with the "sesquiterpene lactone mix:" a marker for contact allergy to Compositae and other sesquiterpene lactone containing plants. Contact Dermatitis 22: 249–252
2. Paulsen E (1992) Compositae dermatitis: a survey. Contact Dermatitis 26: 76–86

3. Wrangsjö K, Ros AM, Wahlberg JE (1990) Contact allergy to Compositae plants in patients with summer exacerbated dermatitis. Contact Dermatitis 22: 148–154
4. Paulsen E, Andersen KE, Hausen BM (1993) Results of routine patch testing with the sesquiterpene lactone mix supplemented with aimed patch testing with extracts and sesquiterpene lactones of Compositae plants. Contact Dermatitis 29: 6–10
5. Paulsen E, Andersen KE (1993) Compositae dermatitis in a Danish dermatology department in one year. II. Clinical features in patients with Compositae contact allergy. Contact Dermatitis 29: 195–201
6. Murphy GM, White IR, Hawk JLM (1990) Allergic airborne contact dermatitis to Compositae with photosensitivity. Photodermatol Photoimmunol Photomed 7: 38–39

Chapter 14
Allergens Related
to Specific Exposures

14.1 Cosmetics and Skin Care Products

ANTON C. DE GROOT and IAN R. WHITE

Contents

14.1.1 What Are Cosmetics?

In current usage, a cosmetic (or toiletry) is any preparation which is applied to the skin, eyes, mouth, hair or nails for the purpose of cleansing, enhancing appearance, giving a pleasant smell or giving protection. Within the definition of a cosmetic may be included:

- Soaps, shampoos, toothpastes, and cleansing and moisturizing creams for regular care
- Colour cosmetics such s eyeshadows, lipsticks and nail varnishes
- Hair colorants and styling agents
- Fragrance products such as deodorants, aftershaves and perfumes
- Ultraviolet light (UV light) screening preparations

We all use cosmetics and, given the enormous volume of sales and the range of products available, there is remarkably little information on the incidence of adverse reactions to them. Most individuals who experience an adverse reaction to a cosmetic have a mild reaction and simply change to another product. Only rarely is an adverse reaction reported to a manufacturer, unless discomfort is marked or significant. Individuals are also unlikely to present to a dermatologist for evaluation, unless an adverse reaction is severe or persistent.

In Europe, the absence of ingredient labelling does not permit adequate evaluation of sources of contact with potential allergens. About 8000 substances are available to the cosmetic scientist for incorporation into cosmetics. Most of these ingredients have had a long and established use and are recognized as being safe or have a low toxicological profile. Some substances, however, pose a significant risk of causing adverse reactions, and for other substances little is known about their safety.

In the general population, a questionnaire survey of 1022 individuals in the United Kingdom found 85 (8.3%) people who claimed to have experienced an adverse reaction related to the use of a cosmetic [1]. Of these 85 individuals, 44 were patch tested and in 11 (1.1%) a significant reaction was obtained to a cosmetic ingredient. In Holland, a survey of 982 individuals attending beauticians found 254 (26%) who claimed to have experienced an adverse reaction to a cosmetic [2]. Evaluation of 150 of this group by patch testing demonstrated 10 individuals, 1% of the total, with an allergic reaction attributable to a cosmetic ingredient. Although not exhaustive, these studies give an idea of the proportion of the population who may have experienced an allergic contact reaction to a cosmetic ingredient at some time.

Detailed information is available on allergy to some cosmetic ingredients in individuals who have been investigated by patch testing because of their eczema of whatever type. The currently employed European standard series of contact allergens [3] includes the following substances which may be used in cosmetics: fragrance mix, balsam of Peru (not used as such in cosmetics but included as an indicator of fragrance sensitivity), formaldehyde, quaternium-15, methylisothiazolinone + methylchloroisothiazolinone (MI/MCI), parabens, wool alcohols, colophony, and p-phenylenediamine. A recent European study of the frequency of hypersensitivity to these agents (except MI/MCI) in a patch-tested population totalling 20791 individuals has shown the incidence of reactions in Table 14.1.1 [4].

Women are more at risk of acquiring hypersensitivity to cosmetic ingredients than men, because of greater product use. The variability in the frequency of the reactions is partially attributable to different patient selection in the various centres. The results of patch testing a consecutive series of 12296 individuals being evaluated for their eczema at St John's Hospital for Diseases of the Skin are shown in Table 14.1.2.

True temporal and geographical variations in the frequency of hypersensitivity to cosmetic ingredients occur, because of differences in ingredient

Table 14.1.1. Frequency of reactions (%; mean from all centres and range) to cosmetic ingredients in the standard series ($n = 20791$) [4]

	Mean	Range
Fragrance mix	7.0	6.4–9.4
Balsam of Peru	5.8	4.0–6.7
Colophony	3.4	1.7–4.7
p-Phenylenediamine	2.8	0.3–4.9
Wool alcohols	2.8	1.2–3.9
Formaldehyde	2.2	1.4–5.2
Parabens	1.1	0.5–2.6
Quaternium-15	0.9	0.3–2.2

Table 14.1.2. Frequency of reactions (%) to cosmetic ingredients in the standard series at St John's Hospital for Disease of the Skin ($n = 12296$) 1984–1989

	Women	Men
Fragrance mix	8.1	5.9
Colophony	4.6	5.6
Formaldehyde	3.6	1.9
Quaternium-15	3.6	1.7
Wool alcohols	1.9	1.5
Balsam of Peru	1.6	2.5
p-Phenylenediamine	1.2	0.8
Parabens	0.5	0.6

use. These differences involve marketing strategies, local product preference and preferred ingredient usage by manufacturers. Additionally, changes in legislation, recommendations on ingredient use and availability are further important factors. A name product with identical appearance and packaging will not necessarily have identical contents either temporally or geographically. As examples, the preservative system in a moisturizer may be different for different national markets and the UV absorber in a suncare preparation may change regularly. Musk ambrette, present in many fragrances, has been removed or reduced without any obvious change in the products, but with a reduction in the incidence of adverse reactions to them.

In the United Kingdom, quaternium-15 (see Sect. 14.1.2.2.3) has been a major cosmetic allergen, but it causes problems infrequently in continental Europe. In various continental European countries, MI/MCI has been an important allergen (see Sect. 14.1.2.2.1), but it rarely causes problems in the United Kingdom. These differences are due totally to population exposure, as measured by usage, and not to any local variations in susceptibility.

14.1.2 The Allergens

14.1.2.1 Fragrances

Fragrances are the most frequent cause of cosmetic allergy [5, 6], both from products primarily used for their perfume (perfumes, colognes, eaux de toilettes, aftershaves, deodorants) and from other scented cosmetics. Patients may react on patch testing to the product and to the fragrance mix in the European standard series and/or to the 'indicator allergens' for fragrance sensitivity: balsam of Peru and colophony. The fragrance mix contains eight very commonly used fragrance materials (each 1%): eugenol, isoeugenol, oak moss absolute, geraniol, cinnamic aldehyde, amyl cinnamaldehyde, hydroxyc-itronellal and cinnamic alcohol, emulsified with sorbitan sesquioleate (Sect. 13.5). This fragrance-mix possibly detects 70–80% of cases of fragrance sensitivity [7]. A perfume may contain 10–300 fragrance compounds. The exact allergen is usually not sought after, but, when it is, most reactions have proved to be caused by the components of the fragrance mix. However, changes in the popularity of ingredients used for new fragrances requires a periodic reappraisal of the composition of the fragrance mix.

Patients allergic to fragrances may use fragrance-free cosmetics. In individuals sensitive to perfumes a fragrance may sometimes be applied to clothing or hair without eliciting an allergic response. However, they should be avoided altogether in fragrance-sensitive individuals who have active eczema. It may be difficult for an individual with hand eczema totally to avoid fragrance contact, and it may be necessary to consider connubial contact with fragrances.

Musk ambrette, used as a fragrance fixer, has been an important cause of photocontact allergy [8]. Its incorporation into new products has been discouraged and its presence in old formulations has been reduced or removed. It is an occult allergen for those already sensitized, with numerous sources of contact remaining in perfumed or flavoured noncosmetic products.

14.1.2.2 Preservatives

Preservatives are added to water-containing cosmetics to inhibit the growth of nonpathogenic and pathogenic microorganisms, which may cause degradation of the product or endanger the health of the consumer. The most commonly used preservatives, their spectra of antimicrobial activity and their use concentrations are listed in Table 14.1.3.

14.1.2.2.1 Isothiazolinones

A mixture of methylisothiazolinone and methylchloroisothiazolinone (MI/MCI) was introduced as a cosmetic preservative in about 1980 [9]. The commercial products of the biocide mixture which are used for cosmetic

Table 14.1.3. Commonly used preservatives [58]

Name	Action spectrum	Use concentration
Methylisothiazolinone + methylchloroisothiazolinone (Kathon CG, Euxyl K100)	Broad spectrum: bacteria, yeast, fungi	3–15 ppm
Formaldehyde	Broad spectrum: fungicide and bactericide	0.05–0.2%
Quaternium-15 (Dowicil 200)	Broad spectrum: bacteria, mould, yeast	0.02–0.3%
Imidazolidinyl urea (Germall 115)	Broad spectrum, especially in combination with parabens	0.05–0.5%
Diazolidinyl urea (Germall II)	Broad spectrum, especially active against Gram-negative bacteria, often combined with parabens or other antifungal preservatives	0.03–0.3%
2-Bromo-2-nitropropane-1,3-diol (Bronopol)	Broad spectrum: most effective against bacteria	0.01–0.1%
Dimethylol dimethyl (DMDM) hydantoin (Glydant)	Broad spectrum, less active against yeast	0.15–0.4%
Parabens	Primarily fungi and Gram-positive bacteria, little active against Gram-negative bacteria	use at maximum solubility (0.3%)

preservation are known as Kathon CG (CG stands for cosmetic grade) and Euxyl K100. Kathon CG contains 1.5% active ingredients in an inert carrier and Euxyl K100 also contains benzyl alcohol. Variations in the mixtures are used in biocides for industrial purposes.

In a Dutch study investigating the allergenic ingredients in cosmetics [6], MI/MCI was noted to be the most frequent cause of cosmetic allergy in the cohort evaluated. Contact allergy to MI/MCI was observed to occur frequently in various European countries in patients suspected of contact dermatitis routinely tested with this preservative system. High prevalence rates have been reported [9–11] from Finland (2.9%), Germany (5.7% and 3.4%), the Netherlands (5.0%), Italy (8.4%), Sweden (4.2%), and Switzerland (3.5%). Lower rates (approximately 1%) have been recorded in the United Kingdom, Denmark and Belgium. Of positive reactions to MI/MCI, 70%–80% have been considered relevant to patients' complaints. Most cases have been caused by leave-on cosmetics, especially skin care products. With few exceptions, the preservative is safe when used in rinse-off products at low concentrations (<5 ppm), but examples have been observed of MI/MCI sensitivity having been induced by shampoos, causing allergic contact dermatitis of the hands in hairdressers.

Because the concentration of MI/MCI in cosmetics is usually below 15 ppm, the products themselves often do not induce positive patch responses in patients allergic to MI/MCI. However, the mixture of MI/MCI at a concentration of 100 ppm in water (which will detect most but not all cases of sensitization) is included in the European standard series [3] (Sect. 13.16).

14.1.2.2.2 Formaldehyde

Formaldehyde is a frequent sensitizer and ubiquitous allergen, with numerous noncosmetic sources of contact (Sect. 13.14). Routine testing in patients with suspected allergic contact dermatitis yields prevalence rates of sensitization of 3% or more [2]. Because of this, the cosmetic industry uses small but effective concentrations, with the amount of free formaldehyde not exceeding 0.2% [13], and restricting its use almost exclusively to rinse-off products. Until recently, most shampoos contained formaldehyde. This practice rarely gave rise to cases of allergic cosmetic dermatitis [14]. In recent years, it has largely been replaced by other preservatives (such as MI/MCI), because formaldehyde (when inhaled as gas) is suspected of being a possible human carcinogen [15]. Some biocides are formaldehyde donors.

14.1.2.2.3 Formaldehyde Donors

Formaldehyde donors are preservatives that, in the presence of water, release formaldehyde. Therefore, cosmetics preserved with such chemicals will contain free formaldehyde, the amount depending on the preservative used, its concentration and the amount of water present in the product. The antimicrobial effects of formaldehyde donors are said to be intrinsic properties of the parent molecules and not related to formaldehyde release. Formaldehyde donors used in cosmetics and toiletries include quaternium-15, imidazolidinyl urea, diazolidinyl urea, 2-bromo-2-nitro-propane-1,3-diol, and dimethylol dimethyl (DMDM) hydantoin. In anionic shampoos the amount of formaldehyde released by such donors increases in the order: imidazolidinyl urea <DMDM hydantoin < diazolidinyl urea < quaternium-15 [16]. Whereas the use of formaldehyde as a preservative has drastically decreased in recent years, the increased popularity of the formaldehyde donors in the cosmetic industry suggests that an increase in the prevalence of sensitivity to them can be expected [17].

Quaternium-15 (Dowicil 200). Patients sensitized to formaldehyde may frequently experience cosmetic dermatitis from using leave-on preparations containing quaternium-15. The threshold for eliciting allergic contact dermatitis for most individuals is approximately 30 ppm formaldehyde [18]. At a concentration of 0.1%, quaternium-15 releases about 100 ppm of free formaldehyde. In some European countries such as Belgium [19] and the Netherlands [10], allergy to quaternium-15 is infrequent. In the United Kingdom, however, routine testing has yielded a prevalence rate of sensitization of 2.6% (3.3% in women, 1.4% in men) [20]. Also in the United Kingdom, 6.9% of female patients with facial dermatitis were allergic to quaternium-15 [21]. Quaternium-15 is included in the European standard series (Sect. 13.15).

Imidazolidinyl Urea (Germall 115). Imidazolidinyl urea releases only small amounts of formaldehyde, and consequently poses little threat to formaldehyde-sensitive subjects. Contact allergy to imidazolidinyl urea occurs occasionally [19, 20]. In 1175 patients tested with the preservative 2% aq. in Belgium, only eight (0.7%) positive reactions were observed, of which one was accompanied by a reaction to formaldehyde [19]. In the United States, where imidazolidinyl urea is part of the routine series, 1.5% of patients patch tested react to the preservative [17]. Cross-reactions to and from the structurally related diazolidinyl urea may be observed [19, 22].

Diazolidinyl Urea (Germall II). Diazolidinyl urea, the newest and most acitve member of the imidazolidinyl urea group, has only been used since 1982. Several case reports of cosmetic allergy from diazolidinyl urea have been published [22, 23]. In a Dutch study of 2142 patients with eczema patch tested with diazolidinyl urea 2% aq, 12 (0.6%) reacted. In 5 of these 12, the patients were also allergic to formaldehyde and formaldehyde donors [24]. The members of the North American Contact Dermatitis Group tested 647 patients with diazolidinyl urea 1% in water, and obtained 12 (1.9%) positive reactions [17]. Patients may become sensitized to diazolidinyl urea without reacting to formaldehyde, but individuals allergic to formaldehyde may experience cosmetic dermatitis from using leave-on preparations preserved with diazolidinyl urea [18]. Cross-reactions to and from imidazolidinyl urea occur [18, 20]. Diazolidinyl urea appears to be a stronger sensitizer than imidazolidinyl urea [25].

2-Bromo-2-Nitropropane-1,3-Diol (Bronopol). Bronopol is not a frequent cause of contact allergy in Europe [6, 19, 20, 26]. In the United States, however, Bronopol was found to be such a common cause of cosmetic allergy from Eucerin cream [27, 28] that the manufacturer decided to replace it. Another concern is that its interaction with amines and amides can result in the formation of nitrosamines or nitrosamides, suspected carcinogens.

Dimethylol Dimethyl Hydantoin (DMDM Hydantoin, Glydant). No cases of cosmetic allergy from DMDM hydantoin have been reported. However, routine testing with DMDM hydantoin 3% aq. in 501 patients resulted in four positive reactions; all four were also allergic to formaldehyde [29]. Subsequent testing in patients allergic to formaldehyde resulted in positive reactions to DMDM hydantoin down to concentrations of 0.3% [30]. Also, repeated open application to the skin of a cream containing 0.25% w/w DMDM hydantoin elicited a positive response in some patients. Consequently, patients sensitized to formaldehyde may experience cosmetic dermatitis from using leave-on products preserved with DMDM hydantoin.

14.1.2.2.4 Parabens

The paraben esters (methyl, ethyl, propyl, butyl) are the most widely used preservatives in cosmetic products. Because the parabens are active primarily against fungi and Gram-positive bacteria, but not against Gram-negative bacteria such as *Pseudomonas*, they are usually combined with other preservatives such as imidazolidinyl urea. With many dermatologists, the parabens have a bad reputation as notorious sensitizers. However, most cases of paraben sensitivity are caused by topical drugs applied to leg ulcers or used on eczematous skin [31]. Routine testing in the European standard series (Sect. 13.13) yields low prevalence rates of sensitization [32]. At the usual concentration of 0.1%–0.3% in cosmetics, parabens rarely cause adverse reactions. Parabens are not included in the North American standard series of contact allergens as the allergen causes problems only uncommonly.

Sensitized individuals may be able to tolerate products containing it, a phenomenon which has been called the paraben paradox. Tolerance is related to concentration, duration and site of application, and skin status.

14.1.2.2.5 Miscellaneous Preservatives

Preservatives which have occasionally caused cosmetic allergy are summarized in Table 14.1.4.

Table 14.1.4. Preservatives and antimicrobials that have caused cosmetic allergy

Acetarsone	Hexachlorophene
Benzalkonium chloride	Mercury
Benzethonium chloride	Phenoxyethanol [61]
Benzoxonium chloride	*o*-Phenylphenol
Benzyl alcohol	Potassium sorbate
Chloroacetamide	Sorbic acid
Chloroxylenol [59]	Sulfiram
Dibromocyanobutane [60]	Thimerosal
Dichlorophene	Triclocarban
Fenticlor	Triclosan
Glutaral	

14.1.2.3 Lanolin and Derivatives

Lanolin and lanolin derivatives are used extensively in cosmetic products as emollients and emulsifiers. Lanolin has a bad reputation among some dermatologists, as routine testing with wool alcohols in the European standard series (Sect. 13.11) reveals many cases of lanolin sensitivity in some centres [12]. However, the majority of individuals have been sensitized by using topical pharmaceutical preparations containing lanolin, especially for treating varicose ulcers and stasis dermatitis (a similar situation to that of parabens) [33]. The presence of lanolin or its derivatives in cosmetics may cause cosmetic dermatitis in lanolin-sensitive individuals, but the risk of sensitization by using such products is small [33]. Chemical modification may enhance its safety [33, 34].

14.1.2.4 Toluenesulphonamide-Formaldehyde Resin

Toluenesulphonamide-formaldehyde resin (Santolite resin) is the usual resin in the majority of nail varnishes (lacquers) and nail hardeners. It is used in preference to the less allergenic polyester resins because it is resistant to chipping. It is a common cause of cosmetic allergy [5, 6, 35].

The diagnosis of a nail lacquer dermatitis should particularly be suspected in patients presenting with a patchy dermatitis on the neck or eyelids, but the pattern of the eczema may be indistinguishable from that of seborrhoeic eczema. Other possible sites of nail lacquer dermatitis include the upper chest, the external auditory meatus, the vulva and the anus.

Sculptured nails based on methyl methacrylate can cause a nail varnish dermatitis and a nail dystrophy in sensitized individuals [36]. Nail adhesives based on *para*-tertiary-butylphenol-formaldehyde resin have caused similar dystrophy [37].

14.1.2.5 *p*-Phenylenediamine and Related Dyes

p-Phenylenediamine and related hair dyes are important sensitizers. Safer permanent dyes with a lower risk of contact allergy, but with the same technical qualities, are not available. Many cases of sensitization were reported in the 1930s and sensitization was considered so great a hazard that its use in hair dyes was prohibited in several countries. Currently, its incorporation in cosmetic products is allowed in the European Community to a maximum concentration of 6% (as free base).

In recent years, the incidence of dermatitis due to hair dyes containing *p*-phenylenediamine (or derivatives) appears to have decreased [38]. This is attributed to the provision of cautionary notices on the product, awareness of the risk, patch testing the product, improvements in the technical quality of the cosmetic product and improvements in the technique of application of these dyes. Nevertheless, *p*-phenylenediamine remains an important cause of cosmetic allergy and is now being seen relatively more in Asian men who dye their hair and beards. These oxidation dyes are also an occupational hazard for hairdressers and beauticians ([39], Sect. 11.16.2). The chemistry of and adverse reactions to oxidation colouring agents have been reviewed [40]. Semipermanent and temporary dyes rarely cause allergic cosmetic dermatitis. Hair colours that have caused cosmetic allergy are listed in Table 14.1.5.

14.1.2.6 Glyceryl Thioglycolate

Glyceryl thioglycolate, a waving agent used in acid permanent waving products, occasionally sensitizes consumers [41], but it is usually an occupational hazard for the hairdresser ([39, 42], Sect. 11.16.2). Glyceryl thioglycolate Is unstable at room temperature, either in water or petrolatum,

Table 14.1.5. Hair colours that have caused cosmetic allergy (adapted from [56])

---

m-Aminophenol
p-Aminophenol
Henna
Lead acetate
2-Nitro-*p*-phenylenediamine
p-Phenylenediamine
N-Phenyl-*p*-phenylenediamine
Pyrocatechol
Resorcinol
Toluene-2,4-diamine
Toluene-2,5-diamine

---

and has a half-life of about 1 year. Prepared dilutions for patch testing (1%) should be refrigerated.

14.1.2.7 UV Filters

Ultraviolet light filters (UV filters) are used in sunscreens to protect the consumer from harmful UV irradiation from the sun and are also incorporated in some cosmetics to inhibit UV photodegradation of the product and thereby increase its shelf life.

UV filters have been identified in increasing frequency as allergens and photoallergens but reactions to them remain uncommon. (Photo)allergic reactions can easily be overlooked, as the resulting dermatitis may be interpreted by the patient/consumer as failure of the product to protect against sunburn or as worsening of the (photo)dermatosis for which the sunscreen was used.

Most reactions are currently caused by dibenzoylmethanes, which are a new class of broad-spectrum UV absorbers, with their main absorption properties in the UVA region (315–400 nm). Several series of patients with (photo) contact allergy to isopropyldibenzoylmethane have been reported [43–45], and its use is now waning. Cross-reactions to other dibenzoylmethanes such as butyl methoxydibenzoylmethane have been observed [45]. Other UV filters that have caused (photo)contact allergy by their presence in cosmetics are listed in Table 14.1.6.

14.1.2.8 Antioxidants

Antioxidants are added to cosmetics to prevent the deterioration of unsaturated fatty acids and are an occasional cause of cosmetic allergy [5, 6], though the actual prevalence may be underestimated [46]. Antioxidants that have caused cosmetic allergy include [10]: BHA (butylated hydroxyanisole) [46], BHT (butylated hydroxytoluene) [46], *t*-butylhydroquinone [46], 2,5-ditert-butylhydroquinone, nordihydroguiaretic acid, propyl gallate [47] and tocopherol.

Table 14.1.6. UV filters that have caused (photo) contact allergy (adapted from [10])

p-Aminobenzoic acid (PABA) [5]
Amyl dimethyl-PABA [43]
Benzophenone-3,4,8,10 [43, 62]
Bornelone
Butyl methoxydibenzoylmethane [43]
β-Carotene
Cinoxate
Drometrizole
Ethoxyethyl-p-methoxycinnamate [43]
Glyceryl-3-(glyceroxy)-anthranilate
Glyceryl-PABA
Homosalate
4-Isopropyldibenzoylmethane [43, 45, 46, 63]
3-(4-Methylbenzylidene)-camphor [43, 45, 46, 63]
Octyl dimethyl-PABA [43]
2-Phenylbenzimidazole-5-sulphonic acid
2-Phenyl salicylate
Witisol

14.1.2.9 Other Allergens

Emulsifiers are very rare causes of cosmetic allergy. Oleamidopropyl dimethylamine, present in a particular baby lotion containing 0.3% of the emulsifier [48], was responsible for allergic contact reactions in many patients in the Netherlands. Other emulsifiers which have caused cosmetic allergy are listed in Table 14.1.7.

Other ingredients of cosmetics which are occasional causes of cosmetic allergy include: cetyl alcohol [49], colophony [50, 51], phenyl salicylate [52], propolis [53, 54], propylene glycol [5] and colours [55]. A comprehensive literature survey on cosmetic allergy is provided in [10] and [56].

14.1.3 Diagnosis

An allergy to a cosmetic product should particularly be suspected in individuals presenting with a dermatitis affecting the face or hands. More widespread problems may be caused by ingredients in products intended for general application to the body. Hypersensitivity to other products such as deodorants usually causes a reaction localized to the site of application.

Most episodes of cosmetic allergy are detected with the allergens included in the European standard series. However, when a cosmetic allergy is suspected it is necessary to test with the patient's own cosmetics and with additional allergens. An example of an extensive 'cosmetic series' (modified from the St John's Hospital for Diseases of the Skin additional cosmetic allergen series) is provided in Table 14.1.8.

Care must be exercised in patch testing with certain cosmetics to avoid false-positive reactions. Detergent-based preparations, such as shampoos,

Table 14.1.7. Emulsifiers and surfactants that have caused cosmetic allergy (adapted from [10])

Cetearyl alcohol [5]
Cetyl alcohol [5]
Cocamide DEA [6]
Cocamidopropyl betaine [6]
Coco-betaine
Diisopropanolamine
Disodium monooleamidosulphosuccinate [5]
Emulgol
Glyceryl stearate [64]
Hydrolysed animal protein [5]
Lauramide DEA [6]
Methyl glucose sesquistearate
Miranol MSA
Myristyl alcohol [65]
Oleamide DEA [5]
PEG-4 dilaurate [6]
PEG-32 stearate [6]
Potassium coco-hydrolysed animal protein [66]
Sodium laureth sulphate
Stearamidoethyl diethylamine
Stearic acid [64]
Sulphated castor oil
TEA-coco-hydrolysed animal protein
TEA-PEG-3 cocamide sulphate
TEA-stearate
Triethanolamine [66, 67]
Trilaureth-4 phosphate

---

should be diluted to 1% aq. before application, but even then toxic patch test reactions are observed regularly and an additional dilution of 0.1% may be needed to corroborate the genuineness of a reaction obtained at 1%. Volatile solvents in waterproof mascaras need to be allowed to evaporate.

A major problem of testing with cosmetics is that false-negative reactions occur. This is because a responsible allergen may be present at too low a concentration to elicit a positive patch test on normal skin. When a product is suspected of being responsible for an allergic contact reaction, but patch tests are noncontributory, a repeated open application test (ROAT) or use test may be necessary (Sect. 10.1.15).

In Europe few cosmetics carry ingredient labelling. In the United States, compulsory labelling has been enforced since 1977 and has been of enormous benefit in advising patients on which cosmetics to avoid when an allergen has been identified [57]. In Europe patients should be instructed to contact the manufacturers of the cosmetic ranges which they prefer and enquire as to which of their products are free of the identified allergens. They should be made aware, however, that formulations change without notification and that products with the same brand name and packaging but purchased in a different country may contain different ingredients.

Table 14.1.8. Cosmetic screening series (adapted from the St John's Hospital for Diseases of the Skin cosmetic series)

1 *Antioxidants*		
BHA (butylated hydroxyanisole)	2%	pet.
Propyl gallate	1%	pet.
2 *Biocides*		
2-Bromo-2-nitropropane-1,3-diol (Bronopol)	0.5%	pet.
Chloroacetamide	0.2%	pet.
Diazolidinyl urea (Germall II)	2%	pet.
Dibromodicyanobutane+phenoxyethanol (Euxyl K400)	1%	pet.
Imidazolidinyl urea (Germall 115)	2%	pet.
Triclosan (Irgasan DP 300)	2%	pet.
3 *Miscellaneous*		
Cetearyl alcohol	30%	pet.
Eucerit	30%	pet.
Hydrogenated lanolin	100%	
Propylene glycol	20%	pet.
Toluenesulphonamide-formaldehyde resin	10%	pet.
Musk ambrette	5%	pet.
4 *UV absorbers*		
p-Aminobenzoic acid (PABA)	2%	pet.
Benzophenone-3 (Oxybenzone)	2%	pet.
Benzophenone-10 (Mexenone)	2%	pet.
Butyl methoxy dibenzoylmethane (Parsol 1789)	2%	pet.
2-Ethoxyethyl-*p*-methoxycinnamate (Cinoxate)	2%	pet.
4-Isopropyldibenzoylmethane (Eusolex 8020)	2%	pet.
3-(4-Methylbenzylidene)-camphor (Eusolex 6300)	2%	pet.
Octyl dimethyl-PABA (Escalol 507)	2%	pet.
Octyl methoxycinnamate (Parsol MCX)	2%	pet.

Allergens in cosmetics may also be present in other consumer items such as detergents, polishes and air fresheners, and patients should be reminded of this.

14.1.4 Cosmetic Ingredient Labelling: The Gap in EC Legislation

European Community regulations do not require that cosmetic manufacturers list all ingredients on their products. Only a very limited number of chemicals must be declared on the label, when present (EEC Cosmetic Directive 76/768/EEC, 10th Adapting Commission Directive 88/233/EEC).

Article 7.3 of the EC Cosmetics Directive provides physicians with the possibility of obtaining information from cosmetic manufacturers: "Furthermore, a Member State may require, for the purposes of prompt and appropriate medical treatment in the event of difficulties, that adequate and sufficient information regarding substances contained in cosmetic products is made available to the competent authority, which shall ensure that this information is used only for the purposes of such treatment." However, contacting manufacturers takes time and may result in considerable delays in diagnosis. Also, the lack of information is a problem to patients allergic to cosmetic ingredients. Compulsory ingredient labelling in the EC would solve these difficulties. Full ingredient labelling will enable the dermatologist adequately to diagnose and treat patients suffering from cosmetic dermatitis, and to advise them on future cosmetic use. Ingredient labelling provides the consumer, who has been instructed which substances to avoid, with the information necessary to purchase products which can be used without the risk of developing recurrences of cosmetic dermatitis. Labelling will enable the early identification of new allergens.

The main problem with ingredient labelling in the EC is the choice of language. The open market renders it impossible for all the various languages of the countries where products are marketed to be used. Therefore, it is suggested that the Dictionary of the US Cosmetic, Toiletry and Fragrance Association (with a European supplement) should be used as a guideline [4].

14.1.5 References

1. Consumers' Association (1979) Reactions of the skin to cosmetics and toiletry products. Consumers' Association, London
2. De Groot AC, Beverdam E, Tjong Ayong C, Coenraads PJ, Nater JP (1988) The role of contact allergy in the spectrum of adverse effects caused by cosmetics and toiletries. Contact Dermatitis 19: 195–201
3. International Contact Dermatitis Research Group (ICDRG) and the European Environmental and Contact Dermatitis Research Group (EECDRG) (1988) Notice. Contact Dermatitis 19: 391
4. De Groot AC (1990) Labelling cosmetics with their ingredients. Br Med J 300: 1636–1638
5. Adams RM, Maibach HI (1985) A five-year study of cosmetic reactions. J Am Acad Dermatol 13: 1062–1069
6. De Groot AC, Bruynzeel DP, Bos JD, van der Meeren HLM, van Joost T, Jagtman BA, Weyland JW (1988) The allergens in cosmetics. Arch Dermatol 124: 1525–1529
7. Larsen WG, Maibach HI (1982) Fragrance contact allergy. Semin Dermatol 1: 85–90
8. Wojnarowska F, Calnan CD (1986) Contact and photocontact allergy to musk ambrette. Br J Dermatol 114: 667–675
9. De Groot AC, Herxheimer A (1989) Isothiazolinone preservative: cause of a continuing epidemic of cosmetic dermatitis. Lancet i: 314–316
10. De Groot AC (1988) Adverse reactions to cosmetics. Thesis, State University of Groningen
11. Frosch PJ, Schulze-Dirks A (1987) Kontaktallergie auf Kathon CG. Hautarzt 38: 422–425
12. Enders F, Przybilla B, Ring J, Burg G, Braun-Falco O (1988) Epicutantestung mit einer Standardreihe. Hautarzt 39: 779–786
13. Cosmetic Ingredient Review (1984) Final report on the safety assessment of formaldehyde. J Am Coll Toxicol 3: 157–184
14. Bruynzeel DP, van Ketel WG, de Haan P (1984) Formaldehyde contact sensitivity and the use of shampoos. Contact Dermatitis 10: 179
15. Council on Scientific Affairs (1989) Formaldehyde. JAMA 261: 1183–1187

16. Rosen M, McFarland AG (1984) Free formaldehyde in anionic shampoos. J Soc Cosmet Chem 35: 157–169
17. Storrs FJ, Rosenthal LE, Adam RM, Clendenning W, Emmett EA, Fisher AA, Larsen WG, Maibach HI, Rietschel RL, Schorr WF, Taylor JS (1989) Prevalence and relevance of allergic reactions in patients patch tested in North America – 1984 to 1985. J Am Acad Dermatol 20: 1038–1045
18. Jordan WP, Sherman WT, King SE (1979) Threshold response in formaldehyde-sensitive subjects. J Am Acad Dermatol 1: 44–48
19. Dooms-Goossens A, de Boulle K, Dooms M, Degreef H (1986) Imidazolidinyl urea dermatitis. Contact Dermatitis 14: 322–324
20. Ford GP, Beck MH (1986) Reactions to quaternium 15, bronopol and Germall 115 in a standard series. Contact Dermatitis 14: 271–274
21. White IR (1986) Prevalence of sensitivity to Dowicil 200 (quaternium-15). Data presented at the 8th International Symposium on Contact Dermatitis, Cambridge, 20–22 March 1986
22. De Groot AC, Bruynzeel DP, Jagtman BA, Weyland JW (1988) Contact allergy to diazolidinyl urea (Germall II). Contact Dermatitis 18: 202–205
23. Kantor GR, Taylor JS, Ratz JL, Evey PL (1985) Acute allergic contact dermatitis from diazolidinyl urea (Germall II) in a hair gel. J Am Acad Dermatol 13: 116–119
24. Perret CM, Happle R (1989) Contact sensitivity to diazolidinylurea (Germall II). In: Frosch PJ, Dooms-Goossens A, Lachapelle J-M, Rycroft RJG. Scheper RJ (eds) Current topics in contact dermatitis. Springer, Berlin Heidelberg New York, pp 92–94
25. Jordan WP (1984) Human studies that determine the sensitizing potential of haptens. Experimental allergic contact dermatitis. Dermatol Clin 2: 533–538
26. Frosch PJ, White IR, Rycroft RJG, Lahti A, Burrows D, Camarasa JG, Ducombs G, Wilkinson JD (1990) Contact allergy to Bronopol. Contact Dermatitis 22: 24–26
27. Storrs F, Bell DE (1983) Allergic contact dermatitis to 2-bromo-2-nitroprane-1,3-diol in a hydrophilic ointment. J Am Acad Dermatol 8: 157–164
28. Peters MS, Connolly SM, Schroeter AL (1983) Bronopol allergic contact dermatitis. Contact Dermatitis 9: 397–401
29. De Groot AC, Bos JD, Jagtman BA, Bruynzeel DP, van Joost T, Weyland JW (1986) Contact allergy to preservatives (II). Contact Dermatitis 15: 218–222
30. De Groot AC, van Joost T, Bos JD, van der Meeren HLM, Weyland JW (1988) Patch test reactivity to DMDM hydantoin. Relationship to formaldehyde. Contact Dermatitis 18: 197–201
31. Wilkinson JD, Hambly EM, Wilkinson DS (1980) Comparison of patch test results in two adjacent areas of England. II. Medicaments. Acta Derm Venereol (Stockh) 60: 245–249
32. Menné T, Hjorth N (1988) Routine testing with paraben esters. Contact Dermatitis 19: 189–191
33. Kligman AM (1983) Lanolin allergy: crisis or comedy. Contact Dermatitis 9: 99–107
34. Edman B, Möller H (1989) Testing a purified lanolin preparation by a randomized procedure. Contact Dermatitis 20: 287–290
35. De Wit FS, De Groot AC, Weyland JW, Bos JD (1988) An outbreak of contact dermatitis from toluenesulfonamide formaldehyde resin in a nail hardener. Contact Dermatitis 18: 280–283
36. Fisher AA (1980) Cross reactions between methyl methacrylate monomer and acrylic monomers presently used in acrylic nail preparations. Contact Dermatitis 2: 345
37. Burrows D, Rycroft RJG (1981) Contact dermatitis from PTBP resin and tricresyl ethyl phthalate in a plastic nail adhesive. Contact Dermatitis 7: 336
38. Cronin E (1980) Contact dermatitis. Churchill Livingstone, Edinburgh, p 121
39. Matsunaga K, Hosokawa K, Suzuki M, Arima Y, Hayakawa R (1988) Occupational allergic contact dermatitis in beauticians. Contact Dermatitis 18: 94–96
40. Zviak C (ed) (1986) The science of hair care. Dekker, New York

41. Tosti A, Melino M, Bardazzi F (1988) Contact dermatitis due to glyceryl monothioglycolate. Contact Dermatitis 19: 71–72
42. Storrs F (1984) Permanent wave contact dermatitis: Contact allergy to glyceryl monothioglycolate. J Am Acad Dermatol 11: 74–85
43. English JSC, White IR, Cronin E (1987) Sensitivity to sunscreens. Contact Dermatitis 17: 159–162
44. De Groot AC, van der Walle HB, Jagtman BA, Weyland JW (1987) Contact allergy to 4-isopropyldibenzoylmethane and 3-(4'-methylbenzylidene)-camphor in the sunscreen Eusolex 8021. Contact Dermatitis 16: 249–254
45. Schauder S, Ippen H (1988) Photoallergisches und allergisches Kontaktekzem durch Dibenzoylmethan-Verbindungen und andere Lichtschutzfilter. Hautarzt 39: 435–440
46. White IR, Lovell CR, Cronin E (1984) Antioxidants in cosmetics. Contact Dermatitis 11: 265–267
47. Wilson AGMcT, White IR, Kirby JDT (1989) Allergic contact dermatitis from propyl gallate in a lip balm. Contact Dermatitis 20: 145–146
48. De Groot AC (1989) Oleamidopropyl dimethylamine. Dermatosen 37: 101–105
49. Hausen BM, Kulenkamp D (1985) Kontaktallergie auf Fludroxycortid und Cetylalkohol. Dermatosen 33: 27–28
50. Fisher AA (1988) Allergic contact dermatitis due to rosin (colophony) in eyeshadow and mascara. Cutis 42: 507–508
51. Hausen BM, Mohnert J (1989) Contact allergy due to colophony. Contact Dermatitis 20: 295–301
52. Calnan CD, Cronin E, Rycroft RJG (1981) Allergy to phenyl salicylate. Contact Dermatitis 7: 208–211
53. Schuler TM, Frosch PJ (1988) Kontaktallergic auf propolis (Bienen-Kittharz). Hautarzt 39: 139–142
54. Hausen BM, Wollenweber E, Senff H, Post B (1987) Propolis allergy (I). Origin, properties, usage and literature review. Contact Dermatitis 17: 163–170
55. English JSC, White IR (1985) Dermatitis from D&C red no 36. Contact Dermatitis 13: 335
56. Nater JP, De Groot AC (1985) Unwanted effects of cosmetics and drugs used in dermatology, 2nd edn. Elsevier, Amsterdam
57. Larsen WG (1989) Why is the USA the only country with compulsary cosmetic labeling? Contact Dermatitis 20: 1–2
58. Decker RL Jr, Wenninger JA (1987) Frequency of preservative use in cosmetic formulas as disclosed to FDA-1987. Cosmet Toilet 102: 21–40
59. Libow LF, Ruszkowski AM, DeLeo VA (1989) Allergic contact dermatitis from para-chloro-meta-xylenol in Lurosep soap. Contact Dermatitis 20: 67–68
60. Senff H, Exner M, Gortz J, Goos M (1989) Allergic contact dermatitis from Euxyl K 400. Contact Dermatitis 20: 38–39
61. Lovell CR, White IR, Boyle J (1984) Contact dermatitis from phenoxyethanol in aqueous cream BP. Contact Dermatitis 11: 187
62. Knobler E, Almeida L, Ruszkowski AM, Held J, Harber L, DeLeo V (1989) Photoallergy to benzophenone. Arch Dermatol 125: 801–804
63. Alomar A, Cerda MT (1989) Contact allergy to Eusolex 8021. Contact Dermatitis 20: 74–75
64. De Groot AC, van der Meeren HLM, Weyland JW (1988) Cosmetic allergy from stearic acid and glyceryl stearate. Contact Dermatitis 19: 77–78
65. De Groot AC, Bruynzeel DP, van Joost T, Weyland JW (1988) Cosmetic allergy from myristyl alcohol. Contact Dermatitis 1: 76–77
66. Dooms-Goossens A, Debusschere K, Dupre K, DeGreef H (1988) Can eardrops induce a shampoo dermatitis? A case study. Contact Dermatitis 19: 143–145
67. Jones SK, Kennedy CTC (1988) Contact dermatitis from triethanolamine in E45 cream. Contact Dermatitis 19: 230

14.2 Topical Drugs

GIANNI ANGELINI

Contents

14.2.1 Incidence

Contact dermatitis induced by topically applied medicaments was common many years ago [1–5] and is still common today [6–9]. It represents, after all, the most common type of skin pathology in the field of drug-induced dermatitis. Its incidence varies considerably from one country to another [3, 10, 11], depending on local prescribing habits, on the number of drugs included in the standard series, and above all on the clinical type of patients tested [5, 6, 8]. Time has seen also considerable changes in the topical medicaments responsible for contact allergy. While dermatitis induced by certain drugs used in the past (penicillin, sulphonamides, preparations of mercury, promethazine) has diminished in frequency, or even disappeared altogether, that attributable to recently introduced agents has gained in significance [8, 12]. In statistical terms, 14%–40% of all cases of allergic contact dermatitis are either caused or complicated by allergy to topical preparations [3, 8, 9, 13, 14]. Problems of contact allergy apply, in particular to patients with eczematous dermatitis due to other causes, to subjects with other dermatoses (especially stasis dermatitis and leg ulcers), to hospital staff and to employees of the pharmaceutical industry.

14.2.2 Factors Favouring Development of Contact Dermatitis

The ease of development of contact dermatitis in response to drugs depends on a number of factors.

Clearly, a most important factor is the intrinsic sensitizing potential of the drug [15]. In this respect it must be pointed out, however, that powerful sensitizers may have a low incidence of sensitization simply because of their infrequent use (e.g. mercury), while, in contrast, a high incidence of sensitization may be associated with much weaker but very widely employed sensitizers (e.g. neomycin). To increase percutaneous absorption and thus the therapeutic activity of an agent, it is often employed in high concentrations and in vehicles, such as dimethyl sulphoxide, capable of inducing structural or chemical changes in the barrier layer of the epidermis. This also increases the chances of inducing irritation or contact allergy. Similarly, the occlusive dressings sometimes employed with topical preparations, which increase drug penetration by a factor of 10 or more, might also favour the development of allergy. However, the most important factor favouring contact allergy to topical preparations is the particular condition of the skin, very often associated with cutaneous pathology and characterized by loss of barrier integrity; this in turn is attributable to various factors, such as damage by alkali or acids, or to exogenous or endogenous skin inflammation present in various skin diseases. For these reasons, contact allergy to drugs arises more frequently in association with preexisting dermatoses and, in particular, in situations where the epidermal barrier is absent, as in cases of erosive, ulcerative or traumatic dermatitis [16–18].

14.2.3 Clinical Patterns

Tissue contact with topical agents applied to the skin or mucous membranes may induce a variety of clinical pictures (Table 14.2.1) of variable pathogenesis, involving either immunological (types I, III and IV) or nonimmunological factors [7, 9, 19–40].

14.2.3.1 Irritant Contact Dermatitis

Irritant contact dermatitis is often induced by chemical agents used for medical purposes (Table 14.2.2), which damage the skin directly at the site of the contact. In addition to the agent's concentration, the duration of its action and its chemical properties, the intensity of the reaction depends on

Table 14.2.1. Eczematous and noneczematous contact dermatitis induced by topical medicaments

Clinical pattern	References
Irritant contact dermatitis	[7, 9, 19–21]
Allergic contact dermatitis	[7, 9, 19, 22–24]
Photoallergic contact dermatitis	[7, 9, 19, 22–24]
Phototoxic contact dermatitis	[23]
Contact urticaria	[23, 25–29]
Airborne irritant contact dermatitis	[30, 31]
Airborne allergic contact dermatitis	[30, 31]
Airborne phototoxic contact dermatitis	[30, 31]
Airborne photoallergic contact dermatitis	[30, 31]
Erythema-multiforme-like eruptions	[32–34, 41–43]
Lichenoid contact dermatitis	[35]
Photocontact urticaria	[36, 37]
Purpuric contact dermatitis	[30]
Acne-folliculitis	[23, 24]
Stinging (subjective irritation)	[19, 23, 129]
Discoloration of the skin	[23]
Lymphomatoid contact dermatitis	[38]
Allergic pustular contact dermatitis	[39, 40]
Contact 'halogenosis'	[24]
Necrosis	[23]
Miscellaneous side-effects	[23]

Table 14.2.2. Topical medicaments that commonly cause irritant contact dermatitis

Oxidizing agents	Hydrogen peroxide, benzoyl peroxide, cantharidin, hypochlorite, potassium permanganate, bromine, free iodine, povidone-iodine
Denaturing agents	Formaldehyde, mercury chloride
Keratolytic drugs	Salicylic acid, resorcinol, pyrogallol
Organic solvents	Alcohols, propylene glycol, ethyl ether, chloroform
Other medicaments	Quaternary ammonium compounds, tar, dithranol (anthralin), thimerosal, gentian violet, hexachlorophene, mercurial compounds, chlorhexidine, capsicum, nonsteroidal antiinflammatory drugs, tretinoin

the individual susceptibility of the subject and various, still largely unknown endogeneous factors. The irritant contact dermatitis induced by topical medicaments is most often of acute type. Clinical lesions develop at the first exposure and within hours of the contact; more rarely they appear after days or months of repeated exposure, depending on the chemical properties of the substance in question and on the structural and functional characteristics of the skin of the site affected (chronic irritant contact dermatitis).

In acute irritant contact dermatitis the cutaneous manifestations, while variable, generally consist of intense erythema and gross oedema with variably-sized blisters.

In some cases, for example, burns, blisters up to the size of a walnut or tangerine may develop. On cessation of the irritant contact, the lesion regresses by rupture of the blister, scab formation, desquamation and then epithelial repair. In some cases the picture may be complicated by secondary bacterial infection with the development of pustules, lymphangitis or lymphadenitis.

14.2.3.2 Allergic Contact Dermatitis

Allergic contact dermatitis is the most common form of contact dermatitis induced by topical drugs and most often arises either as a complication of preexisting eczema induced by other irritants or sensitizers, or as a complication of a dermatosis of a different nature.

In such cases, the superimposed allergy to topical medicaments may manifest itself in various ways, including local exacerbation with increased erythema and pruritus, or by spread to other sites in most cases preceded by local exacerbation. This kind of spread is observed especially in leg ulcers and stasis eczema. Sometimes distant spread of eczematous lesions occurs without the development of local reaction; this is recorded in association with topical preparations containing potent corticosteroids, capable of suppressing the local reaction but not the spread to other sites [9]. A comparable situation has frequently been recorded by ourselves, where eczematous lymphangitis with regional lymphadenopathy occurs as a sign of sensitization in the absence of local reaction.

Another possible complication of allergy to topical medication is persistent generalized erythroderma [7] (Fig. 14.2.1). This is a very serious condition, fortunately rare nowadays, which in our experience most often affects adult or aged men. Generally speaking, these patients are allergic to more than one topical agent (polysensitization) or present group sensitization. Generalized dermatitis is at first conspicuously exudative; subsequently, the erythema acquires a brownish tinge and massive scaling sets in. Laboratory tests show a variety of changes and superficial polylymphadenopathy develops.

In addition to the common types of clinical picture, allergic contact dermatitis induced by topical medicaments may present morphological peculiarities occasionally typical of individual allergens. Sulphonamides, for instance, produce an easily recognizable rash. Primary lesions may suggest the common type of eczema with erythema, vesiculation and exudation, while the secondary lesions, whether surrounding the primary ones or distant, consist of isolated erythemato-papulo-vesicular elements ranging in size from a grain of millet to a lentil, vivid red in colour and with a slightly infiltrated base.

Because of photosensitization, sulphonamide-induced allergic contact dermatitis often presents with typical erythemato-oedematous lesions and blistering in areas exposed to light. Finally, we have frequently

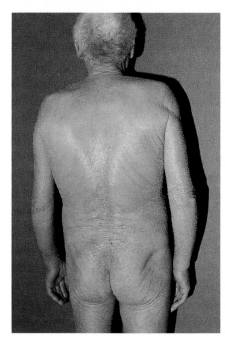

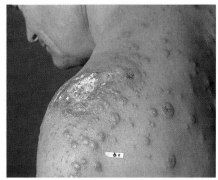

Fig. 14.2.1. Generalized eczematous erythroderma in subject sensitized to penicillin

Fig. 14.2.2. Post-traumatic allergic contact dermatitis of the shoulder due to sulphonamide. Diffuse erythema-multiforme-like secondary eruption

observed a secondary erythema-multiforme-like picture induced by topical sulphonamides [30] (Fig. 14.2.2.).

Light sensitization is also associated with certain topical antihistamines, i.e. promethazine and chemically related compounds. The picture of allergic contact dermatitis develops in exposed areas, with lesions intensely erythematous, oedematous, smooth and shiny, with little exudation and peculiarly red in colour with a slight purple tinge. In addition to this pathognomonic clinical picture, less frequently topical antihistamines may induce blistering, also in exposed areas (Fig. 14.2.3).

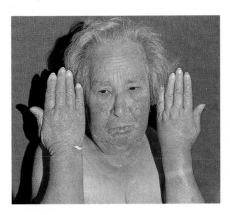

Fig. 14.2.3. Allergic photocontact dermatitis from promethazine

Another topical medicament which produces a pathognomonic clinical picture is pyrrolnitrin, an antimycotic used mainly in Italy, Spain and Japan. It is a common allergen which gives rise almost always to an erythema-multiforme-like picture. The lesions, at first limited to the contact area, spread rapidly to adjacent regions and eventually, in most cases, to the entire skin surface [30, 41, 42]. Mephenesin, a muscle relaxant used primarily by young people after sports injuries, also promotes id-like spread that can take on the aspect of exudative erythema multiforme [43].

Airborne allergic contact dermatitis from medicaments characteristically affects exposed areas. It differs from allergic photocontact dermatitis in involving the upper eyelids (and often the conjunctiva), under the chin, behind the ears, the scalp and the back of the neck [30, 31].

14.2.3.3 Contact Urticaria

Occasionally a drug used topically may induce an immediate urticarial reaction, which, depending on the pathogenic mechanism involved, may be immunological or nonimmunological in type. From the clinical standpoint, drug-induced contact urticaria may be either localized or generalized: occasionally it may be associated with extracutaneous manifestations, such as bronchial asthma and anaphylactoid reactions [26–29]. It is also possible that the same drug may be responsible for both the initial urticarial reaction and the positive delayed response.

14.2.4 Sites and Dermatoses at Risk

Drug-induced contact dermatitis may develop at any cutaneous site. However, certain areas are more at risk than others. This is probably due to the more frequent use of drugs at such sites, to the frequent persistence of skin damage and to specific occluded or semi-occluded skin conditions.

The most vulnerable site is the lower leg in connection with preexisting chronic stasis eczema or ulcers of arterial or mixed type [44–52]. The incidence of contact allergy to topical medicinal preparations ranges in various series from approximately 40% to 90% (mean around 60%). The most commonly responsible allergens are neomycin, benzocaine, parabens, wool alcohols, and bufexamac [53] (Fig. 14.2.4).

Contact allergy to drugs seems also to be particularly high in cases of post-traumatic eczema [5, 8, 54]. Consequently, loss of skin continuity, be it traumatic or vasculopathic, may be taken as representing an 'open door' to sensitization.

Other high-risk sites are the perianal and perineal areas in both sexes [8, 52, 55, 56]. The compounds most often involved are neomycin, benzocaine and ethylenediamine. In our series, the incidence of drug allergy in perianal eczema was 22.8%. This high vulnerability is probably connected with the ease with which erosive lesions develop in this particular area and facilitate

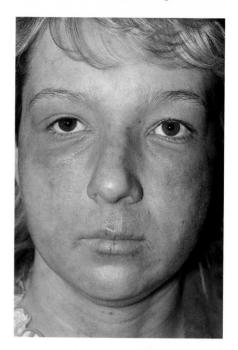

Fig. 14.2.4. Allergic contact dermatitis from bufexamac in a patient with atopic dermatitis. (Courtesy of P.J. Frosch)

percutaneous absorption of allergens. However, other factors must be taken into account, such as the specific anatomy of the site, its high humidity, the thickness of the pseudomucosa and mechanical rubbing.

Sites at more or less moderate risk are the ears and the eyelids, and that in relation to chronic otitis externa and the frequent use of eyedrops [8, 52, 57]. In ophthalmic preparations, thimerosal [58] and phenylephrine [59] seem nowadays to have aetiological significance.

The antibiotics neomycin and gentamicin were the major allergens (13.9% and 9.3%) in a series of 43 patients with suspected adverse reactions to ophthalmic medicaments [60] (Fig. 14.2.5). In order to detect weak sensitizations or cumulative irritant reactions in patients with long-term use of eye medicaments, the authors recommend the use of a method with increased sensitivity, such as the patch test on stripped skin or the scarification technique. Using these methods, the number of positive reactions was higher than that obtained with normal patch tests [60].

Several authors suggest tests designed to assess the drug allergy risk at various sites and in various groups of patients tested [52, 61, 62]. Our data on the incidence of contact allergy to various preparations and their constituents in patients with dermatoses of different types are presented in Table 14.2.3. In agreement with the findings of other authors [52], they show that the hands are a site at very low risk. Schuler and Frosch reported six patients (three men and three women) with contact dermatitis of the hands from propolis: the men had acquired their sensitization in the course of bee keeping, and

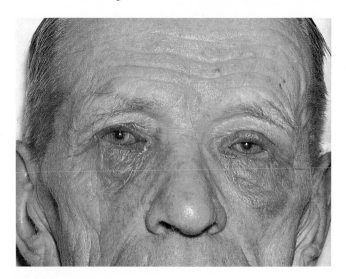

Fig. 14.2.5. Allergic contact dermatitis from neomycin in eyedrops. (Courtesy of P.J. Frosch)

Table 14.2.3. Incidence of contact allergy to medicaments and their components in 22 757 patients with dermatitis (1968–1992)

Dermatitis	Tested	No. Positive	%
Post-traumatic eczema	338	235	59.5
Leg ulcers and stasis eczema	1 204	661	54.9
Perianal and perineal dermatitis	678	125	18.4
Contact dermatitis of the face (including ears and eyelids)	2 459	344	13.9
Pompholyx	1 682	207	12.3
Occupational contact dermatitis (hands)	4 259	515	12.0
Jewellery and apparel dermatitis	2 813	283	10.0
Nummular eczema	338	26	7.6
Atopic dermatitis (90% children)	1 285	76	5.9
Psoriasis	259	7	2.7
Others	7 442	274	3.7
Total	22 757	2753	12.1

the women had been sensitized by propolis contained in ointments of various kinds [63].

The comparatively low incidence of allergy in subjects with chronic forms of dermatitis, such as atopic dermatitis and psoriasis, must also be emphasized. This supports the view that atopic and psoriatic subjects do not easily develop contact allergy, and that in spite of the most abundant use of topical preparations they are not a high-risk group as regards the development of medicament allergy [52, 64, 65].

Table 14.2.4. Cross-sensitizing medicament groups

---

p-Aminophenol compounds (para-group)
Aminoglycoside antibiotics
Phenothiazines
p-Hydroxybenzoic acid esters
Halogenated hydroxyquinolines
Penicillins and breakdown products
Halogenated salicylanilides
Ethylenediamine and related antihistamines
Imidazoles
Quaternary ammonium compounds
Nonsteroidal antiinflammatory drugs
Antiviral agents
Corticosteroids
Hydroquinone derivatives
Piperazine derivatives
Paranitro compounds
Thiuram sulphides (in scabicides and disinfectants)

14.2.5 Cross-Sensitization

In relation to drug-induced dermatitis, if relapses or deterioration with spreading of eczema are to be avoided, knowledge of cross-sensitization is of importance. The phenomenon of cross-sensitization involves various groups of compounds (Table 14.2.4) [9]. A subject sensitized to benzocaine as the primary allergen may cross-react to related drugs (sulphonamides, procaine, tetracaine, butacaine, glyceryl *p*-aminobenzoate) and nondrugs (*p*-phenylenediamine and other *p*-amino dyes).

Other important cross-reacting groups are those of phenothiazines (promazine, promethazine, chlorpromazine), neomycin (kanamycin, framycetin, paromomycin, gentamicin, tobramycin) [66–68] and hydroxyquinolines (vioform, chlorquinaldol, 8-hydroxyquinoline, diiodohydroxyquin). Cross-responses have been reported, though more rarely, between various derivatives of hydroquinone, between imidazoles [69–77], between various parabens [78], between quaternary ammonium compounds, between thiuram sulphides (contained in rubber and in such topical medicaments as scabicides and disinfectants), between nonsteroidal antiinflammatory drugs [79], between halogen salicylanilides and between paranitro compounds [41, 80].

14.2.6 Systemic Contact Dermatitis

An often neglected aetiopathogenic aspect of allergic contact dermatitis is that of its maintenance, or of provocation of recurrence and of spread, of primarily allergic contact dermatitis by systemic administration of the same allergen or of a chemically similar substance. Numerous compounds, especially drugs, may be involved [12, 23, 31, 81, 82]. The drug in question may be taken by mouth, or given intravenously, by inhalation or percutaneously. Generally speaking, the clinical picture of systemic reaction is that of common eczema more or less widespread, with erythematous, vesicular and desquamative lesions. Sometimes specific manifestations are recorded. One of the most common is a dyshydrotic rash of the hands, with or without erythema, limited to the palms and to the palmar aspects of the fingers.

Another is that of an erythematous, oedematous, vesicular rash, either widespread or localized symmetrically to the axillae, eyelids and flexural folds of the elbows, neck and genitals. Occasionally, generalization of contact dermatitis may be recorded, mimicking erythema-multiforme-like, purpuric and vasculitis-like eruptions. In some patients on oral exposure tests we recorded recrudescence of patch test reactions. Under special circumstances systemic manifestations may develop, such as headache, fever, nausea, vomiting and diarrhoea.

The pathogenic mechanism of systemic reactions is still obscure. A provocation test with the responsible hapten promptly produces the reaction, usually within 6–12 h [83, 84]. This, combined with some other clinical observations mentioned above, suggests the operation of a mixed immunological mechanism, types III and IV. However, the few available relevant experimental data have not clarified the problem; the role of circulating immune complexes, raised by several authors, found no confirmation in our study [30].

Usually a systemic reaction arises in a subject previously sensitized by the topical route. The opposite may also occur, i.e. an antibiotic-induced exanthem may be followed by localized dermatitis induced by topical use of the drug (primary endogenic contact eczema) [85]. Table 14.2.5 lists the drugs and chemically related compounds capable of inducing systemic contact dermatitis. The antibiotics relatively frequently used topically are neomycin, chloramphenicol, and, still today in some countries, penicillin. In subjects sensitized to them by topical application, their oral or parenteral administration may cause systemic reaction. In a case of allergic contact dermatitis from penicillin, relapses of the same dermatitis were recorded after ingestion of small amounts of the antibiotic in milk [86].

Recurrences of systemic sulphonamide-induced allergic contact dermatitis, occurring either spontaneously or demonstrated on oral testing, were recorded by us in diabetics treated with sulphonamide derivatives (sulphonylureas: carbutamide, tolbutamide, chlorpropamide). Certain sulphonamide derivatives, such as sulphamethoxazole, must also be avoided in sulphonamide-sensitive persons [83, 87]. In contrast, certain other compounds (diamino diphenylsulphone, salicyl azosulphapyridine) given by mouth to the same patients usually cause no reactions [83, 88].

Nowadays ethylenediamine is one of the most common sensitizers. It is employed in various industrial processes and as a stabilizer in various topical antimycotic and antibiotic preparations, responsible for a large number

Table 14.2.5. Topical medicaments responsible for contact allergy and chemically related systemic medicaments that can produce systemic contact dermatitis

Topical medicament	Related systemic medicaments
Neomycin	Kanamycin
	Paromomycin
	Gentamicin
	Framycetin
Chloramphenicol	Chloramphenicol
Penicillin	Penicillin compounds
Hydroxyquinolines	Iodochlorhydroxyquin
Streptomycin	Streptomycin
Sulphonamide	Procaine
	Para-amino salicylic acid
	Azo dyes in drugs and foods
	Tolbutamide
	Carbutamide
	Chlorpropamide
	Sulphamethoxazole
Glyceryl PABA sunscreens	Same as sulphonamide
Ethylenediamine	Aminophylline
	Ethylenediamine antihistamines
Mercury	Organic and inorganic mercury compounds
Benzocaine	Same as sulphonamide
Promethazine	Phenothiazine antihistamines
Nitroglycerin	Nitroglycerin
Imidazoles	Imidazoles
Nonsteroidal antiinflammatory drugs	Nonsteroidal antiinflammatory drugs
Propylene glycol	Propylene glycol in foods
Capsaicin in ointments and plasters	Capsicum (*Capsicum frutescens*)
Methyl salicylate	Acetylsalicylic acid
Alprenolol	Alprenolol
Clonidine	Clonidine
Corticosteroids	Corticosteroids
Ephedrine	Pseudoephedrine, norephedrine
Nystatin	Nystatin
Acyclovir	Acyclovir

of cases of dermatitis. Ethylenediamine sensitization gives rise to special problems in patients with asthma receiving injections of theophylline [8, 89, 90]. Injectable theophylline is available only in the form of aminophylline, which is a combination of theophylline and ethylenediamine hydrochloride. Certain oral preparations of theophylline also contain ethylenediamine hydrochloride. In subjects with contact allergy to ethylenediamine, either oral or parenteral administration of aminophylline may cause generalized dermatitis.

Of our series of 14884 patients, 445 (3.0%) showed reactions to ethylenediamine. In order to avoid recurrences of preexisting contact dermatitis, patients with allergy to ethylenediamine should also avoid the systemic use of certain antihistamines derived from ethylenediamine, such as tripelennamines, antazoline, methapyrilene, hydroxyzine and pyrilamine [12].

Subjects with contact allergy to nonsteroidal antiinflammatory agents (oxyphenbutazone, bufexamac, ketoprofen), should not be given the same drugs systemically because of the risk of serious generalized cutaneous reactions. The same applies also to cases of hypersensitivity to certain imidazole derivatives, such as miconazole and econazole.

Systemic reactions to drugs may also occur in subjects with allergic contact dermatitis linked to chemically similar nonmedicinal substances. This is observed in patients with contact allergy to tetramethylthiuram disulphide given Antabuse (tetraethylthiuram disulphide) for the treatment of alcoholism [31], and in patients with allergy to paraphenylenediamine after oral administration of azo dyes [83, 91] or of drugs of the para group.

Finally, subjects with allergic contact dermatitis induced by capsaicin, contained in antirheumatic rubefacients (Fig. 14.2.6) and analgesic plasters, are at risk of generalized allergic reactions after ingestion of capsicum-containing foods commonly used in Mediterranean countries [92].

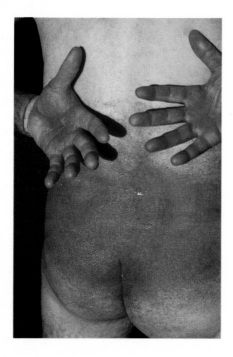

Fig. 14.2.6. Allergic contact dermatitis of the lumbosacral region and palms due to antirheumatic cream containing capsaicin

14.2.7 Sensitizers

Almost all medicaments applied to damaged skin are capable of causing sensitization of variable intensity. The list of topical preparations commonly responsible for such sensitization varies from one country to another, depending on the local customs, and also in time, depending on discoveries made by the pharmaceutical industry and on increasing recognition of the sensitizing potential of topical agents.

Table 14.2.6 shows the incidence of contact allergy to a group of medicaments recorded by us in four different periods (1968–1977, 1978–1983, 1984–1988 and 1989–1992). The changes observed over the years in Italy provide a good idea of the trends in operation. The five most common sensitizers in Italy in the past were sulphonamide, neomycin, benzocaine, promethazine and penicillin. Now the list is headed by ethylenediamine and neomycin. At the same time the increased topical use of new drugs brought to light reactions to other compounds, such as nonsteroidal antiinflammatory agents, some antimycotics, propylene glycol and benzoyl peroxide. Similar points are discussed by Fisher [93] in connection with topical medicaments.

Table 14.2.6. Incidence of contact allergy to some medicaments and components in 22757 patients with dermatitis

Substance	1968–1977 ($n = 3758$)	1978–1983 ($n = 4472$)	1984–1988 ($n = 6654$)	1989–1992 ($n = 7873$)
Sulphonamide	8.2%	0.2%	0.03%	0.02%
Neomycin	7.3%	3.1%	1.6%	1.2%
Benzocaine	6.9%	2.9%	1.1%	0.6%
Promethazine	4.9%	1.6%	0.4%	0.1%
Penicillin	4.6%	0.6%	0.3%	0.1%
Chloramphenicol	2.8%	0.2%	0.4%	0.2%
Ethylenediamine HCl	2.9%	3.3%	3.2%	1.3%
Parabens	2.7%	2.5%	1.1%	0.8%
Wool alcohols	2.6%	2.6%	1.2%	1.0%

Topical drugs capable of inducing allergic contact dermatitis are listed in the Appendix to this section. For a more complete list, the reader is referred to well-known relevant manuals [22–24]. Below, we list only the most common sensitizers divided into groups according to their clinical use and functional characteristics.

Antimicrobials. The substances can induce allergy when applied to healthy skin, as in the case of cosmetic preparations. Yet, sensitization by preservatives arises especially from the use of topical medicaments employed on eczematous or otherwise damaged skin. The most commonly used antimicrobials are parabens, sorbic acid, quaternary ammonium compounds, formaldehyde and formaldehyde-releasing agents, and organic mercury compounds [94].

The parabens (alkyl esters of *p*-hydroxybenzoic acid), the most widely used preservatives, are weak sensitizers and induce allergy more particularly when applied to stasis ulcers [47, 52, 78]. Subjects sensitized by parabens-containing topical medicaments tolerate well parabens-containing cosmetic preparations applied to healthy skin ('parabens paradox') [95].

Less common sensitizers are resorcinol, chlorocresol, chloroacetamide, chlorhexidine, and proflavine.

Merthiolate (thimerosal) is used in vaccines, antitoxins and diluents for the preparation of antigens for prick or intradermal testing, but also in various ophthalmic preparations and contact lens solutions. The allergic reaction may induce conjunctivitis and/or eyelid dermatitis [58].

Antibiotics and Chemotherapeutics. Among antibiotics, the most common sensitizers are neomycin and drugs closely related to it chemically [66–68], and chloramphenicol [96]. Contact allergy to penicillin occurs only in certain countries [8]; in Italy it has become very rare. Sensitization to cephalosporins [97] and semisynthetic penicillins [98] has been reported among health professionals.

Topical exposure to sulphonamide is still possible but is less common than in the past [8]. Streptomycin is not now used topically, but occupational sensitization is possible.

It must be emphasized that the topical use of these antibiotics should be avoided, inasmuch as the development of contact allergy may be very detrimental to the patient when the drug has to be used systemically. The relatively 'safe' topical antibiotics are the tetracyclines, sodium fusidate and erythromycin [99].

Antihistamines. These drugs, still employed topically in certain countries, are potent photoallergens. Particularly active allergens are antihistamines derived from ethylenediamine (antazoline, methapyrilene, pyrilamine, tripelennamine) and phenothiazines (promethazine hydrochloride). The former group also exhibit cross-sensitization within the group, as well as with ethylenediamine and aminophylline. Because of their high and often-exhibited sensitizing potential the topical use of these drugs should be discontinued.

Local Anaesthetics. The principal sensitizers are benzoic acid derivatives (benzocaine, amethocaine, procaine and dibucaine). These are often contained in topical preparation for haemorrhoids, in ointments for the treatment of burns and in eye lotions. They cross-react within the group and with compounds of the para group. Carbocaine has not exhibited sensitizing activity and lidocaine is a rare sensitizer [100].

Positive reactions to benzocaine are not necessarily due to the direct use of the topical anaesthetic and may represent the phenomenon of cross-sensitization with compounds of similar chemical structure. In those cases benzocaine must be considered as a detector of allergy to para group substances.

Antimycotic Agents. The allergic potential of various antimycotic agents is well recognized. They include hydroxyquinolines, esters of hydroxybenzoic acid (parabens), undecylenic acid, halogenated phenol compounds, nystatin, clotrimazole, tolfnaftate and naftifine. Allergic reactions are being reported nowadays to certain imidazole derivatives [69–77], such as miconazole, econazole, sulconazole, oxiconazole, and to pyrrolnitrin [8, 41, 42]. Allergic contact dermatitis from pyrrolnitrin generally develops at the site of tinea cruris and extends secondarily to the trunk and limbs in the form of well-circumscribed lesions of the erythema multiforme type. From 1975 to 1988 we recorded 84 such cases (81 arising in tinea cruris, two in tinea manuum and one in tinea versicolor) and one case of irritant contact dermatitis in a baby of 7 months with napkin dermatitis.

Analgesic and Antiinflammatory Agents. The recent introduction of topical preparations of analgesic and nonsteroidal antiinflammatory agents produced new forms of contact allergy, i.e., to oxyphenbutazone, bufexamac, ibuproxam, ketoprofen, benzydamine hydrochloride and indomethacin. In addition to cross-sensitization within the group, these compounds have a strong photosensitizing potential. The resulting clinical picture is often of the erythema-oedema-vesiculation type or of the erythema multiforme type. Patients sensitized to these drugs by local application are denied their systemic use because of the risk of severe generalized reactions [92].

Corticosteroids. Topical corticosteroids give rise to numerous dermatological complications, but contact sensitization had seemed to be rare. However, the true incidence of such sensitization may have been underestimated for various reasons [101]. The antiinflammatory effect of the corticosteroid may mask contact allergy to the corticosteroid itself or to another constituent of the topical preparation. In such cases the sensitization may manifest itself either in the skin's failure to heal or in the development of distant eczematous lesions. The low concentration of the corticosteroid in the preparation may induce allergic contact dermatitis at the site of its application, but with a negative patch test on intact skin ('cutaneous paradox'). The bioavailability of a corticosteroid in petrolatum is lower than that of commercial preparations; consequently, a corticosteroid contained in a commercial preparation may induce allergic contact dermatitis but the same corticosteroid used in a neutral vehicle may patch test negatively. A further complication is introduced by the absence of vehicle and concentration standardization. It is usually maintained in this respect, however, that a concentration higher (1%–10%) than that in clinical use and special vehicles, such as ethanol, are necessary (Fig. 14.2.7); dilutions in petrolatum can give false-negative reactions. Finally, data on the possibility of corticosteroid cross-allergy are still far from unequivocal.

Contact allergy to corticosteroids must therefore be considered in any case of dermatitis apparently resistant to treatment. In certain cases the dermatitis is localized to the legs and arises in relation to stasis ulcers. The most commonly reported sensitizers among the topical corticosteroids to date are clobetasol propionate, tixocortol pivalate, amcinonide and hydrocortisone [102–104].

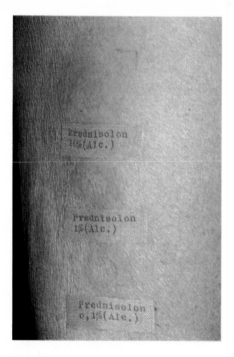

Fig. 14.2.7. Positive patch test reactions to prednisolone in ethanol at three different concentrations. (Courtesy of P.J. Frosch)

Vehicle Constituents. The bases and the various constituents of topical preparations may give rise to contact irritant or allergy. The allergens most often involved are lanolin, balsam of Peru, triethanolamine (in antirheumatic liniments and rubefacients), propylene glycol, and ethylenediamine. Among the additives, dyes and fragrances must not be forgotten.

Propylene glycol (1,2-propanediol) is a viscous hygroscopic liquid used in industry. It is employed also as a wetting agent, solvent, keratolytic and preservative in pharmaceutical preparations for topical (mainly corticosteroid creams and gels) and systemic (syrups, injectable formulations) use. It may induce irritant or allergic reactions [105, 106]. For patch testing, low concentrations (1%–10%) are recommended in order to avoid irritant reactions. Some authors, however, have advocated higher concentrations (20%–50%) propylene glycol in water) in order not to miss cases of contact allergy [107, 108]. Induced and spontaneous systemic reactions after oral administration of propylene glycol have been reported in subjects with preexisting contact dermatitis [12].

Balsams. Various ointments for burns and antirheumatic liniments, plasters and suppositories contain balsamic compounds, such as balsam of Peru, balsam of Tolu and tincture of benzoin. These cross-react among themselves as well as with other balsamic substances.

Tars. Though rarely, tars of both vegetable or mineral origin may induce allergic contact reactions and, in addition, may cause photosensitization.

Benzoyl Peroxide. This antimicrobial and keratolytic agent is used in the treatment of acne, but it is also present in foods and employed in the

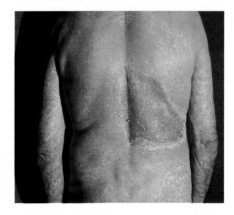

Fig. 14.2.8. Allergic contact dermatitis and secondary generalized eruption due to tromantadine used for treatment of thoracic herpes zoster

production of plastics. It has also proved effective in the treatment of leg ulcers. Its irritant and sensitizing potential is quite well-known [109]. In spite of its very wide use, its incidence of contact allergy in acne is low, but it is much higher in cases of leg ulcers [110].

Antiviral Agents. Allergic reactions have been reported to idoxuridine, acyclovir, and especially to tromantadine (Fig. 14.2.8). The fact that, in spite of their very wide use, reports of allergic reactions are only few suggests that these drugs are rather weak sensitizers [111]. Some possibility exists of cross-reactions between idoxuridine and trifluorthymidine and between tromantadine and amantadine used as an antiparkinsonian agent.

Scabicides. Mesulphen (2,7-dimethylthiantrene) is well-recognized as a cause of contact allergy, but more often it induces contact irritation due to unnecessarily prolonged and inappropriate use by the patient on his or her own initiative. Benzyl benzoate seems to have a minor irritant and sensitizing potential [112].

Adhesive tape. A large majority of adhesive tapes contain colophony, and other allergens include plasticizers, antioxidants and rubber accelerators. Modern tapes may contain acrylic monomers and epoxy resins and hardeners that can cause allergic reactions [24, 113]. Colophony is also contained in some wart removers [114] and in materials used in dental technology [24]. Clinical diagnosis of allergic contact dermatitis from adhesive tape is easy, as the erythematous and vesicular lesions are always more or less limited to the contact area.

Transdermal Drug Delivery Systems. Contact allergy has been reported to nitroglycerin, oestradiol, clonidine and scopolamine in such systems [115]. Excipients or adhesives can sensitize, as well as the active drug.

Other Topical Drugs. In addition to the drugs listed above there exist a great number of other medicaments capable of inducing contact allergy, such as Hirudoid [8, 116], 5-fluorouracil [117], minoxidil [118], salicyclic acid [119], zinc pyrithione [20], dithranol [121], dexpanthenol [122], chlorpromazine [123], polidocanol (Thesit: a topical anaesthetic and antipruritic) [124], tolazoline [125], and ammonium bituminosulphonate [126].

14.2.8 Patch Tests

In addition to the appropriate standard series, patients with contact dermatitis should be tested with all the medicaments that they have applied: consequently, a detailed history is of the utmost importance.

Direct testing with topical commercial preparations may give false-negative reactions, inasmuch as their concentrations of active drugs and of other ingredients are often lower than those required for patch testing. Sometimes, however, the commercial product produces a positive reaction, while the reactions to its individual constituents are negative; this may represent the phenomenon of so-called 'compound allergy' [127].

To facilitate clinical enquiry and to reduce the risk of recurrences, the manufacturers of topical preparations should be required to provide on the container a complete list of the constituents and their concentrations.

14.2.9 Prognosis and Prevention

Drug-induced contact dermatitis generally tends to recur for a variety of reasons. The same drug and, even more so, the same additives are present in various different commercial preparations, which renders prevention difficult. The problem is further complicated by cross-sensitization, especially between aminoglycosides and between compounds of the para group.

It is quite clear that, in order to prevent contact allergy, the topical use of powerful sensitizers and, in particular, of antibiotics such as penicillin must be avoided, especially in the presence of high-risk dermatoses (leg ulcers, injuries). Antibiotics can be used systemically, while local treatments should be restricted to preparations of bland antiseptics, or drugs with low or no sensitizing potential, such as sodium fusidate.

Topical use of sulphonamides and antihistamines should be discontinued: in the latter case their toxicity far exceeds their limited beneficial effects. In many countries these topical agents are available over the counter without prescription.

It is essential, finally, that the patient is given detailed and comprehensive instructions as to the use of topical preparations and is fully informed as to the alternatives to agents to which he or she has become sensitized [128].

14.2.10 Appendix: Topical Drugs Capable of Inducing Allergic Contact Dermatitis

---

Anaesthetics (local)

Amethocaine (tetracaine)	Benzocaine
Amylocaine	Butacaine
Benzamine lactate	Butethamine

Cinchocaine
Dibucaine hydrochloride
Diperocaine
Falicain (propipocaine)
Lignocaine (lidocaine)
Mepivacaine
Pramocaine
Prilocaine
Procaine (novocaine)
Propanidid
Proparacaine

*Antibiotic and antibacterial
compounds*

Acriflavine
Azidamphenicol
Bacitracin
Chloramphenicol
Chlorfenicone
Chlortetracycline
Clindamycin
Cycloheximide
Dihydrostreptomycin
Erythromycin stearate
Framycetin
Fucidin (sodium fusidate)
Gentamicin sulphate
Isonicotinic acid hydrazide
Kanamycin
Lincomycin
Mafenide
Neomycine sulphate
Nitrofurazone
Oxytetracycline
Paromomycin
Penicillin
Polymyxin B
Pristinamycin
Rifamycin
Streptomycin
Sulfonamide
Tetracycline
Tobramycin
Tyrothricin

Virginiamycin
Xanthocillin

Antihistamines

Antazoline
Brompheniramine
Chlorcyclizine
Chlorothen citrate
Chlorpheniramine maleate
Chlorpromazine
Diethylenetriamine
Diphenhydramine
Mepyramine
Methapyrilene hydrochloride
Perphenazine
Pheniramine
Piperazine
Promethazine hydrochloride
Pyribenzamine
Pyrilamine maleate
Tripelennamine

Antimitotic compounds

Chlorambucil
5-Fluorouracil
Mechlorethamine hydrochloride
Nitrogen mustard
Triaziquone

Antimycotic compounds

Benzoic acid
5-Bromo-4-chlorosalicylanilide
Chlordantoin
Chlorphenesin
Chlorquinaldol (Sterosan)
Clophenoxide
Clotrimazole
Croconazole hydrochloride
Dibenzthione
3,5-Dichloro-4-fluoro-
thiocarbanilide
Diiodohydroxyquin
Econazole
Enilconazole

Haloprogin
8-Hydroxyquinoline
Iodochlorhydroxyquin (Vioform)
Isoconazole
Ketoconazole
Miconazole
Naftifine
Nifuratel
Nystatin
Oxiconazole
Pecilocin
Pimaricine
Pyrrolnitrin
Sulconazole nitrate
Tolnaftate
Undecylenic acid
Zinc undecylenate

Antiparasitic drugs

Acetarsol
Benzyl benzoate
Crotamiton
Mesulphen
Monosulfiram

Corticosteriods

Aclomethasone
Amcinonide
Betamethasone
Betamethasone valerate
Budesonide
Clobetasol propionate
Clobetasone butyrate
Cortisone
Desonide
Desoxymethasone
Diflucortolone valerate
Fluocinolone acetonide
Fluocinonide
Fluocortolone
Halcinonide
Hydrocortisone
Hydrocortisone acetate
Hydrocortisone alcohol
Hydrocortisone butyrate

Hydrocortisone succinate
Methylprednisolone
Methylprednisolone acetate
Prednisolone
Prednisone
Tixocortol pivalate
Triamcinolone
Triamcinolone acetonide

Dyes (triphenylmethane)

Brilliant green
Crystal violet
Eosin
Gentian violet
Malachite green
Rosaniline

*Plant-derived substances
in topical drugs*

Abietic acid
Arnica tincture
Balsam of Peru
Balsam of Tolu
Beeswax
Benzoin tincture
Bergamot oil
Chamomile oil
Colophony
Coumarin
Eugenol
Gums (karaya, acacia, tragacanth)
Linseed
Niaouli oil
Storax
Terpineol
Turpentine
Turpentine peroxides
Thyme oil
Wood tar

*Preservatives:
antimicrobials and antioxidants*

Benzyl alcohol
Bismuth

Bithionol
Bronopol
Butylated hydroxyanisole
Butylated hydroxytoluene
Chloroacetamide
Chlorhexidine gluconate
Chlorocresol
Chloroxylenol
Dichlorophene
Ethyl alcohol
Fenticlor
Formaldehyde
Glutaraldehyde
Hexachlorophene
Imidazolidinyl urea
Iodine
Mercurial compounds
    Ammoniated mercury
    Mercuric chloride
    Mercurochrome
    Phenylmercuric acetate
    Phenylmercuric borate
    Phenylmercuric nitrate
Thimerosal
Nitrofural
Parabens
Povidone-iodine
Proflavine
Propyl gallate
Quaternary ammonium compounds
    Benzalkonium chloride
    Benzethonium chloride
    Cetalkonium chloride
Sodium benzoate
Sorbic acid
Tetrachlorsalicylanilide
Triclocarban
Triclosan (Irgasan DP 300)
Usnic acid
Zinc pyrithione

Vehicle constituents

Carbowaxes
Castor oil
Cetyl alcohol

Ethylenediamine hydrochloride
Ethylenediamine tetraacetate
Ethylene glycol
Eucerin
Glycerol
Lanette N
Lanette O
Lanette wax
Lanolin
Oleyl alcohol
Petrolatum
Polyethylene glycol
Propylene glycol
Sesame oil
Sodium lauryl sulphate
Stearyl alcohol
Triethanolamine

Vitamins

Vitamin A acid (retinoic acid)
Vitamin B1 (thiamine)
Vitamin E (tocopherol)
Vitamin K1
Vitamin K3
Vitamin K4

Miscellaneous drugs

Acyclovir
Alprenolol
Ammonium bituminosulphonate
Apomorphine
Benzophenones (sunscreens)
Benzoyl peroxide
Benzydamine hydrochloride
Bufexamac
Capsicum
Cerumenex
Centelase
Cetrimide
p-Chlorobenzenesulphonylglycolic
acid nitrile
Chromonar hydrochloride
Clonidine
Dexpanthenol
Dithranol

Dimercaprol (BAL)
Diphencyprone
Ephedrine
Epinephrine
Furacin
Heparinoid
Hirudoid
Hydroxyphenylbutazone
Ichthyol
Idoxuridine
Indomethacin
Ketoprofen
Meclofenoxate
Mephenesin
8-Methoxypsoralen
Minoxidil
Methyl salicylate
Monobenzyl ether of hydroquinone
Mustard oil
Nitroglycerin
Oestradiol
Oxyphenbutazone
Phenoxybenzamine

Phenylbutazone
Phepzazone
Piperazine
Polidocanol (Thesit)
Practolol
Proflavine
Propolis
Propranolol
Quinidine sulphate
Quinine sulphate
Resorcinol
Salicyclic acid
Scopolamine
Spiramycin
Stilboestrol
Suxybuzone
Tar, coal
Thioxolone
Tolazoline
Triafur
Triton X45
Tromantadine
Tetramethylthiuram disulphide

14.2.11 References

1. Bandmann HJ (1966) Die Kontaktallergie gegen Arzeimittel. Pharmatic 111: 1470–1475
2. Meneghini CL, Rantuccio F, Lomuto M (1971) Additives, vehicles and active drugs of topical medicaments as causes of delayed-type allergic dermatitis. Dermatologica 143: 137–147
3. Bandmann HJ, Calnan CD, Cronin E, Fregert S, Hjorth N, Magnusson B, Maibach HJ, Malten E, Meneghini CL, Pirilä V, Wilkinson DS (1972) Dermatitis from applied medicaments. Arch Dermatol 106: 335–337
4. Meneghini CL, Lomuto M, Angelini G, Rantuccio F (1973) Dermatiti allergiche di tipo eczematoso. G Ital Dermatol 108: 195–208
5. Blondeel A, Oleffe J, Achten G (1978) Contact allergy in 330 dermatological patients. Contact Dermatitis 4: 270–276
6. Wilkinson JD, Hambly EM, Wilkinson DS (1980) Comparison of patch test results in two adjacent areas of England. I. Medicaments. Acta Derm Venereol (Stockh) 60: 245–249
7. Meneghini CL, Angelini G (1982) Le dermatiti da contatto. Lombardo, Rome
8. Angelini G, Vena GA, Meneghini CL (1985) Allergic contact dermatitis to some medicaments. Contact Dermatitis 12: 263–269
9. Wilkinson JD, Rycroft RJG (1986) Contact dermatitis. In: Rook A, Wilkinson DS, Ebling FJG, Champion RH, Burton JL (eds) Textbook of dermatology, 4th edn. Blackwell, Oxford

10. Rudner EJ (1977) North American group results. Contact Dermatitis 3: 208–209
11. Husain SL (1977) Contact dermatitis in the west of Scotland. Contact Dermatitis 3: 327–332
12. Fisher AA (1982) Contact dermatitis from topical medicaments. Semin Dermatol 1: 49–57
13. Dooms-Goossens A (1982) Allergic contact dermatitis to ingredients used in topically applied pharmaceutical products and cosmetics. Thesis, Catholic University of Leuven
14. Edman B, Möller H (1986) Medicament contact allergy. Berufsdermatosen 34: 139–143
15. Dupuis G, Benezra C (1982) Allergic contact dermatitis to simple chemicals. A molecular approach. Dekker, New York
16. Schaefer H, Zesch A, Stüttgen G (1982) Skin permeability. Springer, Berlin Heidelberg New York
17. Barry BW (1982) Dermatological formulations. Percutaneous absorption. Dekker, New York
18. Angelini G, Vena GA (1989) La cute: organo di assorbimento. In: Morganti P, Muscardin L (eds) Dermatologia cosmetologica. Ediemme, Rome
19. Fregert S (1981) Manual of contact dermatitis, 2nd edn. Munksgaard, Copenhagen
20. Marks JG, Rainey MA (1984) Cutaneous reactions to surgical preparations and dressings. Contact Dermatitis 10: 1–5
21. Hostynek JJ, Patrick E, Younger B, Maibach HI (1989) Hypochlorite sensitivity in man. Contact Dermatitis 20: 32–37
22. Cronin E (1980) Contact dermatitis. Livingstone, Edinburgh
23. Nater JP, de Groot AC (1985) Unwanted effects of cosmetics and drugs used in dermatology, 2nd edn. Elsevier, Amsterdam
24. Fisher AA (1986) Contact dermatitis, 3rd edn. Lea and Febiger, Philadelphia
25. Lathi A (1980) Non-immunological contact urticaria. Acta Derm Venereol [Suppl 91] (Stockh) 60: 1–49
26. Von Krogh G, Maibach HI (1981) The contact urticaria syndrome – an updated review. J Am Acad Dermatol 5: 328–339
27. Von Krogh G, Maibach HI (1982) The contact urticaria syndrome. In: Kligman AM, Leyden JJ (eds) Safety and efficacy of topical drugs and cosmetics. Grune and Stratton, New York
28. Von Krogh G, Maibach HI (1982) The contact urticaria syndrome. Semin Dermatol 1: 59–66
29. Lahti A, Maibach HI (1991) Immediate contact reactions: contact urticaria and the contact urticaria syndrome. In: Marzulli FN, Maibach HI (eds) Dermatotoxicology, 4th edn. Hemisphere, Washington
30. Dooms-Goossens A, Deleu H (1991) Airborne contact dermatitis: an update. Contact Dermatitis 25: 211–217
31. Angelini G, Vena GA (1992) Airborne contact dermatitis. Clin Dermatol 10: 123–131
32. Meneghini CL, Angelini G (1981) Secondary polymorphic eruptions in allergic contact dermatitis. Dermatologica 163: 63–70
33. Meneghini CL, Angelini G (1985) Eczémas de contact allergiques et réactions par voie générale á l'allérgéne. Med Hyg 43: 879–886
34. Fisher AA (1986) Erythema multiforme-like eruptions due to topical medications. II. Cutis 37: 198–160
35. Lembo G, Balato N, Patruno C, Pini D, Ayala F (1987) Lichenoid contact dermatitis due to aminoglycoside antibiotics. Contact Dermatitis 17: 122–123
36. Horio T (1975) Chlorpromazine photoallergy; co-existence of immediate and delayed type. Arch Dermatol 111: 1469–1471
37. Lovell CR, Cronin E, Rhodes EL (1986) Photocontact urticaria from chlorpromazine. Contact Dermatitis 14: 290–291

38. Wall LM (1982) Lymphomatoid contact dermatitis due to ethylenediamine dihydro-chloride. Contact Dermatitis 8: 51–54
39. Burkhart CG (1981) Pustular allergic contact dermatitis: a distinct clinical and patho-logical entity. Cutis 27: 630–631, 638
40. De Kort WJA, de Groot AC (1989) Clindamycin allergy presenting as rosacea. Con-tact Dermatitis 20: 72–73
41. Meneghini CL, Angelini G (1975) Contact dermatitis from pyrrolnitrin (an antimy-cotic agent). Contact Dermatitis 1: 288–292
42. Meneghini CL, Angelini G (1982) Contact dermaatitis from pyrrolnitrin. Contact Dermatitis 8: 55–58
43. Degreef H, Bonamie A, van Derheyden D, Dooms-Goossens A (1984) Mephe-nesin contact dermatitis with erythema multiforme features. Contact Dermatitis 10: 220–223
44. Stoltze R (1966) Dermatitis medicamentosa in eczema of the leg. Acta Derm Venereol (Stockh) 46: 54–64
45. Fisher AA (1971) The role of topical medications in the management of stasis ulcers. Angiology 22: 206–210
46. Malten KE, Kuiper JP, van der Staak WBJM (1973) Contact allergic investigations in 100 patients with ulcus cruris. Dermatologica 147: 241–254
47. Rudzki E, Baranoska E (1974) Contact sensitivity in stasis dermatitis. Dermatologica 148: 353–356
48. Angelini G, Rantuccio F, Meneghini CL (1975) Contact dermatitis in patients with leg ulcers. Contact Dermatitis 1: 81–87
49. Breit R (1977) Allergen change in stasis dermatitis. Contact Dermatitis 3: 309–311
50. Fraki JE, Peltonen L, Hopsu-Havu VK (1979) Allergy to various components of topical preparations in stasis dermatitis and leg ulcers. Contact Dermatitis 5: 97–100
51. Kokelj F, Cantarutti A (1986) Contact dermatitis in leg ulcers. Contact Dermatitis 15: 47–49
52. Wilkinson S, Wilkinson JD, Wilkinson DS (1987) Medicament contact dermatitis: risk sites. Boll Dermatol Allerg Prof 2: 21–28
53. Frosch PJ, Raulin C (1987) Kontaktallergie auf Bufexamac. Hautarzt 38: 331–334
54. Angelini G, Vena GA, Giglio G, Fiordalisi F, Meneghini CL (1986) Allergia da con-tatto e cute traumatizzata. Boll Dermatol Allerg Prof 1(2): 24–29
55. Angelini G, Meneghini CL (1975) Allergic contact dermatitis in a group of patients with perianal eczema. Contact Dermatitis 1: 183
56. Vena GA, Giglio G, Angelini G (1988) Allergia da contatto in sede anoperineale e genitale. Boll Dermatol Allerg Prof 3: 55–62
57. Lembo G, Nappa P, Balato N, Pucci V, Ayala F (1988) Contact sensitivity in otitis externa. Contact Dermatitis 19: 64–65
58. Tosti A, Tosti G (1988) Thimerosal: a hidden allergen in ophthalmology. Contact Dermatitis 18: 268–273
59. Ducombs G, de Casamayor J, Verin P, Maleville J (1986) Allergic contact dermatitis to phenylephrine. Contact Dermatitis 15: 107–108
60. Frosch PJ, Weickel R, Schmitt T, Krastel H (1988) Nebenwirkungen von ophthal-mologischen Externa. Z Hautkr 63: 126–136
61. Edman B (1985) Sites of contact dermatitis in relationship to particular allergens. Contact Dermatitis 13: 129–135
62. Edman B (1988) Computerized patch test data in contact dermatitis. Dissertation, University of Lund, Sweden
63. Schuler TM, Frosch PJ (1988) Kontaktallergie auf Propolis (Bienen-Kittharz). Hau-tarzt 39: 139–142
64. Angelini G, Vena GA, Meneghini CL (1987) Psoriasis and contact allergy to propolis. Contact Dermatitis 17: 252–253

65. Meneghini CL, Angelini G (1989) Atopic dermatitis, occupational and contact allergy. In: Maibach HI (ed) Urticaria and the exogenous dermatoses. Saunders, Philadelphia, pp 523–534 (Immunology and allergy of North America, vol 9)
66. Schorr W, Ridgway HB (1977) Tobramycin-neomycin cross-sensitivity. Contact Dermatitis 3: 133–137
67. Pirilä V, Hirvonen M, Rouhunkoski S (1986) The pattern of cross-sensitivity to neomycin. Dermatologica 136: 321–324
68. Rudzki E, Zakrzewski Z, Rebandel P, Grzywa Z, Hudymowicz W (1988) Cross reactions between aminoglycoside antibiotics. Contact Dermatitis 18: 314–316
69. Van Hecke E, Van Bradandt S (1981) Contact sensitivity to imidazole derivatives. Contact Dermatitis 7: 348–349
70. Raulin C, Frosch PJ (1987) Kontaktallergie auf Clotrimazole und Azidamfenicol. Berufsdermatosen 35: 64–66
71. Raulin C, Frosch PJ (1988) Contact allergy to imidazole antimycotics. Contact Dermatitis 18: 76–80
72. Perret CM, Happle R (1988) Contact allergy to miconazole. Contact Dermatitis 19: 75
73. Carmichael AJ, Foulds IS (1988) Imidazole cross-sensitivity to sulconazole. Contact Dermatitis 19: 237–238
74. Motley RJ, Reynolds AJ (1988) Contact allergy to 2,4-dichlorophenylethylimidazole derivatives. Contact Dermatitis 19: 381–382
75. Jelen G, Tennstedt D (1989) Contact dermatitis from topical imidazole antifungals: 15 new cases. Contact Dermatitis 21: 6–11
76. Shono M, Hayashi K, Sugimoto R (1989) Allergic contact dermatitis from croconazole hydrochloride. Contact Dermatitis 21: 225–227
77. Garcia-Bravo B, Maznecos J, Rodriguez-Pichardo A, Navas J, Camacho F (1989) Hypersensitivity to ketoconazole preparations: study of 4 cases. Contact Dermatitis 21: 346–348
78. Menne T, Hjorth N (1988) Routine patch testing with paraben esters. Contact Dermatitis 19: 189–191
79. Figueiredo A, Goncalo S, Freitas JD (1985) Contact sensitivity to pyrazolone compounds. Contact Dermatitis 13: 271
80. Eriksen K (1978) Cross allergy between paranitro compounds with special reference to DNCB and chloramphenicol. Contact Dermatitis 4: 29–32
81. Cronin E (1972) Contact dermatitis. XVII. Reactions to contact allergens given orally or sistemically. Br J Dermatol 86: 104–108
82. Menne T, Hjorth N (1982) Reactions from systemic exposure to contact allergens. Semin Dermatol 1: 15–24
83. Meneghini CL, Angelini G (1978) Gruppensensibilisierung durch photosensibilisierende Medikamente. Z Hautkr 53: 329–334
84. Angelini G, Meneghini CL (1981) Oral tests in contact allergy to paraamino compounds. Contact Dermatitis 7: 311–314
85. Pirilä V (1970) Endogenic contact eczema. Allerg Asthma 16: 15–19
86. Vickers HR, Bagratuni L, Alexander S (1985) Dermatitis caused by penicillin in milk. Lancet 1: 351–352
87. Fisher AA (1982) Systemic contact dermatitis from Orinase and Diabinese in diabetics with paraamino hypersensitivity. Cutis 29: 551–555
88. Angelini G, Meneghini CL, Vena GA (1982) Allergia da contatto e reazioni secondarie ad additivi alimentari. G Ital Dermatol Venereol 117: 195–198
89. Provost TT, Jillson OF (1967) Ethylenediamine contact dermatitis. Arch Dermatol 96: 231–234
90. Mohsenifar Z, Lehrlan S, Carson SA, Tashkin D (1982) Two cases of allergy to aminophylline. Ann Allergy 49: 281–282

91. Baer RL, Leider M (1949) The effects of feeding certified food azodyes in parapheny-lenediamine-hypersensitive subjects. J Invest Dermatol 13: 223–230
92. Meneghini CL, Angelini G (1979) Contact allergy to antirheumatic drugs. Contact Dermatitis 5: 197–198
93. Fisher AA (1982) Topical medicaments which are common sensitizers. Ann Allergy 49: 97–100
94. Hannuksela M, Kousa M, Pirilä V (1976) Allergy to ingredients of vehicles. Contact Dermatitis 2: 105–110
95. Fisher AA (1973) The paraben paradox. Cutis 12: 830–832
96. Van Joost T, Dikland W, Stolz E, Prens E (1986) Sensitization to chloramphenicol; a persistent problem. Contact Dermatitis 14: 176–178
97. Conde-Salazar L, Guimaraens D, Romero LV, Gonzales MA (1986) Occupational dermatitis from cephalosporins. Contact Dermatitis 14: 70–71
98. Moller NE, Nielsen B, von Würden K (1986) Contact dermatitis to semisynthetic penicillins in factory workers. Contact Dermatitis 14: 307–311
99. Fisher AA (1976) The safety of topical erythromycin. Contact Dermatitis 2: 43–44
100. Fregert S, Tegner E, Thelin I (1979) Contact allergy to lidocaine. Contact Dermatitis 5: 185–188
101. Dooms-Goossens A, Verschaeve H, Degreef H, van Berendoncks J (1986) Contact allergy to hydrocortisone and tixocortol pivalate: problems in the detection of corti-costeroid sensitivity. Contact Dermatitis 14: 94–102
102. Guin JD (1984) Contact sensitivity to topical corticosteroids. J Am Acad Dermatol 10: 773–782
103. Reitamo S, Lauerma AI, Stubb S, Käyhkö K, Visa K, Förström L (1986) Delayed hypersensitivity to topical corticosteroids. J Am Acad Dermatol 14: 582–589
104. Coopman S, Dooms-Goossens A (1988) Cross-reactions in topical corticosteroid con-tact dermatitis. Contact Dermatitis 19: 145–146
105. Angelini G, Meneghini CL (1981) Contact allergy from propylene glycol. Contact Dermatitis 7: 197–198
106. Trancik RJ, Maiback HI (1982) Propylene glycol: irritation or sensitization? Contact Dermatitis 8: 185–189
107. Hannuksela M, Salo H (1986) The repeated open application test (ROAT). Contact Dermatitis 14: 221–227
108. Frosch PJ, Pekar U, Enzmann H (1990) Contact allergy to propylene glycol. Do we use the appropriate test concentration? Dermatol Clin 8: 111–113
109. Haustein UF, Tegetmeyer L, Ziegler V (1985) Allergic and irritant potential of ben-zoyl peroxide. Contact Dermatitis 13: 252–257
110. Vena GA, Angelini G, Meneghini CL (1982) Contact dermatitis to benzoyl peroxide. Contact Dermatitis 8: 338
111. Angelini G, Vena GA, Meneghini CL (1986) Contact allergy to antiviral agents. Contact Dermatitis 15: 114–115
112. Meneghini CL, Vena GA, Angelini G (1982) Contact dermatitis to scabicides. Con-tact Dermatitis 8: 285–286
113. Jordan WP (1975) Cross-sensitization patterns in acrylate allergy. Contact Dermatitis 1: 13–15
114. Monk B (1987) Allergic contact dermatitis to colophony in a wart remover. Contact Dermatitis 17: 242
115. Holdiness MR (1989) A review of contact dermatitis associated with transdermal therapeutic systems. Contact Dermatitis 20: 3–9
116. Pecegueiro M, Brandao M, Pinto J, Goncalo S (1987) Contact dermatitis to Hirudoid cream. Contact Dermatitis 17: 290–293
117. Tennstedt D, Lachapelle JM (1987) Allergic contact dermatitis to 5-fluorouracil. Con-tact Dermatitis 16: 279–280

118. Valsecchi R, Cainelli T (1987) Allergic contact dermatitis from minoxidil. Contact Dermatitis 17: 58–59
119. Goh CL, Ng SK (1986) Contact sensitivity to salicylic acid. Contact Dermatitis 14: 114
120. Nigam PK, Tyagi S, Saxena AK, Misra RS (1988) Dermatitis from zinc pyrithione. Contact Dermatitis 19: 219
121. De Groot AC, Nater JP (1981) Contact allergy to dithranol. Contact Dermatitis 7: 5–8
122. Schulze-Dirks A, Frosch PJ (1988) Kontaktallergie auf Dexpanthenol. Hautarzt 39: 375–377
123. Von Ertle T (1982) Beruflich bedingte Kontakt- und Photokontaktallergie bei einem Landwirt durch Chlorpromazin. Berufsdermatosen 30: 120–122
124. Frosch PJ, Schulze-Dirks A (1989) Kontaktallergie durch Polidocanol (Thesit). Hautarzt 40: 146–149
125. Frosch PJ, Albert D, Weickel R (1985) Contact allergy to tolazoline. Contact Dermatitis 13: 272
126. Von Schwale M, Frosch PJ (1983) Kontaktallergie auf Ammoniumbituminosulfonat. Berufsdermatosen 31: 183–186
127. Kellett JK, King CM, Beck MH (1986) Compound allergy to medicaments. Contact Dermatitis 14: 45–48
128. Adams RM, Fisher AA (1986) Contact allergen alternatives: 1986. J Am Acad Dermatol 14: 951–969
129. Frosch PJ, Kligman AM (1977) A method for appraising the stinging capacity of topically applied substances. J Soc Cosmet Chem 28: 197–209

14.3 Clothing

JEAN FOUSSEREAU

Contents

14.3.1 Introduction

In the past 15 years, allergy from clothes and underclothes has become more infrequent, especially contact dermatitis due to textile resins, which used often to be caused by formaldehyde.

In fact, over the years, the patterns of clothing dermatitis have changed greatly owing to changes in fashion and leisure activities and technological developments. For instance, hat wearing having nearly gone completely out of fashion, allergy due to laurel oil used to gloss felt is now only a historical memento. It is the same with allergy to hairnet dyes, which is also no longer observed [1]. By contrast, cases of allergy to diving gear have become not uncommon as leisure activities have changed.

Regarding technology, allergy due to formaldehyde in clothing is now considerably less frequent, perhaps because the use of urea-formaldehyde and melamine-formaldehyde resins is rarer. Indeed, materials treated with dimethyloldihydroxyethylene-urea resins contain formaldehyde at concentrations 10–15 times lower than materials treated with melamine-formaldehyde resins. Moreover, better binding of dyes to textile fibres and the use of automatic washing machines have perhaps combined to make clothing dye allergy less frequent.

In addition, products chosen in industry have an influence on the frequency of clothing dermatitis. Cases of dermatitis from Tinopal CH 3566 [2] are no longer found, this optical brightener which used to be found in detergents for washing clothes no longer being marketed. Nor is allergy to mercaptobenzothiazole from spandex brassieres seen any longer. Spandex is a fibre made from polyurethane elastomer; one of its trade names is Lycra.

Textile fibres themselves, whether they are natural (cellulose based, e.g. cotton; protein based, e.g. silk or wool) or synthetic (e.g. polyamide – Nylon; polyester – Dacron; acrylic – Dralon, Courtelle), are not usually allergenic, though recently allergy has been described to the monomer of Nylon 6, epsilon-aminocaproic acid (EACA) [3]. Clothing or underwear allergies are more usually due to textile resins, dyes, rubber constituents or various other components.

Whenever clothing allergy is suspected, investigation should include both clinical examination of the patient and careful study of the article incriminated. A sample removed from the suspected article may prove useful, in case chemical analysis is needed. However, the article is not always kept by the patient. In 1893, for instance, Puy Le Blanc [4] reported the case of a patient with contact dermatitis from gloves. He had travelled by train the day before for 8 h, wearing his gloves throughout, but, when he arrived at the station, he threw them out of the door of the carriage.

14.3.2 Examination

14.3.2.1 Clinical Examination

Contact dermatitis caused by clothing generally resembles common allergic eczema. The purpuric dermatitis which suggested sensitization to isopropylphenyl p-phenylenediamine (IPPD) reported in 1968 by Batscharov and Minkov [5] in women intolerant to brassieres and girdles is no longer observed.

In the case of dermatitis to brassieres, girdles and sock elastics, the distribution of the lesions – sometimes geometric – is often suggestive. As early as 1899, a patient with foot dermatitis from sock dyes was described by Balzer und Gauchery [6]. The lesions had developed to form regularly spaced parallel bands separated by bands of normal skin. The patient was wearing striped new black socks, with transverse green, red and yellow stripes. The dermatitis lesions corresponding to the black and green stripes were separated by normal skin corresponding to the red and yellow stripes.

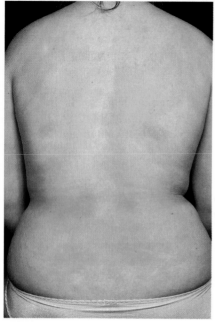

Fig. 14.3.1. Allergic contact dermatitis from clothing dye in black dress

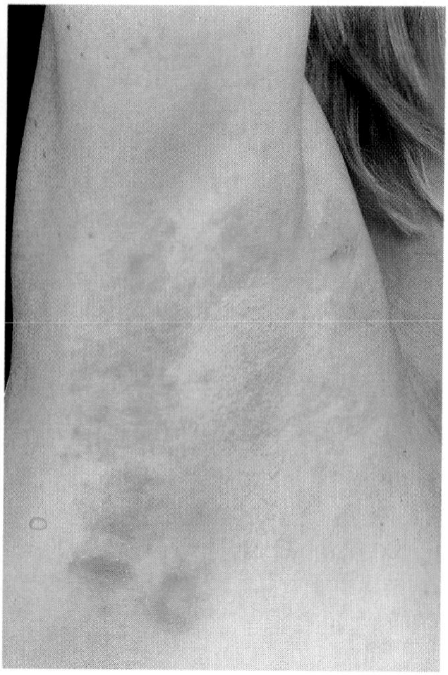

Fig. 14.3.2. Allergic contact dermatitis from clothing resin around axillary borders

Localization is often an important clinical feature: in patients allergic to trousers, dermatitis predominates on the thighs and lower legs. According to Sim-Davies [7], the dermatitis can generalize, and in about one half of patients allergic to trousers, the dorsa of the hands are involved, these areas being in contact with the cloth if the patient has a habit of keeping his hands in his pockets. In 1940, Epstein [8] reported a patient with lesions predominating on the genital area. In cases of allergy to blouses and dresses, the back is selectively affected (Fig. 14.3.1) (as regards dresses, lesions can also involve the posterior aspect of the thigh), with a barrier effect from any girdle or from the brassiere and its straps. According to Epstein [8], dermatitis from dresses predominates in the axillae, especially at their outer borders (Fig. 14.3.2), but it can also involve the neck, forearms and wrists. In cases of allergy to stockings or tights (pantyhose), erythematous, vesicular or even exudative lesions are most marked at sites of friction: popliteal fossae, mimicking atopic dermatitis, and dorsa of the feet or toes. Dermatitis from tights can be localized around the waist. Allergy to underpants is typical, an imprint of the garment being produced on the skin. P.Y. Castelain (1983, personal communication) reported the case of a diver whose linear lesions reproduced previous repairs of his diving suit with a neoprene glue.

In all cases of allergy to clothing, lesions can progress and generalize as long as contact with the allergen is not avoided.

14.3.2.2 Examination of the Garment

Examination of the garment, looking for a useful clue, requires careful thought. In 1953, cases of dermatitis from leather hat bands were reported in Germany. Patch tests with leather from these felt hats were always positive. The agent which was eventually found to be responsible, however, was *Laurus nobilis* oil used to gloss felt. The hats, piled up one upon another in the workshop, were being contaminated by the felt of the hat underneath [9].

14.3.3 The Allergens

14.3.3.1 Formaldehyde from Textile Resins

Two different types of resins are commonly used in the textile industry:
– Urea-formaldehyde resins and melamine-formaldehyde resins, which polymerize within the interstices of the fibres
– Resins obtained from cyclized urea derivatives, which combine directly with the fibre.

In the latter process, methylol (formaldehyde) groups of the resin crosslink with hydroxyl groups of the cellulose to form stable bonds. Compared to

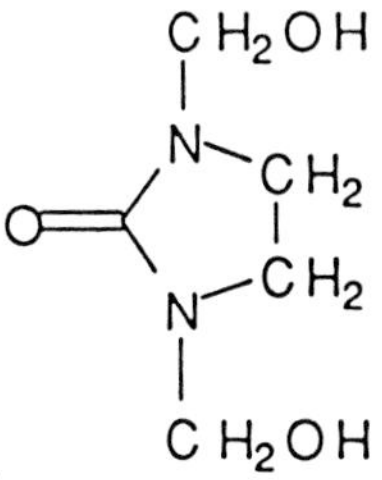

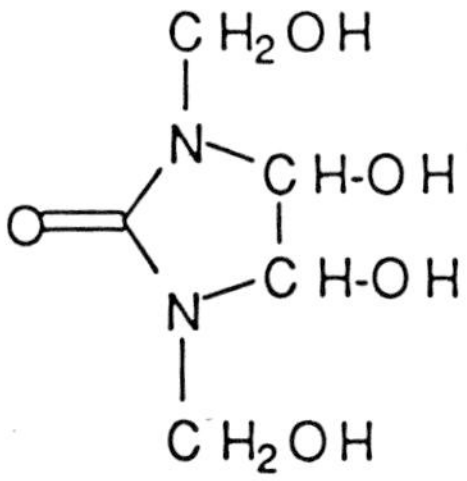

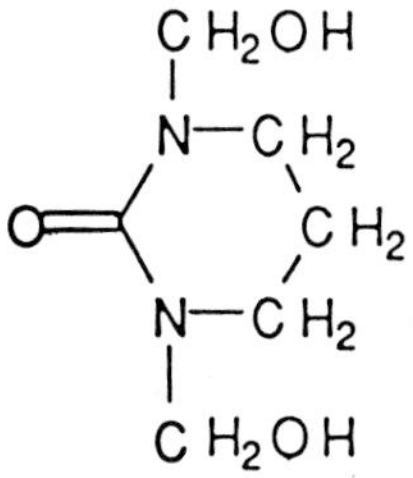

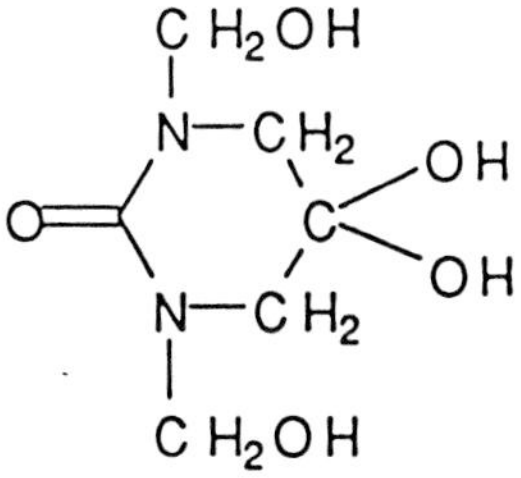

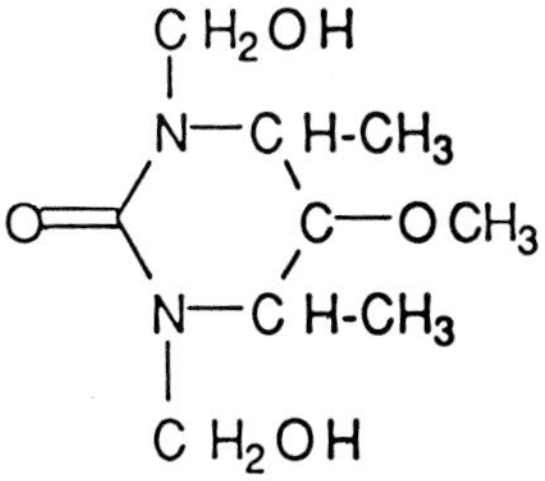

Fig. 14.3.3. Structure of cyclized urea derivatives used as resins

urea-formaldehyde and melamine-formaldehyde resins, a much lower amount of formaldehyde is released from the latter group of resins while manufacturing, storing or wearing the garment. Examples of resins that are cyclized urea derivatives are: dimethylolethylene urea, dimethyloldihydroxyethylene urea, dimethylolpropylene urea, dimethyloldihydroxypropylene urea and dimethylol-4-methoxy-5,5-dimethylpropylene urea (Fig. 14.3.3).

14.3.3.2 Textile Resins Themselves

Formaldehyde-negative patients may be positive to any of the urea-formaldehyde, melamine-formaldehyde or cyclized-urea derived resins.

14.3.3.3 Dyes

General Considerations. Dyes responsible for textile allergies belong, with a few exceptions, to the group of disperse dyes, which are plastosoluble and used for polyesters and acrylics. Disperse dyes causing allergy are classified into two groups: azo dyes and anthraquinone dyes. Azo dyes are characterized by a $R - N = N - R'$ structure and anthraquinone dyes are all based on anthraquinone (Fig. 14.3.4).

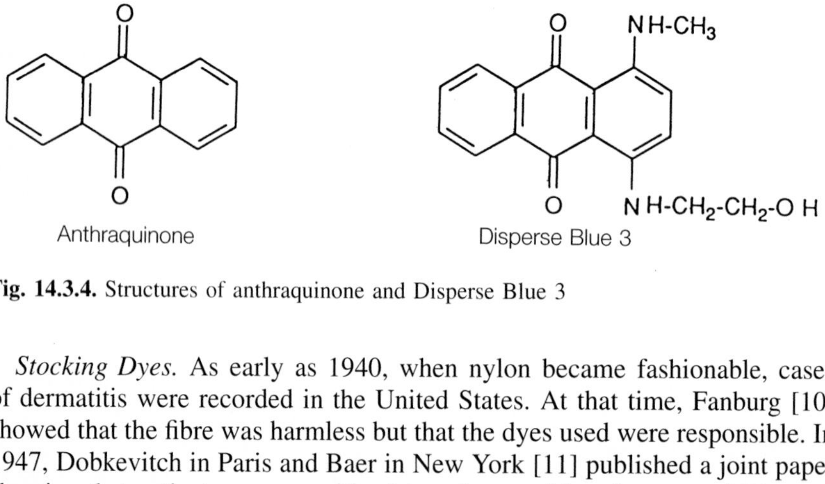

Anthraquinone   Disperse Blue 3

Fig. 14.3.4. Structures of anthraquinone and Disperse Blue 3

Stocking Dyes. As early as 1940, when nylon became fashionable, cases of dermatitis were recorded in the United States. At that time, Fanburg [10] showed that the fibre was harmless but that the dyes used were responsible. In 1947, Dobkevitch in Paris and Baer in New York [11] published a joint paper showing that patients were sensitized to nylon stockings because of Disperse Yellow 3 and Disperse Orange 3 (Fig. 14.3.5). Later on, cases of sensitivity to azo dyes were reported in the United Kingdom [1, 12, 13], Denmark [14], France [15], Finland [16] and Portugal (Menezes Brandão 1985, personal communication).

Cronin [1] found that Disperse Yellow 3, an azo dye, was responsible for stocking allergy in 57 out of 64 female patients tested. Allergy to Disperse Red 1, another azo dye, was detected in 38 out of 57 patients tested and

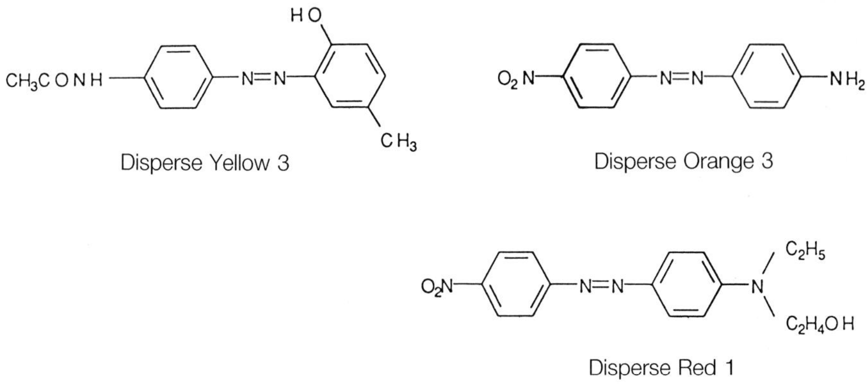

HO

CH₃C O N H ⟨ ⟩ N=N ⟨ ⟩ CH₃

Disperse Yellow 3

O₂N ⟨ ⟩ N=N ⟨ ⟩ NH₂

Disperse Orange 3

O₂N ⟨ ⟩ N=N ⟨ ⟩ N C₂H₅ / C₂H₄OH

Disperse Red 1

Fig. 14.3.5. Structures of three azo dyes. From top left (clockwise): Disperse Yellow 3, Disperse Orange 3, Disperse Red 1.

allergy to Disperse Blue 3, an anthraquinone dye (Fig. 14.3.4), was found in 7 out of 57 patients.

According to Menezes Brandão (1985, personal communication), most of the women with contact dermatitis from stockings (24 out of 28) were allergic to Disperse Orange 3, an azo dye, while Disperse Yellow 3 was a sensitizer in 17 out of 29 patients tested. Four patients were not sensitive to these two dyes; of these four, two reacted to Disperse Red 1 (Fig. 14.3.5). Kousa and Soini [16] reported that out of 12 patients allergic to stockings, nine reacted to Disperse Orange 3 and five to Disperse Yellow 3.

Two women allergic to stockings and to Disperse Orange 3 presented with a relapse of contact dermatitis confined to the retroauricular areas. The relapse was probably caused by the dye present in the plastic arms of their spectacles (Foussereau, unpublished personal cases).

Dyes in Uniforms. Five cases of allergy to Vat Green 1 (Fig. 14.3.6), a dye related to anthraquinone, were reported by Wilson and Cronin [17] in nurses with contact dermatitis from navy blue uniforms. Vat Green 1 was incorporated at 5%–10% concentrations as a shading component. A case of allergy to Disperse Blue 124 (Fig. 14.3.7) in a uniform was observed in a saleswoman working in a department store (Foussereau 1985, unpublished personal case).

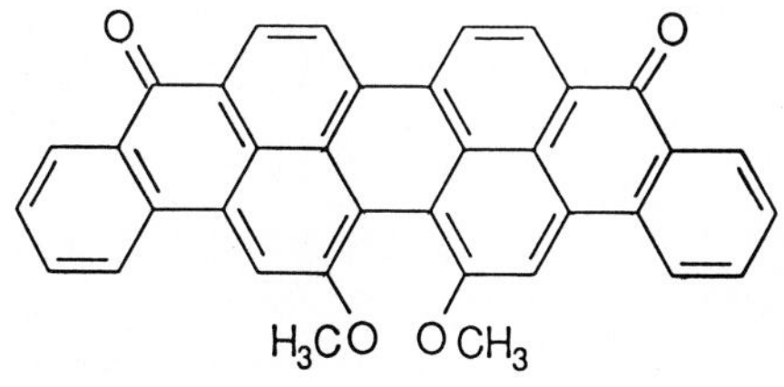

Fig. 14.3.6. Structure of Vat Green 1

H₃CO O CH₃

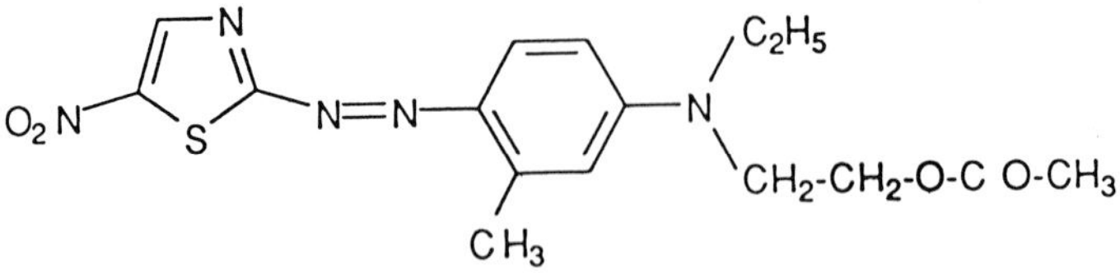

Fig. 14.3.7. Structure of Disperse Blue 124

Dyes in other Garments. According to Cronin [1], the dyes most often responsible for allergy are, in man, Disperse Red 11 (an anthraquinone dye) and Disperse Orange 76 (an azo dye) and, in women, Disperse Blue 124 (an azo dye). Nine cases of allergy to Disperse Blue 106 in women with contact dermatitis from polyester blouses were described by Menezes Brandão et al. [18]. Disperse Blue 106 and Disperse Blue 124 are closely related chemically, the only difference being the presence or absence of an acetate group [19], and are the main cause of allergy to black "velvet" leggings and "bodies".

Concerning trousers (Fig. 14.3.8), Sim Davies [7] reported 14 cases of allergy: half of them were positive to Disperse Yellow 39, a dye belonging to the methine family that is no longer marketed.

14.3.3.4 Rubber

Rubber is not a delayed sensitizer itself, but some of its constituents are allergenic. The main allergens are vulcanization accelerators, e.g. mercaptobenzothiazole, thiurams, thiourea derivatives (diethyl-, dibutyl- and diphenylthiourea) and, less often, antiozonants such as IPPD (see Sect. 13.20).

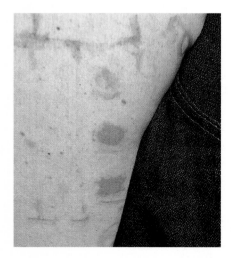

Fig. 14.3.8. Positive patch test reactions to pieces of blue jeans due to clothing dye allergy. (Courtesy of P.J. Frosch)

14.3.3.5 Other Components

Chromium. Chromium, a mordant that fixes dye to cloth, is sometimes used in wool dyeing. Five cases of clothing dermatitis in servicemen from chromium present in their green wool military uniform were described [20].

Cleaners. A case of contact dermatitis of the neck from colophony in a grease and dirt remover containing 1,1,1-trichloroethane at a concentration of 1% was reported [21].

14.3.4 Patch Tests

Patch tests can be performed with a piece cut from the clothing, the material then being moistened. The sample can also be allowed to soak in water for 15 min before patch testing. Patch testing with material previously exposed to steam, as recommended by Sidi and Arouete [22] in dermatitis due to stocking dyes, is not useful. Some authors advise that dyes extracted with solvent from the cloth should be tested; thus, patch tests performed by Fregert [23] were positive to stocking extracts but patch tests with the stocking itself were negative.

As complementary investigations, allergens included in the clothing series 'textile dyes' and 'textile resins' should be tested (Tables 14.3.1, 14.3.2). Dooms-Goossens found Disperse Blue 106 to be the most useful dye of all to test, as it detected 57% of her cases of textile dye dermatitis [24]. Formaldehyde should be tested at a concentration of 1% aq. Higher concentrations may give misleading irritant reactions.

Regarding rubber, the main allergens are mercaptobenzothiazole, thiuram and IPPD. Patch tests with thiourea derivatives (diethyl-, dibutyl- and diphenylthiourea) are important in cases of sensitivity to diving suits.

When carrying out the patch tests, both the garment and its environment are to be considered. Jordan and Bourlas [25] noticed that people sensitized to the rubber present in underwear were intolerant to this rubber only after it had been washed with washing powder containing hypochlorite. The patch tests were negative when the rubber was new and positive after the rubber had been treated with hypochlorite. The rubber incriminated contained zinc dibenzyl dithiocarbamate which, on contact with hypochlorite, was degraded into N, N-dibenzyl carbamate chloride, which gave positive tests.

14.3.5 Cross-reactions

Observations by Dobkevitch and Baer in 1947 [11] showed that 10 out of 10 patients with an allergy to Disperse Yellow 3 showed cross-reactions to

Table 14.3.1. Textile dye allergens

Allergen	Concentration	Vehicle	Comments
Disperse Yellow 3	1%	pet.	Azo dye
Disperse Orange 3	1%	pet.	Azo dye
Disperse Red 1	1%	pet.	Azo dye
Disperse Black 1	1%	pet.	Azo dye
p-Phenylenediamine	1%	pet.	Degradation product of some azo dyes
Aminoazobenzene	0.25%	pet.	Related to some azo dyes
Disperse Blue 3	1%	pet.	Anthraquinone dye
Disperse Blue 124	1%	pet.	Anthraquinone dye
Disperse Blue 106	1%	pet.	Anthraquinone dye, related to Disperse Blue 124

All the allergens listed are available from Chemotechnique (see Chap. 22), except Disperse Black 1

Table 14.3.2. Textile resin allergens

Allergen	Concentration	Vehicle
Formaldehyde	1%	aq.
Urea formaldehyde[a]	10%	pet.
Ethylene urea	10%	pet.
Monomethylol-urea	10%	pet.
Dimethylol-urea	10%	pet.
Melamine-formaldehyde[a]	7%	pet.
Dimethylolpropylene urea[a]	5%	aq.
Dimethylolmethoxypropylene urea[a]	10%	pet.
N,N-Dimethylol-4-methoxy-5,5-dimethylpropylene urea	10%	pet.
Dimethyloldihydroxypropylene urea	10%	pet.
Dimethyloldihydroxyethylene urea	5%	aq.
Tetramethylolacetylene urea	5%	aq.

[a] Available from Chemotechnique (see Chap. 22)

PPD (see Sect. 13.17). According to Cronin [1], PPD is a weak detector of cross-sensitivity to Disperse Yellow 3: out of 27 patients allergic to Disperse Yellow 3, only 7 reacted to PPD.

Concerning women with allergy to Disperse Orange 3, out of 24 patients tested by Menezes Brandão (1985, personal communication), all but 1 proved to be allergic to aminoazobenzene and all but 3 reacted to PPD. Crossreactions between Disperse Orange 3 on the one hand and PPD and aminoazobenzene on the other are not surprising when the formulae of these molecules are considered. Disperse Orange 3 can be degraded into PPD and nitraniline.

14.3.6 Chemical Analyses

When there is a need to define the allergen, chemical analysis of the cloth may be performed, looking for formaldehyde or dyes.

14.3.6.1 Formaldehyde

Formaldehyde present in fabrics can be detected with chromotropic acid diluted in sulphuric acid (see Sect. 10.3). Chromotropic acid powder is stored in the dark, in a refrigerator. 2 g cloth is put into 100 ml distilled water. 24 h later, the extract is filtered. 1 ml is transferred into an Erlenmeyer flask. 5 ml distilled water is added, and then 1 ml 5% chromotropic acid and 5 ml concentrated sulphuric acid [26].

The tests are read after 24 and 48 h, a violet colour indicating the presence of formaldehyde.

This qualitative reaction is very sensitive, since a 0.05% formaldehyde standard solution gives a violet colour. The positivity of the test substance may be compared with the positivity of a formaldehyde control solution placed in a test tube introduced into an Erlenmeyer flask. A solution of 1 drop of formaldehyde in 3 ml water can be used as a control. According to Dahlquist et al. [27], the results are not always significant, as a yellowish, brownish or reddish colour may appear with many substances, e.g. glutaraldehyde, propionaldehyde and acetone.

Formaldehyde can be detected with other methods. For instance, Formalert (Organon Teknika, 5300 S. Portland Avenue, Oklahoma City, OK 73119, USA), a Schiff's reagent (bleached fuchsin + hydrochloric acid) marketed in ready-to-use ampoules, can be employed at room temperature. Other methods of formaldehyde detection have been described [28].

14.3.6.2 Identification of Dyes

Comparative thin-layer chromatography can be carried out with, on one side, dye extracted from the stocking and, on the other side, one or several dyes suspected by the inquiry and the tests and considered as controls.

Disperse Yellow 3 was detected in 51 out of 52 stockings and tights, and Disperse Orange 3 in 17 out of 52 stockings and tights, by Berger et al. [29] in 1984. The colour of the series investigated was beige. Thin-layer chromatography carried out on 23 stockings and tights allowed Hausen and Schulz [30] to identify Disperse Yellow 3 in 22 samples, Disperse Orange 3 in 18 samples, Disperse Blue 3 in 21 samples and Disperse Red 1 in 20 samples.

Thin-layer chromatography, associated with nuclear magnetic resonance spectroscopy and infrared spectrometry, allowed us to discover that BASF Perliton Brown and Ciba JNH Cibacete Brown-the formulae of which were not mentioned in the Colour Index-were, as we suspected, Disperse Yellow 3 [15].

14.3.7 Diagnosis

There are various potential sources of confusion in diagnosis. For instance, allergic contact dermatitis due to diving suits is not to be confused with pressure urticaria and contact dermatitis from stockings predominating in the popliteal fossae may simulate atopic dermatitis.

Eczema confined to the area under trouser pockets can be caused by allergy to the pockets [31] or to the objects contained in the pockets, such as nickel in keys, coins or cigarette lighters, a plastic paper sheath, the leather of a wallet, ballpoint pen inks [32] or a knife contaminated with tulip sap [33], or can be caused by an irritant such as grease or oil impregnating cloth stored in the pocket, such as rags handled by a mechanic.

Indeed, irritation has also to be considered. For instance, an outbreak of dermatitis caused by sock irritation affecting 70 servicemen occurred consequent to the use of tributyltin oxide used as a disinfectant [34]. Hydrofluoric acid used to get rust marks out of linen is caustic and very aggressive to the skin [35]. Dry-cleaning agents can also be irritant, though to a lesser degree [36].

Finally, concerning allergy itself, contamination of cloth by an external agent may occur. Cadot et al. [37] reported an American woman who was aware of sensitization to poison ivy after a picnic. A few months later, her contact dermatitis developed again after she had done some mending on the trousers she had worn for the picnic.

Acknowledgement. My thanks are due to Dr. J.-P. Lepoittevin (Laboratorie de Dermato-Chimie, Strasbourg) for his helpful assistance.

14.3.8 References

1. Cronin E (1980) Contact dermatitis. Churchill Livingstone, Edinburgh
2. Osmundsen PE, Alani MD (1969) Contact allergy due to an optical whitener in washing powders. Br J Dermatol 81: 799–803
3. Tanaka M, Kobayashi S, Miyakawa S (1993) Contact dermatitis from nylon 6 in Japan. Contact Dermatitis 28: 250
4. Puy Le Blanc M (1983) Dermite vésiculeuse des deux mains provoquée par l'usage degants rouges. Ann Dermatol Syph 4: 204–206
5. Batscharov B, Minkov DM (1968) Dermatitis and purpura from rubber in clothing. Trans St Johns Hosp Dermatol Soc 54: 171–182
6. Balzer F, Gauchery P (1989) Dermite eczématiforme des pieds provoquée par lateinture des chaussettes. Ann Dermatol Syph 10: 683–685
7. Sim Davies D (1972) Studies in contact dermatitis, dyes in trousers. Trans St Johns Hosp Dermatol Soc 58: 251–260
8. Epstein E (1940) Eruptions and photosensitivity due to dyed fabrics. Arch Dermatol 41: 1044–1052
9. Gronemeyer W (1953) Hutbanddermatitis. Dtsch Med Wochenschr 78: 232–234
10. Fanburg SJ (1940) Dermatitis following wearing of nylon stockings. JAMA 115: 354–355
11. Dobkevitch S, Baer RL (1947) Eczematous cross-hypersensitivity to azodyes in nylon stocking and to paraphenylenediamine. J Invest Dermatol 9: 203–211

12. Calnan D, Wilson HTH (1956) Nylon stocking dermatitis. Br Med Jest: 147–149
13. Cronin E (1968) Nylon stocking dyes. Trans St Johns Hosp Dermatol Soc 54: 165–169
14. Hjorth N, Rothenborg HW (1967) Zur Häfigkeit der Nylonstrumpfekzem. Z Haut Geschlechtskr 42: 717–722
15. Foussereau J, Tanahashi Y, Grosshans E, Limam-Mestiri S, Khochnevis A (1972) Allergic eczema from Disperse Yellow 3 in nylon stockings and socks. Trans St Johns Hosp Dermatol Soc 58: 75–80
16. Kousa M, Soini M (1980) Contact allergy to a stocking dye. Contact Dermatitis 6: 472–476
17. Wilson HTH, Cronin E (1971) Dermatitis from dyed uniform. Br J Dermatol 85: 67–69
18. Menezes Brandão F, Altermatt C, Pecegueiro M, Bordalo O, Foussereau J (1985) Contact dermatitis to Disperse Blue 106. Contact Dermatitis 13: 80–84
19. Hausen BM (1993) Contact allergy to Disperse Blue 106 and Blue 124 in black "velvet" clothes. Contact Dermatitis 28: 169–173
20. Fregert S, Gruvberger B, Goransson K, Normark S (1978) Allergic contact dermatitis from chromate in military textiles. Contact Dermatitis 4: 223–224
21. Kirk J (1976) Colophony collar dermatitis. Contact Dermatitis 2: 294–295
22. Sidi E, Arouete J (1959) Sensibilisation aux colorants azoïques et au groupe de la para. Presse Med 67: 2067–2069
23. Fregert S (1964) Extraction of allergens for patch testing. Acta Derm Venereol (Stockh) 44: 107
24. Dooms-Goossens A (1992) Textile dye dermatitis. Contact Dermatitis 27: 321–323
25. Jordan WP, Bourlas MC (1975) Allergic contact dermatitis to underwear elastic chemically transformed by laundry bleach. Arch Dermatol 111: 593–595
26. Hovding G (1959) Free formaldehyde in textiles. Acta Derm Venereol (Stockh) 39: 357–368
27. Dahlquist I, Fregert S, Gruvberger B (1980) Reliability of the chromotropic acid method for qualitative formaldehyde determination. Contact Dermatitis 6: 357–358
28. Storrs FJ (1986) Dermatitis from clothing and shoes. In: Fisher AA (ed) Contact dermatitis, 3rd edn. Lea and Febiger, Philadelphia, pp 283–337
29. Berger G, Muslmani M, Menezes Brandão F, Foussereau J (1984) Thin-layer chromatography search for Disperse Yellow 3 and Disperse Orange 3 in 52 stockings and pantyhose. Contact Dermatitis 10: 154–157
30. Hausen BM, Schulz KH (1984) Strumpffarben-Allergie. Dtsch Med Wochenschr 109: 1469–1475
31. Grimalt F, Romaguera C (1981) Contact dermatitis caused by polyamide trouser pockets. Derm Beruf Umwelt 20: 35–39
32. Foussereau J (1985) An allergen in a judo club? Contact Dermatitis 13: 283
33. Foussereau J (1987) Les eczémas allergiques cosmétologiques, thérapeutiques et vestimentaires. Masson, Paris
34. Molin L, Wahlberg JE (1975) Toxic skin reactions caused by tributyltin oxide (TBTO) in socks. Berufsdermatosen 23: 138–142
35. Maleville J, Ducombs G, Pere JC (1985) Dermatoses de contact á un anti-rouille á base d'acide fluorhydrique et de bifluorure d'ammonium. Lettre du GERDA 8: 76–77
36. Storrs FJ (1986) Dermatitis from clothing and shoes. In: Fisher AA (ed) Contact dermatitis, 3rd (edn). Lea and Febiger, Philadelphia, p 303
37. Cadot M, Robin J, Hewitt J (1974) Apparition du poison ivy en France. Bull Soc Fr Dermatol Syphiligr 81: 33–34

14.4 Shoes

Patricia Podmore

Contents

14.4.1 Introduction

Shoe contact dermatitis is typical of many instances of contact dermatitis in that the pattern of presentation suggests the diagnosis but the causative allergen is elusive [1].

However, particularly when dealing with allergic contact dermatitis from shoes, as in many other types of allergic contact dermatitis, the initial pattern of presentation may hold the clue to the causative allergen and should therefore be carefully identified and recorded. This may allow aimed patch testing with specific groups of chemicals.

Dorsal foot dermatitis (Fig. 14.4.1) points to an allergen in the shoe upper, a portion or portions of which should also be patch tested. If the patient presents with a plantar dermatitis (Fig. 14.4.2) sparing the instep and toe creases, allergic contact dermatitis should be suspected, and possible contactants should be looked for in the insole or shoe lining, or perhaps in the constituents of the glue used to hold the insole and shoe lining in place. Again, confirmation should be sought by testing the patient to whatever portion or portions of the shoe are in contact with the area of dermatitis.

Patch test interpretation is made much easier if portions of shoes to be tested are made wafer-thin, smooth-surfaced, regular-edged and large. Since the standard Finn Chamber holds portions no larger than 5 mm^2, many prefer patch testing either with the larger Finn Chamber or without a chamber, but using occlusive tape (not Scanpor) instead. With the last technique, portions

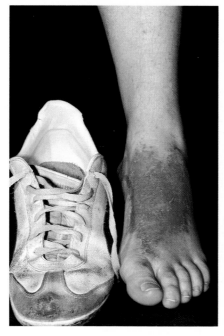

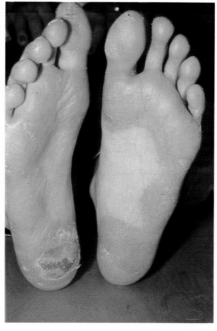

Fig. 14.4.1. Dorsal foot allergic contact dermatitis (Courtesy of P.J. Frosch)

Fig. 14.4.2. Plantar foot allergic contact dermatitis

1 cm^2 or larger may be used to give unequivocal patch test results. Patch testing with scrapings of shoe materials is not recommended.

If the patient's rash is on the instep, which (with exceptions such as modern athletic shoes) is not an area in normal foot posture in contact with the shoe, then one's suspicions should incline more towards an endogenous eczema. A full history of personal and family dermatological status should be sought, and involvement of the skin elsewhere should be looked for. An eczema across the tops of the toes and around the heels should alert one to parts of the shoe called the heel and toe stiffeners or counters. These stiffeners contain a wide variety of chemicals, as discussed below. However, a dermatosis between the toes is more likely to be a microbial infection; toenail clippings and skin scrapings should be examined on a potassium hydroxide mount and cultured for fungus.

Unfortunately, in long-standing or severe cases the initial diagnostic presenting pattern can be obscured, making subsequent diagnosis more difficult. Shoe allergens can migrate to other parts of the shoe or even to stockings, disguising the presenting pattern [2, 3].

Shoes are manufactured from a vast range of potentially sensitizing chemicals. One possible way of tackling shoe dermatitis is to break down all the constituents of the shoes and identify all possible culprits. This task is complicated by the fact that today's shoes are manufactured all over the world,

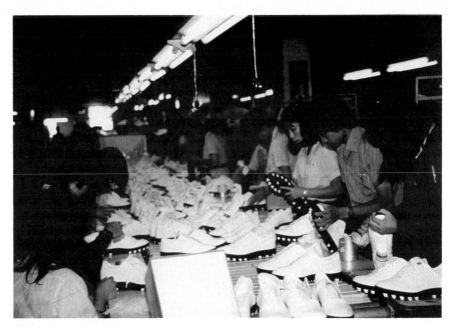

Fig. 14.4.3. Taiwanese shoe factory

often in countries from which information on manufacturing components is not readily available. Another problem can be that different components of the shoe are derived from different countries, their initial country of origin not being recorded [1] (Fig. 14.4.3).

14.4.2 Shoe Uppers

Shoe uppers can be made from traditional materials such as leather or, especially in the case of athletic shoes, rubber or polyurethane. Leather traditionally is chrome-tanned, implicating dichromate as the allergen. However, nowadays, with the high-fashion demand of varied finishes, chrome tanning is a multistep process [4]. Leather is tanned and then retanned. In 95% of cases, primary tanning is with chrome, but other possible processes are vegetable, glutaraldehyde, formaldehyde or synthetic tanning. After tanning, the leather is shaved to a uniform thickness. These shavings are used in athletic shoe uppers after chrome retanning, and therefore athletic shoe uppers also expose wearers to chrome contact dermatitis.

Vegetable tannins are plant or fruit extracts, the most popular of which at present are quebracho, wattle, myrobalans and chestnut. Quebracho is a hardwood from South America. The sawdust of this dense wood contains 25% tannin. Wattle is a catechol-containing tannin derived from the bark of trees of various acacia species. The extract contains 60% tannins. It is often used to retan upper leather. A popular tannin for sole leather is myrobalans, which is obtained from the astringent fruits of the tree *Terminalia chebula.* These fruits are dried nuts with a tannin content of 30%–40%. Myrobalans is a pyrogallol-containing tannin. Another popular shoe leather vegetable tannin is chestnut; the major sources of this extract are France and Italy.

Vegetable tanning is a slow process, taking 3 weeks, compared to a few days involved in chrome tanning. However, it yields a fully resilient hydrophilic leather that is ideal for soles, linings and insoles. It yields a leather which is also chrome-free and therefore indicated for patients who are chromate-allergic.

The other types of tannages are utilized either to decrease the chrome content of factory effluent or to yield particular properties. Tanning with formaldehyde or glutaraldehyde involves a chemical reaction between the aldehyde and the primary amino acid group of the lysinyl residue in the protein side chains of the hide. This yields a soft waterproof leather often used for work shoes. Alum tanning is a tannage under research; sodium and potassium aluminium sulphate are used. Syntanning uses the following synthetic agents: napthalene sulphonic acid and formaldehyde; exchange syntans and phenol, sulphonated and condensed with formaldehyde to give a thermosetting novolac resin (a phenol-terminated resin formed in the presence of excess phenol); and resin syntans, organic nitrogen compounds such as dimethylol urea, dicyandiamide or melamine, reacted with formaldehyde and water to form the *N*-methylol group, which then reacts with an amino group on the hide protein during tannage.

After tanning, the natural oils leached out by tanning are replaced by fat liquoring, using sulphonated and cod-liver oil, synthetic moellon oil (a synthetic fish oil) and sulphonated neatsfoot oil; all of which are biocide preserved. The leather is then dyed. Formerly a rare source of sensitization, dyes are now being manufactured cheaply in Third World countries. Dye manufacture is a complex multistep process, and when a dye is cheaply made, the by-products of the various step reactions are not cleared from the final product but persist as impurities and possible allergens. Chrome-tanned leather is best dyed with acid dyes, and vegetable-tanned leather with basic dyes.

Leather finish gives an attractive but tough outer coat to the leather, in five main steps:

1. Spray stain of metal complex pigments to improve the colour
2. Base coat of acrylic, acrylonitrile or styrene-butadiene resins
3. Protein paste of milk casein protein, egg albumin and vegetable wax solids to give depth of appearance
4. Dry finish coat of nitrocellulose in diisobutyl ketone or in cheaper finish coats, a combination of nitrocellulose and phthalate ester
5. Water-repellent coat of alkenyl succinic acid complex, fluorinated acid chromium complex, stearatochromic chloride complex and silicones

In both the fat liquoring and the finish coat chemicals, biocides are an important additive. It may be difficult to identify the biocides in use in distant countries. Table 14.4.1 lists commonly used biocides.

Table 14.4.1. Common biocides in use

Leather upper

N-octyl-4-isothiazolin-3-one 8% in propylene glycol 92%
  (Kathon LP)

Di-iodomethyl-*p*-tolylsulphone
  (Amical 48)

2-Thiocyanomethyl benzothiazole
  (Busan 30L)

Trichlorophenol ⎫
Pentachlorophenol ⎭ in Taiwan and Korea

Heel and Toe Counter
  Sodium-*o*-phenylphenate
  (Dowicide A)
  1,2-Benzisothiazolin-3-one 10% in
  an aqueous solution of propylene glycol
  (Proxel X L2)

Water-based adhesives
  N-Trichloro-methyl-thiophthalimide
  (Fungitrol 11)
  Copper-8-quinolinolate

Lasting board
  Sodium-*o*-phenylphenate
  (Dowicide A)
  Copper-8-quinolinolate

An alternative upper material to leather is the athletic shoe tricot upper, which consists of rubber or polyurethane foam, flame-bonded to nylon cloth on each side.

Polyurethane is manufactured by a condensation polymerization reaction between two streams of chemicals. Stream A consists of methylene-bis-diisocyanate combined with a polyol, either a polyester or polyether. Stream B contains a mixture of chemicals which dictate the type of reaction to take place and thus the type of polyurethane produced: solid, liquid or foam. During the reaction, gas formation and cross-linking take place. Chain extenders such as butylene glycol are consumed in the reaction. Gas formation is catalysed by tertiary amines to produce a lightweight open-celled foam, whereas organotins catalyse cross-linking to produce a tight, closely packed foam. The two classes of catalyst therefore favour the production of two different types of polymer. Occasionally, heavy metal catalysts such as bismuth neodecanoate substitute for organotins.

To increase the blowing effect in gas formation, foaming agents such as Freon 11, fluorotrichloromethane, are used. The heat generated volatizes the Freon, which condenses at the surface to give an outer skin to the polyurethane. Surfactants, usually organosilicones, are used in the blowing reaction to prevent collapse of the foam cell walls by achieving adequate cell wall tension. The other components in stream B impart final characteristics

Table 14.4.2. Rubber polymers

Polymer	Monomers
Natural rubber	Isoprene
Styrene-butadiene rubber	Styrene, butadiene
Polybutadiene	Butadiene
Synthetic polyisoprene	Synthetic isoprene
Neoprene	Chloroprene
Thermoplastic elastomers	Styrene, isoprene, butadiene
High-styrene resins	Styrene, butadiene
	Isoprene, chloroprene

to the polyurethane. Ultra-violet light stabilizers, hindered phenols, hindered amines and benzotriazoles are present to a level of 0.5%–1% of the final product.

Rubber is a broad term for many different polymers, only one of which is natural rubber (Table 14.4.2). Again, the final characteristics of the polymer are determined by the various chemicals used in its production. All rubbers are polymers of simple hydrocarbon monomers (Fig. 14.4.4) containing one or more double bonds, and, again, during the polymerization process, chain extension, cross-linking and blowing take place [5].

In rubber production, cross-linking is referred to as vulcanization or curing, and this often occurs as an end-stage reaction, where there are sufficient double bonds left in the polymer to allow the process to take place. The catalysts are referred to as vulcanizing agents, and these are primary if they donate sulphur to the reaction, for instance sulphur itself (the original vulcanizing agent), thioureas, carbamates and dithiodimorpholine, or

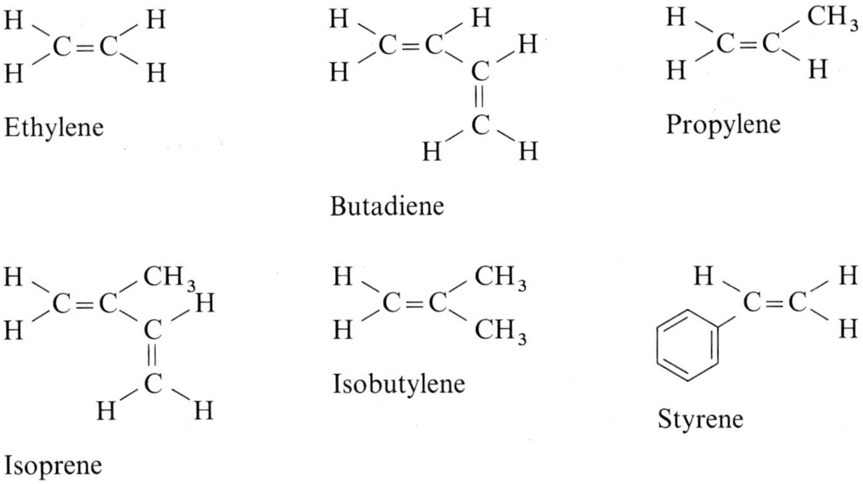

Ethylene

Butadiene

Propylene

Isoprene

Isobutylene

Styrene

Fig. 14.4.4. Rubber monomers

Table 14.4.3. Some less familiar rubber chemicals

Vulcanizers	Diorthotolyl guanidine
	Dicumyl peroxide
Accelerators	Ethylene thiourea
Antioxidants	Octylated diphenylamines
	2,2,4-Trimethyl-1,2-dihydroquinoline
	Butylated hydroxytoluene
	Diphenylamines
Pigment	Titanium dioxide
Resins	Coumarone indene resins
	Terpene phenolic resins
	p-tert-Butylphenol-formaldehyde resin
Blowing agents	Azodicarbonamide
	4,4-Oxybis (benzenesulphonylhydrazide)

secondary if they have low or absent sulphur, such as tellurium, selenium or organic peroxides. Vulcanizing agents usually make up 2%–4% of the reaction mixture.

Accelerators are straightforward catalysts of the polymerization reaction and are of three main classes: thiazoles such as mercaptobenzothiazole; sulphonamides such as 4-morpholinyl-2-benzothiazyl disulphides; or sulphur donors such as dithiocarbamates or thiurams. The other ingredients in the reaction mixture are, again, character-modifying agents (Table 14.4.3).

14.4.3 Shoe Soles

Shoe soles consist mainly of materials discussed above: vegetable-tanned leather, rubber or polyurethane, singly or in combination. The polyurethanes that are used tend to be highly cross-linked, closely packed foams. Natural rubber and polybutadiene are the popular rubbers for soles and heels. Neoprenes are widely used for oil-resistant work soles, utilizing dibenzothiazyl disulphide as the accelerator. Evaflex combines the polymer of ethyl vinyl acetate (EVA) with rubber polymers as another popular shoe soling material.

14.4.4 Shoe Insoles

Similarly, shoe insoles contain the materials as above: rubber, polyurethane and occasionally leather, usually vegetable-tanned. A common cheap insole material is fibreboard. The fibres may be either wood or leather suspended in a biocide-preserved emulsion of various rubber resins, such as neoprene, styrene-butadiene or acrylic resins. The common biocides used are copper-8-quinolinolate or Dowicide A. This mixture is set in sheets, and the insoles are cut out of these sheets. Fibreboard therefore exposes patients to a vast range of allergens and not surprisingly can give positive reactions on patch testing. This fibreboard material is also used in some cases as the lasting board. The lasting board or foundation of the shoe is occasionally thick vegetable-tanned leather, but in cheaper shoes fibreboard tends to be used instead.

14.4.5 Adhesives

The next component of shoes to be considered can be one of the major contributors to the problem of shoe allergic contact dermatitis. Adhesives are used throughout the shoe, often in intimate contact with the foot, as when glueing the shoe insole or shoe lining in place. The main adhesives in use are hot melt, urethane, neoprene and natural rubber adhesive.

Hot melt adhesives, once mentioned, can quickly be dimissed again as unlikely causes of shoe allergic contact dermatitis. These are inert high molecular weight polymers of EVA, polyamides or polyesters in rod, pellet or block form. They are melted down and applied hot to the surface to be stuck, usually in sole or heel attachments.

Latex in common parlance is taken to mean natural rubber. However, in the adhesives industry latex usually means water based, and latex can be urethane, natural or synthetic rubber. Urethane adhesives are simply polyurethane in solution, modified to give the composition tackiness and thus allow it to act as an adhesive. In certain special situations other additives are required: to increase bond strength, isocyanates are added; to stick neoprene, epoxy resins are required; and to stick EVA polymers, tackifiers such as acrylic or phenol-formaldehyde resins are used. Urethanes, a nonrubber adhesive and therefore useful in the presence of rubber allergy, make up 80% of footwear adhesives whereas neoprenes account for less than 20%. Again, urethanes are mainly used for sole and heel attachments.

Table 14.4.4 outlines a typical neoprene formulation. Strong neoprene adhesives contain isocyanates. Isocyanates cause *p-tert*-butylphenol-formaldehyde (PTBP) resin to undergo premature cure, and therefore these strong adhesives either use terpene phenolic resins as tackifiers or consist of two components that are mixed immediately prior to use. Rubber latex adhesives tend to be natural rubber, as synthetic rubber is expensive (Table 14.4.5). They are water based and therefore biocide preserved.

Table 14.4.4. Neoprene formulation

Chlorinated rubber (neoprene)
Phenolic resin (*p-tert*-butylphenol-formaldehyde resin or terpene phenolic resin)
Magnesium oxide
Zinc oxide
Ethylene thiourea
Dioctyl-4-phenylenediamine
Fillers: sodium/calcium silicate
Tetramethylthiuram disulphide
Diorthotolyl guanidine
Sodium dibutyldithiocarbamate

Tackifying resins such as colophony are added. Neoprene and natural rubber latex adhesives are used to glue shoe linings and shoe insoles in place and are therefore in intimate contact with the foot.

14.4.6 Heel and Toe Counters

The final parts of the shoe to be considered as a source of shoe allergic contact dermatitis are the heel and toe stiffeners, or counters (Table 14.4.6). There are five main types, and all serve to strengthen the toes and heels of shoes. The simplest and least problematical type are those found in athletic shoes: a layer of hot melt adhesive. However, the other types are more elaborate, consisting of a web polyester or cotton material impregnated with a variety of resins to give stiffness and support. Counters may therefore contain natural rubber latex, EVA hot melt adhesive, phenol-formaldehyde resin, melamine-formaldehyde resin, urea-formaldehyde resin, pine oil and various biocides, with all the numerous allergens thus implied.

14.4.7 Conclusion

After this intensive look at the shoe structure, an extensive list of allergens can be complied (Table 14.4.7). However, interestingly, common causes of shoe allergic contact dermatitis are allergens in the standard series (see Chap. 13). Despite this knowledge it is difficult to cure patients completely, perhaps because they continue to encounter their allergens in unexpected places. Mercaptobenzothiazole (MBT) and thiurams are rubber chemicals [6] but may not necessarily be only in the rubber soles and heels of shoes. Neoprene adhesives have been shown to contain thiuram, and it is impossible totally to exclude the use of MBT in either synthetic or natural rubber latex. Heel and toe counters, fibreboard lasting boards and leather finish coats all contain rubber resins and therefore MBT or thiurams [7].

Thioureas proved problematical in athletic shoes when they were used as accelerators in the neoprene foam of an athletic shoe insole, and they still sensitize from time to time [8, 9]. Styrenated phenol has recently been identified as an additional allergen in athletic shoe rubber [10].

Diaminodiphenylmethane is a polyurethane percursor and therefore a possible allergen in polyurethane upper foam [11]. Polyurethane foam is distinguishable from neoprene foam in that it tends to look more shiny.

Table 14.4.5. Natural rubber latex formulation

Polyoxyethylene	Phenol
Rosin esters	Formaldehyde
Polymerized wood resin	Parachlorometacresol (Collatone)
Triethanolamine	Fatty acid
Diallyl phenyl sulphone	Caustic potash

Table 14.4.6. Heel and toe counters

Pressed counters
Fireboard coated with urea- or phenol-formaldehyde resin

Glue
Natural rubber latex 95% ethyl vinyl acetate polymer
Hot melt 5%

Thermoplastic counters
Polyvinylchloride impregnated with rubber resins
Surlyn (ethylene methacrylic acid)

Solid styrene
Styrene plasticized with methyl ketone

Thermal counters
Woven fabric coated with rubber or melamine-formaldehyde resins

Glue
Ethyl vinyl acetate hot melts

Three-part counters
1. Woven fabrics impregnated with urea-formaldehyde resin and natural rubber latex
2. Ammonium chloride or sodium acetate
3. Pine oil, sodium-N-methyl-N-oleoyl laurate, dioctyl sodium sulphosuccinate

Table 14.4.7. Shoe chemicals tested and their concentrations

Toluene sulphonamide formaldehyde resin	10% pet.
4,4'-Diaminodiphenylmethane	0.5% pet.
2,2,4-Trimethyl-1,2-dihydroquinoline	1% pet.
1H-Benzotriazole	1% pet.
4,4'-Dithiomorpholine	1% pet.
Coumarone indene resin	20% pet.
Terpene phenolic resin	20% pet.
Tetramethyl butanediamine	1% pet.
N-Octyl-4-isothiazolin-3-one 8% in propylene glycol 92% (Kathon LP)	0.1% pet.
Bismuth neodecanoate	1% pet.
N, N-Diethyl thiourea	1% pet.
Ethylbutyl thiourea	1% pet.
N, N-Dibutyl thiourea	1% pet.
3-Methyl thiazolidine 2-thion (Vulcacit CRU)	1% pet.
Ethylene thiourea	1% pet.
Disperse Orange 3	1% pet.
Disperse Yellow 3	1% pet.
Copper 8-quinolinolate	1% pet.
Diorthotolyl guanidine	1% pet.
Dioctyl phthalate	5% pet.
N-Dodecyl mercaptan	0.1% pet.
Glutaraldehyde	1% aq.
Urea-formaldehyde resin	10% pet.
Dicyandiamide	0.1% aq.
Toluene sulphonhydrazide	0.5% alc.
Dimethylaminoethyl ether (Niax$_1$)	1% pet.
Azodicarbonamide (Azobisformamide)	0.5% pet.

Testing for PTBP resin is complicated. Not all cases of sensitivity are detected by testing with a standard PTBP resin; PTBP itself should also be tested, as well as the actual PTBP resin used in the shoes [12–14]. PTBP resin is the main tackifier used in neoprene adhesive and is therefore found mainly in shoe lining and shoe insole glues. It is also encountered in heel and toe counters as a tackifier.

Colophony, like PTBP resin, is a tackifier occasionally in heel and toe counters, as well as in rubber latex adhesives used to glue shoe insoles and linings in place. Patients sensitive to colophony and PTBP resin should therefore be similarly advised to wear either unlined shoes or leather-lined shoes with the lining stitched, not glued, in place, and shoes with no heel or toe supports.

Nickel trim on shoes can be an unexpected cause of dorsal foot dermatitis.

Shoe contact dermatitis still remains a difficult condition to manage. It is important to search for patients' known allergens in unexpected places in their shoes and to give patients appropriately detailed advice on avoidance. Even then, some cases remain insoluble and must be managed empirically with hypoallergenic footwear, such as plastic shoes or wooden shoes with vegetable-tanned uppers nailed rather than glued in place [15].

14.4.8 References

1. Storrs F (1986) Dermatitis from clothing and shoes. In: Fisher AA (ed) Contact dermatitis, 3rd edn. Lea and Febiger, Philadelphia, p 283
2. Rietschel RL (1984) Role of socks in shoe dermatitis. Arch Dermatol 120: 398
3. Maibach H (1984) Panty hose dermatitis resembling and complicating tinea pedis. Contact Dermatitis 1: 329
4. Thorstensen TC (1985) Practical leather technology, 3rd edn. Krieger, Melbourne
5. Babbit RO (1978) The Vanderbilt rubber handbook. Vanderbilt
6. Lammintausta K, Kalimo K (1985) Sensitivity to rubber. Study with rubber mixes and individual rubber chemicals. Dermatosen 33: 204–208
7. Fogh A, Pock-Steen B (1992) Contact sensitivity to thiram in wooden shoes. Contact Dermatitis 27: 348
8. Roberts JL, Hanifin JM (1979) Athletic shoe dermatitis, contact allergy to ethylbutyl thiourea. JAMA 241: 275–276
9. Roberts JL, Hanifin JM (1980) Contact allergy and cross reactivity to substituted thiourea compounds. Contact Dermatitis 6: 138–139
10. Kaniwa M-A, Momma J, Ikarashi Y, Kojima S, Nakamura A, Nakaji Y, Kurokawa Y, Kantoh H, Itoh M (1992) A method for identifying causative chemicals of allergic contact dermatitis using a combination of chemical analysis and patch testing in patients and animal groups: application to a case of rubber boot dermatitis. Contact Dermatitis 27: 166–173
11. Cronin E (1980) Contact dermatitis. Churchill Livingstone, Edinburgh, p 738
12. Malten K, Seutter E (1985) Allergic degradation products of paratertiary butyl phenol formaldehyde plastic. Contact Dermatitis 12: 222–224
13. Malten KE, Rath R, Pasters HM (1983) Paratertiary butyl phenol formaldehyde and other causes of shoe dermatitis. Dermatosen 5: 149–153
14. Malten KE (1967) Contact sensitizations caused by paratertiary butyl phenol and certain phenol formaldehyde-containing glues. Dermatologica 135: 541–549
15. Mathias TCE, Maibach H (1979) Polyvinylchloride workboots in the management of shoe dermatitis in industrial workers. Contact Dermatitis 5: 249–250

14.5 Pesticides

HANS J. SCHUBERT

Contents

14.5.1 Introduction

14.5.1.1 Definition

Pesticides are farm, garden, forest and household chemicals used against insects, rodents and other animals, fungi, bacteria, viruses, and weeds. Approximately 300 chemicals are currently used in the more than 3000 registered preparations on the market. They are an important source of increasing productivity in farms and horticulture. World production is still increasing.

14.5.1.2 Dangers and Risks

Cutaneous reactions to pesticides are as varied as the chemicals themselves. Most can be categorized as irritants and relatively few are known to be contact allergens or photosensitizers. Despite extensive use, reports of skin diseases from pesticides are not very frequent and mostly of single cases. Disabling skin lesions in farm workers and gardeners are usually attributed to causes other than pesticides, such as poor hygiene, infection, plant allergy, trauma and sunburn. Many general practitioners do not think of the possibility. So the frequency of pesticide-associated dermatitis has probably been underestimated.

In Western and Central Europe, on the other hand, many people only too often suppose that their skin complaints are caused by pesticides –they are afraid of them. But this is only a small part of the world's population and most of them are not at risk, their skin not being exposed directly. They feel endangered and at risk of injury themselves from pest control aeroplanes, which are used to spray and scatter agrochemicals over large areas. In the area of the former German Democratic Republic approximately three-quarters (4.5 million hectares) of the total area in agricultural use was periodically pest-controlled by planes, and sometimes forests too. The other quarter, including gardens, orchards and glasshouses, as well as kitchens, restaurants, food stores, hotels, hospitals and homes, are pest-controlled by man with air-blast sprayers, dusters, watering cans, brushes and other devices, poisonous baits or special equipment for tractors. Wood preservatives are applied by painting, spraying or dipping. Other uses are antifouling paints for ships, decontamination and disinfection of water and soil and slimicides in paper mills.

Contact dermatitis from pesticides is chiefly observed in workers mixing and applying them in the field, as well as among manufacturers and formulators. Persons at risk thus include agricultural workers, dockers (derusters), farmers, florists, gardeners, paper makers, pest control workers, swimming pool service personnel, veterinarians, and weekend gardeners. In several European countries and in the United States, governmental agencies have recommended that workers should not reenter fields and glasshouses treated with pesticides for periods of time specified for each pesticide. This is a commendable system, because field workers and glasshouse gardeners, if allowed to enter too soon, may be contaminated with residues of pesticides. However, the main causes of disease are poor use of protective clothing, often because of the summer heat, and lack of washing facilities at the places of exposure. It is also contributory that safety gloves and other protective clothing do not give complete protection in every case. Their degree of permeability depends on various factors: material and thickness of the gloves, chemical properties of the pesticide and its solvent, concentration, temperature and duration of exposure (contact). The selection of chemically protective gloves is often made without sufficient knowledge as to whether the pesticide can pass through them or not. An inappropriate material can rapidly be penetrated by pesticides: there is no all-round glove protecting from all chemicals. Some gloves give a false sense of security. It is also necessary to know that gloves should be washed frequently during a shift and changed every 4h [1,2]. More information can be obtained from the Swedish data base

DAISY about protective gloves (Aramis Service, S-17184 Solna, Sweden) (see also Table 11.14).

Barrier creams cannot be recommended against pesticides, because certain ointments can trap and accumulate the pesticide and then liberate it for diffusion into the skin, sometimes even enhancing penetration through the horny layer.

There are only a few case reports of photocontact dermatitis from pesticides: dimethyl dichlorinylphosphate, malathion, parathion methyl, phenmedipham, tributyltin oxide, trichlorfon, trichlorometaphos (see below). For handling such pesticides, sun protection has been recommended.

14.5.2 Specific Groups of Pesticides

14.5.2.1 Acaricides

Metam Sodium (Dicid, Nematin, Terra Fume, Vapam). This is a soil fumigant and herbicide (sodium N-methyldithiocarbamate). It is a very strong sensitizer and a toxic vesicant which has caused numerous cases of allergic contact dermatitis due to methyl isothiocyanate, the actual allergen [3].

Patch test concentration: 0.03% aq.

Naled (Bromex, Dibrom). This, too, is an insecticide of the organophosphate group (dimethyl-1,2-dibromo-2,2-dichloroethyl phosphate) and is used on numerous crops and against flies in stables, in kennels and in and around food-processing plants. Occupational dermatitis is rarely seen [4].

Patch test concentration: 0.05% aq.

14.5.2.2 Algicides

Common algicides are irritants such as copper sulphate, copper chelates, quaternary ammonium compounds and organic polyamines. Dinitrochlorobenzene (2,4-DNCB) is a very strong sensitizer, and mercaptobenzothiazole (2-MBT) a weak one. Tributyltin oxide (TBTO), used in marine paints and wood preservatives, is not allergenic but irritant and phototoxic [5].

14.5.2.3 Bactericides

Chloramphenicol (Chloronitrin). This powerful contact allergen in medicine [6] is used against the rot of potatoes and other root vegetables.

Patch test concentration: 1% pet.

Streptomycin. This, too, is a strong contact allergen [7] and is often used in combination with tetracycline to control fireblight in apples and pears and blight of ornamentals (roses, begonias, oleander, etc.).

Patch test concentration: 1% pet. or aq.

14.5.2.4 Fungicides

There are about 40 chemicals used against fungal diseases of plants, their fruits and seeds, and for wood preservation.

Benomyl (Benlate, Chinoin-Fundazol, Product 1991, Tersan). This is a systemic fungicide used worldwide for fruits, nuts, vegetables, bulbs, ornamental plants, and lawns (methyl-1-(butyl-carbamoyl)-2-benzimidazole-carbamate). It is a contact allergen and sometimes a photosensitizer [8–10].

Patch test concentration: 0.1 aq or pet.

Captan (N-trichloromethylmercapto-Δ^4-tetrahydrophthalimide). This is applied on fruits, berries, vegetables, seeds, and ornamental plants. Allergic contact dermatitis is not so rare [11, 12], and urticaria possible.

Patch test concentration: 0.1% aq. or 0.5% pet.

Copper Sulphate and Organic Copper Salts. Copper sulphate and other organic salts (copper abietate, copper naphthenate, copper oleate, copper 8-quinolinolate) are used on ornamentals and can cause irritant contact dermatitis.

Patch test concentration of copper sulphate: 1% aq.

Difolatan (Captafol). This is used for fruits, vegetables, and seeds (N-(1,1,2,2-tetrachloroethylthio)-4-cyclohexene-1,2-dicarboximide) and can cause allergic contact dermatitis and urticaria [13–15].

Patch test concentration: 0.1% pet.

Maneb (Dithane, Manzate; Manganese Ethylene-bis-dithiocarbamate) and Zineb (Dithane 2-78,, Parzate; Zinc Ethylene-bis-dithiocarbamate). These substances, either alone or combined with each other (Fore, Mancozeb, Manzate) or with captan or lindane, are widely used on fruits, vegetables, flowers and lawns. They are weak but frequent sensitizers [8, 16–19] that are related to thiuram and carbamate accelerators for rubber: cross-reactions are seen.

Patch test concentration: 0.5% pet., 1% pet.

Phenylmercuric Acetate. This is used as a seed treatment chemical and against apple scurf. It is an irritant and a contact allergen.

Patch test concentration: 0.06% pet.

Tetrachloroisophthalonitrile (Chlorothalonil, TCPN). This fungicide is used in agriculture and horticulture and also for wood preservation. It is an irritant and a strong contact allergen. Outbreaks in two joinery factories have been seen [20, 21]. Because of its irritancy, if in any doubt patch test with 0.001% in acetone as well.

Patch test concentration: 0.01% pet.

Thiuram (Thiram, TMTD; Tetramethylthiuram Disulphide [22]). This is used on fruits, seeds and lawns, as an animal repellent and rubber accelerator, and in medical soaps. Therefore, reactions are probably more often from the use of protective rubber gloves than from TMTD as a pesticide.

Patch test concentration: 1% pet.

14.5.2.5 Herbicides

Arsenic Compounds. Inorganic arsenic compounds have been replaced by organic arsenic compounds (methane arsenates, cacodylic acid) for use on grasses. They are irritants.

Triazines and Triazoles. Atrazine and other triazines and triazoles (amitrole, anilazine, desmetrine, prometryne, simazine) are widely used weedkillers. Allergic contact dermatitis is occasionally reported [8, 23, 24].

Patch test concentrations:

amitrole	1% aq.
anilazine	0.1% pet.
atrazine	0.05% aq.
ametryne	0.05% aq.
azinphosmethyl	0.25% pet.
simazine	5% aq.

2,4-Dichlorophenoxyacetic Acid (2,4-D) and 2,4,5-Trichlorophenoxyacetic Acid (2,4,5-T). These are selective herbicides against broad-leaved plants and defoliants (Agent Orange of US Army during the Vietnam War). Because of their contamination with dioxin (TCDD), which causes chloracne and porphyria cutanea tarda, and after the Seveso disaster of 1976, their production has largely been stopped. Dissolved in diesel fuel or petroleum, they are strong irritants and contact allergens [8, 25].

Patch test concentration: 0.5% or 1% o.o.

Glyphosate (N-(Phosphonomethyl) Glycine). This is a weedkiller for many indications. The only report of phototoxicity was soon corrected. There is no evidence of irritation, sensitization, phototoxicity or photosensitization [26].

Patch test concentration: 10% aq.

Metam Sodium. This substance (see Sect. 14.5.2.1) is used for chemical selection of potato plants for growing.

Paraquat (1,1'-Dimethyl-4,4'-Dipyridinium). This is a contact herbicide and desiccant and may cause acute irritant bullous dermatitis and fingernail damage [27–29].

Patch test concentration: 0.1% pet.

Propachlor (Ramrod, Satecid 65 WP; 2-Chloro-N-Isopropylacetanilide). This selective preemergence herbicide is used to control grasses and broad-leaved weeds in cabbage, corn, and other crops. It is a strong irritant and sensitizer [30, 31] and related to Alachlor, Lasso and Randox.

Patch test concentration: 0.1–0.5% aq.

Chlorates. Sodium chlorate and potassium chlorate are not selective and are used on paths and waysides. They are not sensitizers but toxic.

14.5.2.6 Insecticides

4,6-Dinitrocresol (Hedolit; DNOC). This is an acaricide, herbicide and defoliant. Jung [17] reported exanthema, urticaria and exfoliative dermatitis due to systemic intoxication, but no allergy. It is an irritant, causing toxic paronychia.
Patch test concentration: 50% aq.

Lindane (HCH; γ-hexachlorocyclohexane). This is widely used in agriculture, in horticulture, in the household, in veterinary medicine and against scabies. Allergic contact dermatitis used to be caused by the δ-isomer [32, 33], now an eliminated impurity. Lindane is well tolerated by the skin.
Patch test concentration: 1% pet.

Malathion (Milon, Fosfotion; O,O-Dimethyl-S-(1,1-Dicarbethoxyethyl)-Dithiophosphate). This common organophosphate is a potent contact and photocontact sensitizer [34]. Despite its extensive use, dermatitis is rarely seen, because the insecticide on the market now seems to be free of the sensitizing contaminant diethyl fumarate [35].
Patch test concentration: 0.5% pet.

Naled. See Sect. 14.5.2.1

Parathion Methyl (Wofatox; O,O-dimethyl-O-p-nitrophenyl-dithiophosphate). This substance, active against plant lice etc., is nowadays more common than parathion ethyl (Parathion). Both are weak sensitizers and may be phototoxic [8, 17, 36]. An erysipeloid-like lesion has also been seen [36].
Patch test concentration: 1% pet.

Pyrethrum and Pyrethroids. Pyrethrum (extract of *Chrysanthemum cinerariaefolium* and *C. coccineum* with pyrethrins, cinerins and jasmolins as active ingredients) and pyrethroids (synthetic substitutes, allethrin and analogs) are very selective contact insecticides for the control of flies and mosquitoes, sometimes mixed with piperonyl butoxide or sulphoxide and lindane as synergists. Allergic pyrethrum dermatitis is very rare. The main allergen is pyrethrosin, a sesquiterpene lactone [37, 38]. Cross-reactions between pyrethrum and several Compositae are possible. A highly characteristic additional side-effect is contact paraesthesia [39].
Patch test concentration: 2% pet.

14.5.2.7 Molluscicides

Metaldehyde is the chemical most used for slug control. There are no reports of skin hazards, and the patch test concentration of this probable contact allergen is unknown.

14.5.2.8 Rodenticides

ANTU (Antirax; 1-(1-Naphthyl)-2-Thiourea). This substance is used against rats and may cause allergic contact dermatitis [40].
Patch test concentration: 1%–2% pet.
Arsenic, Chlorophacinone, Polychlorocamphene, Strychnine Nitrate, Thallium Sulphate and Zinc Phosphide. These are of high systemic toxicity, but there are no reports of skin reactions from cutaneous contact.
Warfarin (3-(α-Acetonylbenzyl)-4-Hydroxycoumarin). This is the most common rat poison. It seems to be well tolerated by the skin.
Patch test concentration: 0.05% pet.

14.5.2.9 Other Pesticides

Other substances are employed as desiccants, nematocides, soil and room fumigants, bird repellents and wood preservatives. Plant growth regulators and fertilizers are other important groups of agricultural chemicals also of special interest to dermatologists.

14.5.3 Patch Testing with Pesticides

In many reports of dermatitis to pesticides, there is no clear differentiation between irritation and allergy, because useful information regarding patch test concentration and vehicle is lacking for most of these chemicals The recommended concentrations in the literature for many pesticides are based on very inadequate data. In many reported cases, the concentration used for patch testing has been too high and therefore irritant. Following such advice, irritant reactions or false-negative reactions might happen. The optimal test concentration is that which gives a minimum of irritant reactions without causing false negativity of allergic reactions. With many pesticides, irritant and allergic reaction levels are very close.

Many of the pesticides sold are mixed preparations of two or three active chemicals of technical grade (with combination products or impurities), solvents (water, lyes, oils, diesel fuel, etc.), surfactants (tensides), fillers (kaolin, silicic acid, milled slate, flour, etc.) and other agents. Some of these components may be irritants. In other cases, the concentration of the allergen in the whole product may be too low to give a positive patch test. Therefore, patch testing should be done with individual chemicals rather than with whole products. Information about the components of a product and the individual pesticide chemicals for patch testing should be requested from the manufacturer or supplier. Commercially available series are marketed by Hermal (Postfach 1228, 21462 Reinbek, FRG) and by Allergie GmbH (Kölner Landstraße 34 a, 40472 Düsseldorf 13, FRG). Confirmed suggestions for patch testing are given by the Dermatology Society of the former GDR [8] and

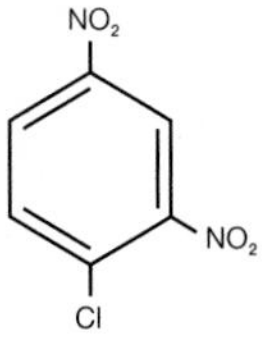

2,4-DNCB

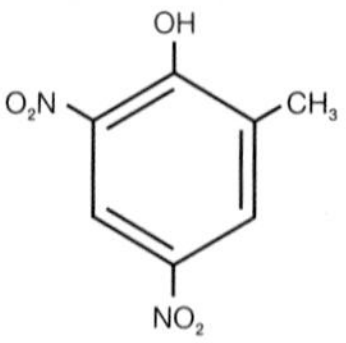

DNOC

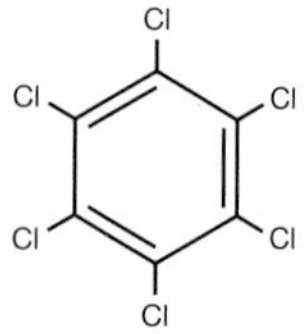

Lindane

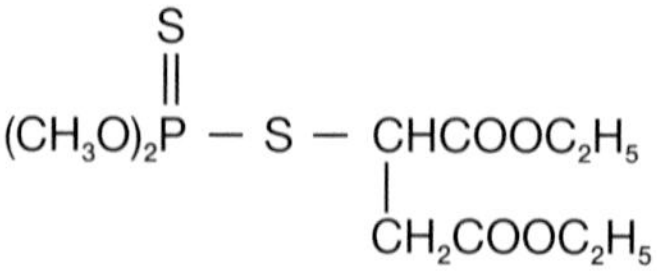

$(CH_3O)_2\overset{\overset{\textstyle S}{\|}}{P} - S - \underset{\underset{\textstyle CH_2COOC_2H_5}{|}}{CH}COOC_2H_5$

Malathion

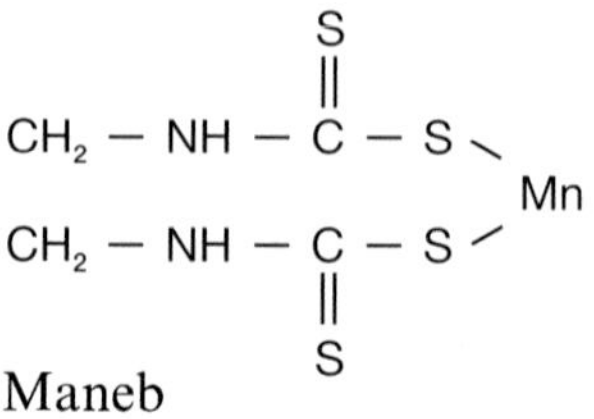

$$CH_2 - NH - \overset{\overset{\textstyle S}{\|}}{C} - S$$
$$CH_2 - NH - \underset{\underset{\textstyle S}{\|}}{C} - S$$
Mn

Maneb

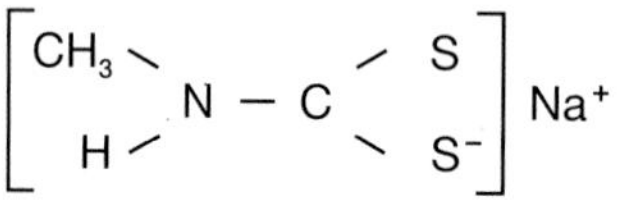

$$\left[\underset{H}{\overset{CH_3}{\diagdown}} N - C \underset{\diagdown}{\overset{\diagup}{}} \overset{S}{\underset{S^-}{}} \right] Na^+$$

Metam sodium

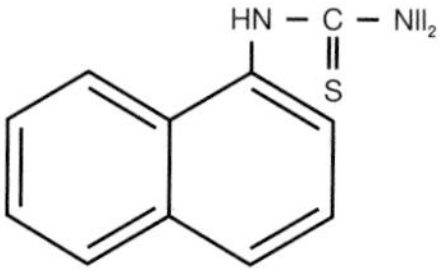

ANTU

$(C_3H_7)HN - C \overset{N=N}{\underset{N-N}{\diagup\diagdown}} C - Cl$

$NH(C_2H_5)$

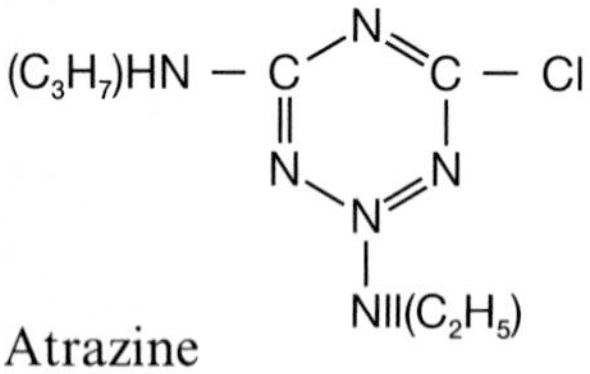

Atrazine

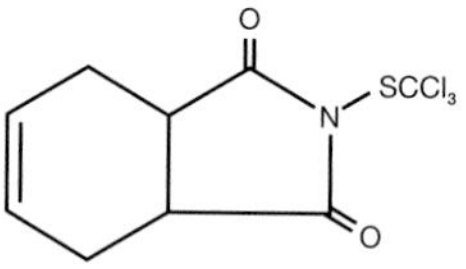

Captan

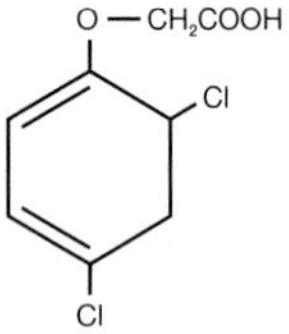

2,4-D

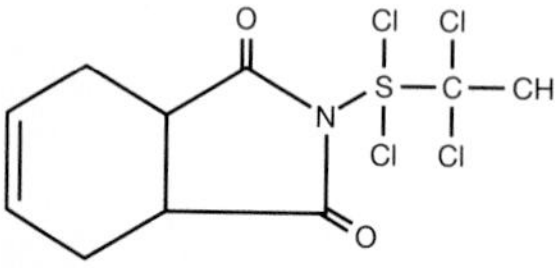

Difolatan

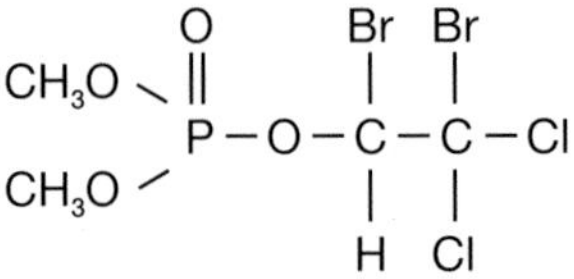

$$\underset{CH_3O}{\overset{CH_3O}{\diagdown\diagup}} \overset{\overset{\textstyle O}{\|}}{P} - O - \underset{\underset{\textstyle H}{|}}{\overset{\overset{\textstyle Br}{|}}{C}} - \underset{\underset{\textstyle Cl}{|}}{\overset{\overset{\textstyle Br}{|}}{C}} - Cl$$

Naled

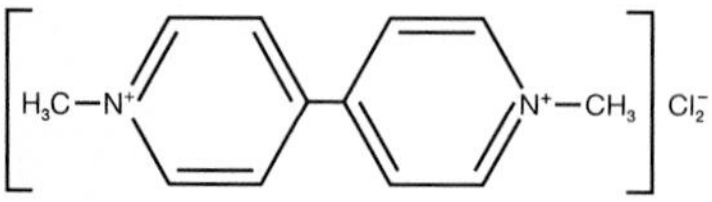

Paraquat

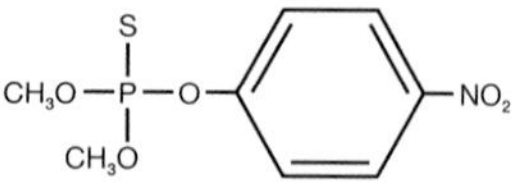

Parathion methyl

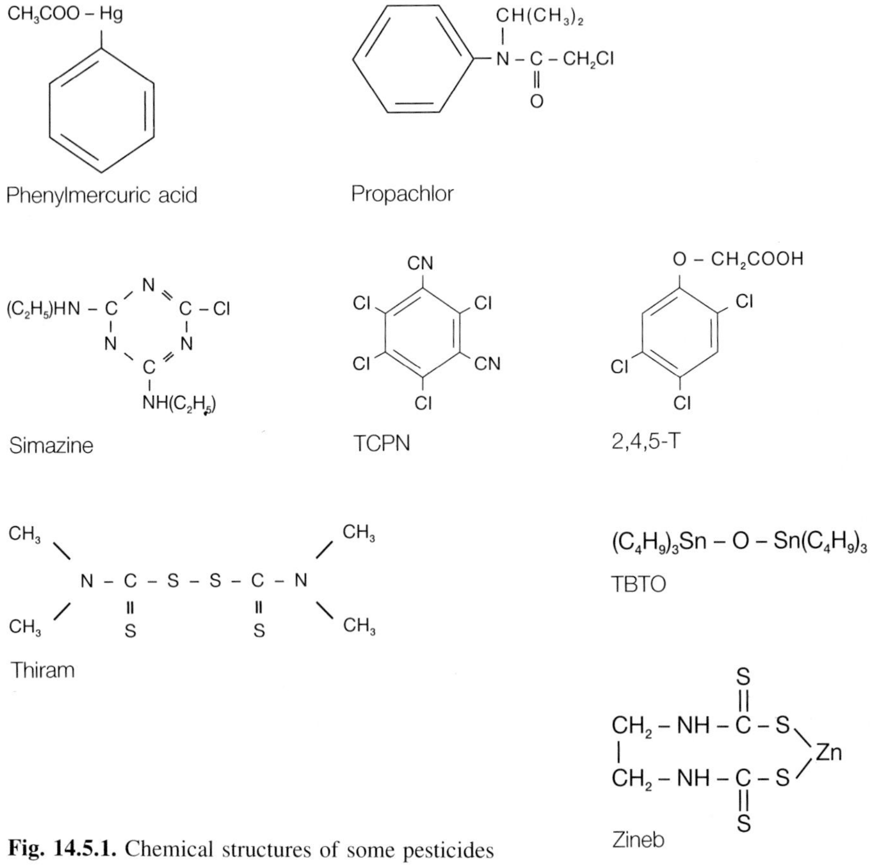

Fig. 14.5.1. Chemical structures of some pesticides

by Lisi et al. [41]. Table 14.5.1 is a summary of these and other reports, and Fig. 14.1.1 shows the chemical structure of some of the important pesticides. The irritant properties of pesticides can be scaled as the ID_{50} or IT_{50} [42, 43], as shown in Table 14.5.2. The ID_{50} is the concentration in percent of a chemical which causes an irritant test reaction after one application in half of the persons or animals on test.

Another question is the safety of patch testing with certain toxic pesticides, the organophosphates for example. They penetrate the skin very well and their median lethal dose (LD_{50}) is low. However, the amounts applied are extremely small (0.25% aq. corresponds to 0.3–0.6 mg per patch), and they will be quickly and completely reduced and their metabolites excreted. Therefore, patch testing with recommended concentrations of pesticides is safe from the toxicological point of view.

Further information may be found in specialized textbooks of occupational dermatology [44–47].

Table 14.5.1. Pesticides: suggested patch test concentrations and vehicles

Alachlor, 0.1% aq. or 1% pet.
Ametryne, 0.05% aq.
Amitrole, 1% aq.
Anilazine, 0.1% pet.
ANTU, 1% or 2% pet.
Atrazine, 0.05% aq.
Azinphos methyl, 0.25% pet.
Benomyl, 0.1% aq. or pet.
Bromophos, 0.025% pet.
Bupirimate, 0.01 or 1% pet.
Butonate, 5% aq.
Captan, 0.1% aq.
Carbaryl, 0.5% or 1% pet.
Carbyne, 10% o.o.
Chloral hydrate, 15% aq.
Chloramphenicol, 1% pet.
Chloridazon, 0.1% or 1% aq. or pet.
Chlormequat, 0.5% aq.
Chlorpropham, 0.5% pet.
Copper sulphate, 0.5% or 1% aq.
2,4-D (techn), 1% aq.
2,4-D/2,4,5-T Mix, 0.5% o.o.
Dalapon, 50% aq. or pet.
Dazomet, 0.1% aq.
2,4-Dichlorophenoxybutyric acid (2,4-DB) 1% aq.
Dichlorodiphenyltrichloroethane (DDT) (techn), 1% pet, or acet.
Demephion-O, 0.25% aq.
Diazinon, 1% pet.
Dichlorophene, 0.5% or 1% pet.
Dichlorprop, 1% aq.
Dichlorphos, 0.05% aq.
Difolatan, 0.1% pet.
Dimethoate, 0.5% or 1% aq.
4,6-Dinitrocresol, 50% aq.
Dinobuton, 1–10% pet.
Dinocap, 1% pet.
Diquat, 0.1% pet.
Ditalimphos, 0.01% pet.
Dithianone, 1% pet.
2,4-DNCB, 0.01% acet. or aq.
Dyrene, 0.1% pet.
Etephon, 1% aq.
Fenazox, 50% aq.
Fentin hydroxide, 0.5% pet.
Folpet, 0.1% pet.
Glyphosate, 10% aq.

Hexachlorocyclohexane (HCH) (techn), 1% pet. or acet.
Lindane, 1% pet. or acet.
Malathion, 0.5% pet.
Mancozeb, 1% pet.
Maneb, 0.5% or 1% pet.
MCPA, 5–10% aq.
Mercaptobenzothiazole (MBT), 2% pet.
Metaldehyde, 1% pet.
Metam sodium, 0.03% aq.
Methidation, 0.5% or 1% pet.
Methomyl, 0.5 or 1% aq.
Molinate, 1% pet.
Naled, 0.5% aq.
Nitrofen, 0.5% pet. or o.o.
Oxydemeton methyl, 0.25% pet.
Paraquat, 0.1% pet.
Parathion ethyl, 1% pet. or aq.
Parathion methyl, 1% pet.
Pentachlorophenol, 1% aq.
Phaltan, 0.05% or 0.1% pet.
Phenmedipham, 0.2% or 0.5% aq.
Pentachloronitrobenzene, 0.5% pet.
Phenylmercuric acetate, 0.05% pet.
o-Phenylphenol, 1% pet.
Phorate, 1% pet.
Pirimiphos methyl, 0.5% pet.
Plondrel, 0.01% pet.
Propachlor, 0.05% or 0.1% aq.
Propanil, 1% pet.
Pyrethrum, 2% pet.
Quintozen, 10% aq.
Randox, 0.01% or 0.1% pet.
Rodannitrobenzene, 1% pet.
Simazine, 5% aq.
Sodium trichloroacetate (TCA), 1% aq.
Streptomycin, 1% pet. or aq.
Tetmosol, 1% pet.
Tetrachloroisophthalonitrile (TCPN), 0.001% or 0.01% acet. or pet.
2,4,5-T, 0.5% o.o.
Thiuram, 1% pet.
Tributyltin oxide (TBTO), 0.001% aq.
Trichlorodinitrobenzene, 0.01% aq.
Trichlorfon, 1% aq.
Warfarin, 0.05% pet.
Zineb, 1% pet.
Ziram, 1% pet.

Table 14.5.2. The ID_{50} of some pesticides in man

Butonate	11%
Carboxin	not irritant
Dalapon	25.6%
Defenuron	100%
DNOC	60%
Fenazox	65.8%
Fenuron	16%
MCPA	6.1%
Propachlor	1.4%
Proximpham	not irritant
Tridemorph	0.05%

14.5.3 References

1. Weber T, Berencesi G (1972) Über die Permeabilität der Schutzhandschuhe für verschiedene Pflanzenschutzmittel. Int Arch Arbeitsmed 30: 23–30
2. Mellström G (1985) Protective effects of gloves compiled in a data base. Contact Dermatitis 13: 162–165
3. Schubert H (1978) Contact dermatitis to sodium N-methyldithiocarbamate. Contact Dermatitis 4: 370–371
4. Edmundsen WF, Davies JE (1967) Occupational dermatitis from Naled. Arch Environ Health 15: 89–91
5. Gammeltoft M (1978) Tributyltinoxide is not allergenic. Contact Dermatitis 4: 238
6. Wüthrich B (1979) Chloramphenikolkontaktallergie. Hautarzt 30: 452–453
7. Marcussen PV (1949) Professional streptomycin hypersensitiveness among hospital staffs. Acta Derm Venereol (Stockh) 49: 410–413
8. Jung HD, Rothe A, Heise H (1987) Zur Epikutantestung von Pflanzenschutz- und Schädlingsbekämpfungsmitteln (Pestiziden). Derm Beruf Umwelt 35: 43–51
9. Savitt LE (1972) Contact dermatitis due to benomyl insecticide. Arch Dermatol 105: 926–927
10. van Joost T, Naafs B, van Ketel WG (1983) Sensitization to benomyl and related pesticides. Contact Dermatitis 9: 153–154
11. Fregert S (1967) Allergic contact dermatitis from pesticides captan and phaltan. Contact Dermatitis 2: 28
12. Marzulli FN, Maibach HI (1973) Antimicrobials: experimental contact sensitizazion in man. J Soc Cosmet Chem 24: 399–421
13. Brown R (1984) Contact sensitivity to difolatan (captafol). Contact Dermatitis 10: 181–182
14. Cushman JR, Street JC (1991) Contact sensitivity to captafol in BALB/c mice. Contact Dermatitis 24: 363–365
15. Cottel WI (1972) Difolatan. Contact Dermatitis 11: 252
16. Adams RM, Manchester RD (1982) Allergic contact dermatitis to Maneb in a housewife. Contact Dermatitis 8: 271
17. Jung HD (1979) Arbeitsdermatosen durch Pestizide. Dtsch Gesundheitswes 34: 1144–1148
18. Manuzzi P, Borrello P, Miscali C, Guerra L (1988) Contact dermatitis due to Ziram and Maneb. Contact Dermatitis 19: 148
19. Nater JP, Terpstra H, Bleumink E (1979) Allergic contact sensitization to the fungicide Maneb. Contact Dermatitis 5: 24–26
20. Meding B (1986) Contact dermatitis from tetrachloroisophthalonitrile in paint. Contact Dermatitis 15: 187

21. Spindeldreier A, Deichmann D (1980) Kontaktdermatitis auf ein Holzschutzmittel mit neuer fungizider Wirksubstanz. Derm Beruf Umwelt 28: 88–90
22. Schulz KH, Hermann WP (1958) Tetramethylthiuramdisulfid, ein Thioharnstoffderivat als Ekzemnoxe bei Hafenarbeitern. Berufsdermatosen 6: 130–135
23. Behrbohm P, Zschunke E (1965) Allergisches Ekzem durch das Antimykotikum "Afungin" (Dibenzthion). Dermatol Wochenschr 151: 1447–1453
24. Schuman SH, Dobson RL (1988) An outbreak of contact dermatitis in farm workers. J Am Acad Dermatol 13: 220–223
25. Jung HD, Wolff F (1977) Kontaktekzeme durch das Herbizid Selest in der Forstwirtschaft. Dtsch Gesundheitswes 32: 1464–1467
26. Maibach HI (1986) Irritation, sensitization, photoirritation and photosensitization assays with a glyphosate herbicide. Contact Dermatitis 15: 152–156
27. Baran RL (1974) Nail damage caused by weed killers and insecticides. Arch Dermatol 110: 467–469
28. Botella R, Sastre A, Castells A (1985) Contact dermatitis to Paraquat. Contact Dermatitis 13: 123–124
29. Howard JK (1979) A clinical survey of paraquat formulation workers. Br J Ind Med 36: 220–223
30. Schubert H (1979) Allergic contact dermatitis due to propachlor. Dermatol Monatsschr 165: 495–498
31. Spencer MC (1966) Herbicide dermatitis. JAMA 198: 169–170
32. Behrbohm P, Brandt B (1960) Allergisches Kontakekzem durch technische und gereinigte Hexachlorcyclohexanpräparate bei der Anwendung im Pflanzenschutz und in der Schädlingsbekämpfung. Berufsdermatosen 8: 95–101
33. Hegyi E, Štóta Z (1965) Zur Frage der Allergenspezifität der Komponenten des technischen Hexachlorcyclohexans. Berufsdermatosen 13: 193–197
34. Kligman AM (1966) The identification of contact allergens by human assay. III. The maximization test: a procedure for screening and rating contact sensitizers. J Invest Dermatol 47: 393–409
35. Hjorth N, Wilkinson DS (1968) Contact dermatitis. Sensitization to pesticides. Br J Dermatol 80: 272–274
36. Svindland HB (1981) Subacute parathion poisoning with erysipeloidlike lesion. Contact Dermatitis 7: 177–179
37. Lisi P (1992) Sensitization risk of pyrethroid insecticides. Contact Dermatitis 26: 349–350
38. Mitchell JC, Dupuis G, Towers GHN (1972) Allergic contact dermatitis from pyrethrum. Br J Dermatol 86: 568–573
39. Flannigan SA, Tucker SB (1985) Variation in cutaneous sensation between synthetic pyrethroid insecticides. Contact Dermatitis 13: 140–147
40. Laubstein H (1962) Kontakekzem durch ein Rodentizid. Berufsdermatosen 10: 154–156
41. Lisi P, Caraffini S, Assalve D (1986) A test series for pesticide dermatitis. Contact Dermatitis 15: 266–269
42. Heise H, Mattheus A, Brust H (1983) Irritationsprüfungen in der Dermatologie – ihre Bedeutung und Aussage. Dermatol Monatsschr 169: 631–637
43. Kligman AM, Wooding WM (1967) A method for the measurement and evaluation of irritants on human skin. J Invest Dermatol 49: 78–94
44. Adams RM (1990) Occupational skin diseases, 2nd edn. Saunders, Philadelphia, pp 546–577
45. Cronin E (1980) Contact dermatitis. Churchill Livingstone, Edingburgh, pp 391–413
46. Hayes WJ (1982) Pesticide studies in man. William and Wilkins, Baltimore
47. Zschunke E (1985) Grundriß der Arbeitsdermatologie. Verlag Volk und Gesundheit, Berlin, pp 110–119

14.6 Plastic Materials

BERT BJÖRKNER

Contents

14.6.1 Introduction

The polymer industry is now one of the most important branches of the chemical industry and uses a wider variety of chemicals than any other. The number of commercially important plastics today is around 50. Application areas for plastics are many and varied; the construction industry, packaging, electronics, recreation, medical, etc. Of the base plastics, 30% are used for packaging and 20% in the construction industry.

There are several ways of classifying polymeric materials. Chemically, they are very large molecules (polymers), formed by the linking up of small molecules (monomers) into large chain-like units. If only one type of monomer is involved in forming the polymer, it is called a homopolymer. If two or more different types are involved, it is called a copolymer.

Polymers can also be classified in other ways. If the monomers simply link up into long chains by joining bonds, and nothing is eliminated in the process, the polymerization is called an *addition* reaction. If two or more different monomers react with each other, thereby eliminating a simple molecule such as water, this polymerization is called a *condensation* reaction.

The words *plastic* and *resin* are often used synonymously. However, strictly, plastics are synthetic macromolecular end products, while the term resin is used to denote all low, medium and high molecular weight intermediate synthetic substances from which plastics are made. Natural rubbers and cellulose do not fit into these definitions because their starting material is of natural origin and not synthetic.

For traditional and practical reasons, plastics can be divided into three major types: *thermoplastic, thermosetting* and *elastomers*. The thermoplastic resins are characterized by softening when exposed to heat and when soft they can be made to flow and assume desired shapes. When cooled, they become hard again. The thermosetting resins, when heated for the first time, undergo further chemical reactions in which cross-links develop between polymer chains, holding them rigid in the desired position. They do not soften on reheating like the original polymer. Examples of thermoplastic resins are polyethylene, polystyrene, polyacrylates, polyvinyl chloride and saturated polyesters. Examples of thermosetting resins are: phenol-formaldehyde resins, epoxy resins and polyurethanes. Examples of elastomers are natural rubbers.

In general, the final plastic products, when *completely* cured or hardened, are considered to be inert and nonhazardous to the skin. Skin problems from plastics are almost exclusively related to ingredients such as monomers, hardeners and other additives, or degradation products of low molecular weight.

14.6.2 Acrylic Resins

The acrylic resins are thermoplastic and are formed by derivatives of acrylic acid (CH_2=CH-COOH). The acrylic group is a vinyl group (CH_2=CH-) and acrylic monomers polymerize in an addition reaction. The monomers in acrylic resins are acrylic acids or methacrylic acids and their esters, cyanoacrylic acid and its esters, acrylamides and acrylonitrile. Thus a great number of different acrylic monomers exist and many different polymers and resins are produced.

Polymerization of acrylic monomers is obtained either at room temperature or by heating. Usually initiators, accelerators and catalysts are added to speed up the process. Polymerization or curing can also be achieved by ultraviolet (UV) light, visible light or electron beams, when no initiators are necessary.

14.6.2.1 Monoacrylates and Monomethacrylates

Mono(meth)acrylates (monoacrylates and monomethacrylates) are used for the production of a great variety of polymers.

Polymethyl methacrylate is the most important plastic in the group of acrylics with the following repeating unit: $[CH_2$-$CH(CH_3)COOCH_3]_n$.

Because of its high transparency this plastic is used in products such as roof windows, houseware, watch glasses, bags, lamp housings and windscreens. In the manufacture of dentures, hearing aids, noise protectors and bone cement in orthopaedic surgery, a two-component system is used. The first component is a prepolymer powder of polymethyl methacrylate with benzoyl peroxide as initiator. The second component is a monomeric liquid of methyl methacrylate containing an accelerator, e.g. N, N-dimethyl-p-toluidine.

Other polymers of the mono(meth)acrylate type are mostly used in industry. Some examples of fields of applications are: leather finishes, adhesives, paints,

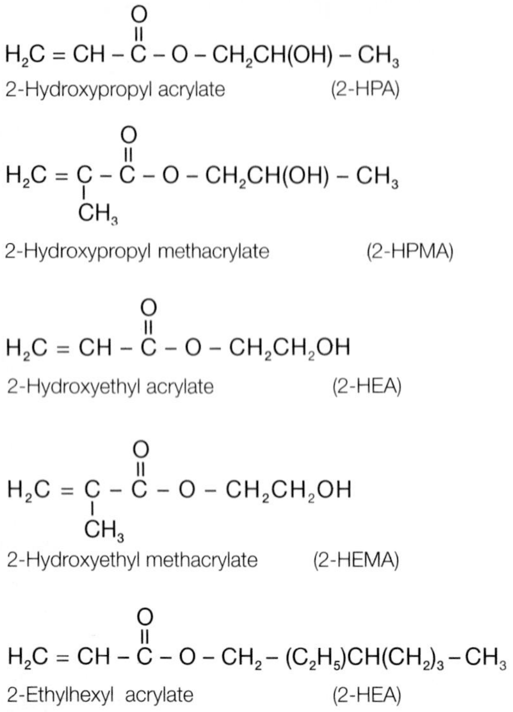

$$\overset{\displaystyle O}{\overset{\displaystyle \|}{H_2C = CH - C - O - CH_2CH(OH) - CH_3}}$$

2-Hydroxypropyl acrylate   (2-HPA)

$$\overset{\displaystyle O}{\overset{\displaystyle \|}{H_2C = C - C - O - CH_2CH(OH) - CH_3}}$$
$$\underset{\displaystyle CH_3}{|}$$

2-Hydroxypropyl methacrylate   (2-HPMA)

$$\overset{\displaystyle O}{\overset{\displaystyle \|}{H_2C = CH - C - O - CH_2CH_2OH}}$$

2-Hydroxyethyl acrylate   (2-HEA)

$$\overset{\displaystyle O}{\overset{\displaystyle \|}{H_2C = C - C - O - CH_2CH_2OH}}$$
$$\underset{\displaystyle CH_3}{|}$$

2-Hydroxyethyl methacrylate   (2-HEMA)

$$\overset{\displaystyle O}{\overset{\displaystyle \|}{H_2C = CH - C - O - CH_2 - (C_2H_5)CH(CH_2)_3 - CH_3}}$$

2-Ethylhexyl acrylate   (2-HEA)

Fig. 14.6.1. Chemical formulae of some monofunctional accrylate compounds in UV-curable acrylate-based paints and lacquers

printing inks and coatings. Butyl acrylate can be used in spectacle frames. 2-Ethylhexyl acrylate is frequently used in pressure-sensitive adhesives but a wide range of other acrylates are also used in this field.

The acrylic monomers preferably used in UV-curable inks and coatings or in the photoprepolymer printing plate procedure are 2-hydroxyethyl acrylate (2-HEA), 2-hydroxypropyl acrylate (2-HPA), 2-hydroxypropyl methacrylate (2-HPMA), 2-hydroxyethyl methacrylate (2-HEMA) and 2-ethylhexyl acrylate (2-EHA) (Fig. 14.6.1). 2-HPMA is also used in UV-sensitive compositions for fissure sealants in dentistry and in Napp printing plates. In waterbased acrylic latex paints, various mono(meth)acrylates can be used. Plastic dispersions of acrylic polymers are used as binders or thickeners. Usually the monomer content is less than 0.3%.

14.6.2.2 Multifunctional Acrylates

Molecules with at least two reactive arcylic groups belong to the class of multifunctional acrylates. These include, for example, di(meth)acrylate esters

Table 14.6.1. Acrylates used in acrylic nail preparations

Methyl methacrylate
Ethyl methacrylate
Butyl methacrylate
Isobutyl methacrylate
Methacrylic acid
Tetrahydrofurfuryl methacrylate
Ethylene glycol dimethacrylate
Diethylene glycol dimethacrylate
Triethylene glycol dimethacrylate
Trimethylol propane trimethacrylate
Urethane methacrylate

of dialcohols or tri- and tetraacrylate esters of polyalcohols. The multifunctional acrylates are used in formulations for UV-curable inks and coatings where they act as cross-linking agents and reactive diluents, becoming a part of the final coating on exposure to UV-light. The multifunctional acrylates are also important compounds in photopolymers, flexographic printing plates and photoresists (an etchresist for printed circuit boards). In acrylic glues, adhesives and anaerobic sealants as well as in artificial nail preparations, the multifunctional acrylate esters are useful (Table 14.6.1). Some of the more commonly used are ethylene glycol dimethacrylate (EGDMA), diethylene glycol dimethacrylate (DEGDMA) and trimethylolpropane trimethacrylate (TMPTMA). Most of the dental composite resin materials and denture base polymers are "diluted" with less viscous "difunctional" acrylates. These are the *meth*acrylic monomers, of which EGDMA, DEGDMA, triethylene glycol dimethacrylate (TREGDMA) and 1,4-butanediol dimethacrylate (BUDMA) are the most extensively used (Figs. 14.6.2, 14.6.3).

The simplest UV-curable ink or coating formulation may consist of only three components, but in practice a typical industrial formulation contains a much higher number of ingredients. The three essential components are a UV-reactive prepolymer, which provides the bulk of the desired properties, a diluent system composed of multifunctional acrylate esters (and at times monofunctional acrylic esters) and a photoinitiator system. The most commonly used multifunctional acrylate in a UV-curable ink or coating formulation is an acrylic acid ester of either

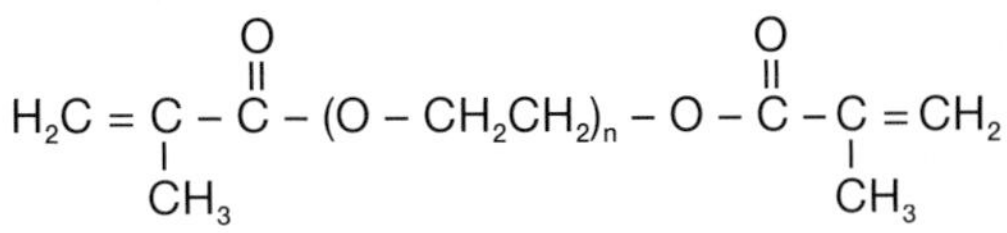

$$H_2C = \underset{\underset{CH_3}{|}}{C} - \overset{\overset{O}{\|}}{C} - (O - CH_2CH_2)_n - O - \overset{\overset{O}{\|}}{C} - \underset{\underset{CH_3}{|}}{C} = CH_2$$

Fig. 14.6.2. Chemical formulae of *n*-ethylene glycol di(meth)acrylates

n=1: Ethylene glycol dimethacrylate   (EGDMA)
n=2: Diethylene glycol dimethacrylate   (DEGDMA)
n=3: Triethylene glycol dimethacrylate   (TREGDMA)

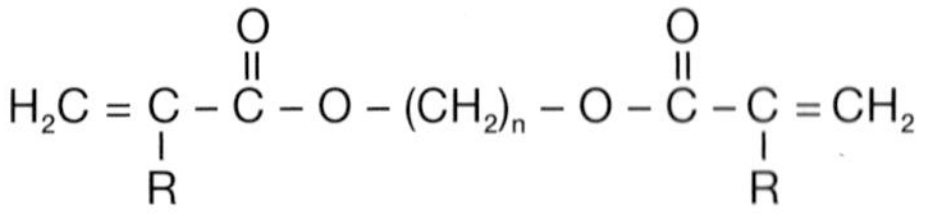

$$H_2C = \underset{\underset{R}{|}}{C} - \overset{\overset{O}{\|}}{C} - O - (CH_2)_n - O - \overset{\overset{O}{\|}}{C} - \underset{\underset{R}{|}}{C} = CH_2$$

R = H &   n = 6:   1,6-Hexanediol diacrylate   (HDDA)
R = CH₃ & n = 4:   1,4-Butanediol dimethacrylate (BUDMA)

Fig. 14.6.3. Chemical formulae of 1,6-hexanediol diacrylate and 1,4-butanediol dimethacrylate

pentaerythritol (PETA), trimethylolpropane (TMPTA) or hexanediol (HDDA) (Figs. 14.6.3, 14.6.4).

In the last decade the use of UV-curable acrylates in inks and coatings has increased tremendously. In the can-coating industry, UV-printing inks are used on beverage and beer cans as well as on bottle tops and aerosol cans. UV-curable acrylate coatings are used as wood finishes, mat varnishes, parquet varnishes and sealers and for varnishing and coating in the furniture industry.

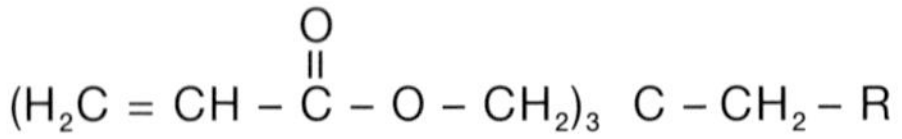

$$(H_2C = CH - \overset{\overset{O}{\|}}{C} - O - CH_2)_3 \; C - CH_2 - R$$

R = OH: Pentaerythritolol diacrylate   (PETA)
R = CH₃: Trimethylolpropane triacrylate (TMPTA)

Fig. 14.6.4. Chemical formulae of two common UV-curable multifunctional acrylates

Both TMPTA and PETA can be used in the production of polyfunctional aziridine, added to paint primer and floor top coatings as a self-curing cross-linker or hardener [1, 2].

Anaerobic acrylic sealants, e.g. Loctite, Treebond and Sta-Lok [3–5], polymerize rapidly in the absence of oxygen and in the presence of metals. The principal components are dimethacrylates. DEGDMA oligomer is most commonly used for screw-thread locking, whereas urethane dimethacrylate is used for retaining and locking flat metal surfaces.

14.6.2.3 Prepolymers

Acrylate resins based on the conventional thermoplastic resins, into which two or more reactive acrylate or methacrylate groups have been introduced, are called prepolymers. The most commonly used prepolymers are acrylated epoxy resins, acrylated polyurethanes, acrylated polyesters and acrylated polyethers.

Epoxy Acrylates. The ß-hydroxyester acrylates are also called epoxy acrylates, because they are usually obtained by reacting epoxy resins or glycidyl derivatives with acrylic acid (Fig. 14.6.5). Both aromatic and aliphatic epoxy acrylates are available, as well as acrylated epoxydized oils. Epoxy acrylates have the most useful applications in the UV-curing field.

BIS-GMA   (2,2-bis[4-(2-hydroxy-3-methacryloxypropoxy)phenyl]-propane) is the addition reaction product between bisphenol A and glycidyl methacrylate or an epoxy resin and methacrylic acid (Fig. 14.6.5). BIS-GMA

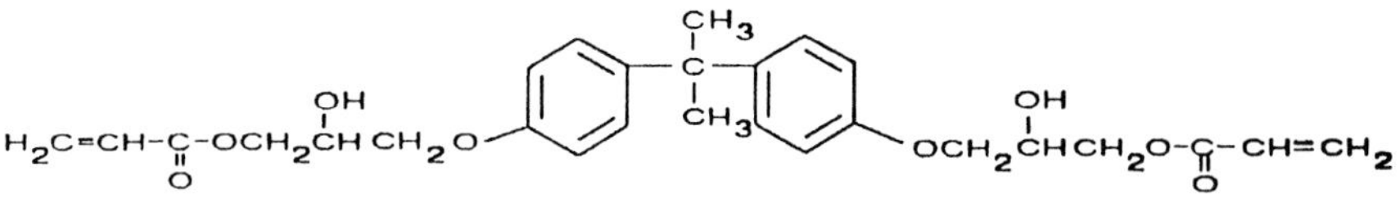

Epoxy Diacrylate

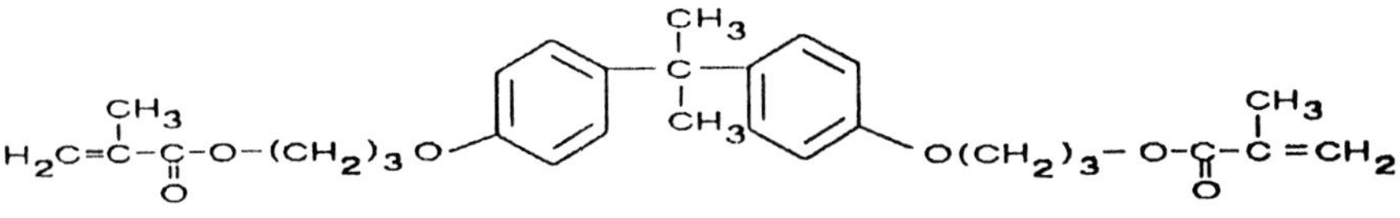

BIS-PMA

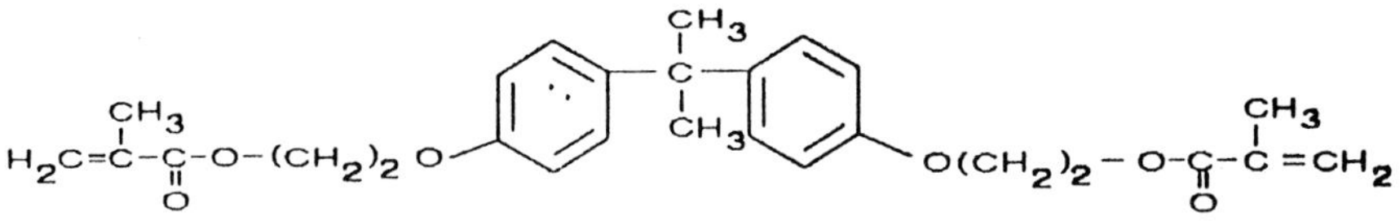

BIS-EMA

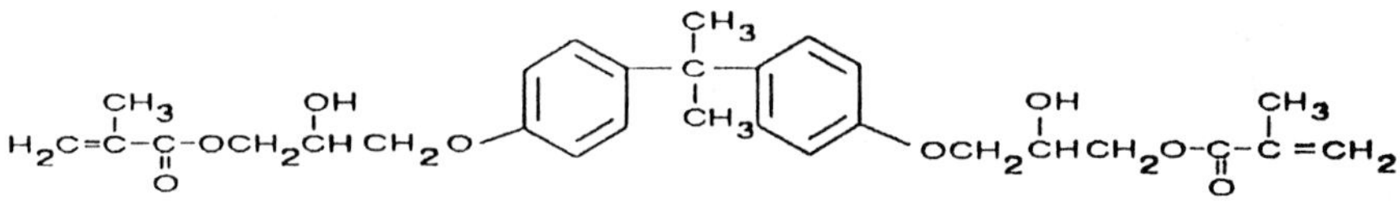

BIS-GMA

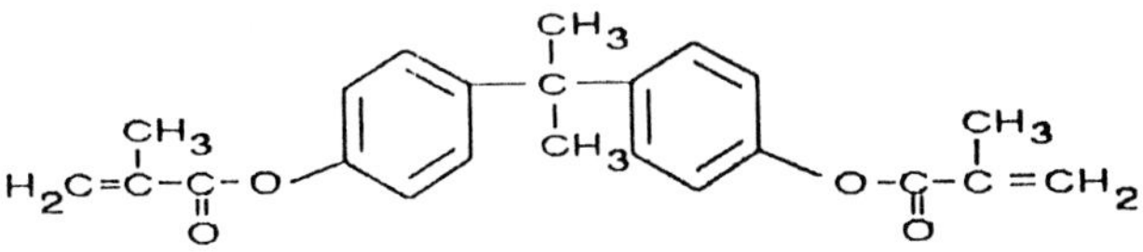

BIS-MA

Fig. 14.6.5. Chemical formulae of di(meth)acrylates based on bisphenol A and epoxy resin

should therefore be classified as a dimethacrylated epoxy. It is the most commonly used prepolymer in dental composite restorative materials. Several similar compounds have also appeared as substitutes for BIS-GMA or in addition to BIS-GMA in dental resins. Such dimethacrylates based on bisphenol A with various chain lengths are BIS-MA (2,2-bis[4-(methacryloxy)phenyl]-propane), BIS-EMA (2,2-bis[4-(2-methacryloxyethoxy)phenyl]-propane) and BIS-PMA (2,2-bis[4-(3-methacryloxypropoxy)phenyl]-propane) (Fig. 14.6.5). The acrylic compounds commonly used in dentistry are listed in Table 14.6.2.

Table 14.6.2. Acrylic compounds used in dental materials

Methyl methacrylate
Triethyleneglycol dimethacrylate
Urethane dimethacrylate
Ethylene glycol dimethacrylate
BIS-GMA
BIS-MA
BIS-EMA
BIS-PMA
2-(Dimethylamino)ethyl methacrylate
Butyl methacrylate
Hydroxyethyl methacrylate
1,6-Hexanediol diacrylate
1,10-Decanediol dimethacrylate
1,4-Butanediol dimethacrylate
1,12-Dodecanediol dimethacrylate
Trimethylpropane trimethacrylate
Phenylsalicylate glycidyl methacrylate
Tetrahydrofurfuryl methacrylate
Benzyl dimethacrylate
Benzaldehyde glycol methacrylate

BIS-GMA resins and the other similar derivatives also find extensive use in industrial applications. Acrylates based on bisphenol A or epoxy resin can be polymerized not only by exposure to electron beams, UV light or even visable light, but also chemically activated by the use of various peroxides.

Urethane Acrylates. There are many types of acrylated urethane on the market. Some are based on aromatic isocyanates while others are of the aliphatic type. The acrylated urethanes are not only used in prepolymers in UV-curable inks or coatings, for instance in vinyl flooring, but also as resins with dental applications. The acrylated urethanes used in dentistry are mostly of the methacrylated types.

Polyester Acrylates. There are also various types of polyester acrylates and they are mostly used in UV-curable laquers and printing inks for wood and paper coatings.

14.6.2.4 Effects on the Skin of Acrylate Esters

Investigations of the skin irritating potential of various acrylic monomers have shown that the diacrylates are strong irritants, monoacrylates are weak to moderate irritants, and monomethacrylates and dimethacrylates are non irritant or weak irritants to guinea pig skin [6–10]. Multifunctional acrylates, as well as acrylated preopolymers, seem to be more skin irritating than the corresponding methacrylates. These effects have been seen when patch testing both humans and guinea pigs [11]. Bullous irritant skin reactions in workers exposed to tetramethylene glycol diacrylate have been reported [12]. A peculiar delayed irritation from butanediol diacrylate and hexanediol diacrylate has been observed by Malten et al. [13]. Tetraethylene glycol diacrylate can cause delayed cutaneous irritant reactions as well as allergic contact dermatitis [14].

The sensitizing potential in guinea pigs of many mono(meth)acrylates, multifunctional (meth)acrylates and acrylated resins has been thoroughly investigated by various authors [6–9, 11, 15]. Monoacrylates are strong sensitizers while monomethacrylates have a weak to moderate sensitizing potential. Thus the introduction of a methyl group reduces the sensitizing potential of monoacrylates. Of the multifunctional acrylates, the di- and triacrylic compounds should be regarded as potent sensitizers. The methacrylated multifunctional acrylic compounds are weak sensitizers.

Among the various di(meth)acrylates based on bisphenol A or epoxy resin, the allergenicity seems to diminish if the acrylates have three or more methylene groups in the molecular chain [16, 17]. The sensitizing capacity of the various prepolymers on the market is more difficult to predict. Epoxy acrylates are strong sensitizers and their sensitizing capacity is due to the entire molecule, thereby excluding the epoxide group as the sole sensitizing part of the compounds. There may be free epoxy resin present in epoxy acrylates, which may sensitize separately or simultaneously. Probably, the whole molecular structure of polyester acrylate acts as an allergen as well. However, the reactive terminal acrylate or methacrylate groups seem to be of great importance for antigen formation and sensitization [18]. It seems that the aliphatic urethane acrylates are more potent sensitizers than the aromatic ones, while the aliphatic urethane methacrylate commonly used in dental resins is a weak sensitizer [19, 20].

There are many reports about contact allergy to mono(meth)acrylates in humans. Contact dermatitis due to 2-HPMA in printers exposed to printing plates, as well as to UV-curing inks, has been reported [21, 22]. Contact allergy to 2-HEMA, one of the ingredients in a photoprepolymer mixture, has been described [23]. Contact dermatitis from 2-EHA in an acrylic-based adhesive tape has been reported [24]. Orthopaedic surgeons, surgical technicians, nurses and dental technicians are exposed to methyl methacrylate monomer when preparing bone cement and dentures. Contact allergy to methyl methacrylate monomer is very rare in patients undergoing hip surgery [25, 26].

In the last decade, many reports about contact allergy caused by various multifunctional acrylic compounds have been published [27–38]. People at risk of developing contact allergy to multifunctional tri- and diacrylates are those working with UV-curable inks or coatings, while contact allergy to dimethacrylates is more commonly seen in dentistry, in those working with anaerobic acrylic sealants and in those exposed to acrylic nails [39, 40]. There are some reports of allergic contact reactions to dimethacrylates based on bisphenol A or epoxy resin in dental composite materials. At risk of developing contact dermatitis are dentists and dental technicians, as well as dental patients. Some patients allergic to BIS-GMA also react to epoxy resin MW 340 [17, 41]. It is uncertain whether any residual epoxy resin monomer is left unreacted or whether it is formed in the synthesis of the BIS-GMA monomer.

Methyl methacrylate can penetrate the skin and produce paraesthesia of the fingers for months after discontinuation of contact with the monomer. Such as effect on the peripheral nervous system has also been described for acrylamide, but it might also occur with other acrylic monomers [42].

14.6.2.5 Acrylonitrile

Acrylonitrile ($H_2C=CH-CN$) is used as a copolymer in approximately 25% of all synthetic fibers. It is further used for synthetic rubbers and for the production of acrylonitrile – butadiene – styrene plastics and styrene – acrylonitrile plastics. These ter- and copolymers are used in the automobile industry and in the production of household wares, electrical appliances, suitcases, food packaging and disposable dishes. Acrylonitrile can also be a constituent in fabrics and paints [43].

Skin Problems from Acrylonitrile. There are only a few reports about contact allergy to the acrylonitrile monomer [44–46].

14.6.2.6 Acrylamide and Derivatives

Acrylamide ($H_2C=CH-CO-NH_2$) is used as a paper making strengthener, as an emulsion thickening agent and in biochemistry in gel electrophoresis. Polyacrylamide is used for the separation of solids suspended in water, as in cleaning of sewage. Acrylamide, as well as structurally related substances, is also used as a copolymer in adhesives and water-based paints. Acrylamide and its derivatives are also used in the production of photopolymer printing plates [47].

Skin Problems from Acrylamide and Derivatives. Polyacrylamide is inert to the skin but the monomer can be irritating and cause contact allergy. Skin problems are seen among printers exposed to photopolymerizing printing plates. Acrylamide and the acrylamide compounds N, N'-methylene-bis-acrylamide and N-methylolacrylamide have been described as allergens [21, 48, 49]. N-methylolacrylamide sensitization has also been observed in workers making PVA-acrylic copolymers for paints. Paraesthesia in the exposed fingers from acrylamides and some of its analogues has been reported [50]. Acrylamide, N-hydroxymethylacrylamide and N, N'-methylene-bis-acrylamide are moderate sensitizers when tested in guinea pigs [9].

14.6.2.7 Cyanoacrylates

Cyanoacrylates ($H_2C=C(CN)$-COOR), often called "superglues", are used as adhesives for plastics, rubber, glass, and metals and in medicine to bind tissues and to seal wounds. They polymerize rapidly when exposed to water.

Skin Problems from Cyanoacrylates. Cyanoacrylates are known to be irritating to the eyes and respiratory tract when vaporized. Irritation and discomfort of the face and eye irritation may occur in workers due to associated low humidity [51]. Contact sensitization to cyanoacrylates is considered extremely rare, because of the immediate bonding of the cyanoacrylate to the surface keratin [52].

14.6.2.8 Preventive Methods When Handling Acrylic Resins

To protect the hands from the various acrylic compounds, gloves are recommended. However, it has been demonstrated that methyl methacrylate, as well as other acrylic monomers such as butyl acrylate and acrylamide, easily penetrates rubber latex gloves [9, 53]. All vinyl gloves appeared to provide poorer protection.

Polyethylene gloves give the best protection against methyl methacrylate diffusion [9]. This material, however, is not sufficiently elastic, and is easily perforated by a sharp edge or a rough surface. Nitrile gloves give better protection than neoprene gloves against UV-curable acrylate resins [11, 54]. New multilayered glove materials have been shown to have especially good chemical resistance. An example is a Danish laminated glove in which ethylene vinyl alcohol copolymer is laminated with polyethylene on both sides [55].

Most of the acrylic compounds used in UV-curable acrylic resins should be regarded as irritants and relatively potent sensitizers and care should be taken accordingly to minimize their contact with the skin. Certain measures that seem effective in preventing the occurrence of dermatitis include the use of impervious protective gloves and protective clothing. Face shields and goggles are recommended whenever there is a risk of splattering. Contaminated skin should be washed with soap and water and contaminated clothing immediately removed. Separation of clean and contaminated clothing is necessary. Careful education of employees about skin hazards is also recommended.

14.6.2.9 Patch Testing

In general, a patch test concentration of 2% pet. is recommended for the methacrylated monomers and 0.1% pet. for the acrylated monomers, to avoid patch test sensitization [56].

14.6.3 Epoxy Resin Systems

Epoxy (or ethoxylin) resins are plastics of the thermosetting type. They are produced by polycondensation of a polyhydroxy compound and epichlorohydrin in the presence of caustic soda. The chemical binding of 2 carbon and 1 oxygen atom into an epoxy group is characteristic of all epoxy resins. This group is chemically very reactive. About 90% of epoxy resins are diglycidyl ethers of the bisphenol A type, formed by combining epichlorohydrin and disphenol A, which is the commercial name of 2,2-bis(4-hydroxyphenyl)propane. By varying the proportion of epichlorhydrin and bisphenol A during the manufacturing process, different amounts of low and high molecular weight resins can be formed in the mixture. The final product is a polymer with the chemical structure shown in Fig. 14.6.6.

The repeating unit has a molecular weight (MW) of 284. When $n = 0$, a low molecular product that is the major constituent of commercial low molecular weight epoxy resins is obtained, diglycidyl ether of bisphenol A (DGEBA). Commercial epoxy resins are mixtures of oligomers of different molecular weights, 340 ($n = 0$), 624 ($n = 1$), 908 ($n = 2$), 1192 ($n = 3$), etc. Low molecular weight epoxy resin has an average molecular weight below 1000, with a high amount of the MW 340 oligomer. Epoxy resin with an average molecular weight exceeding 1000 contains less MW 340 oligomer [57]. Those epoxy resins with an average molecular weight exceeding 908 are solid, and those with lower average molecular weight are semisolid or liquid.

Apart from the resin and hardener or curing agent, epoxy systems sometimes also contain reactive diluents. Other components which can be added to the basic raw materials are colorants, fillers, tar, UV-light absorbers, flame retardants, solvents, reinforcement agents and plasticizers. Epoxy resins may also be blended with formaldehyde resins based on phenol, urea and melamine.

Epoxy resin is used for casting of models, as glue for metal, rubber, plastics and ceramics, as electrical insulation, in floor coverings, for anti-corrosion protection of metals, for mending of cracks in concrete, and for laminates and composites. Most of the epoxy resins are used for paints and coatings. High molecular weight epoxy resins in various solvents are used for painting

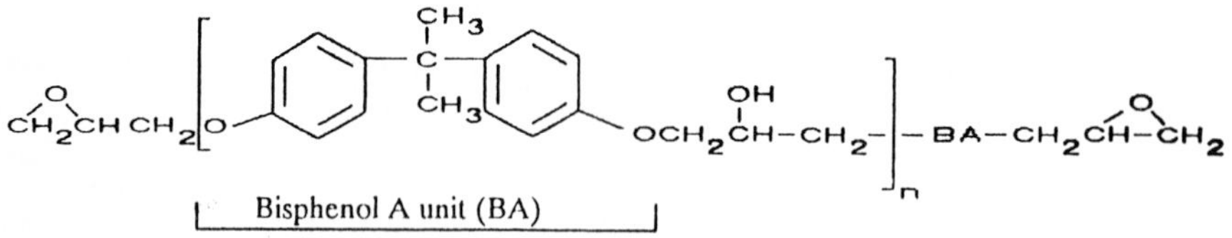

MW	n
340	0
624	1
908	2
1192	3

Fig. 14.6.6. Diglycidyl ether of bisphenol A (DGEBA epoxy resin)

and as powders for electrostatic hard coating of metal. Preimpregnated glass fibre ("prepreg") is used as a reinforcement in the plastics industry and in electronic circuit boards [58, 59].

Instead of using bisphenol A in the epoxy resin system, other polyhydroxy compounds can be used, e.g. resorcinol, glycerol, ethylene glycol, pentaery-thritol and bisphenol F (DGEBF).

Fibres of carbon, glass and nylon, etc., impregnated with epoxy resin systems are increasingly used as composite materials where great strength is required. However, there are difficulties concerning adherence to carbon fibres with epoxy resins of the bisphenol A type, so other epoxy systems have been developed: diglycidyl ether of tetrabromobisphenol A (4Br-DGEBA), tetraglycidyl-4,4'-methylenedianiline (TGMDA), triglycidyl derivative of *p*-aminophenol (TGPAP) and *o*-diglycidyl phthalate. 4Br-DGEBA is often used as flame retardant in these systems.

Aliphatic epoxy resins are used in paints. Epoxy acrylates, usually obtained by reacting epoxy resin with acrylic acid, are commonly used as prepolymers in UV-curable printing inks and coatings. Both aromatic and aliphatic epoxy acrylates are available, as well as acrylated epoxydized oils.

14.6.3.1 Hardeners

There are many curing agents or hardeners on the market. These hardeners may act at either room (cold curing) or elevated temperatures (thermal curing). The cold curing hardeners are mostly polyamines, polyamides or isocyanates. The hardeners used for thermal curing are acids and anhydrides or aldehyde condensation products, e.g. phenol-formaldehyde resins, melamine-formaldehyde resins and urea-formaldehyde resins.

The most commonly used hardeners for the DGEBA resin system are listed in Table 14.6.3. Common hardeners for composite epoxy resins are diamino-diphenyl sulphone (DDS), methylenedianiline, boron trifluorine monoethyl-amine complex and dicyandiamide [60]. The polymerization of epoxy resins can be speeded up by adding accelerators, e.g. tertiary amines.

14.6.3.2 Epoxy Reactive Diluents

Reactive diluents containing one or more epoxide groups react with the hardener at approximately the same rate as the resin. They are used primarily for reducing the viscosity of resins. There are many reactive diluents on the market and most of them are used in the cold curing process. They are blended in commercial epoxy resin at concentrations of 10%-30% [61].

The epoxy reactive diluents are either aromatic, like phenyl and cresyl glycidyl ether, or aliphatic, e.g. butyl and allyl glycidyl ether or other alkyl glycidyl ethers with longer carbon chains (C_8-C_{14}). Examples are Epoxide 7 and Epoxide 8.

Table 14.6.3. The most commonly used hardeners in the DGEBA resin system

Aliphatic Polyamines	*Cycloaliphatic Polyamines*
Ethylenediamine (EDA)	Isophoronediamine (IDP)
Diethylenetriamine (DETA)	*N*-Aminoethylpiperazine
Triethylenetetramine (TETA)	3,3'-Dimethyl-4,4'-diaminodicyclohexyl-
Dipropylenetriamine (DPTA)	methane
Tetraethylenepentamine (TEPA)	
Diethylaminopropylamine (DEAPA)	
Trimethylhexamethylenediamine	
(TMDA)	
Aromatic amines	*Polyaminoamides*
p, p'-Diaminodiphenylmethane (DDM)	Based on polyamines, e.g. TEPA, TETA
m-Phenylenediamine (MPDA)	
p, p'-Diaminodiphenyl sulphone (DDS)	
Dimethylaminomethyl phenol (DMP)	
Adducts	*Imidazoline compounds*
Based on the reaction between aliphatic	Based on amines, e.g. DETA and dibasic
or aromatic amines and epoxy resin,	acids
epoxy reactive diluents, ethylene oxide	
etc.	
Acid anhydrides	*Dicyanodiamide (Dicy)*
Pththalic acid anhydride (PA)	1-Cyanoguanidine
Maleic acid anhydride (MA)	
Methyltetrahydrophthalic acid anhydride	
Hexahydrophthalic acid anhydride	
	Isocyanates
	Di- and polyisocyanates
Polymercaptans	*Polyphenols*

14.6.3.3 Skin Problems from Epoxy Resin Systems

Epoxy resins have been found to be one of the most frequent causes of occupational allergic contact dermatitis in some countries [62]. Contact allergy usually develops within a few months. In many cases allergic epoxy dermatitis develops after accidental contact with epoxy resin, and frequent causative agents for epoxy dermatitis are paints and the raw materials for paints [62]. However, it is not unusual to find a positive patch test reaction to epoxy resin where the cause of the sensitization is unknown. Dermatitis caused by epoxy resin systems is localized mostly to the hands and forearms but sometimes the face is also involved. If the face and eyelids are involved the dermatitis may be caused by airborne sensitization to hardeners or reactive diluents. These compounds are very volatile compared to epoxy resin [63].

It is mainly the epoxy resin oligomer of MW 340 that is responsible for epoxy resin allergy. The oligomer of MW 624 is also a sensitizer but weaker than the MW 340 oligomer. The sensitizing capacity of epoxy resin decreases as the average molecular weight increases [57, 64].

High molecular weight epoxy resin in solvents for painting, or epoxy resin powder for electrostatic coating of metals, rarely cause sensitization because of the low content of MW 340 oligomer.

Even if the epoxy resin is believed to be cured, up to 25% of it can remain unhardened, particularly when cured at room temperature [58]. Contact dermatitis may thus be elicited in previously sensitized individuals. Traces of nonhardened epoxy resin have been found in twist-off caps, film cassettes, furniture, metal pieces, sign boards, textile labels, stoma pouches, polyvinylchloride plastic, nasal cannulas, haemodialysis sets, cardiac pacemakers, fibreglass, brass doorknobs and tool handles, among other products [65].

Methods used to detect the presence of epoxy resins of the bisphenol A type have been described by Fregert and Trulsson [65, 66]. Resins based on bisphenol F are also sensitizers. They probably cross-react with resins based on bisphenol A.

The composite epoxy resins linke o-diglycidyl phthalate, tetraglycidyl-4,4'-methylenedianiline (TGMDA) and diglycidyl ether of tetrabromobisphenol A (4Br-DGEBA) are considered to be strong sensitizers in humans [60, 67]. Contact allergy to the composite epoxy resins is not revealed by testing with DGEBA epoxy resin. DGEBA, TGMDA and o-diglycidyl phthalate do not cross-react [60, 68].

The hardeners have usually been found to be responsible for less than 10% of allergic contact dermatitis due to epoxy-related compounds [69]. The most potent sensitizers among the hardeners are the aliphatic polyamines (see Table 14.6.3) [58, 69, 70]. The cycloaliphatic polyamines (e.g. isophorone-diamine, and N-aminoethylpiperazine) are also strong sensitizers [69, 71, 72]. Hardeners of the polyaminoamide type are not sensitizers. However, polyaminoamides may contain aliphatic amines. The adducts are nonsensitizers providing they do not contain free amine. The aliphatic polyamines are also strong skin irritants.

Contact urticaria caused by the epoxy resin hardener methylhexahydrophthalic anhydride has also been reported [62]. The reactive diluents are strong sensitizers [61, 73–75]. Contact dermatitis due to epichlorohydrin has been reported [76, 77]. There is controversy about the sensitizing capacity of bisphenol A [78].

14.6.3.4 Patch Testing

As about 90% of contact allergy caused by epoxy resin systems is due to epoxy resin of the bisphenol A type (DEGBA), a patch test with a low molecular weight epoxy resin containing a high amount of oligomer MW 340 is adequate in most cases. The International Contact Dermatitis Research

Group has recommended testing with epoxy resin 1% pet. and this allergen is included in the European standard series. Patients should also be tested with their own resins at a corresponding concentration. There are too many hardeners and reactive diluents on the market to be used in routine testing. However, if sensitivity to the hardeners or reactive diluents is suspected, it is necessary to get information and samples from the manufacturer concerning the ingredients and test them separately. The recommended test concentration for hardeners and reactive diluents is 0.1%–1% in petrolatum, acetone or ethanol.

14.6.3.5 Prevention

Both the management and the workers in contact with the epoxy resin systems should be advised to take steps to avoid skin contact. This can be achieved by the strict use of aprons and disposable gloves and regular cleaning and maintenance of all contaminated equipment. Also recommended in order to reduce the allergenic properties of epoxy compounds is to use the MW 340 oligomer at the lowest possible concentration and to use high molecular weight reactive diluents. The hardeners should be of the polyaminoamide type or adducts not containing aliphatic polyamines. High molecular weight epoxy resins should also be regarded as potential sensitizers, and they should be marked with labels specifying the amount of MW 340 oligomer. Epoxy resins penetrate plastic and rubber gloves. Good protection is obtained with heavy duty vinyl gloves [79]. However, new multilayered glove material (4H-Glove) has demonstrated even better protection against epoxy resins [55]. Barrier creams may perhaps provide protection against epoxy resins for some hours [80–82].

14.6.4 Phenol-Formaldehyde Resins

Phenol-formaldehyde resins are polymers formed by the interaction of a phenol, or a mixture of phenols, and formaldehyde. The polymerization is a polycondensation type reaction. When phenol reacts with an excess of formaldehyde under alkaline conditions, a *resol* resin is produced. As formaldehyde is in excess in the process, various methylol phenol compounds are formed. These are 2-methylol phenol (2-MP), 4-methylol phenol (4-MP), 2,4-dimethylol phenol (2,4-MP), 2,6-dimethylol phenol (2,6-MP), 2,4,6-trimethylol phenol (2,4,6-MP) and, to a limited extent, 3-methylol phenol (3-MP) (Fig. 14.6.7) [83]. The resol resins are formable, fusible and soluble. They can be considered as prepolymers and may be transformed into the final stage simply by heating the resol.

Resins formed when formaldehyde reacts with an excess of phenols under acidic conditions are called *novolak* resins. Methylol phenols are also generated in novolaks but they are present only in very small concentrations.

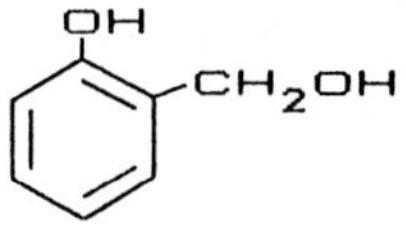

Fig. 14.6.7. Chemical formulae of various methylol phenols

2-Methylol phenol

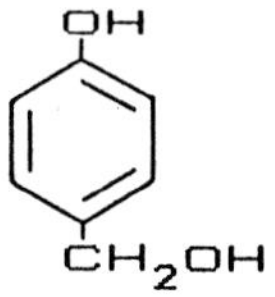

4-Methylol phenol

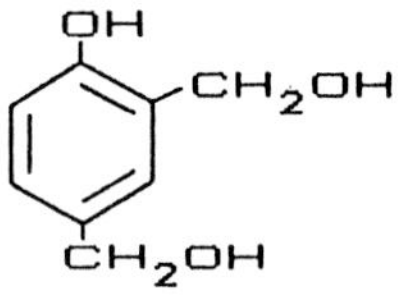

2,4-Dimethylol phenol

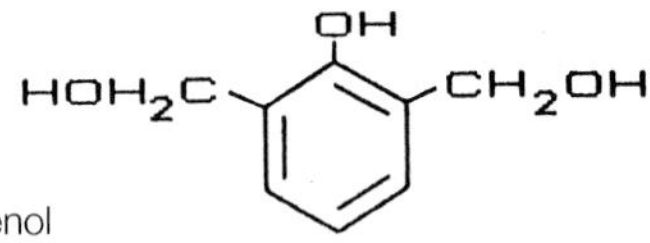

2,6-Dimethylol phenol

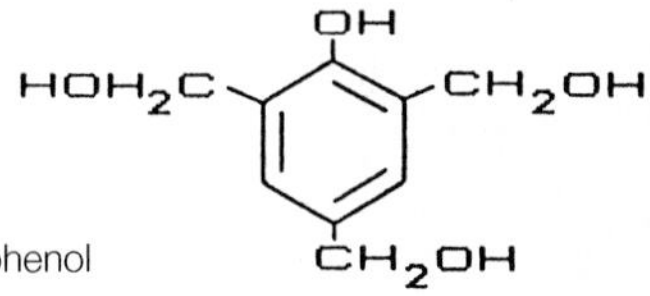

2,4,6-Trimethylol phenol

Mainly, three dihydroxydiphenyl methanes (HPM, bisphenol F isomers) are generated: 2,2'-HPM, 4,4'-HPM and 2,4'-HPM. The novolak resins are also formable, fusible and soluble. For final curing, formaldehyde, *p*-formaldehyde or hexamethylenetetramine are necessary as well as heating. The final cured polymer for both novolaks and resols is called resite or C-stage resin.

Commercially, phenol-formaldehyde resins are most commonly based on phenol itself but other phenols such as cresols, xylenols, resorcinol, bisphenol A, and *p-tert*-butylphenol and nonylphenol can be used. Other aldehydes besides formaldehyde have also been used, e.g. furfural.

Resins based on formaldehyde are widely used. Impregnated textiles and paper are used for the production of decorative equipment and integrated cirucits for the electronics industry. Surface-coating resins are based on alkyl-substituted phenols or modified phenol-formaldehyde resins. They are used as protective and isolating varnishes for packing, as they are not water soluble. Modified resins may also be used in inks and as binders for powder on typewriting correction paper. *p-tert*-Butylphenol-formaldehyde resin is used in adhesives based on neoprene and in other rubber adhesives used in shoes, automobile interiors, upholstery, furniture and hobbies. They are also used as adhesives for leather, artificial fingernails and labels. Adhesives based on phenol-formaldehyde resins are also used for glass and mineral fibres in the production of insulating material. Their binding and adhesive properties result in their presence in foundry sand moulds, brake linings and clutch facings.

14.6.4.1 Skin Problems from Phenol-Formaldehyde Resins

The raw materials may cause irritation on the skin and phenols may cause chemical burns. Another adverse reaction to certain phenol-formaldehyde resins is depigmentation, and the causative compounds seem to be simple phenols [84]. Contact dermatitis is the most frequent adverse reaction in workers handling phenol-formaldehyde resins [85, 86]. *p-tert*-Butylphenol-formaldehyde resin is the most common allergen and is considered a potent sensitizer. Reviews on occupational eczema from *p-tert*-butylphenol-formaldehyde resin have been published [83, 86, 87].

There are fewer reports of sensitivity to phenol-formaldehyde resins other than *p-tert*-butylphenol-formaldehyde resins [88, 89]. *p-tert*-Butylphenol-formaldehyde resin is included in the European standard series [83, 90]. However, phenol-formaldehyde resin has only occasionally been included in previous patch test series and thus contact dermatitis from phenol-formaldehyde resins has probably been missed. *p-tert*-Butylphenol-formaldehyde resin and resins based on other types of phenols and formaldehyde do not necessarily contain the same sensitizers [83, 90]. It has also been shown that formaldehyde is not a main sensitizer in phenol-formaldehyde resins. Simultaneous reactions to phenol-formaldehyde resins, colophony/hydroabietyl alcohol and balsam of Peru/fragrance mix, are possible [91]. Resins and products based on phenol-formaldehyde resins have been resolved by Bruze into 14 contact sensitizers. These are various methylol phenols and dihydroxydiphenyl methanes. The 4,4'-dihydroxy-(hydroxymethyl)-diphenyl methanes were the most potent allergens [83, 92, 93].

14.6.4.2 Patch Testing

Bruze found 2.5 times more patients with contact allergy to phenol-formaldehyde resins when routinely patch tested with a resin based on phenol and formaldehyde (P-F-R-2) in addition to *p*-tert-butylphenol-formaldehyde resin [90]. P-F-R-2 is therefore recommended for routine patch testing, preferably as a separate patch test but otherwiese as a mix with *p-tert*-butylphenol-formaldehyde resin [90].

14.6.5 Polyurethane Resins

These plastics are formed by the reaction between diisocyanates and poly-hydroxy compounds (polyols). The polyurethanes are of the thermosetting type of plastic and the polymerization is a polyaddition reaction. The poly-hydroxy compounds used are mainly polyalchohols, polyesters or polyethers, but isocyanates can also react with other molecules if they bear active hydroxyl groups. The isocyanates used in the production of polyurethane plastics are shown in Fig. 14.6.8. Toluene diisocyanate (TDI) is the most commonly used diisocyanate, often as mixtures of the isomers 2,4-TDI and 2,6-TDI. Diphenylmethane-4,4'-diisocyanate (MDI) is industrially used as crude MDI, which is a mixture of 4,4'-MDI with 2,4'-MDI and 2,2'-MDI. Crude MDI is also named polymethylene polyphenyl isocyanate (PAPI or PMPPI). Phenyl isocyanate is usually a contaminant in MDI. 1,6-Hexamethylene diisocyanate (HDI) is the most commonly used diisocyanate in lacquers, coatings and paints. Trimethyl hexamethylene diisocyanate (TMDI) is a mixture of the 2 isomers 2,2,4- and 2,4,4-TMDI.

Many diisocyanates are used in a prepolymerized form. These prepolymers are synthesized by adding a small amount of the isocyanate to a polyol. The various prepolymers can be extended by adding water.

Polyurethanes occur in many forms, such as coatings, paints, one- or two-component glue, elastomers, castings, foams, fibres and synthetic rubbers. Flexible polyurethane foams are used for mattresses, cushions, dashboards and packaging. Recommended patch test concentrations for diisocyanates are 0.1–1.0% pet. or acet.

14.6.5.1 Skin Problems from Polyurethane Resins

Most at risk of developing dermatitis from polyurethane resins are workers with industrial exposure, such as those manufacturing polyurethanes, car painters, adhesive workers and insulation installers. The polyols are not sensitizers and contact allergy to the various isocyanates is rare in spite of their extensive use. However, there are rigorous rules to follow when working with polyurethanes to minimize the effect that the isocyanate monomers may have on the respiratory tract and thus the skin hazards as well. Contact allergy to TDI, MDI, IPDI (isophorone diisocyanate), HDI, TMDI and DMDI (dicyclohexylmethane-4,4'-diisocyanate) has been reported [52, 94–98]. MDI-positive patients may also react to 4,4'-diaminodiphenylmethane. However, it is not certain if MDI is the actual allergen as MDI and water form 4,4'-diaminodiphenylmethane.

Unreacted isocyanate monomer may remain in surplus inside polyurethane foams even after curing. This can create a health hazard due to isocyanate exposure when polyurethane dust is produced during machining or cutting. If polyurethanes are heated to above 250°C, they decompose into isocyanates and nitrogen oxides and might again cause dermatitis.

Toluene diisocyanate (2,4- & 2,6- TDI)

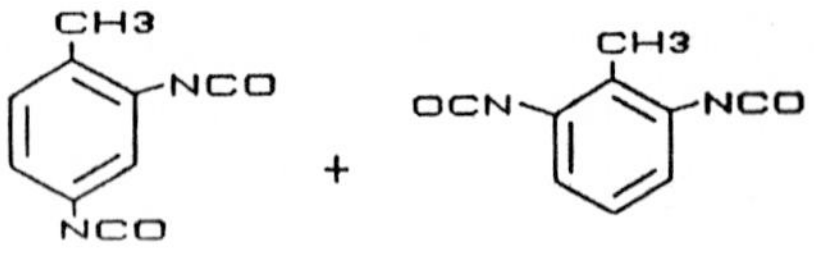

Diphenylmethane-4,4'-diisocyanate (MDI)

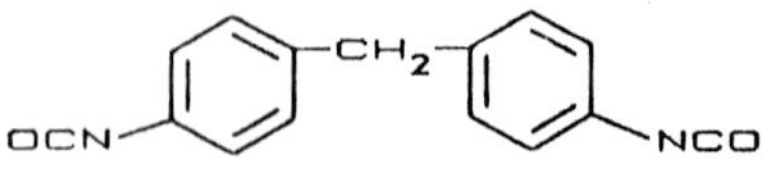

Dicyclohexylmethane-4,4'-diisocyanate (DMDI)

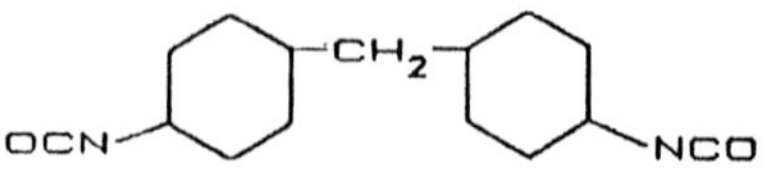

Polymethylene polyphenyl
isocyanate (PAPI)

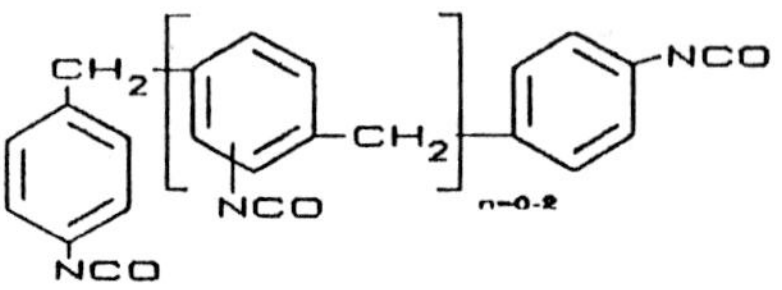

1,6-Hexamethylene diisocyanate (HDI)

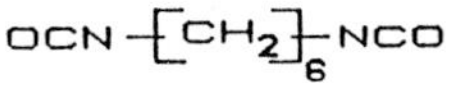

Trimethylhexamethylene diisocyanate

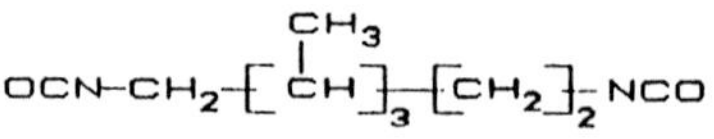

Isophorone diisocyanate (IPDI)

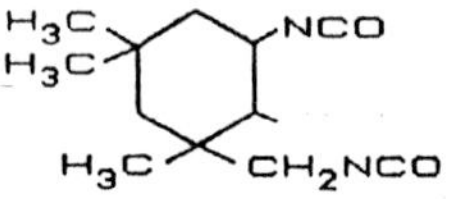

Triphenylmethane-4,4',4''-triisocyanate

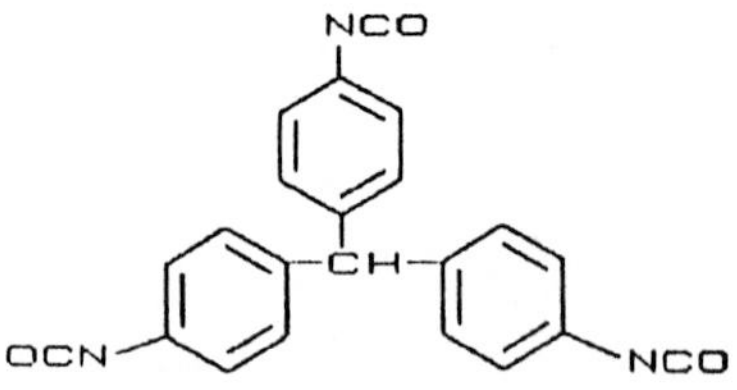

Fig. 14.6.8. Chemical formulae of various isocyanates used in the production of polyurethane plastics

Animal experiments with guinea pigs and mice have been performed and MDI, TDI and HDI found to be sensitizers. Skin irritation from isocyanates has also been reported [99–101].

14.6.6 Amino Plastics

Amino plastics is the common name for plastics formed by the reaction between an aldehyde and a compound with one or more amino groups. The most common aldehyde is formaldehyde but sometimes hexamethylenetetramine, which is a formaldehyde releaser, can be used. The most common amino-containing compounds are urea (carbamide; $H_2N-CO-NH_2$) and melamine (2,4,5-triamino-1,3,5-triazine), and their reaction with formaldehyde produces urea-formaldehyde and melamine-formaldehyde resins. The polymerization between the aldehyde and the amine is of the polycondensation type, forming a thermosetting resin. In amino plastics there is always an excess of formaldehyde. The amino resins are cured by heat, commonly with an inorganic acid as catalyst. Although both resins are quite similar in appearance, the melamine-formaldehyde resins have superior water resistance to cured urea-formaldehyde resins. Both amino plastics are relatively unaffected by common organic solvents, oils and greases and are widely used as laminating and bonding materials in the wood and furniture industry. They are used as wood glues and surface coatings. They are also utilized to improve the wet strength of paper and crease resistance of textiles. Powders from urea-formaldehyde resins can be moulded and used as containers for cosmetic products, electrical fittings and bottle tops. Urea-formaldehyde foams have found application as insulation in refrigerators and within the walls of houses. Other typical uses of urea-formaldehyde resins are clock cases, lavatory seats and buttons. Tableware, such as plates and cups moulded from powders filled with α-cellulose, are very common articles made of melamine-formaldehyde resins. In addition, high-quality decorative laminates are made of melamine-formaldehyde resins. These resins are often used in conjunction with fillers and reinforcements such as glass mat and cloth, silica, cotton fabrics and certain synthetic fibres.

14.6.6.1 Skin Problems from Amino Plastics

Primary sensitization usually does not occur from the finished product but occasionally from the uncured material. Textile dermatitis caused by urea- and melamine-formaldehyde resins is rare. Formaldehyde can be released from amino plastics andd contact allergy to urea- and melamine-formaldehyde resins is often combined with formaldehyde allergy. Urea and melamine do not cause contact allergy. Occupational irritant contact dermatitis from fibre-board containing urea-formaldehyde resin has been reported [102].

14.6.7 Polyester Resins

Polyester resins are polycondensation thermosetting compounds. They are made in two different forms, saturated and unsaturated.

The *saturated polyesters* are produced from dicarboxylic acids, usually phthalic acid or its anhydride, and polyalcohols, usually glycerol, pentaery-thritol or trimethylolpropane. The saturated polyesters synthesized in this way are also termed unmodified alkyd resin, which is a macromolecule commonly used as a plasticizer for other plastic materials. Alkyd resins are formed by modification with oils containing fatty acids, which bind to free hydroxyl groups on the polyfunctional alcohol. In this form the resin is often used in modern water-based paints and surface coatings.

Unsaturated polyesters are produced through esterification of organic acids, e.g. maleic acid anhydride, fumaric acid and phthalic acid anhydride, with diols, e.g. diethylene glycol or 1,2-propylene glycol. The unsaturated polyester is cured by cross-linking between parts of the linear macromolecule. The cross-linking agent most commonly used is styrene, but vinyl toluene and methyl methacrylate are also used. To start the cross-linking process an initiator or catalyst is always required. The catalyst is usually a peroxide such as benzoyl peroxide or methyl ethyl ketone peroxide. Accelerators or activators are necessary only for curing at room temperature. The accelerators are metal salts, e.g. cobalt naphthenate, or tertiary amines such as dimethylaniline, diethylaniline and dimethyl-*p*-toluidine. The peroxide-cured unsaturated polyesters have been used commercially for many years, but unsaturated polyesters cured by UV light have equivalent properties. The UV-curable polyester system is used in the furniture industry as top coats for furniture, doors, panels, etc. During recent years orthopaedic casts cured by UV light have been increasingly used. Usually they consist of an unsaturated polyester with vinyl toluene as the cross-linking agent and a benzoin-ether molecule as photoinitiator. The resin is impregnated into woven glass fibre. Reactive (meth)acrylate groups can be attached to be molecular backbone of the unsaturated polyesters through functional groups such as hydroxyl and anhydride, forming acrylated polyesters used in UV-curable inks or coatings for wood and paper.

Unsaturated polyesters combined with glass fibre have many applications as a reinforced plastic used in the motor industry, piping, bath tubs, roof panels and other applications. They are also used as protective coatings, finishes, lacquers and fillers.

14.6.7.1 Skin Problems from Polyester Resins

Irritant or allergic contact dermatitis from *saturated polyesters* appears to be very rare. Triglycidyl isocyanurate (TGIC), a trifunctional epoxy compound used as cross-linker in heat-cured polyester paints, has been described as a contact sensitizer [103]. Alkyd resins are not sensitizing.

Contact dermatitis from *unsaturated polyester* resins is also very rare. Those at risk are workers employed in manufacturing industry, with few exceptions [104]. In most cases the dermatitis is irritant and not allergic. Contact allergy to unsaturated polyester in a boat builder has been reported [105]. According to Malten, unsaturated polyester no longer appears to have sensitizing capacity, presumably because the formation of sensitizing free maleic acid esters is prevented by the avoidance of monoalcoholic impurities [96]. Should the diols contain monoalcohols like ethanol and butanol, then diethyl maleate and dibutyl maleate can be formed, which are strong contact sensitizers. Diethyl maleate was reported to be a sensitizer in four men working with unsaturated polyester resins [106]. Sometimes contact allergy from additives in unsaturated polyester resins can occur. Examples of such additives are cobalt compounds, allylphthalate, organic peroxides, dimethylaniline, dimethyl-*p*-toluidine and the inhibitor in styrene, e.g. *p-tert*-butylcatechol or hydroquinone.

The irritant effects of unsaturated polyesters are mostly due to glass fibre, solvents, styrene and other additives.

14.6.8 Polyvinyl Resins

The chemical structure of a vinyl compound is $CH_2=CH-R$, where $CH_2=CH-$ is the vinyl group and R represents many different chemical groups. Some examples of vinyl compounds used to synthesize polyvinyl resins are vinyl chloride (R=Cl-), vinyl acetate (R=CH_3COO-), vinyl acetal (R=$CH_3(CH_2)_n$-O-, $n = 0,1,3$), vinyl alcohol (R=OH-) and vinylidene chloride ($CH_2=CCl_2$). The polyvinyl resins are polymerized through a polyaddition reaction and belong to the group of thermoplastics. Vinyl chloride ($CH_2=CH-Cl$) is a gaseous monomer, polymerized by suspension, emulsion, solution or bulk processes, and as initiators potassium persulphate, benzoyl peroxide, lauryl peroxide, percarbonate and some azo-compounds can be used. The repeating unit of polyvinyl chloride (PVC) is -CH_2-CHCl-.

PVC is one of the most inexpensive thermoplastics and is the most used widely plastic after polyethylene. The presence of chlorine in the hydrocarbon backbone gives rigidity and toughness to the polymer but PVC liberates hydrogen chloride when exposed to high temperatures. To prevent this, stabilizers are added to the polymer. The toughness and rigidity of hard PVC give rise to applications in sewage systems, agricultural products, drinking water pipes, furniture, window frames, dishes and packages of various shapes.

Plasticizers, mainly phthalates, are added to PVC to impart flexibility to the finished products and to improve processibility of the melt. To almost all PVC, plasticizers are added. Hard PVC contains approximately 10% and soft PVC up to 60% –70% plasticizers. The plasticizers are mostly in the form of phthalic acid esters, most commonly di(2-ethylhexyl) phthalate (DEHP), often termed dioctyl pthalate (DOP). However, more than one plasticizer is usually used when properties other than flexibility are also required in the end product. Sometimes uncured epoxy resin is added as a plasticizer and stabilizer to PVC. Soft or plasticized PVC is very popular in applications such as artificial skin, wallpapers, laminated table cloths, carpets, toys, garden hoses, wire coatings for electric cables, shower curtains, adhesive plasters, foils, bandages, casts and protective gloves.

14.6.8.1 Skin Problems from Polyvinyl Resins

Workers processing PVC plastics can develop contact dermatitis [107, 108]. Cured PVC usually does not contain any remaining monomer, but in fresh batches of PVC granulates, trapped monomer is likely to remain. Contact dermatitis from identification bracelets made of PVC plastics has been reported. The reactions were believed to be irritant due to some unknown chemical in the bracelets. Additives can migrate out of the plastic and sensitization may occur but seems to be rare.

Allergic contact reaction to epoxy resin in PVC plastic film and to diphenylthiourea and phenylisothiocyanate in PVC adhesive tape has been reported [109, 110]. Diphenylthiourea is a heat stabilizer in PVC and is partly decomposed to phenylisothiocyanate.

14.6.9 Polystyrene Resins

Polystyrene is a hard transparent plastic. It is manufactured by polyaddition polymerization of styrene ($CH_2=CH-C_6H_5$) using a peroxide initiator. Polystyrene resin is one of the thermoplastics, with the repeating unit -$CH_2CH(C_6H_5)$-. As a foam, polystyrene plastic is very important in the fields of packaging and insulation. Modified polystyrene plastics with a co- or ter-polymer structure have been developed. Examples of these are the styrene-butadiene, styrene-acrylonitrile and acrylonitrile-butadiene-styrene plastics. These materials are used in household utensils, toys, electronic and electrical appliances, recreational articles, handles, bags and pipes. Polystyrene products can usuallay be identified by their metallic sound when dropped on a hard surface. Polystyrene products are also widely used in food packaging and disposable tableware.

To increase the light stability of styrene-based plastics, stabilizers such as benzophenones, benzotriazoles and organic nickel compounds are usually added.

14.6.9.1 Skin Problems from Polystyrene Resins

Contact allergy to styrene is extremely rare. One patient, sensitive to styrene, cross-reacted at patch testing to 2-, 3- and 4-vinyltoluene (2-,3- and 4-methylstyrene) and to the metabolites styrene epoxide and 4-vinylphenol (4-hydroxy-styrene). It is assumed that styrene is a prohapten metabolized in the skin by aryl hydrocarbon hydroxylase to styrene epoxide, which acts as the true hapten. Styrene occurs both in nature and as a synthetic product and vinyl toluenes (methylstyrenes) occur as synthetic products in plastics [111].

14.6.10 Polyolefins

Polyolefins belong to a group of thermoplastics polymerized through polyaddition reaction of olefins (unsaturated hydrocarbons). The most important are ethylene (ethene, $CH_2=CH_2$), which gives polyethylene, and propylene (propene, $CH_2=CHCH_3$), which gives polypropylene.

Polyethylene is the most important plastic of all by volume and was already known half a century ago. The repeating unit of polyethylene is -CH_2-CH_2-. Polymerization is produced at high or low pressures, aided by catalysts and initiators. According to their density, polyethylenes are grouped into three main categories; low-density polyethylenes, linear low-density polyethylenes and high-density polyethylenes. All of these types are lighter than water and they are amongst the most inexpensive of plastics. Films and sheets for packaging uses are the most widespread forms of polyethylene plastics. Because low-density polyethylene is soft and flexible, transparent and nontoxic due to the absence of plasticizers, it is used as food packaging. In addition, shopping bags and sacks are among the most popular applications of low-density polyethylenes. Linear low-density polyethylene is, because of its greater mechanical strength, the main plastic on the film manufacturing industry. Because low-density polyethylene has outstanding chemical and frost resistance, its main applications are for hoses, coatings of electric cables and wires, and many kinds of household utensils such as jars, containers, deep-freeze boxes and cases. High-density polyethylenes are used mainly for bottles and containers, but also for shopping bags and pipes.

Polypropylene has the repeating unit -CH_2-$CH(CH_3)$-. It is similar to high-density polyethylene, but slightly harder and tougher. In addition to filament applications, such as home furnishings, nonwoven products and carpets, polypropylene is generally used for pipes and films.

14.6.10.1 Skin Problems from Polyolefins

Contact dermatitis from polyethylene and polypropylene is extremely rare. It is most likely to be caused by added ingredients such as catalysts and initiators. If heated, polyolefins will degrade and form aldehydes, ketones and acids, among other chemicals, which may cause airborne contact dermatitis.

14.6.11 Polyamides

The polyamides are thermoplastics manufactured by condensation polymerization of adipic acid (HOOC-(CH$_2$)$_4$-COOH) and hexamethylenediamine (N$_2$N-(CH$_2$)$_6$-NH$_2$). The resulting polymer has a linear structure, with the repeating unit -OC-(CH$_2$)$_4$CONH-(CH$_2$)$_6$-NH-. Other polyamides can be polymerized from caprolactam and water.

The polyamides are made into fibres and are known as nylons. The transparency of polyamide films make them very useful for packaging purposes. Hospital wares made of polyamide plastics have high stability at sterilization temperatures and combined films of laminates are used, for example, in vacuum packaging of meat.

14.6.11.1 Skin Problems from Polyamides

Contact dermatitis from polyamides is rare.

14.6.12 Polycarbonates

A polycarbonate plastic is characterized by the -O-CO-O- group. It can be made from phosgene ($COCl_2$) and bisphenol A (4,4'-dihydroxydiphenyl-2,2-propane) and has the structure $-O-(C_6H_4)-C(CH_3)_2-(C_6H_4)-O-CO-$. Bisphenols other than bisphenol A can also be used. Polycarbonate plastic is a very transparent, tough and inert material and is very resistant towards sunlight and weather. It is used among other things in safety helmets, bulletproof windows, shields, doors, bottles and lamp globes. However, the plastic is relatively expensive and therefore has limited applications.

14.6.12.1 Skin Problems from Polycarbonates

Contact dermatitis from polycarbonates is rare.

14.6.13 Other Plastic Materials

Other plastics of less dermatological importance are coumarone-indene polymers, cellulose polymers and cyclohexanone resins. It is not fully known if monomers, additives or impurities are the cause of dermatitis in reported cases [112, 113].

14.6.14 Additives in Synthetic Polymers

The major classes of additives to plastics are plasticizers, flame retardants, heat stabilizers, antioxidants, UV light absorbers, blowing agents, initiators, lubricants and flow control agents, antistatic agents, curing agents, colorants, fillers and reinforcements, solvents and optical brighteners. There are nearly 2500 individual chemicals or mixtures that are utilized in the above major classes of additives.

14.6.14.1 Plasticizers

Plasticizers constitute a broad range of chemically and thermally stable products of a variety of chemical classes that are added to improve the flexibility, softness and processibility of plastics. Their principal use is in thermoplastic resins. Approximately 450 plasticizers are commercially available. Many are esters of carboxylic acids (e.g. phthalic, isophthalic, adipic, benzoic, abietic, trimellitic, oleic and sebacic acids) or phosphoric acid. Although there are about 100 phthalates that have been employed as plasticizers, around 14–15 phthalates account for over 90% of commercial phthalate production. The major phthalates utilized are di(2-ethylhexyl) phthalate (DEHP) (often named dioctyl phthalate, DOP), diisononylphthalate (DINP), diisodecylphthalate (DIDP) and butyl benzylphthalate (BBP).

14.6.14.2 Flame Retardants

Flame retardants are required for high-performance thermoplastic resins because of their use in electrical and high-temperature applications. There are many and varied chemicals used as flame retardants, of which chlorine- and bromine-containing aliphatic, cycloaliphatic and aromatic compounds are the most widely used. By brominating bisphenol A in epoxy resins to tetrabromobisphenol A a more fire-resistant epoxy resin can be produced.

14.6.14.3 Heat Stabilizers

Plastics, particularly chlorine-containing polymers, are susceptible to thermal decomposition when exposed to high temperatures or prolonged heat. The major chemical classes of stabilizers include metal salts and epoxidized oils and esters.

14.6.14.4 Antioxidants

Oxidative degradation of polymers during the manufacturing process or during their useful lifetimes is a major industrial concern. Examples of antioxidants are alkylated phenols and polyphenols (e.g. butylated hydroxytoluenes and 4-*tert*-butylcatechol), esters, organic phosphates, hydroquinones and triazoles.

14.6.14.5 Ultraviolet Light Absorbers

Radiation from the sun or fluorescent lightning is responsable for the rapid degradation of most plastics. The most widely used UV absorbers belong to six distinct chemical classes:
1. Benzophenones
2. Benzotriazoles
3. Salicylates
4. Acrylates
5. Organonickel derivatives
6. Hindered amines

The most widely used UV absorbers are 2-hydroxybenzophenones, 2-hydroxyphenylbenzotriazoles and 2-cyanodiphenylacrylate.

14.6.14.6 Initiators

Most commercial synthetic polymers are produced by a chain reaction polymerization process. Some of the many initiators used are various peroxides, e.g. benzoyl peroxide, di-*tert*-butyl peroxide, cyclohexanone peroxide and methyl ethyl ketone peroxide. There are more than 65 commercially available organic peroxides in over 100 formulations.

14.6.14.7 Curing Agents

The usefulness of a number of plastics such as unsaturated polyester, epoxy and phenolic resins is limited unless their linear polymer chains are cross-linked or cured. The various curing agents and compounds used as initiators (accelerators or catalysts) are discussed under the various plastics.

14.6.14.8 Colorants (Dyes and Pigments)

Pigments are inert and, unlike dyes, insoluble in the medium in which they are incorporated. Both inorganic and organic pigments are used in plastics.

Most colorants are inorganic pigments, with titanium dioxide being the most commonly used and iron oxides the second most common.

14.6.14.9 Skin Problems from Additives

Contact allergy to various additives is briefly mentioned in connection with the various plastics. As there are so many additives to plastics, more detailed information will be found in the dermatological literature. Rare sensitizers are phthalates, for example, dibutyl, dioctyl, tricresyl, triphenyl, *o*-diglycidyl and tricresyl ethyl phthalate. Contact allergy to UV light absorbers like 2-hydroxy benzophenone, resorcinol monobenzoate, 2-(2'-hydroxy-5'-methyl-phenyl-benzotriazole (Tinuvin P) and bis-(2,2,6,6)-tetramethyl-4-piperidyl sebacate has been found [114]. Organic pigments, mostly of the azo type, are potentially sensitizing additives in plastics [115].

Other additives of dermatological importance are hydroquinone, *p-tert*-butyl-catechol, cobalt naphthenate, benzoyl peroxide, dimethylaniline, methyl 4-toluene-sulphonate, *p*-tolydiethanolamine, and dimethyl-, diethyl- and diphenylthiourea.

14.6.15 References

1. Dahlquist I, Fregert S, Trulsson L (1983) Contact allergy to trimethylolpropane triacrylate (TMPTA) in an aziridine plastic hardener. Contact Dermatitis 9: 122–124
2. Cofield BG, Storrs FJ, Strawn CB (1985) Contact allergy to aziridine paint hardener. Arch Dermatol 121: 373–376
3. Dempsey KJ (1982) Hypersensitivity to Sta-Lok and Loctite anaerobic sealants. J Am Acad Dermatol 7: 779–784
4. Ranchoff RE, Taylor JS (1985) Contact dermatitis to anaerobic sealants. J Am Acad Dermatol 13: 1015–1020
5. Conde'-Salazar L, Guimaraens D, Romero LV (1988) Occupational allergic contact dermatitis from anaerobic acrylic sealants. Contact Dermtitis 18: 129–132
6. Van der Walle HB (1982) Sensitizing potential of acrylic monomers in guinea pig. Thesis, Catholic University of Nijmegen
7. Van der Walle HB, Clecak G, Geleick H, Bensink T (1982) Sensitizing potential of 15 mono(meth)acrylates in the guinea pig. Contact Dermatitis 8: 223–235
8. Van der Walle HB, Waegemaekers T, Bensink (1983) Sensitizing potential of 12 di(meth)acrylates in the guinea pig. Contact Dermatitis 9: 10–20
9. Waegemaekers T (1985) Some toxicological aspects of acrylic monomers, notably with reference to the skin. Thesis, Katholieke Universiteit te Nijmegen
10. Cavelier C, Jelen G, Herve-Bazin B, Fossereau J (1981) Irritation et allergic aux acrylates et methacrylates. Premiere partie. Monoacrylates et monomethacrylates simples. Ann Dermatol Venereol 108: 549–556
11. Björkner B (1984) Sensitizing capacity of ultraviolet curable acrylic compounds. Thesis, University of Lund
12. Beurey J, Mougeolle J-M, Weber M (1976) Accidents cutanés des résines acryliques dans l'imprimerie. Ann Dermatol Syphiligr 103: 423–430
13. Malten KE, den Arend JACJ, Wiggers RE (1979) Delayed irritation: hexanediol diacrylate and butanediol diacrylate. Contact Dermatitis 5: 178–184

14. Nethercott JR, Gupta S, Rosen C,, Enders LJ, Pilger CW (1984) Tetraethylene glycol diacrylate. A cause of delayed cutaneous irritant reaction and allergic contact dermatitis. J Occup Med 26: 513–516

15. Parker D, Turk JL (1983) Contact sensitivity to acrylate compounds in guinea pigs. Contact Dermatitis 9: 55–60

16. Björkner B (1981) Sensitization capacity of acrylated prepolymers in ultraviolet curing inks tested in the guinea pig. Accta Derm Venereol (Stockh) 61: 7–10

17. Björkner B, Niklasson B, Persson K (1984) The sensitizing potential of di(meth)acrylates based on bisphenol A or epoxy resin in the guinea pig. Contact Dermatitis 10: 286–304

18. Björkner B (1982) Sensitization capacity of polyester methacrylate in ultraviolet curing inks tested in the guinea pig. Acta Derm Venereol 62: 153–182

19. Björkner B (1984) Sensitizing potential of urethane (meth)acrylates in the guinea pig. Contact Dermatitis 11: 115–119

20. Nethercott JR, Jakubovic HR, Pilger C, Smith JW (1982) Allergic contact dermatitis due to urethane acrylate in ultraviolet cured inks. Br J Ind Med 40: 241–250

21. Bang Pedersen N, Senning A, Otkjaer Nielsen A (1983) Different sensitizing acrylic monomers in NAPP printing plate. Contact Dermatitis 9: 459–464

22. Björkner B (1984) Contact allergy to 2-hydroxypropyl methacrylate (2-HPMA) in an ultraviolet curable ink. Acta Derm Venereol (Stockh) 64: 264–267

23. Malten KE, Bende WJM (1979) 2-Hydroxy-ethyl-methacrylate and di-and tetraethylene glycol dimethacrylate: contact sensitizers in a photoprepolymer printing plate procedure. Contact Dermatitis 5: 214–220

24. Whittington CW (1981) Dermatitis from UV acrylate in adhesive. Contact Dermatitis 7: 203–204

25. Monteny E, Oleffe J, Donkerswolke M (1978) Methylmethacrylate hypersensitivity in a patient with cemented endoprosthesis. Acta Orthop Scand 49: 554–556

26. Fregert S (1983) Occupational hazards of acrylate bone cement in orthopedic surgery. Acta Orthop Scand 54: 787–789

27. Smith WDL (1977) Allergic contact dermatitis due to a triacrylate in ultraviolet cured inks. Contact Dermatitis 3: 312–314

28. Emmett EA, Kominsky JR (1977) Allergic contact dermatitis from ultraviolet cured inks. J Occup Med 19: 113–115

29. Emmett EA (1977) Contact dermatitis from polyfunctional acrylic monomers. Contact Dermatitis 3: 245–248

30. Nethercott JR (1978) Skin problems associated with multifunctional acrylic monomer in ultraviolet curing inks. Br J Dermatol 98: 541–552

31. Malten KE (1979) Recently reported causes of contact dermatitis due to synthetic resins and hardeners. Contact Dermatitis 5: 11–23

32. Björkner B, Dahlquist I (1979) Contact allergy caused by UV-cured acrylates. Contact Dermatitis 5: 403–404

33. Björkner B (1980) Allergic contact dermatitis from acrylates in ultraviolet curing inks. Contact Dermatitis 6: 405–409

34. Björkner B (1980) Allergenicity of trimethylol propane triacrylate in ultraviolet curing inks in the guinea pig. Acta Derm Venereol (Stockh) 60: 528–531

35. Malten KE (1982) Old and new, mainly occupational dermatological problems in the production and processing of plastics. In: Maibach HI, Gellin AG (eds) Occupational and industrial dermatology. Year Book, Chicago, pp 237–283

36. Björkner B (1984) The sensitizing capacity of multifunctional acrylates in the guinea pig. Contact Dermatitis 11: 236–246

37. Björkner B, Maibach HI (1987) Allergenicity of ultraviolet curable acrylic compounds and product development. Medical Device and Diagnostic Industry, April 1987

38. Taylor JS (1989) Acrylic reactions –ten-years' experience. In: Frosch PJ, Dooms-Goossens A, Lachapelle J-M, Rycroft RJG, Scheper RJ (eds) Current topics in contact dermatitis. Springer, Berlin Heidelberg New York, pp 346–351

39. Fisher AA (1980) Cross reactions between methyl methacrylate monomer and acrylic monomers presently used in acrylic nail preparations. Contact Dermatitis 6: 345–347

40. Kanerva L, Estlander T, Jolanki R (1989) Occupational allergic contact dermatitis from acrylates: observations concerning anaerobic acrylic sealants and dental composite resins. In: Frosch PJ, Dooms-Goossens A, Lachapelle J-M, Rycrof RJG, Scheper RJ (eds) Current topics in contact dermatitis. Springer, Berlin Heidelberg New York, pp 352–359

41. Kanerva L, Estlander T, Jolanki R (1989) Allergic contact dermatitis from dental composite resins due to aromatic epoxy acrylates and aliphatic acrylates. Contact Dermatitis 20: 201–211

42. Fries IB, Fischer AA, Salvati EA (1975) Contact dermatitis in surgeons from methylmethacrylate bone cement. J Bone Joint Surg [Am] 57: 547–549

43. Jordan WP (1975) Cross-sensitization patterns in acrylate allergies. Contact Dermatitis 8: 13–15

44. Balda BR (1971) Allergic contact dermatitis due to acrylonitrile. Contact Dermatitis Newslett 9: 219

45. Balda BR (1975) Akrylonitril als Kontaktallergen. Hautarzt 26: 599

46. Romaquera C, Grimalt F, Vilaplana J (1985) Methyl methacrylate prosthesis dermatitis. Contact Dermatitis 12: 172

47. Malten KE (1987) Printing plate manufacturing process. In: Maibach HI (ed) Occupational and industrial dermatology, 2nd edn. Year Book, pp 351–366

48. Malten KE, van der Meer-Roosen CH, Seutter E (1978) Nyloprint-sensitive patients react to N, N'-methylene-*bis*-acrylamide. Contact Dermatitis 4: 214–222

49. Pedersen NB, Chevallier M-A, Senning A (1982) Secondary acrylamides in nyloprint printing plate as a source of contact dermatitis. Contact Dermatitis 8: 256–262

50. Edwards PM (1975) Neurotoxicity of acrylamide and its analogues and effects of these analogues and other agents on acrylamides neuropathy. Br J Ind Med 31–38

51. Calnan CD (1979) Cyanoacrylate dermatitis. Contact Dermatitis 5: 165–167

52. Malten KE (1982) Old and new, mainly occupational dermatological problems in the production and processing of plastics. In: Maibach HI, Gellin GA (eds) Occupational and industrial dermatology. Year Book, pp 237–283

53. Pegum JC, Medhurst FA (1971) Contact dermatitis from penetration of rubber gloves by acrylic monomer. Br Med J 2: 141–143

54. Rietschel RL, Huggins R, Levy N, Pruitt PM (1984) In vivo and in vitro testing of gloves for protection against UV-curable acrylate resin systems. Contact Dermatitis 11: 279–282

55. Roed-Petersen J (1989) A new glove material protective against epoxy and acrylate monomer. In: Frosch PJ, Dooms-Goossens A, Lachapelle J-M, Rycroft RJG, Scheper RJ (eds) Current topics in contact dermatitis. Springer, Berlin Heidelberg New York, pp 603–606

56. Kanerva L, Estlander T, Jolanki R (1988) Sensitization to patch test acrylates. Contact Dermatitis 18: 10–15

57. Thorgeirsson A, Fregert S (1977) Allergenicity of epoxy resins in the guinea pig. Acta Derm Venereol (Stockh) 57: 253–356

58. Fregert S (1981) Manual of contact dermatitis, 2nd edn. Munksgaard, Copenhagen

59. Fregert S (1987) Contact dermatitis from epoxy resin systems. In: Maibach HI (ed) Occupational and industrial dermatology, 2nd edn. Year Book, Chicago, pp 341–345

60. Burrows D, Fregert S, Campbell H, Trulsson L (1984) Contact dermatitis from the epoxy resins tetraglycidyl-4,4'-methylene dianiline and o-diglycidyl phthalate in composite material. Contact Dermatitis 11: 80–82

61. Thorgeirsson A, Fregert S, Magnusson B (1975) Allergenicity of epoxy-reactive diluents in the guinea pig. Berufsdermatosen 23: 178–183
62. Jolanki R, Estlander T, Kanerva L (1987) Occupational contact dermatitis and contact urticaria caused by epoxy resins. Acta Derm Venereol Suppl (Stockh) 134: 90–94
63. Dahlquist I, Fregert S (1979) Allergic contact dermatitis from volatile epoxy hardeners and reactive diluents. Contact Dermatitis 5: 406–407
64. Fregert S, Thorgeirsson A (1977) Patch testing with low molecular oligomers of epoxy resins in humans. Contact Dermatitis 3: 301–303
65. Fregert S (1988) Physiochemical methods for detection of contact allergens. In: Taylor JS (ed) Occupational dermatoses. Saunders, Philadelphia, pp 97–104 (Dermatological clinics, vol 6)
66. Fregert S, Trulsson L (1978) Simple methods for demonstration of epoxy resin of bisphenol A type. Contact Dermatitis 4: 69
67. Jolanki R, Sysilampi M-L, Kanerva L, Estlander T (1989) Contact allergy to cycloaliphatic epoxy resins. In: Frosch PJ, Dooms-Goossens A, Lachapelle J-M, Rycroft RJG, Scheper RJ (eds) Current topics in contact dermatitis. Springer, Berlin Heidelberg New York, pp 360–367
68. Lembo G, Balato N, Cusano F, Baldo A, Ayala F (1989) Contact dermatitis to epoxy resins in composite material. In: Frosch PJ, Dooms-Goossens A, Lachapelle J-M, Rycroft RJG, Scheper RJ (eds) Current topics in contact dermatitis. Springer, Berlin Heidelberg New York, pp 377–380
69. Thorgeirsson A (1978) Sensitization capacity of epoxy resin hardeners in the guinea pig. Acta Derm Venereol (Stockh) 58: 332–336
70. Mathias CGT (1987) Allergic contact dermatitis from a nonbisphenol A epoxy in a graphite fiber reinforced epoxy laminate. J Occup Med 29: 754–755
71. Lachapelle JM, Tennstedt D, Dumont-Fruytier M (1978) Occupational allergic contact dermatitis to isophorone diamine (IPD) used as an epoxy resin hardener. Contact Dermatitis 4: 109–112
72. Dahlquist I, Fregert S (1979) Contact allergy to the epoxy hardener isophoronediamine (IPD). Contact Dermatitis 5: 120–121
73. Thorgeirsson A (1978) Sensitization capacity of epoxy reactive diluents in the guinea pig. Acta Derm Venereol (Stockh) 58: 329–331
74. Dahlquist I, Fregert S (1979) Contact allergy to Cardura ^{R}E, an epoxy reactive diluent of the ester type. Contact Dermatitis 5: 121–122
75. Rudzki E, Krajewska D (1979) Contact sensitivity to phenolglycidyl ether. Derm Beruf Umwelt 27: 42–44
76. Lovell CR, Rycroft RJG, Mahood J (1984) Isolated cardura E10 sensitivity in an epoxy resin chemical process. Contact Dermatitis 11: 190–191
77. Prens EP, de Jong G, van Joost T (1986) Sensitization to epichlorohydrin and epoxy system components. Contact Dermatitis 15: 85–90
78. Van Joost T (1988) Occupational sensitization to epichlorohydrin and epoxy resin. Contact Dermatitis 19: 278–280
79. Pegum JS (1979) Penetration of protective gloves by epoxy resin. Contact Dermatitis 5: 281–283
80. Blanken R, Nater JP, Veenhoff E (1987) Protection against epoxy resins with glove materials. Contact Dermatitis 16: 46–47
81. Blanken R, Nater JP, Veenhoff E (1987) Protective effect of barrier creams and spray coatings against epoxy resins. Contact Dermatitis 16: 79–83
82. Estlander T, Jolanki R (1988) How to protect the hands. In: Taylor JS (ed) Occupational dermatoses. Saunders, Philadelphia, pp 105–114 (Dermatological clinics, vol 6)
83. Bruze M (1985) Contact sensitizers in resins based on phenol and formaldehyde. Acta Derm Venereol Suppl (Stockh) 119: 1–83

84. Stevenson CJ (1981) Occupational vitiligo: clinical and epidemiological aspects. Br J Dermatol 105: [Suppl] 51–56
85. Bruze M, Almgren G (1988) Occupational dermatoses in workers exposed to resins based on phenol and formaldeyhde. Contact Dermatitis 19: 272–277
86. Foussereau J, Cavelier C, Selig D (1976) Occupational eczema from para-tertiary-butylphenol formaldehyde resins: a review of the sensitizing resins. Contact Dermatitis 2: 254–258
87. Schubert H, Agatha G (1979) Zur Allergennatur der para-tert. Butylphenolformalde-hydeharze. Derm Beruf Umwelt 27: 49–52
88. Högberg M, Wahlberg JE (1980) Health screening for occupational dermatoses in house painters. Contact Dermatitis 6: 100–106
89. Fregert S (1981) Contact allergy to phenoplastics. Contact Dermatitis 7: 170
90. Bruze M (1988) Patch testing with a mixture of 2 phenol-formaldehyde resins. Contact Dermatitis 19: 116–119
91. Bruze M (1986) Simultaneous reactions to phenol-formaldehyde resins colophony/hy-droabietyl alcohol and balsam of Peru/perfume mixture. Contact Dermatitis 14: 119–120
92. Bruze M, Zimerson E (1985) Contact allergy to 3-methylol phenol, 2,4-dimethylol phenol and 2,6-dimethylol phenol. Acta Derm Venereol (Stockh) 65: 548–551
93. Bruze M (1986) Sensitizing capacity of 4,4'-dihydroxy-(hydroxymethyl)-diphenyl methanes in the guinea pig. Acta Derm Venereol (Stockh) 66: 110–116
94. Lubach D (1978) Erkrankung durch Diisocyanate, pt 1: Schaden der Atemwege und der Haut. Derm Beruf Umwelt 26: 184–187
95. White IR, Stewart JR, Rycroft AJ (1983) Allergic contact dermatitis from an organic di-isocyanate. Contact Dermatitis 9: 300–303
96. Malten KE (1984) Dermatological problems with synthetic resins and plastics in glues, part I. Derm Beruf Umwelt 32: 81–86
97. Malten KE (1984) Dermatological problems with synthetic resins and plastics in glues, part II. Derm Beruf Umwelt 32: 118–125
98. Tanaka K, Takeoka A, Nishimura F, Hanada S (1987) Contact sensitivity induced in mice by methylene bisphenyl diisocyanate. Contact Dermatitis 17: 199–204
99. Cronin E (1980) Contact dermatitis. Churchill Livingstone, Edinburgh, pp. 575–663
100. Adams RM (1990) Occupational skin disease, 2nd ed n. Saunders, Philadelphia, pp. 387–394
101. Fisher AA (1986) Contact dermatitis, 3rd edn. Lea and Febiger, Philadelphia, pp 546–565
102. Vale PT, Rycroft RJG (1988) Occupational irritant contact dermatitis from fibreboard containing urea-formaldehyde resin. Contact Dermatitis 19: 62
103. Mathias CGT (1988) Allergic contact dermatitis from triglycidyl isocyanurate in polyester paint pigments. Contact Dermatitis 19: 67–68
104. Mac Farlane AW, Curley RK, King CM (1986) Contact sensitivity to unsaturated polyester resins in a limb prosthesis. Contact Dermatitis 15: 301–303
105. Lidén C, Löfström A, Storgards-Hatam K (1984) Contact allergy to unsaturated polyester in a boatbilder. Contact Dermatitis 11: 262–263
106. Malten KE, Zielhuis RL (1964) Industrial toxicology and dermatology in the production and processing of plastics. Elsevier, New York
107. Vidović R, Kansky A (1985) Contact dermatitis in workers processing polyvinyl chloride plastics. Derm Beruf Umwelt 33: 104–105
108. Schulsinger C, Möllegaard K (1980) Polyvinyl chloride dermatitis not caused by phthalates. Contact Dermatitis 6: 477–480
109. Fregert S, Meding B, Trulsson L (1984) Demonstration of epoxy resin in stoma pouch plastic. Contact Dermatitis 10: 106
110. Fregert S, Trulsson L, Zimerson E (1982) Contact allergic reaction to diphenylth-iourea and phenylisothiocyanate in PVC adhesvie tape. Contact Dermatitis 8: 38–42

111. Sjöborg S, Fregert S, Trulsson L (1984) Contact allergy to styrene and related chemicals. Contact Dermatitis 10: 94–96

112. Bruze M, Boman A, Bergqvist-Karlsson A, Björkner B, Wahlberg JE, Voog E (1988) Contact allergy to cyclohexanone resin in humans and guinea pigs. Contact Dermatitis 18: 46–49

113. Heine A, Laubstein B (1990) Contact dermatitis from cyclohexanone-formaldehyde resin (L_2 resin) in a hair lacquer spray. Contact Dermatitis 22: 108

114. Niklasson B, Björkner B (1989) Contact allergy to the UV-absorber Tinuvin P in plastics. Contact Dermatitis 21: 330–334

115. Jolanki R, Kanerva L, Estlander T (1987) Organic pigments in plastics can cause allergic contact dermatitis. Acta Derm Venereol Suppl (Stockh) 134: 95–97

14.7 Health Personnel

José G. Camarasa

Contents

14.7.1 Introduction

Health personnel carry out a wide spectrum of jobs, all of them susceptible to different forms of contact dermatitis. In this respect, a hospital is like a large factory. Many factors can be dangerous to the skin of health workers. All the potential biological and physical causes cannot be considered in this chapter. Radiation and viral, fungal, bacterial or animal factors may all cause occupational dermatoses in health personnel, but rarely of the contact dermatitis type.

Nevertheless, protective measures and general prevention must be organized as in a major industry [1].

14.7.1.1 Range of Occupations

Health personnel can be divided into three main groups. The first of these includes physicians, surgeons, medical specialists, radiologists, laboratory specialists and dental personnel. The second group includes nurses, clinical assistants, laboratory and radiology technicians, biologists, pharmacists, physiotherapists and dialysis workers. The third group includes office personnel, technical services workers, kitchen and laundry workers, cleaners and disinfection area and sterilization area workers. Veterinarians deserve special attention because of their wide spectrum of work.

14.7.1.2 Irritant Contact Dermatitis

The most common type of contact dermatitis in health personnel is irritant contact dermatitis. The frequent use of disinfectant solutions, detergents and soaps for hand washing produces dryness of the hands and then fissured eczema. Irritant contact dermatitis readily provokes allergic sensitization, because a considerable number of substances with sensitizing potential are also used.

14.7.1.3 Atopy as a Risk Factor

Atopy is a risk factor. The presence of atopy in health personnel or their relatives favours the development of hand dermatitis. Hand dermatitis occurred in 65% of persons with atopic symptoms and in 75% of those who had unusually dry skin and atopic relatives. Among the remaining workers, only 33% had had eczema elsewhere on the skin or on the hands [2, 3].

14.7.1.4 Wet Work

Hospital wet work also increases the risk of hand eczema. Previous irritant contact dermatitis produced by wet working predisposes to allergic reactions, mostly to nickel, fragrances or rubber chemicals. Of persons with allergic contact dermatitis 55% had suffered irritant hand dermatitis previously, compared to 44% of those without positive patch test reactions. Of those with sensitivity to fragrance 70% had suffered from hand dermatitis [4].

14.7.1.5 Hand Dermatitis

As many as 75% of the occupational skin diseases in hospital cleaning women were irritant contact dermatitis of the hands, 21% were allergic contact dermatitis and 4% were candidosis of the finger webs. The causes of irritant contact dermatitis were detergents, alkaline soaps, acids, sodium perborate and hypochlorite and hypobromite compounds [5–7].

Local and general prophylactic measures must be extended in order to reduce occupational hand dermatitis among hospital workers, including nurses, cleaning personnel, kitchen workers, and clinical assistants, among many others.

14.7.2 Dental Personnel

Hand dermatitis in dentists is often a combination of irritant and allergic contact dermatitis [8]. Clinical examination of the patients usually does not help the differential diagnosis. Dentists are working increasingly in rubber gloves and wash their hands very often. Moreover, they have contact with irritants and sensitizers of great potency (Table 14.7.1). The result can be a chronic dry fissured dermatitis of the fingertips and palms, which very commonly changes into a pruritic erythematous scaling dermatitis, or even into a relapsing vesicular eczema, invading the dorsum of the hands and the skin of the fingers with a severe periungual reaction.

14.7.2.1 Local Anaesthetics

Local anaesthetics as a solution, spray or injection are widely used in dentistry and dentists are frequently sensitized to them. *Benzocaine* and *amethocaine* are both *para*-substituted benzene derivatives and have a strong sensitizing capacity. Many dentists become sensitized from contact with local anaesthetic on the fingers when injecting into the buccal mucosa [9–10].

Amethocaine (tetracaine) is used in odontology and as a topical anaesthetic in urology, ophthalmology and otolaryngology. Curtacain, Anethaine, Decicain, Pantocain and Tanexol are amongst the trade names. Of patients allergic to the caine mix in the standard series, 19% were allergic to amethocaine. Five of these were odontologists and the allergy was the sole explanation of their dermatitis. The frequency of simultaneous cross-sensitivity between amethocaine and other anaesthetics of the group is low: procaine 1 out of 16 cases, benzocaine 5 out of 16 cases. Only cyclomethycaine is important: 7 out of 12 cases, perhaps due to its closer chemical structure [11].

Table 14.7.1. Allergens for dentists [1–21]

	test
Antiseptics	
Cresol	1% pet.
Formaldehyde	1% aq.
Hexachlorophene	1% pet.
Ammoniated mercury	1% pet.
Thymol	2% pet.
Benzalkonium chloride	0.1 and 0.01% aq.
Ethanol	as is
Local anaesthetics	
Amethocaine	5% pet.
Amylocaine	5% pet.
Benzocaine	5% pet.
Cyclomethycaine	5% pet.
Cinchocaine	5% pet.
Lidocaine (xylocaine)	5% pet.
Procaine	1% pet.
Proxymetacaine	5% pet.
Metals	
Cr, Ni, Co, Hg, Pt, Pd, potassium dicyanoaurate	0.001% aq.
Sodium thiosulphatoaurate	0.5% pet.
Rubber	
Mercapto mix	2% pet.
Thiuram mix	1% pet.
Resins	
Methyl methacrylate	2% pet.
Epoxy resin	1% pet.
Triethyleneglycol dimethacrylate (TEGDMA)	2% pet.
Urethane dimethacrylate (UEDMA)	2% pet.
Ethyleneglycol dimethacrylate (EGDMA)	2% pet.
BIS-GMA	2% pet.
N,N-Dimethyl-p-toluidine	5% pet.
2-Hydroxy-4-methoxybenzophenone	2% pet.
BIS-MA	2% pet.
Methyl dichlorobenzene sulphonate	0.1% alc.
p-Tolyldiethanolamine	2% alc.
2-Hydroxyethyl methacrylate (2-HEMA)	2% pet.
Essential oils	
Eugenol	1% pet.
Cinnamon oil	1% pet.
Menthol	1% pet.
Eucalyptus oil	1% pet.
Clove oil	1% pet.
Balsam of Peru	25% pet.
Others	
Antibiotics (neomycin), sulphonamides, hydrazine, wax (Carnauba), colophony (20% pet.)	

14.7.2.2 Resins

Acrylic resin is a mixture of the acrylic monomer methyl methacrylate with a powder of polymethyl methacrylate. Most dentures are made of acrylic resin. Acrylic monomer itself is a very strong sensitizer but the fully cured resin does not sensitize. Persons sensitized to acrylic monomer can sustain allergic contact dermatitis after touching acrylics in which residual acrylic monomer remains, when resins are not well heat-cured. Exposure of the skin of the hands of dental personnel to acrylic monomer produces allergic contact dermatitis from this material. Because of its defatting power and its strong solvency power, it penetrates rubber gloves easily, making this protection insufficient.

Patch testing with acrylic monomer may be performed at 2% pet. [12]. Some resins contain benzoyl peroxide (test 1% pet.) or hydroquinone (test 2% pet.), which can cause confusion as to the real sensitizer.

Formaldehyde is widely used as a disinfectant for sterilization of dental instruments. Dentists and many other health personnel become allergic to formaldehyde, which is used because of its efficiency as a disinfectant and also as a fixative for tissues. It is a strong irritant in high concentrations and a sensitizer even in weak solutions. The nails are also affected, losing their colour and hardness, and paronychia may be produced from contact with formaldehyde on the fingers. Its high sensitization power can result in it producing disseminated skin symptoms from only local skin contact or inhalation in very sensitive persons (test 1% aq.).

BIS-GMA (2,2-bis [4-(2-hydroxy-3-methacryloxypropoxy) phenyl] propane) [13,14] and *2-HEMA* (2-hydroxyethyl methacrylate) [14] are sensitizers in UV-cured dental bonding materials (BIS-GMA, test 2% pet.; 2-HEMA, test 2% pet.).

14.7.2.3 Impression Materials and Tooth Sealants

Dental impression materials and tooth sealants cause allergic contact dermatitis on the fingers of dentists. Two substances have mainly been reported: methyl dichlorobenzene sulphonate, used as a catalyst [15–17], and methyl *p*-toluenesulphonate, also a catalyst [18] (methyl dichlorobenzene sulphonate, test 0.1% acet.; methyl *p*-toluenesulphonate, test 1% acet.).

Colophony may constitute approximately 10% of dental impression materials, a source that explains why some dentists become allergic to colophony [19].

14.7.2.4 Essential Oils

Dentists are exposed to several different essential oils:
– Eugenol is used in antiseptics and many pharmaceutical products. It is a
  contact irritant and also a sensitizer (test 1% pet.).

- Cinnamon oil is a flavouring agent and also an antiseptic used in dentistry. It is a common sensitizer (test 1% pet.).
- Menthol or synthetic mints are also sensitizing flavours much employed in dental products (test 1% pet.).
- Balsam of Peru is also used as a component of dental cement. Its sensitization capacity is very well known (test 25% pet.).

Allergies to balsam of Peru may occur with other different essential oils, variously present in dental cements, solvents or antiseptic solutions. Among others must be considered eucalyptus oil (test 1% alc. or 2% pet.) and clove oil (test 2% pet.) [20, 21].

14.7.3 Nurses, Clinical Assistants and Cleaners

Nurses, clinical assistants and cleaners commonly have their hands exposed to irritants, and so often suffer irritant contact dermatitis of the hands. As a result of this, the risk of sensitization is high. Some pharmaceutical products have special relevance for them (Table 14.7.2).

Table 14.7.2. Special allergens for nurses [1]

	Test
Phenothiazines (chlorpromazine)	1% pet.
Glutaraldehyde	1% aq. or pet.
Streptomycin	1% pet.
Penicillin	10000 IU/g pet.[a]
Ampholyt G	1% aq.
Tego 103 G	0.1% aq.
Chloramine-T	0.05% aq.

[a] See text, Sect. 14.7.3.1

14.7.3.1 Medicaments

Streptomycin is a specially important contact sensitizer, because of the severity of the reaction, the minimal contact needed to elicit reactions, and the persistence of the symptoms long after avoiding contact with the antibiotic (test 1% pet.) [22].

Penicillin sensitizes by contact during injections, but contact allergy to penicillin may be associated with generalized immediate reactions of the anaphylactic type. So general measures for preventing anaphylactic shock must also be taken in persons with penicillin contact dermatitis. Testing with penicillin must be done with extreme care. To date, in vivo tests for allergy to penicillin have not been developed. Because of the risk of severe acute generalized reactions, testing with penicillin must be done only in hospitals. An open test with penicillin should be made prior to any other. A closed patch test should be carried out only when an open test is negative, and should be removed immediately any generalized reaction is observed. If the history of contact allergy to penicillin is obvious and severe, no closed patch test should be done, even if the open test is negative. There is no general agreement on a penicillin patch test concentration. Penicillin 10000 IU/g pet. is used in my practice and at St John's Dermatology Centre, London. Patch testing can also detect generalized immediate allergies to penicillin, without contact dermatitis from this antibiotic [23, 24].

Chlorpromazine causes allergic contact dermatitis in nurses who inject or give out the drug in tablet form to patients, thus handling it with their fingers. This happens particularly from pulverizing the tablets. This drug can sensitize by itself or in combination with photoallergic mechanisms (test 1% pet. or photopatch test if unexpected negative results appear) [25, 26].

Maclofenoxate is an analeptic of the central nervous system that may also sensitize nurses who inject it into patients [27].

Cyanamide (carbodiimide) is still used in some countries such as Spain for the treatment of alcoholism. Nurses can be sensitized from contact with pills containing this drug, when handling them in psychiatric wards [28]. In many other countries tetraethylthiuram disulphide (Antabuse) represents a similar risk to nurses.

Potassium chloride has been reported as causing allergic contact dermatitis in a nurse handling it in solution [29].

The cephalosporin *cefotiam hydrochloride* [30] and the antipneumocystis drug *pentamidine isethionate* [31] have both been described as causes of immunological contact urticaria in nurses.

14.7.3.2 Glutaraldehyde

1,5-Pentanedial (glutaraldehyde) is a pharmacological agent used for hyperhidrosis, as an antifungal, and for the treatment of warts and some bullous diseases such as Weber-Cockayne syndrome, porphyria cutanea tarda, and epidermolysis bullosa acquisita. It has also been recommended for herpes zoster, herpes simplex and *Pseudomonas* infections.

It causes brown discoloration of the skin, is very unstable and is a contact irritant and sensitizer, especially in nurses who use instruments sterilized with glutaraldehyde. It is an aliphatic dialdehyde, soluble in water, alcohol and many other solvents. At 2% it is employed as a cold sterilizer for many instruments in hospitals (for bronchoscopy, cytoscopy, anaesthetics, renal dialysis, etc.). Unbuffered solutions of glutaraldehyde are stable and have little antimicrobial potential. When sodium bicarbonate is added, an alkaline pH of 8.0 results and a strong antimicrobial is obtained. Its antiviral, fungicidal and bactericidal activity is enhanced, but it remains stable only for 10–15 days. Activated glutaraldehyde (Cidex) retains the allergenic contact capacity of 1,5-pentanedial [32, 33].

Mainly nurses, clinical assistants and cleaning workers in hospitals suffer allergic contact dermatitis from glutaraldehyde. Cases of hand eczema produced by this biocide are increasing and the clinical symptoms often show some chronicity, possibly because glutaraldehyde is also employed as a leather-tanning agent, in wallpaper, in photographic film and in other industries. Although glutaraldehyde and formaldehyde do not seem to cross-react [34, 35], some patients show positive allergic reactions to both substances [36, 37] (test 1% aq. or pet., but beware false-positive reactions [38]).

14.7.3.3 Ampholytics, Surfactants, Soaps

Desimex, Ampholyt G and Tego 103 G are dodecyldiaminoethylglycine hydrochloride. Tego 103 G also contains small quantities of formaldehyde and benzyl alcohol. Ampholyt G contains neither additional substance. Tego contains four active ingredients: 9-lauryl-3,6,9-triazanonanoic acid, 7-lauryl-1,4,7-triazaheptane, 6,9-dilauryl-3,6,9-triazanonanoic acid and 7-dilauryl-1,4,7-triazaheptane.

Ampholytics are used as disinfectants in many different places but have recently been widely used by hospital personnel. Some cases of allergic contact dermatitis have been described. Because of the chemical nature of these substances, some patients could also be reactive to ethylenediamine, though this special cross-reaction can be implicated only in a minority of cases [39, 40]

Some other substances used by nurses for topical treatment of various dermatoses may cause severe allergic contact dermatitis, some of them with a chronic course and persistent lesions. The use of protective gloves and systematic prevention of contact must be recommended. Dinitrochlorobenzene, nitrogen mustards and squaric acid diethylester are clear examples of such substances.

Antiseptics that commonly cause contact dermatitis to nurses, clinical assistants and cleaners are widely used in the different hospital wards. The majority of exposures occur in dental and surgical personnel (see Sects. 14.7.2, 14.7.4).

More recently, chloramine-T (sodium p-toluenesulphonchloramine) has been described as a sensitizer for nurses [41]. Chloramine-T is used as sterilizer, disinfectant, antiseptic and chemical reagent (test 0.05% aq.).

Allergic contact dermatitis from undecylenamide diethanolamide in a liquid soap has been described in a hospital employee [42].

14.7.4 Surgeons

14.7.4.1 Gloves

Chemical components of rubber gloves commonly cause allergic contact dermatitis of the hands and forearms in surgeons. Although many different substances can sensitize, the most frequent are those tested in the thiuram mix of the standard series. Less frequent are mercaptobenzothiazole and others tested in mercapto mix. Release of thiurams and carbamates from rubber gloves varies between brands [43]. The role of glove powder remains debatable [44].

Immunological contact urticaria of the hands, also produced by rubber gloves, is less frequent but must be recognized. Allergy to a natural protein contained in rubber latex coming from the *Hevea* tree has been identified. Moreover contact allergy from surgical rubber gloves can produce, besides contact urticaria, a generalized anaphylactic reaction. This type of contact urticaria can be demonstrated by cutaneous tests and an in vitro radioallergosorbent test (RAST; IgE) (latex – *Hevea braziliensis* Phadebas RAST allergen discs, MK82, no. 61682, Pharmacia). Those allergic to natural rubber gloves can develop episodes of urticaria, bronchospasm or intestinal spasms from eating banana, peach, avocado or chestnut [45].

Cutaneous tests include a use test of surgical rubber gloves with wet hands, for a few minutes, until any allergic contact urticaria appears, and an open application test with gentle rubbing of the skin. The open application test can be done on normal skin, advisedly on the dorsum of the hand, since on other skin areas the test may be negative. Usually the weal reaction appears quickly and is intense. Therefore a closed patch, prick or scratch test is in the first instance not recommended, in order to avoid undesirable and dangerous generalized reactions (see also Sect. 2.3.2).

Surgeons allergic to components of rubber may use other types of glove. Elastyren gloves (Danpren, DK-2620 Alberslund, Denmark) do not contain thiuram allergens and are useful for those surgeons allergic to rubber chemicals.

The use of disposable polythene gloves (e.g. Disposaglove) underneath latex gloves can prevent contact urticaria in sensitive patients. Others use vinyl undergloves to prevent dermatitis. Still others improve using hypoallergenic latex surgical gloves (Ansell Gammex; Ansell Rubber Co., Malacca, Malaysia) [46–48].

Acrylic bone cement is used, amongst other things, for fixation of prostheses to the bone of the hip joint. Bone cement contains methyl methacrylate monomer and polymethyl methacrylate. The monomer is a strong lipid solvent. The hand dermatitis caused by allergy to it is usually a dry, pruriginous, fissured, chronic eczema of the fingertips, sometimes with paraesthesia and tingling or burning sensations. Gloves usually do not protect the hands from acrylic bone cement. Indeed, even if two pairs of rubber gloves are worn, the sensitized surgeon may suffer from contact with acrylic cement, because enough acrylic penetrates both pairs if he or she has contact for sufficient time [49–51].

14.7.4.2 Antiseptics

Some substances used because of their antiseptic power are present in surgical scrubbing agents in the preoperating room. Some surgeons contract chronic, dry, pruritic, irritant contact dermatitis of the dorsum of the hands from such agents. It is not infrequent for superimposed allergic contact dermatitis to appear, because these substances also have allergic capacity. The most commonly employed are: hexachlorophene G 11 (test 1% pet.), dichlorophene G 4 (test 1% aq.), tribromosalicylanilide (TCSA) (test 0.5% pet.), dibromosalicylanilide (test 1% pet.), triclosan (Irgasan DP 300) (test 2% pet.), Fentichlor (test 1% pet.), chlorhexidine (test both acetate and gluconate 0.5% aq.) [52], cresol (test 1% aq.), Dowicides (phenolic substances) (test 1% pet.), imidazolidinyl urea (test 2% pet.), sodium hypochlorite (test 0.5% aq.), sodium hyposulphite (test 0.5% aq.), and benzydamine hydrochloride (test 0.5% aq.) [53].

Some quaternary ammonium compounds are of special interest. The most common and widely used is benzalkonium chloride (alkylbenzyldimethylammonium chloride), a cationic detergent used as a preoperative skin disinfectant, and also for surgical instruments. Its presence in cosmetics, soaps, medicaments and its capacity for sensitize are well-known. People allergic to benzalkonium chloride must avoid any quaternary ammonium compounds, because of cross-reactions [54, 56]. Patch testing with 0.1% aq. can also provoke irritant reactions. True allergic responses are obtained testing with 0.01% aq.

14.7.5 Laboratory Personnel

Laboratories use many different substances capable of producing contact dermatitis in their personnel [1]. Some are listed in Tables 14.7.3 and 14.7.4.

In pharmaceutical laboratories, mainly in product synthesis areas, contact dermatitis may arise in the pharmacologists who synthesize such products. Very often the sensitizers are not the final compounds. Sensitizations have been published as individual case reports, and substances mentioned include vitamin K_3 sodium bisulphite [57, 58], codeine [59], cephalosporins, cytosine arabinoside [60], 3,4-dicarbethoxyhexane-2,5-dione [61], 2-aminophenyl disulphide [62], ethyl-2-bromo-p-methoxyphenylacetate [63], ethyl chloro oximido acetate [64], and pyridine in Karl Fischer reagent [65].

Contact dermatitis caused by alcohols is of special interest. Amyl, butyl, ethyl, methyl, and isopropyl alcohols cause allergic contact dermatitis, but rarely. Contact allergy to alcohols may cause a generalized allergic reaction when alcohol is ingested. Nevertheless, contact reactions to alcohol do

Table 14.7.3. Histology laboratory allergens

	Test		Test
Potassium dichromate	0.5% pet.	Sudan III-IV	2% pet.
Formaldehyde	1% aq.	Aniline	1% pet.
Epoxy resin	1% pet.	Congo red	2% pet.
Glutaraldehyde	1% aq. or pet.	Picric acid	1% pet.
DPPD	1% pet.		

DPPD, N, N'-Diphenyl-p-phenylenediamine

Table 14.7.4. Biochemistry laboratory allergens

	Test		Test
Ammoniated mercury	1% pet.	Picric acid	1% pet.
Phenylhydrazine	1% pet.	Potassium dichromate	0.5% pet.
Methyl Orange	2% pet.	PPD base	1% pet.

PPD, *p*-phenylenediamine

not necessarily signify that a systemic reaction will develop after drinking alcoholic liquor [66, 67]. Alcohols can be patch tested undiluted. Two types of response may appear: an immediate wealing reaction in 15 min or a common eczematous patch in 2–4 days. Sometimes a combination of both reactions has been described [68].

14.7.6 Veterinarians

Veterinarians are exposed to many organic, biological and chemical substances that may produce allergic contact dermatitis. Sensitized veterinarians can suffer asthma, rhinitis and contact dermatitis from dander, hair, bristles, or saliva from cows, horses, cats or dogs [69]. Specific IgE and scratch tests are diagnostic. Clinically, allergic contact urticaria, allergic contact dermatitis or both reactions can be observed [70].

14.7.6.1 Antibiotics

Certain antibiotics are more often used in veterinary than in human medicine. Spiramycin, tylosin and benzyl penicillin diethylaminoethylester (penethamate) are the most important. Spiramycin and tylosin are used to treat pigs with enteritis, mastitis in cows, and respiratory infections in household pets [71]. Penethamate hydriodide is used for local or intralesional treatment of mastitis in cows. It cross-reacts with penicillin [72].

14.7.6.2 Feed Additives and Other Medicaments

Hormones, vitamins, minerals, antibiotics, growth stimulants, preservatives, metals, antioxidants and certain other substances are present in animal feeds (Table 14.7.5). Health personnel who handle these additives may experience allergic contact dermatitis. For example, vitamin A and vitamin D_3 contain 5% ethoxyquin as an antioxidant preservative. Ethoxyquin (6-ethyl-1,2-dihydro-2,2,4-trimethylquinoline) is a contact sensitizer. Quindoxin, a growth promoting factor, is a common sensitizer and also induces photodermatitis [73, 74]. Halquinol, a chlorinated derivative of 8-hydroxquinoline, is added to animal feeds for prevention of *Escherichia coli* and *Salmonella* infections. Halquinol causes irritant, allergic and photoallergic dermatitis, and sometimes allergic contact urticaria and airborne contact dermatitis [75].

Table 14.7.5. Animal feed additives [81, 82]

	Function	Test
Amprolium	Growth promoter	10% aq.
Arsanilic acid	Growth promoter	10% pet.
Bacitracin zinc	Growth promoter	20% pet.
Chlortetracycline hydrochloride	Growth promoter	3% pet.
Sulphacetamide	Growth promoter (prevents enteral infections)	1% pet.
Tylosin tartrate	Growth promoter (prevents Gram-negative infections)	5% pet.
Diethylstilbestrol	Fattening cattle	0.1% eth.
Ethoxyquin	Antioxidant preservative	1% pet.
Ethylenediamine	Antiseptic	1% pet.
Medroxyprogesterone acetate	Abortions	1% pet.
Neomycin sulphate	Prevention of dysentery	20% pet.
Nitrofurazone	Prevention of *Salmonella*	1% pet.
Penicillin	Prevention of mastitis	10000 IU/g[a]
Thiabendazole	Worm control	1% pet.
Piperazine	Worm control	1% pet.
Phenothiazines	Worm control	1% pet.

[a] see text, Sect. 14.7.3.1

Table 14.7.6. Patch test series for veterinarians [79, 80]

Penicillin	10000 IU(g pet.[a])	Formaldehyde	1% aq.
Streptomycin	1% pet.	Mercaptobenzothiazole	2% pet.
Dihydrostreptomycin	0.1% pet.	Merthiolate	0.1% pet.
Erythromycin base	1% pet.	Pierazine	1% aq.
Oxytetracycline	10% pet.	Tuberculin	10% aq.
Penethamate	1% pet.	Bovine tuberculin	10% aq.
Spiramycin (Rovamycin)	10% pet.	Ethoxyquin	1% pet.
Tylosin (tartrate)	5% pet.	Quindoxin	0.1% pet.
Procaine	2% aq.	Chlorpromazine	0.5% pet.
Benzocaine	5% pet.		

[a]See text, Sect. 14.7.3.1

Dinitolmide, which is used to control coccidiosis in chicken factories [76], and nitrofurazone, used for treatment of salmonellosis in pigs and as a growth promoting factor for cattle and swine, can also cause allergic contact dermatitis in veterinarians [77].

Chloropromazine and other phenothiazine derivatives are used by veterinarians and farmers for the sedation of animals. Contact and photodermatitis in a farmer due to chlorpromazine used for sedation of pigs suggest that this type of medicament should be included in a patch test series for veterinarians (Table 14.7.6) [78].

Occupational contact allergy to lincomycin and spectinomycin in chicken vaccinators has been documented [83].

14.7.7 References

1. Camarasa JG, Conde Salazar L (1988) Occupational dermatoses in sanitary workers. In: Orfanos CE, Stadler R, Gollnick H (eds) Dermatology in five continents. Proceedings of the XVII World Congress of Dermatology, Berlin, May 24–29, 1987. Springer, Berlin Heidelberg New York, pp 1045–1048
2. Lammintausta K, Kalimo K (1981) Atopy and hand dermatitis in hospital wet work. Contact Dermatitis 7: 301–308
3. Nilsson E, Mikaelsson B, Andersson S (1985) Atopy, occupation and domestic work as risk factors for hand eczema in hospital workers. Contact Dermatitis 13: 216–223
4. Lammintausta K, Kalimo K, Havu VK (1982) Occurrence of contact allergy and hand ecezmas in hospital wet work. Contact Dermatitis 8: 84–90
5. Hansen KS (1983) Occupational dermatoses in hospital cleaning women. Contact Dermatitis 9: 343–351
6. Singgih SIR, Lantinga H, Nater JP, Woest TE, Kruyt-Gaspersz JA (1986) Occupational hand dermatoses in hospital cleaning personnel. Contact Dermatitis 14: 14–19
7. Gawkrodger DJ, Lloyd MH, Hunter JAA (1986) Occupational skin disease in hospital cleaning and kitchen workers. Contact Dermatitis 15: 132–135
8. Oshima H, Kawahara D, Kosugi H, Nakamura M, Sugai T, Tamaki T (1991) Epidemiologic study on occupational allergy in the dental clinic. Contact Dermatitis 24: 138–139
9. Samitz MH, Schmunes E (1969) Occupational dermatoses in dentists and allied personnel. Cutis 5: 180
10. Calnan CD, Stevenson CJ (1963) Studies in Contact Dermatitis. XV. Dental materials. Trans St Johns Hosp Dermatol Soc 18: 24
11. Garcia Perez A, Conde Salazar L, Guimaraens D, Garcia Bravo B, Lopez Correcher B (1981) La sensibilidad de contacto a la Ametocaina. Actes Dermosifiliográficas 72: 441–448
12. Fisher AA (1954) Allergic sensitization of the skin and oral mucosa to acrylic denture materials. JAMA 156: 238
13. Fisher AA (1986) Contact dermatitis in health personnel. In: Contact dermatitis, 3rd edn. Lea and Febiger, Philadelphia
14. Kanerva L, Estlander T, Jolanki R, Tarvainen K (1993) Occupational allergic contact dermatitis caused by exposure to acrylates during work with dental prostheses. Contact Dermatitis 28: 268–275
15. Van Ketel WG (1977) Reactions to dental impression materials. Contact Dermatitis 3: 55
16. Groeningen GV, Nater JP (1975) Reaction to dental impression materials. Contact Dermatitis 1: 373–376
17. Nally FS, Storrs J (1973) Hypersensitivity to a dental impression material. Br Dent J 134: 244
18. Malten KE (1979) Recently reported causes of contact dermatitis due to synthetic resins and hardeners Contact Dermatitis 5: 11–23
19. Dawson TAJ (1977) Colophony sensitivity in dentistry. Contact Dermatitis 3: 343
20. Axell T, Björkner B, Fregert S, Niklasson B (1983) Standard patch test series for screening of contact allergy to dental materials. Contact Dermatitis 9: 82–84
21. Aberer W, Holub H, Strohal R, Slavicek R (1993) Palladium in dental alloys - the dermatologists' responsibility to warn? Contact Dermatitis 28: 163–165
22. Sidi E, Longueville R, Hincky M (1958) Occupational eczema in therapists. Thomas, Springfield, p 196
23. Blanton WB, Blanton FM (1953) Unusual penicillin hypersensitivities. J Allergy 24: 405
24. Pecegueiro M (1990) Occupational contact dermatitis from penicillin. Contact Dermatitis 23: 190–191

25. Calnan CD, Frain-Bell W, Cuthbert JW (1962) Occupational dermatitis from chlorpromazine. Trans St Johns Hosp Dermatol Soc 48: 49
26. Camarasa JG (1976) Contact dermatitis to phenothiazines Nemactil® and Decentan®. Contact Dermatitis 2: 123
27. Foussereau J, Lautz JP (1972) Allergy to maclofenoxate in nurses. Contact Dermatitis Newslett 6: 231
28. Conde Salazar L, Guimaraens D, Romero L, Harto A (1981) Allergic contact dermatitis to Cyanamide (carbodiimide) Contact Dermatitis 7: 329–330
29. Zabala R, Aguirre A, Eizaguirre X, Diaz Perez JL (1993) Contact dermatitis from potassium chloride. Contact Dermatitis 29: 218–219
30. Miyahara H, Koga T, Imayama S, Hori Y (1993) Occupational contact urticaria syndrome from cefotiam hydrochloride. Contact Dermatitis 29: 210–211
31. Belsito DV (1993) Contact urticaria from pentamidine isethionate. Contact Dermatitis 29: 158–159
32. Sanderson KV, Cronin E (1968) Glutaraldehyde and contact dermatitis. Contact Dermatitis Newslett 4: 79
33. Lyon TC (1971) Allergic contact dermatitis due to Cidex. Oral Surg 32: 895
34. Neering H, van Ketel WG (1974) Glutaraldehyde and formaldehyde allergy. Contact Dermatitis Newslett 16: 518
35. Maibach HI (1975) Glutaraldehyde: cross reaction to formaldehyde. Contact Dermatitis 1: 326
36. Nethercott JR, Holnes DL, Page E (1988) Occupational contact dermatitis due to glutaraldehyde in health care workers. Contact Dermatitis 18: 193–197
37. Hansen KS (1983) Glutaraldehyde occupational dermatitis. Contact Dermatitis 9: 81–82
38. Hansen EM, Menné T (1990) Glutaraldehyde: patch test, vehicle and concentration. Contact Dermatitis 23: 369–370
39. Foussereau J, Samsoen M, Hecht MTh (1983) Occupational dermatitis to Ampholyt G in hospital personnel. Contact Dermatitis 9: 233–234
40. Suhonen R (1980) Contact allergy to dodecyldi (aminoethyl)glycine-Desimex I. Contact Dermatitis 6: 290–291
41. Lombardi P, Gola M, Acciai MC, Sertoli A (1984) Unusual occupational allergic contact dermatitis in a nurse. Contact Dermatitis 20: 302
42. Christersson S, Wrangsjö K (1991) Contact allergy to undecylenamide diethanolamide in a liquid soap. Contact Dermatitis 27: 191–192
43. Knudsen BB, Larsen E, Egsgaard H, Menné T (1993) Release of thiurams and carbamates from rubber gloves. Contact Dermatitis 28: 63–69
44. Milković-Kraus S (1992) Glove powder as a contact allergen. Contact Dermatitis 26: 198
45. Crisi G, Belsito DV (1993) Contact urticaria from latex in a patient with immediate hypersensitivity to banana, avocado and peach. Contact Dermatitis 28: 247–248
46. Nutter AF (1979) Contact uriticaria by rubber. Br J Dermatol 101: 597–598
47. Turjanmaa K (1987) Incidence of inmediate allergy to latex gloves in hospital personnel. Contact Dermatitis 5: 270–275
48. Taylor JS, Cassettari J, Wagner W, Helm Th (1989) Contact urticaria and anaphylaxis to latex. Am Acad Dermatol [Suppl] 21: 874–876
49. Pegum J, Medhurst FA (1971) Contact dermatitis from penetration of rubber gloves by acrylic monomer. Br Med J 2: 141
50. Fries JB, Fisher AA, Salvati EA (1975) Contact dermatitis in surgeons from methylmethacrylate bone cement. J Bone Joint Surg [Am] 57: 547
51. Fisher AA (1979) Paresthesia of the fingers accompanying dermatitis due to methylmethacrylate bone cements. Contact Dermatitis 5: 56
52. Knudsen BB, Avnstorp C (1991) Chlorhexidine gluconate and acetate in patch testing. Contact Dermatitis 24: 45–49
53. Foti C, Vena GA, Angelini G (1992) Occupational contact allergy to benzydamine hydrochloride. Contact Dermatitis 27: 328–329

54. Afzelius H, Thulin H (1979) Allergic reactions to Benzalkonium Chloride. Contact Dermatitis 5: 60
55. Fisher AA, Stillman MA (1972) Allergic contact sensitivity to benzalkonium chloride. Arch Dermatol 106: 169–171
56. Wahlberg JE (1962) Two cases of hypersensitivity to quaternary ammonium compounds. Acta Derm Venereol (Stockh) 42: 230
57. Romaguera C, Grimalt F, Conde Salazar L (1980) Occupational dermatitis from vitamin K_3 sodium bisulfite. Contact Dermatitis 6: 355
58. Camarasa JG, Barnadas M (1982) Occupational dermatosis by vitamin K_3 sodium bisulfite. Contact Dermatitis 8: 268
59. Romaguera C, Grimalt F (1983) Occupational dermatitis from codeine. Contact Dermatitis 9: 170
60. Conde Salazar L, Guimaraens D, Romero L (1984) Occupational dermatitis from cytosin arabinoside synthesis. Contact Dermatitis 1: 44
61. Niklasson B, Björkner B (1990) Contact allergy to 3,4-dicarbethoxyhexane-2,5-dione. Contact Dermatitis 23: 46–47
62. Tomb RR, Lepoittevin J-P, Caussade P (1991) Contact allergy to 2-aminophenyl disulfide. Contact Dermatitis 25: 196–197
63. Kanzaki T, Sakakibara N (1992) Occupational allergic contact dermatitis from ethyl-2-bromo-p-methoxyphenylacetate. Contact Dermatitis 26: 204–205
64. Hausen BM (1992) Occupational allergic contact dermatitis from ethyl chloro oximido acetate. Contact Dermatitis 27: 277–278
65. Knegt-Junk C, Geursen-Reitsma L, van Joost T (1993) Allergic contact dermatitis from pyridine in Karl Fischer reagent. Contact Dermatitis 28: 252
66. Fregert S, Kokanson R, Rosman H et al. (1963) Dermatitis from alcohols. J Allergy 34: 404
67. Martin-Scott I (1960) Contact dermatitis from alcohol. Br J Dermatol 72: 372
68. van Ketel WG, Tan Lim KN (1979) Contact dermatitis from ethanol. Contact Dermatitis 1: 7
69. Camarasa JG (1986) Contact eczema from cow saliva. Contact Dermatitis 2: 117
70. Prahl P, Roed-Petersen J (1979) Type I allergy from cows in veterinary surgeons. Contact Dermatitis 5: 33–36
71. Hjorth N, Weissmann K (1972) Occupational dermatitis among veterinary surgeons caused by spiramycin and tylosin. Contact Dermatitis Newslett 12: 320
72. Hjorth N (1967) Occupational dermatitis among veterinary surgeons caused by Penethamate. Berufsdermatosen 15: 163
73. Melhorn HC, Beetz D (1971) Das Antioxydant Aethoxyquin als berufliches Ebenzatogen bei einem Futtermitteldosierer. Berufsdermatosen 19: 84
74. Burrows D (1975) Contact dermatitis in animal feed mill workers. Br J Dermatol 92: 167
75. Caplan RM (1973) Contact dermatitis from animal feed additives (letter to editor) Arch Dermatol 107: 918
76. Bleumink E, Nater JP (1973) Allergic contact dermatitis to dinitolmide (letter to editor). Arch Dermatol 108: 423–424
77. Nelder KM (1972) Contact dermatitis from animal feed additives. Arch Dermatol 106: 722–723
78. Ertle VT (1982) Beruflich bedingte Kontakt- und Photokontaktallergie bei einem Landwirt durch Chlorpromazin. Dermatosen 4: 120–122
79. Hjorth N (1975) Battery for testing veterinary surgeons. Contact Dermatitis 1: 122
80. Rudzki E, Rebandel P, Grzywa Z, Pomorski Z, Jakiminska B, Zawisza E (1982) Occupational dermatitis in veterinarians. Contact Dermatitis 8: 72
81. Malten KE (1978) Therapeutics for pets as neglected causes of contact dermatitis in housewives. Contact Dermatitis 4: 296–299
82. Fisher AA (1973) Allergic contact dermatitis in animal feed handlers. Cutis 16: 201
83. Vilaplana J, Romaguera C, Grimalt F (1991) Contact dermatitis from lincomycin and spectinomycin in chicken vaccinators. Contact Dermatitis 24: 225–226

14.8 Plants and Plant Products

GEORGES DUCOMBS and RICHARD J. SCHMIDT

Contents

14.8.1 Introduction

Contact dermatitis from plants or plant products may occur by several mechanisms. Irritant reactions may be mechanically or chemically induced; these are not commonly seen. The most common dermatoses seen in dermatology clinics comprise delayed and immediate contact reactions of allergic aetiology. Photoirritant reactions also occur quite commonly, but photoallergic reactions seem to be very rare. Reactions of mixed aetiology do occur - thus, irritant and allergic reactions are often superimposed, while mechanical plus chemical irritant effects are evoked by, for example, stinging nettles. These mechanisms are discussed more fully in [1] and [2] as well as in Chap. 2. Unusually, some plants and plant products may evoke dermatoses (including photodermatoses) following ingestion or internal administration by other means. Such reactions are, however, beyond the scope of this chapter.

There are no statistics available to establish the actual incidence of dermatitis from plants and plant products (the so-called phytodermatoses). The problem may in fact be a good deal commoner than the literature would suggest. A number of patients may either self-medicate following self-diagnosis or diagnosis by pharmacist, relative, etc. or attend their family doctor, who prescribes palliative treatment without necessarily ascertaining the cause of the skin reaction. In either instance, the case fails to reach the dermatologist. Fregert [3] reported a study involving 1752 patients considered to have occupational dermatoses; among these patch-tested patients, he found 8% of women and 6% of men reacting to plant-derived products. We estimate that perhaps 5%–10% of all cases of contact allergy seen in European dermatology clinics are caused by plants or plant products.

In Europe, a high proportion of phytodermatoses are occupationally acquired. Persons most at risk are florists, gardeners, horticulturalists, foresters, farmers, cooks and others involved in food preparation, and woodworkers but hobby gardeners, housewives and others who handle or come into contact with plant materials nonoccupationally are also at risk. Indeed, any persons enjoying leisure pursuits in the garden or countryside (children playing, campers, walkers, etc.) are likely to come into contact with plant material with the potential to evoke a contact dermatitis.

14.8.2 Clinical Aspects

14.8.2.1 Irritant Contact Dermatitis

14.8.2.1.1 Mechanical Irritation

A number of plants can provoke 'macrotraumatic' injury by mechanical means because of their armament of prickles, spines or thorns. Others, because of the knife-like morphology of their leaf edges, may lacerate the skin. Although typically a trivial and self-limiting event, such mechanical damage may lead to the development of sores and granulomatous lesions which may develop insidiously some time after the initial trauma has been forgotten. In arid regions of the Americas, for example, cacti (family Cactaceae) are responsible for injuries that may become granulomatous [4] (Fig. 14.8.1).

Certain plants are injurious because of their bristles or barbs (trichomes or glochids) which can cause 'microtrauma'. These structure can penetrate the outer layer of skin and cause a papular dermatitis, prurigo and even urticaria. In Israel, Shanon and Sagher [5] have described 'sabra dermatitis' from handling the prickly pear or Indian (or Barbary) fig (*Opuntia vulgaris* Miller, *O. ficus-indica* Miller, family Cactaceae). This dermatitis simulates chronic eczema or scabies and is caused by the penetration of the skin by glochids from the spine cushions of the plants and their fruit. Microtrauma from calcium oxalate needle crystals (raphides) also evokes a characteristic

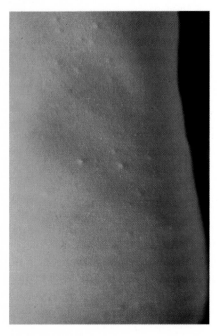

Fig. 14.8.1. Granulomatous lesions on a child's arm from cactus. (Courtesy of F. Vakilzadeh)

dermatitis resembling that caused by glass fibre [6]. Penetration of the skin by such raphides may be accompanied by an intracutaneous injection of plant sap. This can result in an irritant or allergic skin reaction to one or more of the sap constituents. Thus, the preparation of the tubers of various aroids for food use (for example, the cocoyams, *Xanthosoma* spp., family Araceae) carries with it the risk of dermatitis from the calcium oxalate needle crystals and the saponins that they contain [7]. Similarly, calcium oxalate raphides in dumbcanes (*Dieffenbachia* spp., family Araceae), which are commonly grown as decorative house plants, are responsible for an urticarial dermatitis or bullous and oedematous stomatitis in people who have handled damaged plant material or accidently chewed the leaves. The reaction in the mouth renders the victim speechless (hence the common name of the plant) and may be life threatening if the airway becomes obstructed. The severity of the reaction is consistent with the finding that the plant sap contains a protease, named dumbcain, which contributes to the irritant reaction [8].

14.8.2.1.2 Chemical Irritation

Many plants are capable of eliciting an irritant skin reaction without the need for preliminary or concomitant mechanical irritation. The irritants involved vary from weakly irritant compounds, which require repeated exposure and some skin abrasion to exert their effects, to some of the most irritant compounds known to man, which can elicit inflammation in microgram quantities (see Sect. 14.8.3.7). Such potent skin irritants are also mucous membrane irritants, which can cause violent purgation and intense ocular irritation that may lead to blindness.

Acute dermatitis lasts several hours, sometimes less. Chronic dermatitis develops after repeated contact with the irritant agent or occurs on the background of previous contact with weakened skin. These irritant dermatoses manifest themselves only at sites of contact, such as the hands, forearms, mucous membranes, perioral regions, buttocks, etc.

The clinical presentation of irritant contact dermatitis is polymorphic, varying from simple dryness of the skin, cracking and hyperkeratosis to inflammatory reactions with oedema, erythema, papules and vesicles. If the irritant is very strong, as with spurges (*Euphorbia* spp., family Euphorbiaceae) for example, there may be bullae, superficial necrosis or ulceration. Pain rather than itching is also a feature.

14.8.2.2 Allergic Contact Dermatitis

Allergic contact dermatitis from plants can present in many forms, depending both upon the allergen and the method of exposure: 'typical' acute eczema, periungual allergic contact dermatitis, airborne contact dermatitis, contact urticaria and erythema-multiforme-like eruptions.

14.8.2.2.1 Acute Eczema

The normal presentation is that of an allergic contact dermatitis, typically involving exposed parts such as the hands, forearms, eyelids and sometimes even the genitals if the allergen can be conveyed by the hands or clothing. The initial erythematovesicular eruption may develop into a full-blown erythroderma as, for example, with *Frullania* dermatitis.

14.8.2.2.2 'Tulip Fingers'

A number of examples of (usually) occupationally acquired periungual eczema of the finger tips have been described. This takes the form of a fissured, hyperkeratotic and painful eruption, of which the best-known example is 'tulip fingers' seen in tulip pickers (*Tulipa* spp. and cultivars, family Liliaceae); similar reactions may arise in persons handling daffodil and narcissus bulbs (*Narcissus* spp. and cultivars, family Amaryllidaceae), alstroemeria flowers (*Alstroemeria* spp. and cultivars, family Alstroemeriaceae (Fig. 14.8.2), garlic (*Allium sativum* L., family Alliaceae), etc. Although nominally an immunologically mediated reaction, tulip fingers and related eruptions (especially 'daffodil itch' or 'lily rash' in daffodil bulb/flower handlers; see [9]) may arise in part from mechanical and/or chemical irritation.

14.8.2.2.3 Airborne Contact Dermatitis

Hjorth et al. [10] have well described airborne contact dermatitis of plant origin, that is, dermatitis arising from contact with airborne plant particles

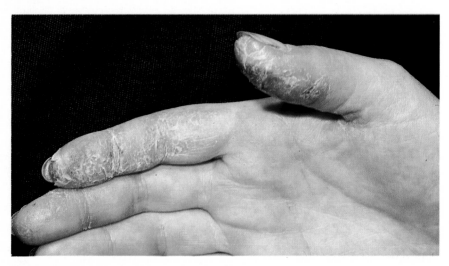

Fig. 14.8.2. Allergic contact dermatitis in a nursery gardener from alstroemeria. (Courtesy of P.J. Frosch)

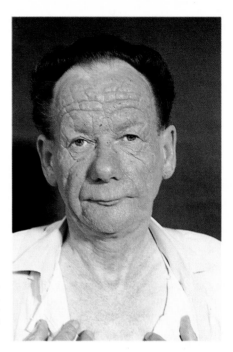

Fig. 14.8.3. Airborne contact dermatitis in a farmer from Compositae. Note marked infiltration on forehead and sharp upper border due to wearing hat. (Courtesy of N. Hjorth)

and resembling a photodermatitis. Airborne contact dermatitis may be differentiated from a true photodermatitis, which normally spares the upper eyelids and the triangle of skin behind the earlobe (see Sect. 2.4.3.1). Although pollens are usually incriminated as the causative agent, Arlette and Mitchell [11] believe that finely pulverized material derived from dead plants is the more likely aetiological agent in the case of ragweeds (*Ambrosia* spp.) and related members of the Compositae family (Fig. 14.8.3). Similarly, Foussereau et al. [12] noted that innocently walking in a forest may bring on an attack of eczema in patients who are sensitized to liverworts of the genus *Frullania* (family Jubulaceae), suggesting that either particles of liverwort (spores?) or vapourized allergen is the causative agent. Thune and Solberg [13] described airborne contact dermatitis from lichen particles, whilst Schmidt [14] believes that vaporized allergen may be responsible for airborne contact dermatitis in florists exposed to chrysanthemums (*Dendranthema* cultivars, family Compositae). In North America and elsewhere it is recognized that the smoke from burning poison ivy (*Toxicodendron* spp.) and related plants in the Anacardiaceae family may sensitize if the allergenic oleoresin is vaporized rather than pyrolyzed [15].

14.8.2.2.4 Contact Urticaria

This type of reaction differs from those described in Sects. 14.8.2.2.2 and 14.8.2.2.3 above in that it belongs to the class of immediate (as opposed

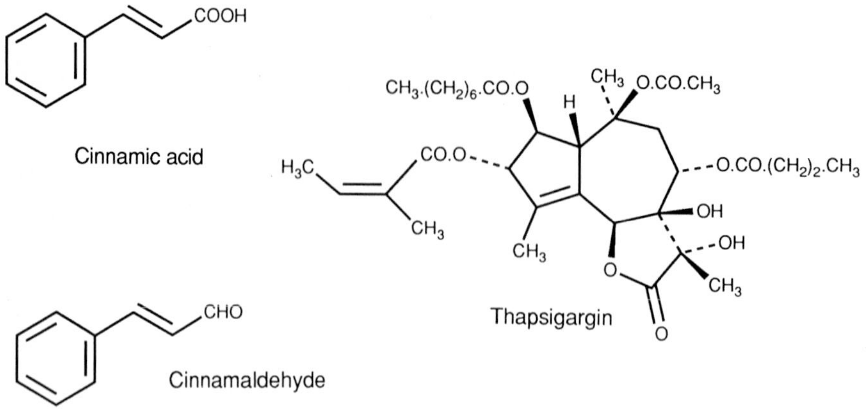

Fig. 14.8.4. Examples of contact urticants from plants and plant products

to delayed) immune responses; nonimmunologic urticarial reactions are also known. Thus, protein contact dermatitis is a well-documented occupational urticaria seen in persons who handle foods [16–19]. Among nonprotein elicitors of urticaria are balsam of Peru and the cinnamic acid derivatives contained therein [20], and thapsigargin from *Thapsia garganica* L. (family Umbelliferae) [21–22]. The structures of cinnamic acid, cinnamaldehyde and thapsigargin are given in Fig. 14.8.4. The mechanism by which nonimmunologic urticants elicit their effect, at least in the case of those listed, appears to involve the release of histamine from mast cells. As with eczemas of delayed allergic aetiology, urticarias may also spread from the initial site of contact and become generalized.

An airborne contact urticaria in a warehouseman, resulting from exposure to dust derived from cinchona bark (*Cinchona* spp., family Rubiaceae), has been reported by Dooms-Goossens et al. [23].

14.8.2.2.5 Erythema-multiforme-like Eruption

Bonnevie [24] described an erythema-multiforme-like rash which developed after contact with leaves of *Primula obconica* Hance (family Primulaceae). The clinical picture resembles that of a drug eruption. Holst et al. [25] described a similar reaction following contact with certain tropical woods (Rio rosewood, *Dalbergia nigra* Allemão; pao ferro, *Machaerium scleroxylon* Tul., family Leguminosae) (Fig. 14.8.5) as did Martin et al. [26] and, more recently, Irvine et al. [27]. Schwartz and Downham [28] provided a case report of erythema multiforme associated with poison ivy dermatitis.

We have seen a pemphigoid-like reaction in the wife of a woodworker who had been helping her husband work with bois d'olon, a kind of satinwood (*Fagara heitzii* Aubrév. and Pellegrin, family Rutaceae)

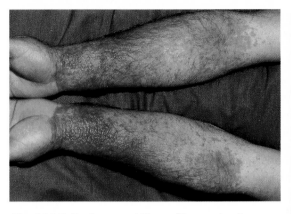

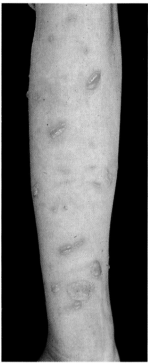

Fig. 14.8.5. Erythema-multiforme-like reaction in a carpenter caused by wood dust (pao ferro). (Courtesy of P.J. Frosch)

Fig. 14.8.6. Phototoxic dermatitis from forocoumarin-containing plants. (Courtesy of P.J. Frosch)

14.8.2.3 Phytophotodermatitis

14.8.2.3.1 Phototoxic Dermatitis

Oppenheim first described dermatitis bullosa striata pratensis or meadow dermatitis in 1926 [29, 30]. The condition develops only under particular circumstances. The individual, having been out in the sun for some time, with areas of bare skin and having been sunbathing on damp grassy vegetation, notices the appearance, over several hours, of pruriginous erythemato-bullous rash in a distribution pattern mimicking the shape of the grass or the veins of leaves (Fig. 14.8.6). Damp vegetation may be replaced by atmospheric humidity or perspiration. The linear, figurate and vesiculo-bullous nature of the lesions on sun-exposed skin leads one to suspect the phototoxic nature of the dermatosis. Healing occurs after a variable period and is accompainied by postinflammatory hyperpigmentation. The so-called strimmer rash [31, 32] appears to be a variant of this condition, having a diffuse rather than striated or figurate presentation: a strimmer (string *timmer*) is an ingenious hand-held device for cutting vegetation with a mechanically whirled string (now nylon or plastic).

Meadow dermatitis and associated conditions are commonly ascribed to contact with members of the plant family Umbelliferae which grow in grassy meadows; in Europe in late summer these plants are in fact a common cause of bullous dermatitis, which may present in a wide variety of circumstances. For example, Quadripur and Gründer [33] described Oppenheim's dermatitis in 58 soldiers on exercise in open country whilst Campbell et al. [34] almost mistook extensive linear and blistering skin lesions on the back of an 8-year-old girl for signs of whipping by her father.

Another form of phototoxic contact dermatitis has been described under the name of berloque dermatitis. This is induced by some perfumes or cosmetics, in particular those such as the classic eau-de-Cologne which contain oil of bergamot. Berloque dermatitis normally begins with erythema at the site where perfume runs down the skin and is irradiated by the sun. Again, this is normally followed by postinflammatory hyperpigmentation which may last many months. Mitchell and Rook [35] provide an extensive review of this subject.

These phototoxic dermatoses are apparently caused by furocoumarins (synonym, psoralens) which are present in the implicated plants. They cause exaggeration of the burning potential of sunlight or artificial ultraviolet light. Pathak et al. [36] provide a detailed review of the various psoralen-containing plants: they have a limited distribution in the plant kingdom, the most important sources being the Leguminosae, Moraceae, Rutaceae and Umbelliferae. Figure 14.8.7 gives the structures of psoralen, the most active naturally occurring furocoumarin, and the related xanthotoxin and bergapten. It should also be noted that Kitchevatz [37] provided evidence that chlorophyll itself, when irradiated on the skin, could produce the lesions of meadow dermatitis.

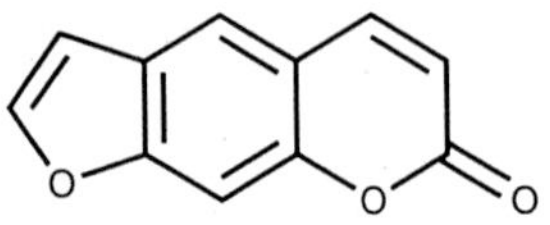

Psoralen 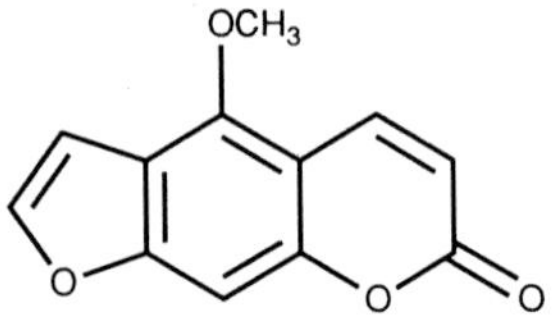   Bergapten (5-Methoxypsoralen; 5-MOP)

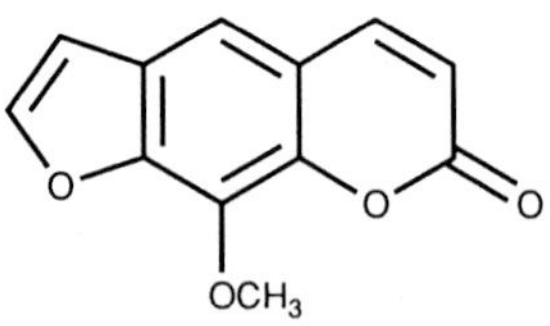

Xanthotoxin (8-Methoxypsoralen; 8-MOP)

Fig. 14.8.7. Furocoumarins (psoralens) with phototoxic properties

14.8.2.3.2 Photoallergic Dermatitis

Plant- or plant-product-induced photoallergic dermatitis occurs only very rarely. Perhaps the only well-authenticated cases are a reaction to *Parthenium hysterophorus* L. (family Compositae) described by Bhutani and Rao [38] and photoallergy to psoralens described by Ljunggren [39]. However, experimentally induced photoallergy to psoralens and to other coumarins known to occur naturally has been described [39, 40]. It is difficult to differentiate between a photoaggravated contact dermatitis and a true photoallergy. Photoaggravation of an allergic contact dermatitis is a more likely diagnosis than true photoallergy when plant material is implicated as the cause of a photosensitivity reaction of the skin, as has been demonstrated in a study by Thune and Solberg [13] in lichen pickers with a history of photosensitivity. A rather different relationship between contact allergy and photosensitivity is seen in the photosensitivity dermatitis and actinic reticuloid syndrome, as described by Frain-Bell and Johnson [41] in which allergic (but not photoallergic) contact sensitivity to oleoresins from members of the plant family Compositae is seen in patients with a marked photosensitivity that expresses itself even in the absence of exposure to the plant material. In this disease, it appears that an initial contact sensitization progresses to a generalized photosensitivity state (see Sect. 2.4.6).

14.8.3 Dermatologically Important Plants

It is not possible to consider here the total panorama of plants liable to evoke contact dermatitis, but those most often incriminated are described below.

14.8.3.1 Alliaceae

Members of the genus Alliaceae are widely grown and used for culinary purposes. In addition, garlic (*Allium sativum* L.) has both a contemporary and a long folkloric history of use as a medicinal agent.

Whilst the lachrymatory properties of onions (*Allium cepa* L.) are widely appreciated, they are rarely discussed in the medical literature. Most commonly reported are occupational dermatoses from garlic and to a lesser extent from onion; these include both immediate and delayed reactions [16, 42–47]. A typical presentation is a circumscribed irritable hyperkeratotic eczema on the fingers of one or both hands, sometimes the thumb, index and middle fingers of the left hand, which may be used to grasp the garlic bulb whilst the knife is held in the right hand [48, 49]. Less distinct patterns of eczema have been reported by Edelstein [50] and Inman [51]; sensitization can be found more frequently than the 'typical' distribution described above.

Garlic and other *Allium* species have often been reported to have both irritant and allergenic properties; the irritancy of the plants and of extracts prepared from them makes patch testing a little difficult, and this has led to a variety of suggestions for the preparation of extracts suitable for patch testing. The situation is further complicated by the fact that the phytochemicals responsible for the irritancy and allergenicity are not present in undamaged plant material but are released as a response to damage. Although never studied in detail, each different extraction procedure undoubtedly affects the manner in which the irritants/allergens are released in a different way, making it virtually impossible to produce a standard extract. For all these reasons, case reports in which plant extracts or plant material 'as is' are used in patch testing have to be interpreted with some caution. Mitchell [52] discussed some of the problems in patch testing with garlic.

Cross-reactions between garlic and onion have occasionally been described but are inconstant and unreliable because of the frequent occurrence of irritancy. Furthermore, concomitant sensitivity to both garlic and onion cannot easily be ruled out.

The irritant and allergenic compounds in garlic and onion are derived from a variety of sulphur-containing amino acids present in the intact plants. Although the disproportionation reactions in both onion and garlic are essentially similar, a minor structural difference between the principal precursor compounds results in the formation of lachrymatory thiopropanal-*S*-oxide from onion but allicin and diallyldisulphide from garlic [53]. These reactions are shown in Fig. 14.8.8. Papageorgiou et al. [54] identified diallyldisulphide, allylpropyldisulphide and allicin as the principal low molecular weight allergens of garlic. Diallyldisulphide 5% pet. [47] seems to be a suitable preparation for the investigation of garlic dermatitis, though 1% pet. may have less risk of irritancy.

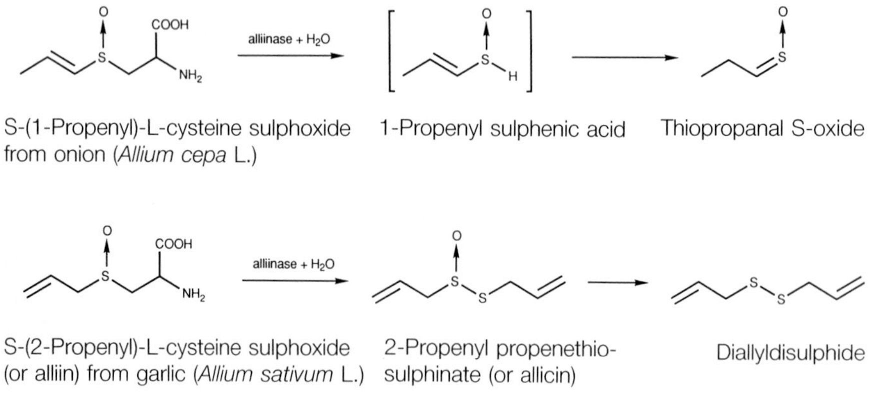

S-(1-Propenyl)-L-cysteine sulphoxide   1-Propenyl sulphenic acid   Thiopropanal S-oxide
from onion (*Allium cepa* L.)

S-(2-Propenyl)-L-cysteine sulphoxide   2-Propenyl propenethio-   Diallyldisulphide
(or alliin) from garlic (*Allium sativum* L.)   sulphinate (or allicin)

Fig. 14.8.8. Formation of volatile irritants and allergens from sulphur-containing amino acids in onions and garlic

14.8.3.2 *Alstroemeriaceae* and *Liliaceae*

These two families are considered together because members of the genera *Alstroemeria* and *Bomarea* (family Alstroemeriaceae) and of *Tulipa* (family Liliaceae) release the allergen tulipalin A when plant material is damaged [55–57]. Tulipalin A, otherwise known as α-methylene-γ-butyrolactone, is released from a glucoside precursor known as tuliposide A. Hausen et al. [58] believe the precursor to be 1-tuliposide A, but Santucci et al. [59] reported that in *Alstroemeria ligtu* L. only 6-tuliposide A can be detected (Fig. 14.8.9). There is evidence that the tuliposide itself can elicit allergic contact dermatitis [56, 59], but this may be the outcome of some spontaneous degradation to tulipalin A on the skin [60]. Tulips contain a second glucoside, tuliposide B [61]. Patients sensitive to tulip reportedly do not react to either tuliposide B or tulipalin B. However, Barbier and Benezra [62] have shown that tulipalin B (β-hydroxy-α-methylene-γ-butyrolactone) is a sensitizer in guinea pigs, and that cross-reactivity between tulipalins A and B does occur.

Garden tulips are available both as 'species tulips' and as cultivars of hybrid origin. Dermatitis among bulb handlers and florists is an important and common occupational hazard. It seems certain that both irritant and allergic contact dermatitis occurs. Bulb collectors, sorters and packers develop a characteristic dermatitis called tulip fingers (see also Sect. 14.8.2.2.2), a painful dry fissured hyperkeratotic eczema, at first underneath the true margin

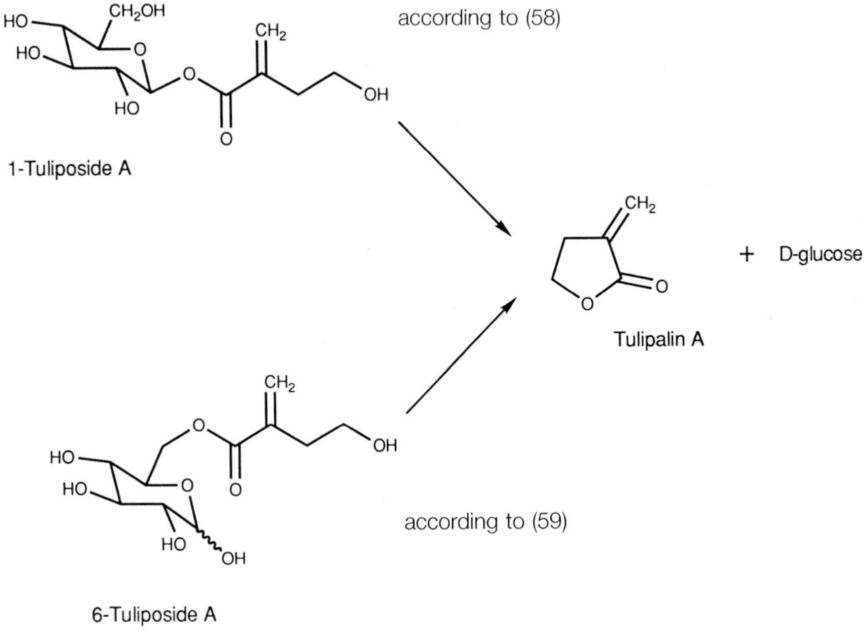

Fig. 14.8.9. Formation of the allergenic tulipalin A from a glycosidic precursor

of the nails, spreading to the periungual regions, fingers and hands [63]. Sometimes an irritable dermatitis spreads to the face, foreams and genital region. Tulip fingers is common in the Netherlands and other parts of Europe. The allergen is found mainly in the epidermis of the bulb, but contact dermatitis is possible also from handling cut-flowers.

Alstroemeria hybrids are popular in the cut-flower trade. Horticulturalists and florists are at risk of both irritant and allergic contact dermatitis. Handling of cut-flowers provokes a dermatitis affecting mainly the fingertips, which is similar to tulip fingers [64–66]. Depigmentation may follow the resolution of alstroemeria dermatitis [67]; patch tests with alstroemeria can also lead to depigmentation.

In the preparation of plant material for patch testing, it should be remembered that the various cultivars of *Alstroemeria* and *Tulipa* do not necessarily contain similar levels of tuliposide A. *Tulipa* cv Rose Copeland, for example, is said to be a notorious sensitizer [68] whereas *Tulipa fosteriana* Hoog cv Red Emperor has been found to contain very much less tuliposide than other cultivars [56]. For patch testing, Hjorth and Wilkinson [63] recommended either a filtered 96% ethanol extract of the bulb of *Tulipa* cv Apeldoorn or an 80% acetone extract of the bulbs diluted with 70% ethanol immediately prior to use. Hausen et al. [58] found that short ether extracts of alstroemerias were so rich in tulipalin A that they carried the risk of active sensitization. They preferred to use a tuliposide-rich methanolic extract incorporated into petrolatum. Santucci et al. [59] found that 50-μl applications of 6-tuliposide A at 0.01% and α-methylene-γ-butyrolactone at 0.001% in ethanol gave positive patch test reactions in alstroemeria-sensitive patients.

14.8.3.3 Amaryllidaceae

The Amaryllidaceae family comprises some 1100 species of plant in 85 genera, many of which are cultivated for their showy flowers. Amongst these, daffodils, narcissi, and jonquils (*Narcissus* spp. and cultivars) constitute a significant dermatological hazard because of their irritant and allergenic properties. An important bulb and cut-flower industry exists in the Netherlands and the Isles of Scilly, and with it the occupational diseases known as daffodil itch or lily rash [63, 68].

The rash has long been ascribed in part to the calcium oxalate needle crystals present both in the dry outer scales of the bulbs and in the sap exuding from cut flower stems [59]. Klaschka et al. [70] recognized that the dermatitis from *Narcissus* is probably always caused in part by an allergic mechanism and in part by irritant effects. Recently, Gude et al. [9] have identified two allergenic alkaloids from *N. pseudonarcissus* L., namely masonin and homolycorin (Fig. 14.8.10), but considered that irritancy caused by any of a number of other alkaloids also present in the plant was at least as important in the aetiology of the lily rash.

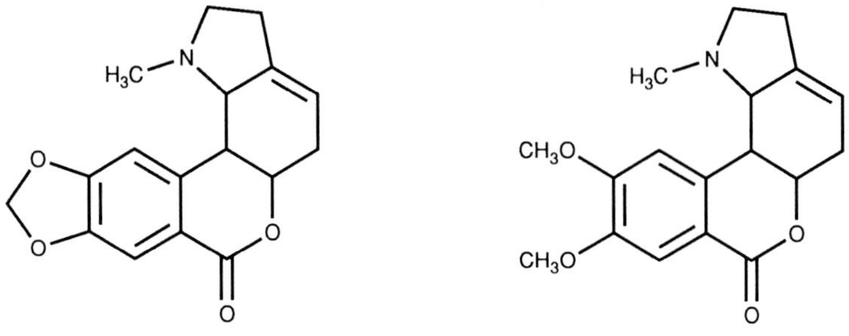

Masonin   Homolycorin

Fig. 14.8.10. Allergenic alkaloids from daffodils (*Narcissus pseudonarcissus* L.)

14.8.3.4 Anacardiaceae, Ginkgoaceae and Proteaceae

These plant families are considered together because they contain similar contact allergens and hence evoke similar dermatoses. Nevertheless, the clinical picture may vary depending upon the precise mode of contact.

The Anacardiaceae family includes some 600 species in its 60 genera and is considered by Mitchell and Rook [15] to cause more dermatitis than all other plant families combined. Some tropical species are of economic importance: *Mangifera indica* L. provides mangoes; *Anacardium occidentale* L. yields cashew nuts and also cashew nut shell oil which is used in the manufacture of brake linings; *Semecarpus anacardium* L.f. is the Indian marking nut tree, from which an indelible marking ink may be prepared; *Toxicodendron vernicifluum* F. Barkley is the Japanese lacquer tree. Although these and many other species in the Anacardiaceae are dermatologically hazardous, perhaps the most important genus is *Toxicodendron,* which includes the poison ivies, oaks, and sumacs of North America and elsewhere. According to Kligman [71] over half the population of the United States is sensitive to poison ivy and its relatives. In contrast, because the plants are not a part of the natural flora, poison ivy dermatitis is virtually unknown in Europe [72].

Early literature refers to poison ivy and its relatives as species of *Rhus.* Gillis [73] discussed the relationships between *Rhus* and the related genus *Toxicodendron* and concluded that these plants were more appropriately classified as species and subspecies of *Toxicodendron.* This distinction was made on morphological grounds, but there appears also to be a phytochemical distinction, since none of the remaining *Rhus* species is a significant dermatological hazard. [However, Ippen [72] has observed a case of a woman who had become sensitized to poison ivy or poison oak (*Toxicodendron* spp.) whilst in the United States and subsequently showed apparent cross-reactions to *Rhus copallina* L., *R. semialata* Murray (syn. *R. javanica* L.), and *R. trichocarpa* Miq.] Not unexpectedly, there is a good deal of nomenclatural confusion in the dermatological literature, especially with regards to the multitude of synonyms that exist. The Appendix provides an extensive list of correct names and their synonyms in an attempt to clarify the situation. (It should recognized that even these 'correct' names are not immutable and could again change in the future as new information emerges.)

Few if any dermatological reports referring to individual subspecies of *Toxicodendron* have appeared in the literature, largely because case reports of poison ivy dermatitis hardly warrant publication, but also because of the problems involved in identifying the plants precisely as to sub-species. Guin et al. [90] and Guin and Beaman [91] provide maps showing the distribution of various *Toxicodendron* species and sub-species in the United States. Gillis [73] also provides this information.

Ginkgo biloba L., the ginkgo tree, is the sole representative of the family Ginkgoaceae and, being known from fossil records, is regarded as one of the world's oldest surviving tree species. Contact dermatitis from ginkgo tree fruit has been reported in localities in which female ginkgo trees grow, either through inadvertent contamination of the skin with the fruit pulp [92] or through collecting and using the nut within the fruit in cooking [93, 94] or in children through playing with the fallen fruit as marbles. Allergic reactions occur following contact only with the fruit pulp and not with the leaves [95].

The lesions consist of erythematous papules and vesicles, with swelling in more severe cases, usually affecting the face, forearms and thighs; the penis and scrotum may also be affected [96]. Stomatitis, cheilitis and proctitis following ingestion of ginkgo fruit was described by Becker and Skipworth [97], who recommended patch tests with fruit pulp 1% acet.

Sowers et al. [92] described cross-reaction between ginkgo fruit pulp and poison ivy, and also between ginkgo and cashew nut. This may be rationalized on the basis that similar alkylbenzene derivatives are found in all these plant species. Recently, however, Lepoittevin et al. [98] reported a study in guinea pigs in which no clear cross-reactions were observed between the ginkgolic acids found in *Ginkgo* fruits and urushiols from *Toxicodendron*.

In Australasia, members of the family Proteaceae are the cause of a poison-ivy-like dermatitis. The best known are probably *Grevillea robusta* Cunn., the silky or silver oak, and related *Grevillea* species and cultivars. Contact with the wild and cultivated plants, as well as with objects made from the wood, have been recorded [99–102].

The allergenic agents in all these members of the Anacardiaceae, Ginkgoaceae and Proteaceae are mono- or dihydroxybenzene derivatives, mostly with C_{15} or C_{17} alk(en)yl side chains. More specifically, they are alk(en)yl derivatives of phenol, catechol, resorcinol or salicylic acid. The alkenyl catechols are also known as urushiols; other trivial names such as cardanol, grevillol and anacardic acid have been applied to the alk(en)yl phenols, resorcinols and salicylic acids, respectively. A representative selection of these compounds is given in Fig. 14.8.11. Because of the fact that

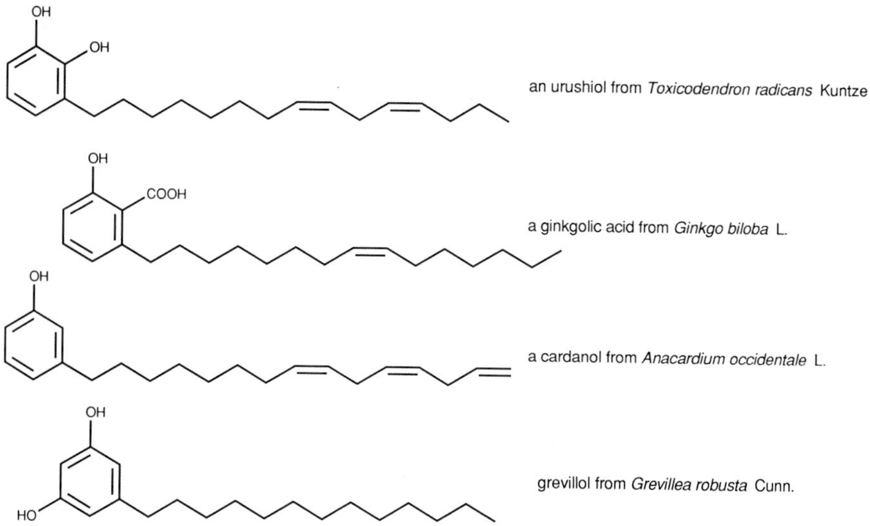

Fig. 14.8.11. Urushiols and related allergenic mono- and dihydroxyalk(en)ylbenzenes from the Anacardiaceae, Ginkgoaceae and Proteaceae

the allergenic material is invariably a mixture of closely related compounds, and because of the close similarity between individual compounds from a variety of botanical sources, there is the possibility of cross-sensitization between different species throughout the world [103].

14.8.3.5 Compositae (or Asteraceae) and Liverworts

This very large family, second only in size to the Orchidaceae, comprises some 13000 species (20000 according to some estimates) in over 900 genera. Representatives are found throughout the world, the majority being herbaceous plants.

The family provides a number of food plants: lettuce, endive, chicory, dandelion, salsify, scorzonera, artichoke, etc. Very many more are grown for their decorative flowers: chrysanthemums, dahlias, heleniums, etc. Others are widespread and common weeds. It is therefore difficult to avoid contact with these plants. Additionally, some species such as arnica, chamomile and feverfew are used medicinally, the first two by application to the skin.

The variety of Compositae-induced dermatoses reflects the variety of plants found in the family. This has been reviewed by Schmidt [14]. The most important dermatosis is the sesquiterpene-lactone-induced allergic contact dermatitis, but this can present in a number of different ways. Accidentally exposed subjects develop acute eczema. Continuous occupational exposure frequently leads to acute dermatitis, which often relapses and later becomes chronic and lichenified. When the dermatosis is localized to the elbow or knee flexures, it can simulate atopic dermatitis. The eczema, initially localized to the face, hands and genitals, can become generalized as an erythroderma, which can even be fatal [11]. Alternatively, exposure to the sesquiterpene lactones may occur through contact with airborne material – to produce a so-called airborne contact dermatitis.

In hot and dry regions of the United States or Australia, for example, the pulverized remains of dead plant material may become windborne and induce a dermatosis of exposed skin that can be mistaken for a photodermatitis [11]. In the United States, this is known as ragweed dermatitis [104] because it is largely caused by ragweeds, which are species of *Ambrosia*. An alternative name for the condition is weed dermatitis [105], this being used in regions where other composite weeds such as *Ambrosia, Artemisia, Helenium* and *Iva* species predominte. In Australia, the same condition is described as bush dermatitis [106]; the plants implicated are species of *Arctotheca, Conyza, Cynara* and *Dittrichia*. Yet another variant of the condition has in recent years spread through India. This has been termed parthenium dermatitis [107] after the offending plant (*Parthenium hysterophorus* L.).

The environmental conditions favouring ragweed dermatitis and its variants in hot and arid climates are not normally encountered in the temperate climate of Europe. Nevertheless, there are also European variants of ragweed dermatitis which have been described in rather specialized circumstances. The plants responsible include *Tanacetum parthenium* Schultz-Bip. [108, 109], *Cichorium intybus* L. [110], liverworts of the genus *Frullania* [12] and the chrysanthemums of florists [14].

Contact dermatitis from ragweed particularly affects male subjects and spares women and children [11], but the reason for this sex discrimination has not been determined.

The allergens are sesquiterpene lactones, a common feature of which is the presence of a γ-butyrolactone ring bearing an exocyclic α-methylene group, as originally noted by Mitchell and Dupuis [111]. A selection of typical structures is given in Fig. 14.8.12. Because the range of structures encountered among the known contact allergenic sesquiterpene lactones is very wide, and because each individual species contains a more or less complex mixture of these compounds, cross-sensitivity between various species in the Compositae is common but neither complete nor predictable. This unpredictability may be exemplified by the fact that individual cultivars of, for example, the autumn-flowering chrysanthemums (*Dendranthema* cultivars) do not necessarily cross-react [14, 112] whilst cross-reactions between members of the Compositae and liverworts of the genus *Frullania* (family Jubulaceae), laurel (*Laurus nobilis* L.) of the family Lauraceae, and various members of the family Magnoliaceae have been reported [12, 113–116].

A vast number of species in the Compositae have been described either as causes of contact dermatitis or as elicitors of positive patch test reactions. Many more may be regarded as potential contact allergens on the basis of

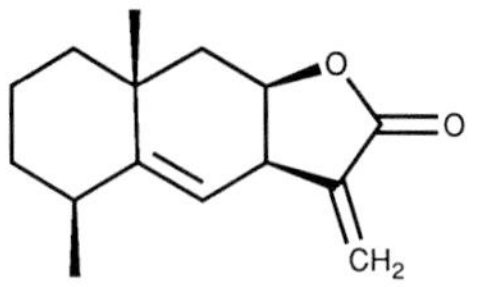

Alantolactone
from *Inula helenium* L.

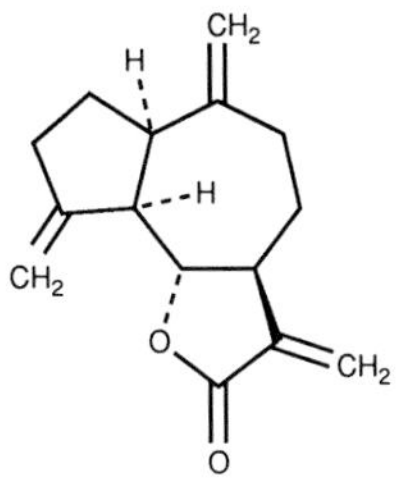

Dehydrocostus lactone
from *Saussurea lappa* C.B. Clarke

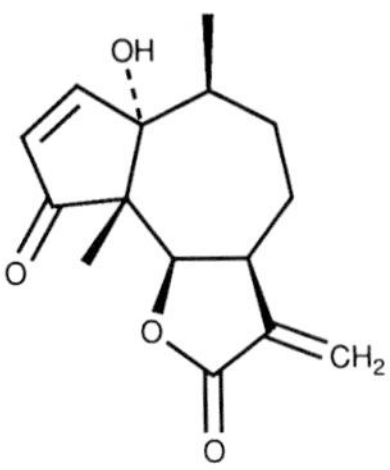

Parthenin
from *Parthenium hysterophorus* L.

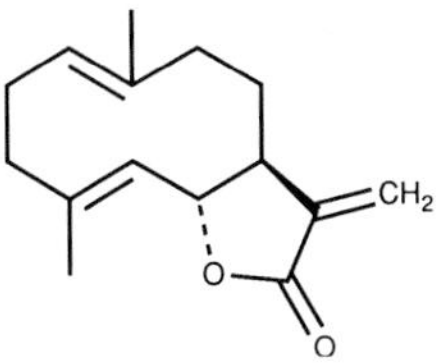

Costunolide
from *Saussurea lappa* C.B. Clarke

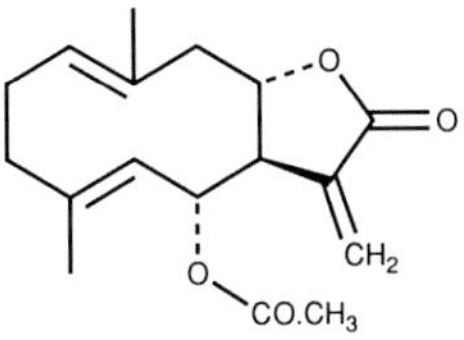

Laurenobiolide
from *Laurus nobilis* L.

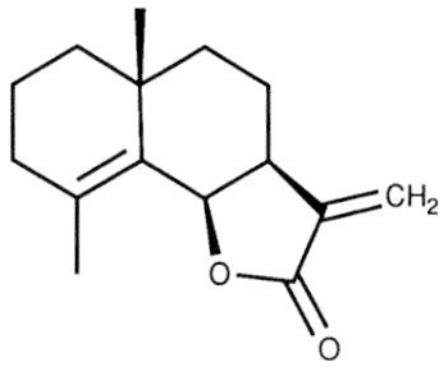

(−)-Frullanolide
from *Frullania tamarisci* Dum.

Fig. 14.8.12. Structures of some allergenic sesquiterpene lactones from Compositae, Lauraceae and liverworts

their reported content of sesquiterpene lactones bearing an α-methylene-γ-butyrolactone ring. The Allendix provides the common and botanical names of those species which may be regarded as the most likely causes of contact dermatitis.

Liverworts, together with mosses and hornworts, comprise a group of small, nonvascular plants known as bryophytes. Typically they grow in damp locations, although they can withstand periods of dessication. Of the liverworts, only a few species of *Frullania* have been described as causes of allergic contact dermatitis. These are found growing epiphytically on tree trunks, and hence have been recognized in areas of Canada (Vancouver Island, British Columbia), the United States (Oregon) and France (Bordeaux) as the cause of occupational contact dermatitis in forest workers and woodcutters [147]. *Frullania dilatata* Dum., *F. tamarisci* Dum. and *F. tamarisci* Dum. ssp. *nisquallensis* Hatt. are the most aggressive species. Instances of cross-sensitivity reactions between *Frullania* species and members of the Compositae are accounted for by the occurrence of structurally similar sesquiterpene lactones in the plants concerned [148] – *Frullania* species are a source of (+)- and (−)-frullanolide [149].

14.8.3.6 Cruciferae (or Brassicaceae)

This large family of about 3200 species in 375 genera, together with the smaller families Cleomaceae and Capparidaceae, characteristically contain compounds known as glucosinolates which, in many species, release mustard oils (isothiocyanates) when the plant material is damaged. These mustard oils impart a pungency to the plants that contributes to the value of many as food plants: cabbages, kale, cauliflower, brussels sprouts, broccoli, radish, mustard, cress, turnips, kohlrabi, etc. all belong to the Cruciferae [150].

The mustard oils are known to be irritant, and this has led to their use in folkloric medicine as counterirritants and in rubefacient ointments. Most commonly used for this purpose has been the oil from black mustard seed (*Brassica nigra* Koch), which is principally allyl isothiocyanate.

Notwithstanding the irritant properties of mustard oils and pharmaceutical preparations made therefrom, Coulter [151] noted that he had observed no irritant reactions following rough handling of members of the Cruciferae. Clinically, these plants are more commonly found to be responsible for allergic contact dermatitis in food handlers: Mitchell and Jordan [152] reported dermatitis of the fingers in a waitress who chopped radishes (*Raphanus sativus* L.); Leoni and Cogo [153] described occupational contact dermatitis from cabbage (*Brassica oleracea* L. var. *capitata* Alef.); and Sinha et al. [44] found that cabbage juice produced positive patch test reactions in 5 out of 53 patients with hand dermatitis suspected to have been caused by vegetables.

To avoid irritant reactions, patch test concentrations in the range 0.1%–0.05% pet. should be prepared [154, 155]. Allyl, phenyl and benzyl isothiocyanates are most commonly implicated as causes of allergic contact dermatitis. Patients sensitized to benzyl isothiocyanate appear not to cross-react to phenyl isothiocyanate [152, 156]. Methyl isothiocyanate [157] should be tested if plants belonging to the Capparidaceae are suspected as the cause of dermatitis. Positive patch test reactions to all four of these isothiocyanates have been reported in various circumstances.

Figure 14.8.13 shows the structures of methyl, allyl, phenyl and benzyl isothiocyanates and the process by which allyl isothiocyanate is produced from its glucosinolate precursor sinigrin [158], by the action of an enzyme named myrosinase, when the plant material is damaged.

14.8.3.7 Euphorbiaceae

The Euphorbiaceae comprises some 5000 species in about 300 genera which, with the exception of the polar regions, are found throughout the world. The largest and most widely distributed genus is *Euphorbia.* In Europe, euphorbias are small weeds known as spurges; tropical species are shrubs or trees, often resembling cacti in arid parts of Africa. They contain a latex which, in very many species, is a skin irritant. The irritant compounds are diterpene esters belonging to three general classes: the tiglianes, ingenanes and daphnanes. These irritant diterpenes are also found in other genera of the Euphorbiaceae and, interestingly, in the unrelated family Thymelaeaceae. Schmidt [159] and

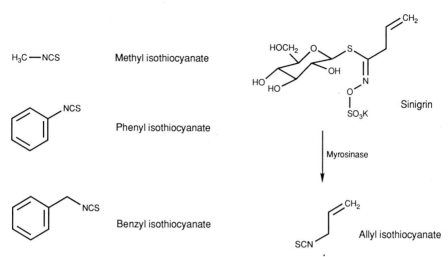

H_3C—NCS   Methyl isothiocyanate

NCS   Phenyl isothiocyanate

Sinigrin

Myrosinase

NCS   Benzyl isothiocyanate

Allyl isothiocyanate

Fig. 14.8.13. Structures of some irritant and allergenic mustard oils; formation of allyl isothiocyanate from sinigrin, its precursor glucosinolate

Webster [160] provide reviews of the distribution of these compounds in the two families; Evans [161] discusses their irritant properties in the context of their tumour-promoting and other biologically hazardous properties.

Clinically, cases of irritant contact dermatitis from members of the Euphorbiaceae and Thymelaeaceae are only rarely seen in Europe. It is likely that accidental skin contact occurs quite frequently but the irritant reaction resolves spontaneously within 1–2 days and is therefore unlikely to present in a dermatology clinic. Thus, whilst there is an extensive anecdotal literature supported by numerous scientific studies of the irritant compounds, clinical studies and case reports are rare: Satulsky and Wirts [162] described 60 cases of irritant contact dermatitis from the notorious manchineel tree (*Hippomane mancinella* L.) of tropical America; Rook [163] recorded a case of irritant contact dermatitis from *Synadenium grantii* Hook. f. in a gardener; Calnan [164] observed an irritant patch test reaction to the petty spurge (*Euphorbia peplus* L.), a garden weed presented by the patient as a house plant; Strobel et al. [165] described perioral dermatitis from *Euphorbia tirucalli* L., the pencil tree; Worobec et al. [166] described the irritant properties of *Euphorbia hermentiana* Lemaire (the friendship cactus), following the use of this plant by a bank as an inducement to open a savings account; Hickey et al. [167] examined the irritant properties of a number of tigliane, ingenane and daphnane polyol esters in humans; Pinedo et al. [168] described a case of an 8-year-old girl who developed irritation and swelling of the face and eyelids as a result of a fight in which she was beaten with *Euphorbia marginata* Pursh (snow-on-the-mountain) by a boy.

Elpern [169] noted that, in Hawaii in the period 1981–1982, contact dermatitis accounted for about 20% (305 cases) of all diagnoses in the dermatology clinic on Kauai. Of these, 61 cases were attributable to plant contact, for which mango (*Mangifera indica* L., family Anacardiaceae), the euphorbias and mokihana (*Pelea anisata* H. Mann, family Rutaceae) were most frequently blamed. Although he noted that mango evokes an allergic contact dermatitis, and mokihana a photoirritant dermatitis, the aetiology of the reactions to the euphorbias was not stated. It is possible therefore that he may have observed allergic reactions to euphorbias. Allergic rather than irritant contact dermatitis is well documented for two commonly grown ornamental plants belonging to the Euphorbiaceae: *Codiaeum variegatum* Blume var. *pictum* Muell. Arg. (the croton) and *Euphorbia pulcherrima* Willd. (the poinsettia) [170–174]. The allergens have not yet been characterized.

It should be remembered that the irritant properties of these plants are sometimes utilized in popular remedies, for example, for treating warts and basal cell carcinomas [175]. The potential for use of euphorbias to produce dermatitis artefacta should also be recognized.

The structures of representative irritants from the Euphorbiaceae and Thymelaeaceae are shown in Fig. 14.8.14. 12-Deoxyphorbol-13-phenylacetate, an example of a tigliane polyol ester, is found in *Euphorbia helioscopia* L., the common sun spurge [176]; resiniferatoxin, an example of a daphnane polyol ester and one of the most irritant compounds known to man, is found in *Euphorbia resinifera* Berg [177, 178]; 3-*O*-hexadecanoylingenol, an example of an ingenane polyol ester, is found in *Euphorbia lathyris* L.,

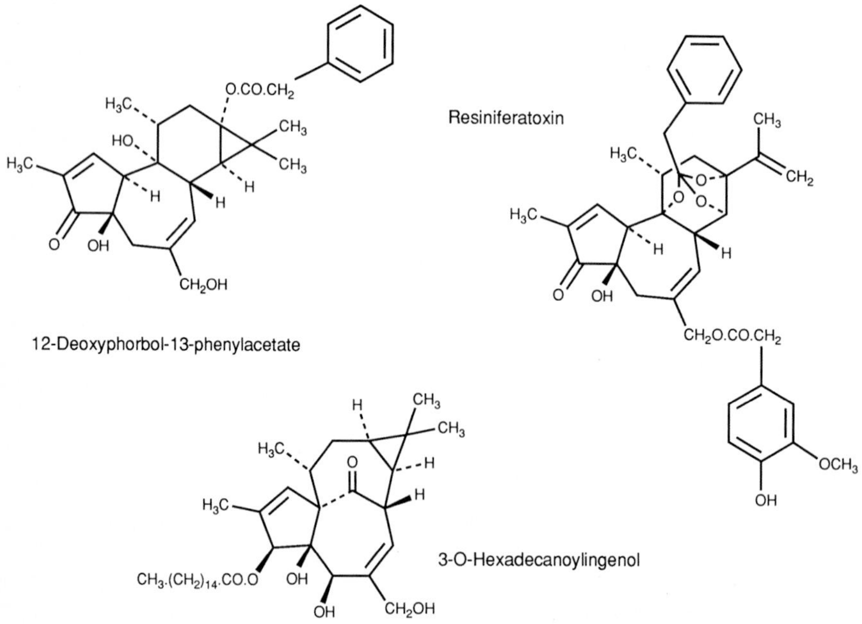

Fig. 14.8.14. Examples of irritant diterpene esters found in the Euphorbiaceae

the caper spurge [179]. Readers interested in a comprehensive survey of the occurrence of such compounds in the Euphorbiaceae and Thymelaeaceae are referred to [180–182].

14.8.3.8 Lichens

Lichens are rather interesting organisms, consisting of a fungus and an alga growing together in symbiosis. They are found growing on walls, roofs, trees, and rocks.

Several species are sensitizing. Those most often found as causes of contact dermatitis are species of *Parmelia, Evernia, Cladonia* and *Usnea.* Contact dermatitis usually affects forestry workers and lichen pickers, and appears on the hands, forearms, face and other exposed areas [183, 184]. Allergy to lichens may also be observed following exposure to perfumes containing oak moss, which is derived from *Evernia prunastri* Ach. and related species [185, 186]. A history of abnormal photosensitivity seems to predispose to lichen-induced contact allergy; irradiation of patch tests to lichens and their extracts may elicit enhanced responses [13, 187–190]. An airborne contact dermatitis simulating photodermatitis has also been suggested to contribute to the clinical features seen in patients with lichen allergy [13].

Champion [191] described immediate allergy (asthma and urticaria) following inhalation of, or direct contact with, algae from lichens.

Lichens can be tested 'as is' but irritant reactions may occur. Oak moss present in the fragrance mix of the European standard series is a mixture of *Evernia prunastris* Ach., *Pseudevernia fufuracea* Zopf., and *Parmelia furfuracea* Ach. Lechen-derived compounds such as atranorin, usnic acid, evernic acid, etc. can be tested at 0.1% or 1% pet. (Structures of some lichen-derived compounds are given in Fig. 14.8.15). Whether or not cross-sensitization between structurally related lichen compounds occurs is not clear. Concomitant sensitization is certainly possible, because of the common occurrence of some of the lichen compounds in a number of species [183, 184].

14.8.3.9 Primulaceae

Although a moderately large family of cosmopolitan distribution, only the primula (*Primula obconica* Hance) presents a significant dermatological hazard. (However, other species of *Primula* are also known to be able to sensitize [192]). *P. obconica* is popularly grown in Europe as a house and greenhouse plant for its showy and long-lasting flowers. For a number of years, this species was the most common cause of plant-induced contact dermatitis in Europe but has become less of a problem in recent years as its reputation has stimulated a widespread avoidance response. In the United Kingdom and elsewhere, this plant has reappeared for sale in department

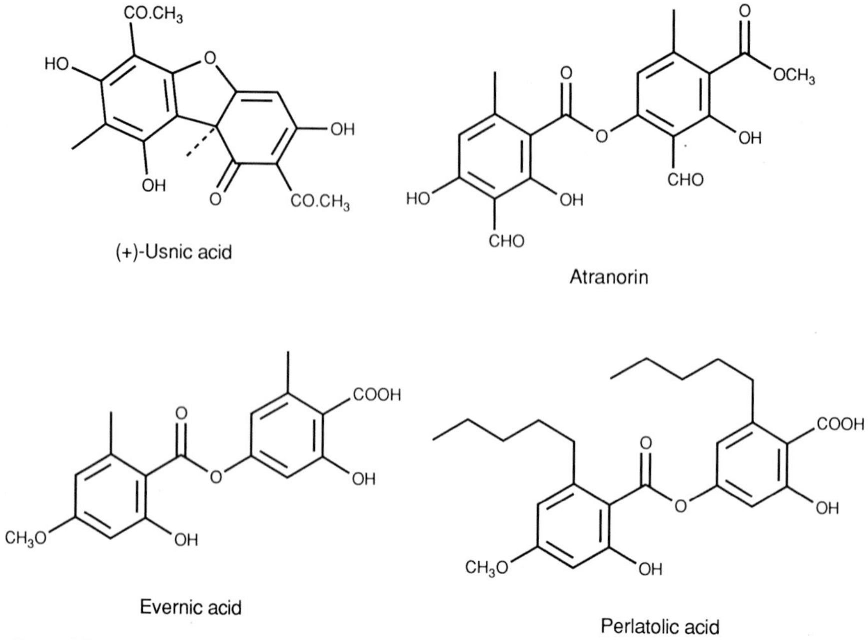

Fig. 14.8.15. Some allergenic lichen compounds

stores and garden centres, and it may be supposed that the incidence of primula dermatitis will rise again as a new generation of unsuspecting young adults becomes exposed.

Hundreds of literature reports pertaining to primula dermatitis have appeared since the first reports in the late nineteenth century. Similarly, a number of reviews have been published, to which readers are referred [193, 194].

The eyelids, face, neck, fingers, hands, and arms are most often affected (Figs. 14.8.16, 14.8.17). *P. obconica* can also cause conjunctivitis and an erythema-multiforme-like eruption.

The most important allergen of primula is primin (Fig. 14.8.18), a quinone [195]. The presence of another allergen has been suggested [194, 196]; this would appear to be the quinhydrone formed from primin and miconidin, its quinol derivative [193], although miconidin itself is surely allergenic.

Patch testing with the commercially available synthetic primin carries the real risk of active sensitization if concentrations greater than 1:10000 are used; a solution of 1:50000 is considered adequate for patch testing [197]. Because the content of primin in the leaves varies with the season, method of cultivation and cultivar identity [198, 199], the outcome of using fresh plant material 'as is' for patch testing varies from the occurrence of false negatives during the winter months [197] to active sensitization between the months of April to August, when primin levels are at their highest [199, 200]. Agrup

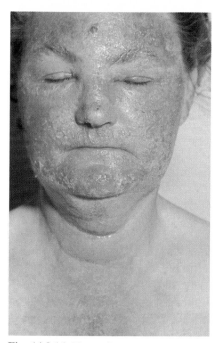

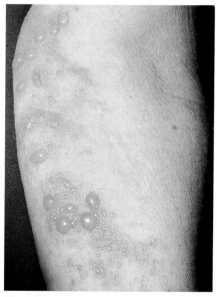

Fig. 14.8.17. Streaky and bullous primula dermatitison the forearm. (Courtesy of P.J. Forsch)

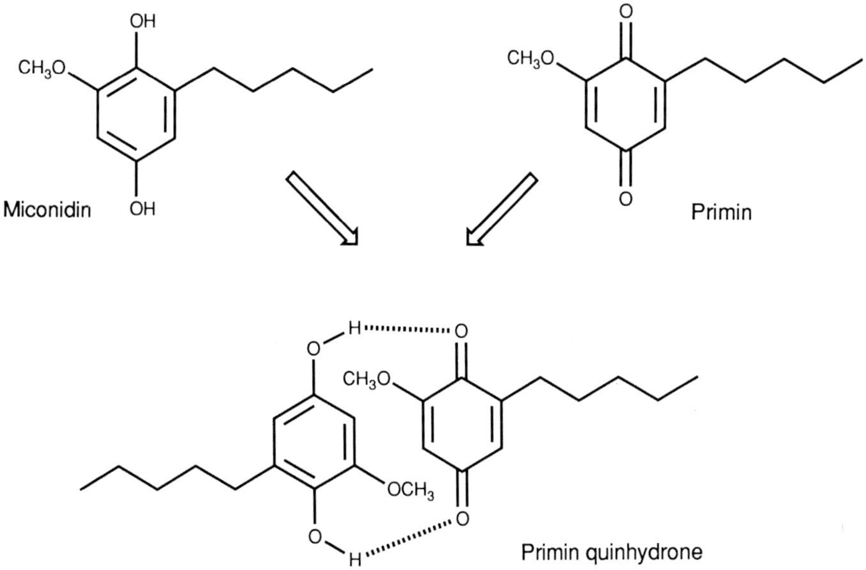

Fig. 14.8.16. Unusually severe exudative oedematousprimula dermatitis on the face. (Courtesy of N. Hjorth)

Miconidin

Primin

Primin quinhydrone

Fig. 14.8.18. Primin, the allergenic quinone of *Primula obconica* Hance

et al. [201] recommended the use of an ether extract of the levels harvested in spring (60 g fresh weight dipped in 100 ml ether before concentrating to 50 ml at room temperature).

14.8.3.10 Ranunculaceae

Many members of this family can cause irritation when crushed on the skin [202]. This has led to the use of poultices of the plants as counterirritants in traditional medicine for the treatment of rheumatic joints, etc., perhaps most commonly in eastern Europe. Overtreatment reactions may occasionally present in dermatology clinics [203–207].

The following plants are representative members of the Ranunculaceae that may be regarded as likely causes of irritant contact dermatitis: *Anemone nemorosa* L. (wood anemone); *Actaea spicata* L. (baneberry, herb Christopher); A. *alba* Miller (white baneberry); *Caltha palustris* L. (marsh marigold, kingcup); *Clematis vitalba* L. (traveller's joy, old man's beard); *Pulsatilla patens* Miller (synonym *Anemone patens* L.; prairie crocus); *P. vulgaris* Miller (synonym *Anemone pulsatilla* L.; Pasque flower); *Ranunculus acris* L. (synonym R. *acer* auct.; common meadow buttercup); *R. arvensis* L. (corn buttercup); *R. bulbosus* L. (bulbous buttercup); and *R. repens* L. (creeping buttercup).

The irritant agent is protoanemonin, which is released from its precursor compound ranunculin by simple enzymatic cleavage when the plant material

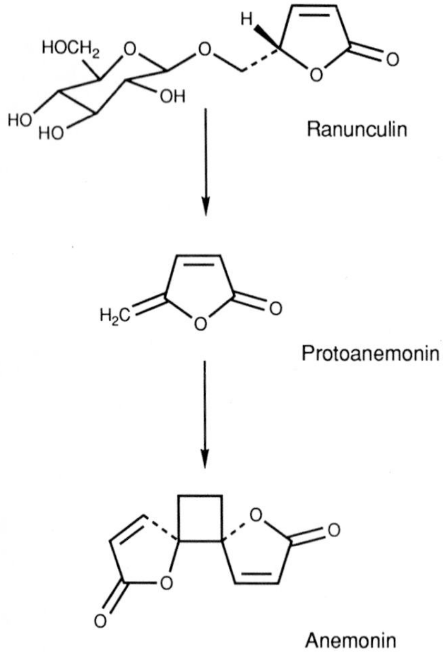

Ranunculin

Protoanemonin

Anemonin

Fig. 14.8.19. Formation of the irritant protoanemonin from ranunculin and its subsequent dimerization to the nonirritant anemonin

is damaged [208–211]. It rapidly loses its irritant properties by dimerizing to form anemonin (Fig. 14.8.19).

14.8.3.11 Umbelliferae, Rutaceae and Moraceae

Members of these families are most commonly encountered as causes of phototoxic contact dermatitis. The phototoxic agents are psoralens (see Sect. 14.8.2.3.1; Fig. 14.8.7). Children using the stems of hogweeds (*Heracleum mantegazzianum* Somm. and Lev. and *H. sphondylium* L.) as toy telescopes or peashooters in late summer typically develop bullous and erythematous lesions around the eyes and mouth [212, 213]; other exposed areas of skin may be affected if contact with the sap occurs during energetic play in stands of these plants, which are weeds of uncultivated land along roads, railways and streams [32].

Because several members of the Moraceae, Rutaceae and Umbelliferae are important sources of food (fig, citrus fruits, parsnip and celery), phototoxic reactions may occasionally be observed following occupational or nonoccupational contact on the hands and arms and around the mouth. Similarly, rue (*Ruta graveolens* L., family Umbelliferae), grown as a herb in gardens, may elicit phototoxic reactions following picking, as can perfumes containing bergamot oil (from *Citrus bergamia* Risso and Poit., family Rutaceae) following their application to sun-exposed skin. Table 14.8.1 provides a list of plants known to elicit phototoxic contact dermatitis ascribable to their psoralen content. The word psoralen actually derives from the name of the babchi plant (*Psoralea corylifolia* L., family Leguminosae), the seeds of which have a long history of use in the treatment of vitiligo.

Although allergic reactions to psoralens seem not to have been described, photoallergic reactions can occur [39, 40]. However, a number of psoralen-containing plants may also sensitize as a result of other compounds that they contain. For example, citrus oils are generally weakly allergenic but also irritant and some are phototoxic [241]. Similarly, carrots (*Daucus carota* L., family Umbelliferae) have sensitized workers in the canning industry [242–244], but there is no convincing evidence that they may elicit phototoxic reactions, although weak phototoxicity has been observed experimentally by van Dijk and Berrens [245]. Thus, if an allergic reaction is suspected, it is important to realize that irritancy and photoaggravation may occur during patch testing.

14.8.3.12 Woods

Although woods are not derived from a botanically homogeneous source, they may be considered together because of the special circumstances surrounding their exploitation as natural products.

Table 14.8.1. Some psoralen-containing plants known to elicit phototoxic contact dermatitis

Common name(s)	Botanical name	Synonym(s)	Reference to dermatitis
Leguminosae			
	Psoralea spp.		[214]
Moraceae			
Fig	*Ficus carica* L.		[215–218]
Rutaceae			
Lime	*Citrus aurantifolia* Swingle		[36, 219]
Bergamot orange	*Citrus bergamia* Risso and Poit.		[220, 221]
Sweet orange	*Citrus sinensis* Osbeck	*Citrus aurantium* L. var. *sinensis* L.	[222, 223]
Gas plant	*Dictamnus albus* L.	*Dictamnus fraxinella* Pers.	[36, 224, 225]
Mokihana	*Pelea anisata* H. Mann		[226, 227]
Blister bush	*Phebalium argenteum* Smith		[228]
	Ruta chalepensis L.	*Ruta bracteosa* DC.	[229]
Garden rue	*Ruta graveolens* L.		[230, 231]
Umbelliferae			
Bishop's weed	*Ammi majus* L.		[232]
Angelica	*Angelica archangelica* L.		[233, 234]
Celery	*Apium graveolens* L. var. *dulce* Pers.		[235–237]
Palm of Tromsø	*Heracleum stevenii* Manden.	*Heracleum laciniatum* Hornem.	[238]
Giant hogweed	*Heracleum mantegazzianum* Somm. and Lev.		[32, 213]
Hogweed	*Heracleum sphondylium* L.		[239]
Parsnip	*Pastinaca sativa* L.	*Peucedanum sativum* Benth. and Hook	[34, 224, 240]

Most dermatoses from contact with woods are occupational and are seen in carpenters, joiners, cabinet makers and in associated tradespersons. Less common are dermatoses in end-users of finished wood products, such as violin chin-rests, bracelets, knife handles, etc. (It should also be remembered that dermatoses following contact with liverworts and lichens growing on trees may be observed in forestry workers. These are considered in Sects. 14.8.3.5 and 14.8.3.8). The higher incidence of dermatitis in woodworkers than in end-users of wooden products is related to their exposure to airborne sawdust, which may drift inside loosely fitting protective clothing and adhere to sweaty areas of skin. Thus, dermatoses of the axillae, waistband, groin and ankles may be observed, in addition to those of the hands and arms, face and neck and of the scalp in bald men. The additional hazards of asthma, adenocarcinoma, and Hodgkin's disease associated with the inhalation of the sawdust of certain woods, as well as of systemic symptoms if the wood contains pharmacologically active constituents, have also been described by Hausen [246] and Willis [247].

A number of extensive reviews of wood-induced dermatoses have been published [246, 248–251], to which readers are referred for more detailed information.

The most common contact allergens found in woods are the quinones. Because of the wide occurrence of quinones such as 2,6-dimethoxy-1,4-benzoquinone, cross-sensitivity between woods may be expected to occur; indeed, in studies with guinea pigs, cross-reactivities between primin, deoxylapachol, various dalbergiones, mansonones, and other quinones have been observed [246]. Interestingly, cross-sensitivity between primin and various wood quinones does not seem to occur in humans [252]. In addition to quinonoid allergens, a number of other types of low molecular weight allergens have been identified from woods, reflecting the variety of botanical sources from which exploitable woods are obtained. Structures of some of the best-known wood allergens are given in Fig. 14.8.20.

The most highly sensitizing woods are of tropical and subtropical origin, but it should be realised that woods derived from trees growing in temperate regions have also been known to sensitize. Thus, Weber [253] reported dermatitis from alder (*Alnus* sp.), ash (*Fraxinus* sp.), beech (*Fagus* sp.), birch (*Betula* sp.) and poplar (*Populus* sp.) woods.

The most extensively grown and exploited trees in temperature regions are the pines (*Pinus* spp.), spruces (*Picea* spp.), firs (*Abies* spp.), and related conifers (family Pinaceae). These are only rarely implicated as causes of allergic contact dermatitis but are sources of oil of turpentine and of

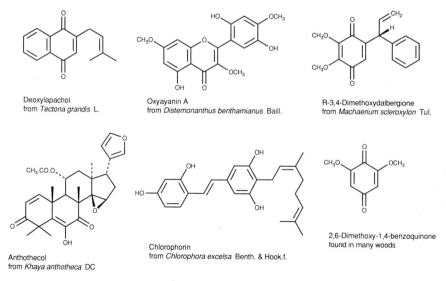

Deoxylapachol
from *Tectona grandis* L.

Oxyayanin A
from *Distemonanthus benthamianus* Baill.

R-3,4-Dimethoxydalbergione
from *Machaerium scleroxylon* Tul.

Anthothecol
from *Khaya anthotheca* DC

Chlorophorin
from *Chlorophora excelsa* Benth. & Hook.f.

2,6-Dimethoxy-1,4-benzoquinone
found in many woods

Fig. 14.8.20. Some allergenic compounds from tropical woods

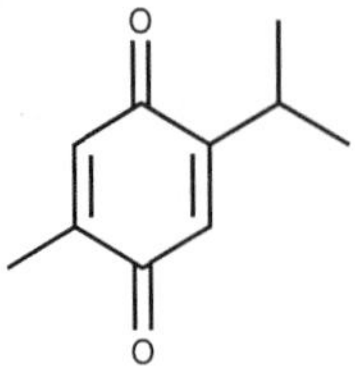

Thymoquinone
from *Calocedrus decurrens* Florin

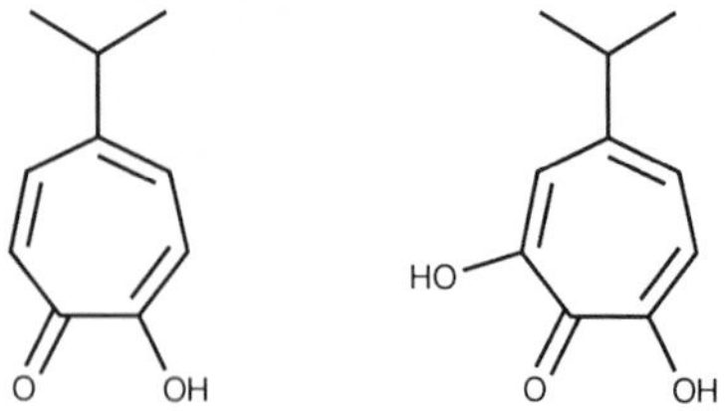

γ-Thujaplicin and 7-hydroxy-4-isopropyltropolone
from *Thuja plicata* D. Don

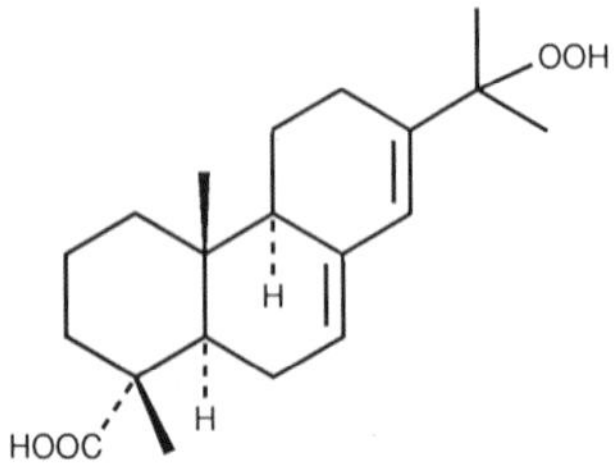

15-Hydroperoxyabietic acid
from colophony

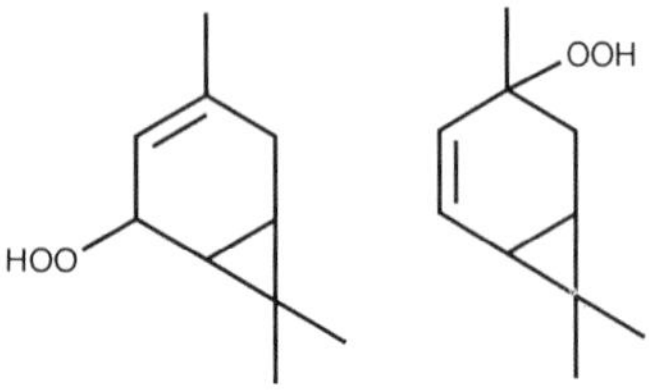

Δ3-Carene hydroperoxides
from turpentine oil

Fig. 14.8.21. Allergenic compounds from various conifers and from turpentine oil and colophony

colophony, both of which are well-known sensitizers. In both of these wood-derived products, the actual sensitizers are believed to be the hydroperoxidic air-oxidation products that are present together with the major constituents from which they are formed. Abietic acid, for example, has long been incriminated as the cause of colophony dermatitis, when, in fact, if rigorously purified, it appears to be neither a sensitizer nor an elicitor of colophony dermatitis – whereas 15-hydroperoxyabietic acid is a potent sensitizer [254, 255]. Similarly, hydroperoxides of $\triangle^3$-carene and not $\triangle^3$-carene itself are believed to be the allergens of oil of turpentine [256, 257]. The structures of these sensitizers are shown in Fig. 14.8.21. The quinonoid sensitizers from incense cedar and Western red cedar, two coniferous woods belonging to the family Cupressaceae (respectively, *Calocedrus decurrens* Florin and *Thuja Plicata* D. Don) are also shown.

Woods provide some rather significant problems with their identification. Most are transported under a trivial rather than botanical name, and it is not unusual for these trivial names to be misapplied either inadvertently or deliberately. It is imperative, if patch testing is to be meaningful, that a solid sample of a wood believed to be a cause of contact dermatitis (or any other pathological lesion) is sent to a wood anatomist for identification [246]. Its origin and any available trade names should also be made known to the wood anatomist. Once identified, patch testing with the freshly made sawdust, 10% pet., may be carried out on both the patient(s) and on several control subjects, because of the high incidence of irritancy [248]. When purified isolates from woods are available for patch testing, these may be prepared according to the recommendations of Hausen [250].

14.8.4 Diagnosis

Finding the source of a plant-induced contact dermatitis is often difficult. A provisional diagnosis may be made by questioning patients about their occupation, their hobbies, and their recent excursions during which plant contact may have occurred. It is often necessary to enlist the help of a botanist to identify plants brought in by patients. Certainly, if the results of an investigation of a plant-induced dermatosis are to be published, it is essential to identify the plant precisely. Whilst photographs of plants are helpful, they are usually less helpful than accurate drawings showing features that enable similar species to be distinguished one from another. There is no substitute for a botanist who is familiar with the taxonomic literature on the plant concerned, but just as there are specialties in the medical profession, no one botanist is an expert on all plants.

14.8.4.1 Patch Testing

14.8.4.1.1 Tests Using Plants

Once a plant has been incriminated and identified, reference to the literature should reveal whether or not it has a track record as an allergenic plant. It is helpful to consider not only the plant species itself but also its generic and familial identity. This is because the genetic information that groups plants into species, genera and families also determines to a large extent the nature of the so-called secondary plant metabolites. Thus, sesquiterpene lactones are a common feature of members of the family Compositae whilst mono- and dihydroxy alk(en)ylbenzenes are commonly found in members of the family Anacardiaceae. The phytochemical knowledge base of the plant kingdom is now so extensive that it is becoming increasingly unlikely that an unknown class of phytochemicals remains to be discovered as an inducer of allergic contact dermatitis.

If further investigation of the suspected plant-induced dermatosis is indicated, it is often possible to carry out tests with plant material 'as is' or with extemporaneously prepared extracts. Whilst a diagnosis of a plant-induced contact dermatitis can usually be established with a few grammes of fresh plant material, identification of the phytochemical(s) responsible requires either a supply of the purified sensitizers known to be present in the plant or a fairly laborious extraction, isolation, purification, and characterization procedure using, ideally, several kilogrammes of fresh plant material. It is important to use, whenever possible, the actual plant material (even the actual plant part) that is believed to be responsible for the contact dermatitis under investigation. This is because distinct chemical races may exist in outwardly identical plants, resulting in one specimen containing the allergen whilst the second does not. As noted in Sects. 14.8.3.2 and 14.8.3.5, cultivars of plants such as tulips and chrysanthemums are also known to exhibit varying propensities to induce and elicit allergic contact dermatitis. If an inappropriate sample of plant material is tested, the risk of a missed diagnosis clearly exists (although a positive patch test reaction may well be relevant, albeit fortuitously). Care should be taken with plants known to contain either irritant compounds (such as *Euphorbia* spp.) or highly allergenic compounds (such as primulas), where the past experiences of other dermatologists as reported in the literature should be heeded.

14.8.4.1.2 Plant Extracts

As a general rule, if the allergen is a low molecular weight secondary plant metabolite that is capable of penetrating intact skin, it is likely to be soluble in acetone, ethanol or ether. Thus, a filtered acetone or ethanol extract of dried plant material, or a 'short ether extract' of fresh material, usually produces a solution suitable for preliminary patch testing. It is not rational to produce water extracts of fresh plant material, although this is often carried out and often produces active extracts. However, a consideration of the possible complexities regarding the presence of more or less inactive precursor compounds releasing allergenic or irritant compounds when plant material is damaged (see Sects. 14.8.3.1, 14.8.3.2, 14.8.3.6, 14.8.3.10), shows that a 'rational' approach is not necessarily the best approach. If for no other reason, water extracts are not recommended because they cannot be stored for more than 1–2 days because they are susceptible to microbial and chemical degradation. Extracts in organic solvents are generally more stable, but even they should not be regarded as having an indefinite shelf life. Incorporating an evaporated extract into petrolatum represents a standard means of preparing material for patch testing, but it is questionable whether this extra manipulation of the extract confers any benefit over the application of a known volume of the extract onto a standard occlusive patch such as a Finn Chamber.

14.8.4.1.3 Available Allergens

Unfortunately, relatively few plant constituents are available commercially for patch testing (Hermal and Chemotechnique have lists of plant allergens). Those that are available should ideally be purified before use (if they have not already been incorporated into petrolatum) because they may be only of technical grade and hence contain perhaps 20% of unidentified impurities. Volatile oil constituents – the aromatic oils of plants – are notoriously unstable to air oxidation and are generally virtually impossible to purify (except through derivatization and resynthesis) if liquid at room temperature – but it should also be remembered that the air oxidation products themselves may in fact be the sensitizers.

There is an ongoing search to identify mixtures of compounds that can be used reliably to detect particular common types of plant- or plant-product-induced dermatoses. Thus, various authors have recommended mixtures to detect colophony allergy, sesquiterpene lactone allergy (see Sect. 10.5.3.1), lichen allergy, etc. It is likely that none of these mixtures will ever be regarded as an absolutely certain means of detecting the group allergy in question.

14.8.4.1.4 Photopatch Testing

Contact dermatitis from plants can closely simulate a photocontact dermatitis, but plant-induced photoallergy is actually very rare (see Sects. 14.8.2.3.2 and 14.8.3.8). Photoaggravation of patch test reactions may be indicative of an underlying acquired photosensitivity state that may or may not be causally associated with contact with the plant material being investigated (see Sect. 10.5.4).

14.8.4.1.5 Results and Relevance

Patch testing with numerous plants or extracts can cause an 'angry back'; each plant part or plant extract must then be tested again separately. The interpretation of patch test results must not overlook the possibility of irritant reactions or the possibility of contact urticaria, although both of these effects could subside before the first reading is made.

The validity and relevance of patch test results is often difficult to determine. Positive reactions to plant material applied 'as is' do not necessarily prove that the plant is responsible for the dermatosis being investigated – the reaction may have arisen from contamination of the plant material with pesticides or other agricultural/horticultural chemicals, or from fungal contamination. Another cause of false-positive reactions is the use of too high a concentration of an extract, whereby a subclinical sensitivity may be evoked. The possibility of active sensitization to the material being tested should also not be overlooked. False-negative reactions may arise if an inappropriate sample of plant material is tested (see Sect. 14.8.4.1.1), or if the extract contains an insufficient concentration of the allergen, perhaps as a result of using an aged extract. The relevance of positive test reactions can be difficult to determine because the patient may have handled several plants over a period of time and become sensitized to some or all. The phenomenon of cross-sensitization adds a further dimension to the problem of relevance.

14.8.4.1.6 Cross-sensitization

Cross-sensitization may arise when the patient is sensitized to a particular compound in one plant and then reacts to another plant containing the same compound; alternatively, a cross-reaction may occur if two different compounds are metabolized to the same ultimate hapten; or, if following sensitization to the primary allergen, the immune surveillance process misidentifies the second compound because of its structural similarity to the primary sensitizer. Thus, cross-reactions may occur to plants not previously encountered by the patient, as well as to isolates that are not actually present in the sensitizing plant. Clearly, cross-reactions are almost impossible to detect with certainty in man because the primary sensitizer cannot easily be determined.

14.8.5 Therapy

Therapy of acute contact dermatitis or chronic eczema is symptomatic. Fresh water can be used in compresses. Local or systemic corticosteroids are useful, but the risk of sensitization to the corticosteroid if used locally [258] should be considered. As soon as the plant responsible for contact dermatitis has been identified, steps should be taken to avoid further contact. If the plant is encountered in the workplace, the patient may have to consider a change of occupation. However, work practice and occupational hygiene measures should first be reviewed because of the employer's legal responsibility to provide a safe working environment (see Chap. 11).

Hyposensitization measures have been attempted with limited success when avoidance of contact is impracticable – such as with poison ivy in certain outdoor occupations. These have been reviewed by Watson [259]. Currently, there is no scientific basis behind this practice, and the risk of toxic side effects should be borne in mind. Induction of tolerance in naive subjects appears to be a more successful strategy than desensitization of those already sensitized [260].

14.8.6 Appendix Correct Names and Synonyms of Some Dermatologically Hazardous Members of the Anacardiaceae and Compositae

Common name(s)	Botanical name	Synonym(s)	Reference to dermatitis
Anacardiaceae			
Cashew nut tree, acajou	*Anacardium occidentale* L.		[74]
Christmas bush, poison ash	*Comocladia dodonaea* Urban	*Comocladia ilicifolia* Sw., *Ilex dodonaea* L.	[75]
	Gluta laccifera Ding Hou	*Melanorrhoea laccifera* Pierre	[76]
East coast rengas, ape-nut	*Gluta renghas* L.		[77]
Burmese lacquer tree, theetsee	*Gluta usitata* Ding Hou	*Melanorrhoea usitata* Wallich	[78]
	Holigarna ferruginea March		[79]
Litre, aroeira	*Lithraea caustica* Hook. and Arn.	*Lithraea venenosa* Miers	[80]
Mango	*Mangifera indica* L.		[81]
Poisonwood, coral sumac, Honduras walnut	*Metopium toxiferum* Krug and Urban	*Rhus metopium* L.	[82]
Indian marking nut tree, bhilawa	*Semecarpus anacardium* L.	*Anacardium orientale* auct.	[83]
Um-tovane, tovana, rainbow leaf	*Smodingium argutum* E. Meyer		[84]
Western poison oak	*Toxicodendron diversilobum* Greene	*Rhus diversiloba* Torrey and A. Gray, *Rhus toxicodendron* L. ssp. *diversiloba* Engl.	[85]
	T. radicans L. ssp. *barkleyi* Gillis	*Rhus villosum* Sessé and Mociõo	
	T. radicans L. ssp. *divaricatum* Gillis	*T. divaricatum* Greene, *Rhus divaricata* Greene	
	T. radicans L. ssp. *eximium* Gillis	*T. eximium* Greene, *Rhus eximia* Standley	
Taiwan tsuta-urushi	*T. radicans* L. ssp. *hispidum* Gillis	*Rhus toxicodendron* L. var. *hispida* Engl., *Rhus intermedia* Hayata	
	T. radicans L. ssp. *negundo* Gillis	*T. negundo* Greene, *T. aborigunum* Greene	
Tsuta-urushi	*T. radicans* L. ssp. *orientale* Gillis	*T. orientale* Greene, *Rhus orientalis* Schneider	
	T. radicans L. ssp. *pubens* Gillis	*Rhus toxicodendron* L. var. *pubens* Engelm.	
Poison ivy, poison vine, markweed	*T. radicans* L. ssp. *radicans*	*T. radicans* Kuntze, *Rhus radicans* L., *Rhus toxicodendron* L.	[86]
	T. radicans L. ssp. *verrucosum* Gillis	*T. verrucosum* Greene, *Rhus verrucosa* Scheele	
Rydberg's poison ivy	*T. rydbergii* Greene	*T. radicans* Kuntze var. *rydbergii* Erskine, *Rhus toxicodendron* L. var. *rydbergii* Garnett, *Rhus rydbergii* Small	

14.8.6 Appendix Continued

Common name(s)	Botanical name	Synonym(s)	Reference to dermatitis
Manzanillo, hinchador	*Toxicodendron striatum* Kuntze	*Rhus striata* Ruiz and Pavón, *Rhus juglandifolia* Wild.	[87]
Japanese wax tree	*Toxicodendron succedaneum* Kuntze	*Rhus succedanea* L.	[88]
Eastern poison oak, oak leaf ivy	*Toxicodendron toxicarium* Gillis	*T. quercifolium* Greene, *T. toxicodendron* L. Britten, *Rhus quercifolia* Steudel, *Rhus toxicodendron* L. var. *quercifolium* Michx., *Rhus toxicarium* Salisb.	[86]
Japanese lacquer tree	*Toxicodendron vernicifluum* F. Barkley	*Rhus verniciflua* Stokes, *Rhus vernicifera* DC.	[89]
Poison sumac, poison elder	*Toxicodendron vernix* Kuntze	*Rhus vernix* L., *Rhus venenata* DC.	[86]
Compositae			
Yarrow, nosebleed, milfoil, thousand leaf	*Achillea millefolium* L.	*Achillea lanulosa* Nutt.	[115, 117]
False ragweed	*Ambrosia acanthicarpa* Hook.	*Franseria acanthicarpa* Cov.	[104, 117]
Short ragweed, common ragweed	*Ambrosia artemisifolia* L.	*Ambrosia elatior* L.	[104, 117]
Western ragweed, perennial ragweed	*Ambrosia psilostachya* DC.		[118]
Giant ragweed, tall ragweed	*Ambrosia trifida* L.	*Ambrosia aptera* DC.	[119]
Corn chamomile	*Anthemis arvensis* L.		[120]
Stinking mayweed, dog chamomile	*Anthemis cotula* L.	*Maruta cotula* DC.	[121]
Capeweed	*Arctotheca calendula* Levyns	*Arctotis calendulacea* L.	[106, 122]
Arnica, mountain tobacco, wolf's bane	*Arnica montana* L.		[123]
Prairie sage	*Artemisia ludoviciana* Nutt. ssp. *typica* Keck	*Artemisia ludoviciana* Nutt.	[18, 124–126]
Common mugwort	*Artemisia vulgaris* L.		
Australian dogwood	*Cassinia aculeata* R.Br.		
Roman chamomile, dog fennel	*Chamaemelum nobile* All.	*Anthemis nobilis* L.	[121, 127]
Endive	*Cichorium endivia* L.		[128]

Common name	Scientific name	References
Chicory	*Cichorium intybus* L.	[128, 129]
Fleabane	*Conyza bonariensis* Cronq. *Erigeron bonariensis* L.	[122, 130]
Wild artichoke, cardoon	*Cynara cardunculus* L.	[106]
Globe artichoke	*Cynara scolymus* L.	[106]
Dahlia	Dahlia cultivars	[131, 132]
Autumn flowering chrysanthemum	Dendranthema cultivars *Chrysanthemum x hortorum* W. Miller, *Chrysanthemum morifolium* Ramat.	[125, 133–135]
Stinkwort	*Dittrichia graveolens* Greuter *Inula graveolens* Desf., *Erigeron graveolens* L.	[106, 122]
Showy gaillardia	*Gaillardia pulchella* Foug. *Gaillardia picta* Sweet	[105]
Sneezeweed, false sunflower	*Helenium autumnale* L.	[136]
Sneezeweed, bitterweed	*Helenium amarum* H. Rock *Helenium tenuifolium* Nutt., *Gaillardia amara* Raf.	[105, 137–140]
Sunflower	*Helianthus annuus* L.	
Elecampane, scabwort	*Inula helenium* L.	[105]
Narrow-leaf marshelder	*Iva angustifolia* Nutt.	[118, 124, 136]
Marshelder	*Iva xanthifolia* Nutt.	[128, 129]
Lettuce	*Lactuca sativa* L.	[115, 136]
Marguerite, ox-eye daisy	*Leucanthemum vulgare* Lam. *Tanacetum leucanthemum* Schultz-Bip., *Chrysanthemum leucanthemum* L.	
German chamomile, wild chamomile	*Matricaria chamomilla* L. var. *recutita* Grierson *Matricaria Chamomilla* L., *Matricaria recutita* L., *Chamomilla recutita* Rauschert	[121]
Guayule	*Parthenium argentatum* A. Gray	[141]
Feverfew, congress grass, whitetop	*Parthenium hysterophorus* L.	[107]
Costus	*Saussurea lappa* C.B. Clarke *Saussurea costus* Lipsch.	[140, 142]
Small-flowered marigold, stinking roger	*Tagetes minuta* L. *Tagetes glandulifera* Schrank	[143]
Pyrethrum	*Tanacetum cinerariifolium* Schultz-Bip. *Chrysanthemum cinerariifolium* Vis., *Pyrethrum cinerariifolium* Trevir.	[144]
Feverfew	*Tanacetum parthenium* Schultz-Bip. *Chrysanthemum parthenium* Bernh., *Matricaria parthenium* L.	[108, 115]
Tansy	*Tanacetum vulgare* L.	[127]
Dandelion	*Taraxacum officinale* Weber	[145]
Cocklebur, spiny clotbur	*Xanthium spinosum* L.	[106]
Noogoora Burr	*Xanthium strumarium* L.	[117, 146]
Californian Burr	*Xanthium strumarium* L. ssp. *italicum* D. Löve *Xanthium californicum* Greene, *Xanthium italicum* Moretti	[106]

624   Georges Ducombs and Richard J. Schmidt

14.8.7 References

1. Mitchell J, Rook A (1979) Botanical dermatology. Greengrass, Vancouver, pp 26–39
2. Evans FJ, Schmidt RJ (1980) Plants and plant products that induce contact dermatitis. Planta Med 38: 289–316
3. Fregert S (1975) Occupational dermatitis in 10-year material. Contact Dermatitis 1: 96–107
4. Karpman RR, Spark RP, Fried M (1980) Cactus thorn injuries to the extremities: their management and etiology. Ariz Med 37: 849–851
5. Shanon J, Sagher F (1956) Sabra dermatitis. An occupational dermatitis due to prickly pear handling simulating scabies. Arch Dermatol 74: 269–275
6. Snyder DS, Harfield GM, Lampe KF (1979) Examination of the itch response from the raphides of the fishtail palm *Caryota mitis.* Toxicol Appl Pharmacol 48: 287–292
7. Morton JF (1972) Cocoyams (*Xanthosoma caracu, X. atrovirens* and *X. nigrum*), ancient root- and leaf-vegetables, gaining in economic importance. Proc F1 State Hortic Soc 85: 85–94
8. Walter WG, Khanna PN (1972) Chemistry of the aroids. I. *Dieffenbachia sequine, amoena,* and *picta.* Econ Bot 26: 364–372
9. Gude M, Hausen BM, Heitsch H, König WA (1988) An investigation of the irritant and allergenic properties of daffodils (*Narcissus pseudonarcissus* L., Amaryllidaceae). A review of daffodil dermatitis. Contact Dermatitis 19: 1–10
10. Hjorth N, Roed-Peterson J, Thomsen K (1976) Airborne contact dermatitis from Compositae oleoresins simulating photodermatitis. Br J Dermatol 95: 613–620
11. Arlette J, Mitchell JC (1981) Compositae dermatitis. Current aspects. Contact Dermatitis 7: 129–136
12. Foussereau J, Muller JC, Benezra C (1975) Contact allergy to *Frullania* and *Laurus nobilis:* cross-sensitization and chemical structure of allergens. Contact Dermatitis 1: 223–230
13. Thune PO, Solberg YJ (1980) Photosensitivity and allergy to aromatic lichen acids, Compositae oleoresins and other plant substances. Contact Dermatitis 6: 64–71, 81–87
14. Schmidt RJ (1986) Compositae. Clin Dermatol 4: 46–61
15. Mitchell J, Rook A (1979) Botanical dermatology. Greengrass, Vancouver, pp 63–97
16. Hjorth N, Roed-Petersen J (1976) Occupational protein contact dermatitis in food handlers. Contact Dermatitis 2: 28–42
17. Hannuksela M, Lahti A (1977) Immediate reactions to fruits and vegetables. Contact Dermatitis 3: 79–84
18. Kaupinnen K, Kousa M, Reunala T (1980) Aromatic plants-a cause of severe attacks of angio-edema and urtucaria. Contact Dermatitis 6: 251–254
19. Veien NK, Hattel T, Justesen O, Nørholm A (1983) Causes of eczema in the food industry. Derm Beruf Umwelt 31: 84–86
20. Forsbeck M, Skog E (1977) Immediate reactions to patch tests with balsam of Peru. Contact Dermatitis 3: 201–205
21. Brøgger Christensen S, Norup E, Rasmussen U (1984) Chemistry and structure-activity relationship of the histamine secretagogue thapsigargin and related compounds. In: Krogsgaard-Larsen P, Brøgger Christensen S, Kofod H (eds) Natural products and drug development, Alfred Benzon Symposium 20. Munksgaard, Copenhagen, pp 405–418
22. Norup E, Smitt UW, Brøgger Christensen S (1986) The potencies of thapsigargin and analogues as activators of rat peritoneal mast cells. Planta Med 52: 251–255
23. Dooms-Goossens A, Deveylder H, Duron C, Dooms M, Degreef H (1986) Airborne contact urticaria due to cinchona. Contact Dermatitis 15: 258

24. Bonnevie P (1939) Ätiologie und Pathogenese der Ekzemkrankheiten. Barth, Leipzig
25. Holst R, Kirby J, Magnusson B (1976) Sensitisation to tropical woods giving erythema multiforme-like eruptions. Contact Dermatitis 2: 295–296
26. Martin P, Bergoend H, Piette F (1980) Erythema multiforme-like eruption from Brasilian rosewood. 5th international symposium on contact dermatitis, Barcelona
27. Irvine C, Reynolds A Finlay AY (1988) Erythema multiforme-like reaction to "rosewood". Contact Dermatitis 19: 224–225
28. Schwartz RS, Downham TF (1981) Erythema multiforme associated with *Rhus* contact dermatitis. Cutis 27: 85–86
29. Oppenheim M (1932) Dermatite bulleuse striée, consécutive aux bains de soleil dans les prés. (Dermatitis bullosa striata pratensis). Ann Dermatol Syphiligr 3 (1): 1–7
30. Kissmeyer A (1933) Dermatite bulleuse striée des prés. Bull Soc Fr Dermatol Syphiligr 40: 1486–1489
31. Freeman K, Hubbard HC, Warin AP (1984) Strimmer rash. Contact Dermatitis 10: 117–118
32. Ippen H (1984) Photodermatitis bullosa generalisata. Derm Beruf Umwelt 32: 134–137
33. Qadripur S-A, Gründer K (1975) Kasuistischer Beitrag über Gruppenerkrankung mit Photodermatitis bullosa striata pratensis (Oppenheim). Hautarzt 26: 495–497
34. Campbell AN, Cooper CE, Dahl MGC (1982) "Non-accidental injury" and wild parsnips. Br Med J 284: 708
35. Mitchell J, Rook A (1979) Botanical dermatology. Greengrass, Vancouver, 614–617
36. Pathak MA, Daniels F, Fitzpatrick TB (1962) The presently known distribution of furocoumarins (psoralens) in plants. J Invest Dermatol 39: 225–239
37. Kitchevatz M (1933) Photodermite actino-calorique chlorophyllienne. Note préliminaire. Bull Soc Fr Dermatol Syphiligr 40: 761–764
38. Bhutani LK, Rao DS (1978) Photocontact dermatitis caused by *Parthenium hysterophorus.* Dermatologica 157: 206–209
39. Ljunggren B (1977) Psoralen photoallergy caused by plant contact. Contact Dermatitis 3: 85–90
40. Kaidbey KH, Kligman AM (1981) Photosensitization by coumarin derivatives. Arch Dermatol 117: 258–263
41. Frain-Bell W, Johnson BE (1979) Contact allergic sensitivity to plants and the photosensitivity dermatitis and actinic reticuloid syndrome. Br J Dermatol 101: 503–512
42. Bleumink E, Doeglas HMG, Klokke AH, Nater JP (1972) Allergic contact dermatitis to garlic. Br J Dermatol 87: 6–9
43. Bleumink E, Nater JP (1973) Contact dermatitis to garlic: cross reactivity between garlic, onion, and tulip. Arch Dermatol Forsch 247: 117–124
44. Sinha SM, Pasricha JS, Sharma RC, Kandhari KC (1977) Vegetables responsible for contact dermatitis of the hands. Arch Dermatol 113: 776–779
45. van Ketel WG, de Haan P (1978) Occupational eczema from garlic and onion. Contact Dermatitis 4: 53–54
46. Campolmi P, Lombardi P, Lotti T et al. (1982) Immediate and delayed sensitization to garlic. Contact Dermatitis 8: 352–353
47. Cronin E (1987) Dermatitis of the hands in caterers. Contact Dermatitis 17: 265–269
48. Burks JW (1954) Classic aspects of onion and garlic dermatitis in housewives. Ann Allergy 12: 592–596
49. Borda JM, Bozolla C (1961) Queratosis de pulpejos de dedos por contacto de Liliáceas. Arch Argent Dermatol 11: 293–299
50. Edelstein AJ (1950) Dermatitis caused by garlic. Arch Dermatol Syphilol 61: 111
51. Inman PM (1965) Dermatitis in a crisp factory. Acta Derm Venereol (Stockh) 45: 295–296

52. Mitchell JC (1980) Contact sensitivity to garlic (*Allium*). Contact Dermatitis 6: 356–357
53. Freeman GG, Whenham RJ (1976) Nature and origin of volatile flavour components of onion and related species. Int Flavours Food Addit 7: 222–227, 229
54. Papageorgiou C, Corbet J-P, Menezes-Brandao F, Pecegueiro M, Benezra C (1983) Allergic contact dermatitis to garlic (*Allium sativum* L.). Identification of the allergens: the role of mono-, di-, and trisulfides present in garlic. A comparative study in man and animal (guinea-pig). Arch Dermatol Res 275: 229–234
55. Brongersma-Oosterhoff UW (1967) Structure determination of the allergenic agent isolated from tulip bulbs. Recl Trav Chim Pays-Bas 86: 705–708
56. Verspyck Mijnessen GAW (1969) Pathogenesis and causative agent of "tulip finger". Br J Dermatol 81: 737–745
57. Slob A, Jekel B, de Jong B, Schlatmann E (1975) On the occurrence of tuliposides in the Liliiflorae. Phytochemistry 14: 1997–2005
58. Hausen BM, Prater E, Schubert H (1983) The sensitizing capacity of *Alstroemeria* cultivars in man and guinea pig. Remarks on the occurrence, quantity and irritant and sensitizing potency of their constituents tuliposide A and tulipalin A (α-methylene-γ-butyrolactone). Contact Dermatitis 9: 46–54
59. Santucci B, Picardo M, Iavarone C, Trogolo C (1985) Contact dermatitis to *Alstroemeria*. Contact Dermatitis 12: 215–219
60. Beijersbergen JCM (1972) A method for determination of tulipalin A and B concentrations in crude extracts of tulip tissues. Recl Trav Chim Pays-Bas 91: 1193–1200
61. Slob A (1973) Tulip allergens in *Alstroemeria* and some other Liliiflorae. Phytochemistry 12: 811–815
62. Barbier P, Benezra C (1986) Allergenic α-methylene-γ-butyrolactones. Study of the capacity of β-acetoxy and β-hydroxy-α-methylene-γ-butyrolactones. to induce allergic contact dermatitis in guinea pigs. J Med Chem 29: 868–871
63. Hjorth N, Wilkinson DS (1968) Contact dermatitis. IV. Tulip fingers, hyacinth itch and lily rash. Br J Dermatol 80: 696–698
64. Rycroft RJG, Calnan CD (1981) Alstroemeria dermatitis. Contact Dermatitis 7: 284
65. Rook A (1981) Dermatitis from *Alstroemeria:* altered clinical pattern and probable increasing incidence. Contact Dermatitis 7: 355–356
66. Marks JG (1988) Allergic contact dermatitis to *Alstroemeria*. Arch Dermatol 124: 914–916
67. Björkner BE (1982) Contact allergy and depigmentation from alstroemeria. Contact Dermatitis 8: 174–184
68. van der Werff PJ (1959) Occupational diseases among workers in the bulb industries. Acta Allerg 14: 338–355
69. Walsh D (1910) Investigation of a dermatitis among flower-pickers in the Scilly Islands, the so-called "lily rash". Br Med J ii: 854–856
70. Klaschka F, Grimm WW, Beiersdorff HU (1964) Tulpen-Kontaktekzem als Berufsdermatose. Hautarzt 15: 317–321
71. Kligman AM (1958) Poison ivy (*Rhus*) dermatitis. An experimental study. Arch Dermatol 77: 149–180
72. Ippen H (1983) Kontaktallergie gegen Anacardiaceae. Übersicht und Kasuistik zur "Poison Ivy" -Allergie in Mitteleuropa. Derm Beruf Umwelt 31: 140–148
73. Gillis WT (1971) The systematics and ecology of poison-ivy and the poison-oaks (Toxicodendron, Anacardiaceae). Rhodora 73: 72–159, 161–237, 370–443, 465–540
74. Marks JG, DeMelfi T, McCarthy MA, Witte EJ, Castagnoli N, Epstein WL, Aber RC (1984) Dermatitis from cashew nuts. J Am Acad Dermatol 10: 627–631
75. Pardo-Castello V (1923) Dermatitis venenata: a study of tropical plants producing dermatitis. Arch Dermatol Syphilol 7: 81–90

76. Bertrand G, Brooks G (1934) Recherches sur le latex de l'arbre à laque du Camboge (*Melanorrhoea laccifera* Pierre). Bull Soc Chim Fr (5) 1: 109–114
77. Ridley HN (1911) Rengas-poisoning. Malay Med J 9 (2): 7
78. Watt G (1906) Burmese lacquer ware and Burmese varnish. Kew Bull (5): 137–147
79. Srinivas CR, Kulkarni SB, Menon SK, Krupashankar DS, Iyengar MA, Singh KK, Sequeira RP, Holla KR (1987) Allergenic agent in contact dermatitis from *Holigarna ferruginea*. Contact Dermatitis 17: 219–222
80. Sprague TA (1921) Plant dermatitis. J Botany 59: 308–310
81. Kirby-Smith JL (1938) Mango dermatitis. Am J Trop Med 18: 373–384
82. Jackson WPU (1946) Plant dermatitis in the Bahamas. Br Med J ii: 298
83. King DF, Wolfish PS, Heng MCY (1983) The much-maligned dhobie. J Am Acad Dermatol 8: 258
84. Findlay GH, Whiting DA, Eggers SH, Ellis RP (1974) Smodingium (African 'poison ivy') dermatitis. History, comparative plant chemistry and anatomy, clinical and histological features. Br J Dermatol 90: 535–541
85. Corbett MD, Billets S (1975) Characterization of poison oak urushiol. J Pharm Sci 64: 1715–1718
86. Gross M, Baer H, Fales HM (1975) Urushiols of poisonous Anacardiaceae. Phytochemistry 14: 2263–2266
87. Hurtado I de (1965) Contact dermatitis caused by the "manzanillo" (*Rhus striata*) tree. Int Arch Allergy Appl Immunol 28: 321–327
88. Nakamura T (1985) Contact dermatitis to *Rhus succedanea*. Contact Dermatitis 12: 279
89. Powell SM, Barrett DK (1986) An outbreak of contact dermatitis from *Rhus verniciflua (Toxicodendron vernicifluum)*. Contact Dermatitis 14: 288–289
90. Guin JD, Gillis WT, Beaman JH (1981) Recognizing the toxicodendrons. J Am Acad Dermatol 4: 99–114
91. Guin JD, Beaman JH (1986) Toxicodendrons of the United States. Clin Dermatol 4: 137–148
92. Sowers WF, Weary PE, Collins OD, Cawley EP (1965) Ginkgo-tree dermatitis. Arch Dermatol 91: 452–456
93. Nakamura T (1985) Ginkgo tree dermatitis. Contact Dermatitis 12: 281–282
94. Tomb RR, Foussereau J, Sell Y (1988) Mini epidemic of contact dermatitis from ginkgo tree fruit. Contact Dermatitis 19: 281–283
95. Mitchell JC, Maibach HI, Guin J (1981) Leaves of *Ginkgo biloba* not allergenic for *Toxicodendron* sensitive subjects. Contact Dermatitis 7: 47–48
96. Bolus M, Raleigh NC (1939) Dermatitis venenata due to ginkgo berries. Arch Dermatol Syphilol 39: 530
97. Becker LE, Skipworth GB (1975) Ginkgo tree dermatitis, stomatitis, and proctitis. J A M A 231: 1162–1163
98. Lepoittevin J-P, Benezra C, Asakawa Y (1989) Allergic contact dermatitis to *Ginkgo biloba* L.: relationship with urushiol. In: Frosch PJ, Dooms-Goossens A, Lachapelle J-M, Rycroft RJG, Scheper RJ (eds) Current topics in contact dermatitis. Springer, Berlin Heidelberg New York, pp 158–162
99. Occolowitz JL, Wright AS (1962) 5-(10-Pentadecenyl)resorcinol from *Grevillea pyramidalis*. Aust J Chem 15: 858–861
100. Ridley DD, Ritchie E, Taylor WC (1968) Chemical studies of the Proteaceae. II. Some further constituents of *Grevillea robusta* A. Cunn.; experiments on the synthesis of 5-*n*-tridecylresorcinol (grevillol) and related substances. Aust J Chem 21: 2979–2988
101. Hoffman TE, Hausen BM, Adams RM (1985) Allergic contact dermatitis to "silver oak" wooden arm bracelets. J Am Acad Dermatol 13: 778–779
102. Menz J, Rossi ER, Taylor WC, Wall L (1986) Contact dermatitis from *Grevillea* "Robyn Gordon'. Contact Dermatitis 15: 126–131

103. Benezra C, Ducombs G (1987) Molecular aspects of allergic contact dermatitis to plants. Derm Beruf Umwelt 35: 4–11

104. Mitchell JC, Roy AK, Dupuis G, Towers GHN (1971) Allergic contact dermatitis from ragweeds (*Ambrosia species.*) The role of sesquiterpene lactones. Arch Dermatol 104: 73–76

105. Shelmire B (1939) Contact dermatitis from weeds; patch testing with their oleoresins. J A M A 113: 1085–1090

106. Burry JN, Kuchel R, Reid JG, Kirk J (1973) Australian bush dermatitis: Compositae dermatitis in South Australia. Med J Aust i: 110–116

107. Towers GHN, Mitchell JC, Rodriguez E, Bennett FD, Subba Rao PV (1977) Biology & chemistry of *Parthenium hysterophorus* L., a problem weed in India. J Sci Ind Res 36: 672–684

108. Hausen BM (1981) Berufsbedingte Kontaktallergie auf Mutterkraut (*Tanacetum parthenium* (L.) Schultz-Bip.; Asteraceae). Derm Beruf Umwelt 29: 18–21

109. Mensing H, Kimmig W, Hausen BM (1985) Airborne contact dermatitis. Hautarzt 36: 398–402

110. Malten KE (1983) Chicory dermatitis from September to April. Contact Dermatitis 9: 232

111. Mitchell JC, Dupuis G (1971) Allergic contact dermatitis from sesquiterpenoids of the Compositae family of plants. Br J Dermatol 84: 139–150

112. Schmidt RJ (1985) When is a chrysanthemum dermatitis not a *Chrysanthemum* dermatitis? The case for describing florists' chrysanthemums as *Dendranthema* cultivars. Contact Dermatitis 13: 115–119

113. Asakawa Y, Benezra C, Ducombs G, Foussereau J, Muller JC, Ourisson G (1974) Cross-sensitization between *Frullania* and *Laurus nobilis:* the allergen laurel. Arch Dermatol 110: 957

114. Fernández de Corres L, Corrales Torres JL (1978) Dermatitis from *Frullania,* Compositae and other plants. Contact Dermatitis 4: 175–176

115. Hausen BM, Osmundsen PE (1983) Contact allergy to parthenolide in *Tanacetum parthenium* (L.) Schulz-Bip. (feverfew, Asteraceae) and cross-reactions to related sesquiterpene lactone containing Compositae species. Acta Derm Venereol (Stockh) 63: 308–314

116. Mitchell J, Rook A (1979) Botanical dermatology. Greengrass, Vancouver, 456–458

117. Mitchell JC (1975) Botanical basis of geographic ecology, p 2. Int J Dermatol 14: 301–321

118. Brunsting LA, Williams DH (1936) Ragweed (contact) dermatitis. Observations in forty-eight cases and report of unsuccessful attempts at desensitization by injection of specific oils. J A M A 106: 1533–1525

119. O'Quinn SE, Isbell KH (1969) Influence of oral prednisone on eczematous patch test reactions. Arch Dermatol 99: 380–389

120. Möslein P (1963) Pflanzen als Kontakt-Allergene. Berufsdermatosen 11: 24–28

121. Hausen BM, Busker E, Carle R (1984) Über das Sensibilisierungsvermögen von Compositenarten VII. Experimentelle Untersuchungen mit Auszügen und Inhalts- stoffen von *Chamomilla recutita* (L.) Rauschert und Anthemis cotula L. Planta Med 50: 229–234

122. Burry JN (1979) Dermatitis from fleabane: Compositae dermatitis in South Australia. Contact Dermatitis 5: 51

123. Hausen BM (1980) Arnikaallergie. Hautarzt 31: 10–17

124. Brunsting LA, Anderson CR (1934) Ragweed dermatitis. A report based on eighteen cases. J A M A 103: 1285–1290

125. Mitchell JC, Geissman TA, Dupuis G, Towers GHN (1971) Allergic contact dermatitis caused by *Artemisia* and *Chrysanthemum* species. J Invest Dermatol 56: 98–101

126. Maiden JH (1909) On some plants which cause inflammation or irritation of the skin, pt II. Agric Gaz NSW 20: 1073–1082

127. Hausen BM (1979) The sensitizing capacity of Compositae plants. III. Test results and cross-reactions in Compositae-sensitive patients. Dermatologica 159: 1–11

128. Vail JT, Mitchell JC (1973) Occupational dermatitis from *Cichorium intybus, C. endivia,* and *Lactuca sativa* var. *longifolia.* Contact Dermatitis Newslett 14: 413

129. Friis B, Hjorth N, Vail JT, Mitchell JC (1975) Occupational contact dermatitis from *Cichorium* (chicory, endive) and *Lactuca* (lettuce). Contact Dermatitis 1: 311–313

130. Burry JN, Kloot PM (1982) The spread of composite (Compositae) weeds in Australia. Contact Dermatitis 8: 410–413

131. Vryman LH (1933) Dahlienwurzelrinden-Dermatitis. Arch Dermatol Syph 168: 233

132. Calnan CD (1978) Sensitivity to dahlia flowers. Contact Dermatitis 4: 168

133. Olivier J, Renkin A (1954) Eczéma par sensibilité à une seule variété de chrysanthémes. Arch Belg Dermatol Syphiligr 10: 296–297

134. Rook AJ (1961) Plant dermatitis. The significance of variety-specific sensitization. Br J Dermatol 73: 283–287

135. Hausen BM, Schulz KH (1976) Chrysanthemum Allergy. III. Identification of the allergens. Arch Dermatol Res 255: 111–121

136. Mackoff S, Dahl AO (1951) A botanical consideration of the weed oleoresin problem. Minn Med 34: 1169–1173

137. Hausen BM, Spring O (1989) Sunflower allergy. On the constituents of the trichomes of *Helianthus annuus* L. (Compositae). Contact Dermatitis 20: 326–334

138. Gougerot, Burnier, Boulle (1933) Purpura réticulé et eczéma généralisé à la suite d'application de feuille d'aunée (¡¡ Inula Helenium ¿¿); sensibilisation. Bull Soc Fr Derm Syphiligr 40: 1702–1704

139. P'iankova ZP, Nugmanova ML (1975) Dermatit ot deviasila. [Dermatitis due to elecampane]. Vestn Dermatol Venereol (12): 52–54

140. Marzulli FN, Maibach HI (1980) Further studies on effects of vehicles and elicitation concentration in contact sensitization testing in humans. Contact Dermatitis 6: 131–133

141. Rodriguez E, Reynolds GW, Thompson JA (1981) Potent contact allergen in the rubber plant guayule (*Parthenium argentatum.*) Science 211: 1444–1445

142. Cheminat A, Stampf J-L, Benezra C, Farrall MJ, Fréchet JMJ (1981) Allergic contact dermatitis to costus: removal of haptens with polymers. Acta Derm Venereol (Stockh) 61: 525–529

143. Verhagen AR, Nyaga JM (1974) Contact dermatitis from *Tagetes minuta.* A new sensitizing plant of the Compositae family. Arch Dermatol 110: 441–444

144. Mitchell JC, Dupuis G, Towers GHN (1972) Allergic contact dermatitis from pyethrum (*Chrysanthemum* spp.). The roles of pyrethrosin, a sesquiterpene lactone, and of pyrethrin II. Br J Dermatol 86: 568–573

145. Hausen BM (1982) Taraxinsaüre-1'-O-β − D-glucopyranosid das Kontaktallergen des Löwenzahns (*Taraxacum officinale* Wiggers). Derm Beruf Umwelt 30: 51–53

146. Maiden JH (1918) Plants which produce inflammation or irritation of the skin. Agric Gaz NSW 29: 344–345

147. Mitchell JC (1986) *Frullania* (liverwort) phytodermatitis (woodcutter's eczema). Clin Dermatol 4: 62–64

148. Mitchell JC, Fritig, B, Singh B, Towers GHN (1970) Allergic contact dermatitis from *Frullania* and Compositae. The role of sesquiterpene lactones. J Invest Dermatol 54: 233–239

149. Knoche H, Ourisson G, Perold GW, Foussereau J, Maleville J (1969) Allergenic component of a liverwort: a sesquiterpene lactone. Science 166: 239–240

150. Mitchell J, Rook A (1979) Botanical dermatology Greengrass, Vancouver, pp 227–236

151. Coulter S (1904) The poisonous plants of Indiana. Proc Indiana Acad Sci: 51–63

152. Mitchell JC, Jordan WP (1974) Allergic contact dermatitis from the radish, *Raphanus sativus.* Br J Dermatol 91: 183–189
153. Leoni A, Cogo R (1964) Dermatite professionale da contatto con cavolo capuccio. Minerva Dermatol 39: 326–327
154. Gaul LE (1964) Contact dermatitis from synthetic oil of mustard. Arch Dermatol 90: 158–159
155. Mitchell J, Rook A (1979) Botanical dermatology. Greengrass, Vancouver, p 229
156. Fregert S, Dahlquist I, Trulsson L (1983) Sensitization capacity of diphenylthiourea and phenylisothiocyanaté. Contact Dermatitis 9: 87–88
157. Richter G (1980) Allergic contact dermatitis from methyl isothiocyanate in soil disinfectants. Contact Dermatitis 6: 183–186
158. Ettlinger MG, Lundeen AJ (1956) The structures of sinigrin and sinalbin; an enzymatic rearrangement. J Am Chem Soc 78: 4172–4173
159. Schmidt RJ (1986) Biosynthetic and chemosystematic aspects of the Euphorbiaceae and Thymelaeaceae. In: Evans FJ (ed) Naturally occurring phorbol esters. CRC Press, Boca Raton, pp 87–106
160. Webster GL (1986) Irritant plants in the spurge family (Euphorbiaceae). Clin Dermatol 4: 36–45
161. Evans FJ (1986) Environmental hazards of diterpene esters from plants. In: Evans FJ (ed) Naturally occurring phorbol esters. CRC Press, Boca Raton, pp 1–31
162. Satulsky EM, Wirts CA (1943) Dermatitis venenata caused by the manzanillo tree. Further observations and a report of sixty cases. Arch Derm Syphilol 47: 797–798
163. Rook AJ (1965) An unrecorded plant irritant, *Synadenium grantii.* Br J Dermatol 77: 284
164. Calnan CD (1975) Petty spurge (*Euphorbia peplus* L.) Contact Dermatitis 1: 128
165. Strobel M, N'Diaye B, Padonou F, Marchand JP (1978) Les dermites de contact d'origine végétale (à propos de 10 cas observés à Dakar). Bull Soc Méd Afr Noire Lang Fr 23: 124–127
166. Worobec SM, Hickey TA, Kinghorn AD, Soejarto DD, West D (1981) Irritant contact dermatitis from an ornamental, *Euphorbia hermentiana.* Contact Dermatitis 7: 19–22
167. Hickey TA, Worobec SM, West DP, Kinghorn AD (1981) Irritant contact dermatitis in humans from phorbol and related esters. Toxicon 19: 841–850
168. Pinedo JM, Saavedra V, Gonzalez-de-Canales F, Llamas P (1985) Irritant dermatitis due to *Euphorbia marginata.* Contact Dermatitis 13: 44
169. Elpern DJ (1985) The dermatology of Kauai, Hawaii, 1981–1982. Int J Dermatol 24: 647–652
170. D'Arcy WG (1974) Severe contact dermatitis from poinsettia. Arch Dermatol 109: 909–910
171. Hausen BM, Schulz KH (1977) Occupational contact dermatitis due to croton (*Codiaeum variegatum* (L.) A. Juss var. *pictum* (Lodd.) Muell. Arg.). Sensitization by plants of the Euphorbiaceae. Contact Dermatitis 3: 289–292
172. Schmidt H, Ølholm Larsen P (1977) Allergic contact dermatitis from croton (*Codiaeum*). Contact Dermatitis 3: 100
173. Cleenewerck M-B, Martin P (1989) Occupational contact dermatitis due to *Codiaeum variegatum* L., *Chrysanthemum indicum* L., *Chrysanthemum* × *hortorum* and *Frullania dilatata* L. In: Frosch PJ, Dooms-Goossens A, Lachapelle J-M, Rycroft RJG, Scheper RJ (eds) Current topics in contact dermatitis. Springer, Berlin Heidelberg New York, pp 149–157
174. Santucci B, Picardo M, Cristaudo A (1985) Contact dermatitis from *Euphorbia pulcherrima.* Contact Dermatitis 12: 285–286
175. Weedon D, Chick J (1976) Home treatment of basal cell carcinoma. Med J Aust i: 928

176. Schmidt RJ, Evans FJ (1980) Skin irritants of the sun spurge (*Euphorbia helioscopia* L.). Contact Dermatitis 6: 204–210

177. Adolf W, Sorg B, Hergenhahn M, Hecker E (1982) Structure-activity relations of polyfunctional diterpenes of the daphnane type. I. Revised structure for resiniferatoxin and structure-activity relations of resiniferonol and some of its esters. J Nat Prod 45: 347–354

178. Schmidt RJ, Evans FJ (1979) Investigations into the skin-irritant properties of resiniferonol ortho esters. Inflammation 3: 273–280

179. Fürstenberger G, Hecker E (1972) Zum Wirkungsmechanismus cocarcinogener Pflanzeninhaltsstoffe. Planta Med 22: 241–266

180. Evans FJ (1986) Phorbol: its esters and derivatives. In: Evans FJ (ed) Naturally occurring phorbol esters. CRC Press, Boca Raton, pp 171–215

181. Schmidt RJ (1986) The daphnane polyol esters. In: Evans FJ (ed) Naturally occurring phorbol esters. CRC Press, Boca Raton, pp 217–243

182. Schmidt RJ (1986) The ingenane polyol esters. In: Evans FJ (ed) Naturally occurring phorbol esters. CRC Press, Boca Raton, pp 245–269

183. Mitchell JC (1965) Allergy to lichens. Arch Dermatol 92: 142–146

184. Mitchell JC, Shibata S (1969) Immunologic activity of some substances derived from lichenized fungi. J Invest Dermatol 52: 517–520

185. Dahlquist I, Fregert S (1980) Contact allergy to atranorin in lichens and perfumes. Contact Dermatitis 6: 111–119

186. Thune P, Solberg Y, McFadden N, Staerfelt F, Sandberg M (1982) Perfume allergy due to oak moss and other lichens. Contact Dermatitis 8: 396–400

187. Tan KS, Mitchell JC (1968) Patch and photopatch tests in contact dermatitis and photodermatitis: a preliminary report of investigation of 150 patients, with special reference to "cedar-poisoning". Can Med Assoc J 98: 252–255

188. Thune P (1977) Allergy to lichens with photosensitivity. Contact Dermatitis 3: 213–214

189. Thune P (1977) Contact allergy due to lichens in patients with a history of photosensitivity. Contact Dermatitis 3: 267–272

190. Salo H, Hannuksela M, Hausen B (1981) Lichen pickers dermatitis (*Cladonia alpestris* (L.) Rab.). Contact Dermatitis 7: 9–13

191. Champion RH (1971) Atopic sensitivity to algae and lichens. Br J Dermatol 85: 551–557

192. Mitchell J, Rook A (1979) Botanical dermatology. Greengrass, Vancouver, pp 546–553

193. Hausen BM (1979) Primelallergie. Hintergründe und Aspekte. Mater Med Nordmark 31 (3/4): 57–76

194. Hjorth N (1979) Primula dermatitis. In: Mitchell J, Rook A (ed) Botanical dermatology. Greengrass, Vancouver, pp 554–564

195. Schildknecht H (1957) Struktur des Primelgiftstoffes. Z Naturforsch 22B: 36–41

196. Cairns RJ (1964) Plant dermatoses: some chemical aspects and results of patch testing with extracts of *Primula obconica*. Trans St. John's Hosp Derm Soc 50: 137–143

197. Fregert S, Hjorth N, Schulz K-H (1968) Patch testing with synthetic primin in patients sensitive to *Primula obconica*. Arch Dermatol 98: 144–147

198. Hjorth N (1966) Primula dermatitis: sources of error in patch testing and patch test sensitization. Trans St John's Hosp Derm Soc 52: 207–219

199. Hjorth N (1967) Seasonal variations in contact dermatitis. Acta Derm Venereol (Stockh) 47: 409–418

200. Fernández de Corres L, Leanizbarrutia I, Muñoz D (1987) Contact dermatitis from Primula obconia Hance. Contact Dermatitis 16: 195–197

201. Agrup G, Gregert S. Hjorth N, Övrum P (1968) Routine patch tests with ether extract of *P. obconica*. Br J Dermatol 80: 497–502

202. Mitchell J, Rook A (1979) Botanical dermatology. Greengrass, Vancouver, pp 572–588
203. Frenzl F (1937) Artificial dermatitis caused by *Anemone nemorosa* Cas Lék Cesk 76: 1831–1835
204. Spengler F (1946) Die therapeutische Verwendung der Anemone nemorosa, des Buschwindröschens. Pharmazie 1: 222–223
205. Rodziewicz J, Wlodarczyk S (1961) Zmiany skórne wywoł ane działaniem jaskru. Przegl Dermatol 48 [Suppl]: 429–434
206. Aaron TH, Muttitt ELC (1964) Vesicant dermatitis due to prairie crocus (*Anemone patens* L.). Arch Dermatol 90: 168–171
207. Rudzki E, Dajek Z (1975) Dermatitis caused by buttercups (Ranunculus). Contact Dermatitis 1: 322
208. Kipping FB (1935) The lactone of γ-hydroxyvinylacrylic acid, protoanemonin. J Chem Soc: 1145–1147
209. Hill R, van Heyningen R (1951) Ranunculin: the precursor of the vesicant substance of the buttercup. Biochem J 49: 332–335
210. Moriarty RM, Romain CR, Karle IL, Karle J (1965) The structure of anemonin. J Am Chem Soc 87: 3251–3252
211. Boll PM (1968) Naturally occurring lactones and lactames. I. The absolute configuration of ranunculin, lichesterinic acid, and some lactones related to lichesterinic acid. Acta Chem Scand (B) 22: 3245–3250
212. Drever JC, Hunter JAA (1970) Giant hogweed dermatitis. Scot Med J 15: 315–319
213. Camm E, Buck HWL, Mitchell JC (1976) Phytophotodermatitis from *Heracleum mantegazzianum.* Contact Dermatitis 2: 68–72
214. Innocenti G, Dall'Acqua F, Guiotto A, Caporale G (1977) Investigation on skin-photosensitizing activity of various kinds of *Psoralea.* Planta Med 31: 151–155
215. Zaynoun ST, Aftimos BG, Abi Ali L, Tenekjian KK, Khalidi U, Kurban AK (1984) Ficus carica; isolation and quantification of the photoactive components. Contact Dermatitis 11: 21–25
216. Ippen H (1982) Phototoxische Reaktion auf Feigen. Hautarzt 33: 337–339
217. Kitchevatz M (1934) Etiologie et pathogénèse de la dermatite des figues. Bull Soc Fr Dermatol Syphiligr 41: 1751–1759
218. Houloussi-Behdjet D (1933) Dermatite des figues et des figuiers. Bull Soc Fr Dermatol Syphiligr 40: 787–796
219. Sams WM (1941) Photodynamic action of lime oil (*Citrus aurantifolia*). Arch Derm Syphilol 44: 571–587
220. Opdyke DLJ (1973) Monographs on fragrance raw materials. Food Cosmet Toxicol 11: 1031–1033
221. Girard J, Unkovic J, Delahayes J, Lafille C (1979) Étude expérimentale de la phototoxicité de l'essence de bergamote; corrélation entre l'homme et le cobaye. Dermatologica 158: 229–243
222. Volden G, Krokan H, Kavli G, Midelfart K (1983) Phototoxic and contact toxic reactions of the exocarp of sweet organges: a common cause of cheilitis? Contact Dermatitis 9: 201–204
223. Fisher JF, Trama LA (1979) High-performance liquid chromatographic determination of some coumarins and psoralens found in citrus peel oils. J Argic Food Chem 27: 1334–1337
224. Sommer RG, Jillson OF (1967) Phytophotodermatitis (solar dermatitis from plants). Gas plant and the wild parsnip. N Engl J Med 276: 1484–1486
225. Möller H (1978) Phototoxicity of *Dictamnus alba.* Contact Dermatitis 4: 264–269
226. Elpern DJ, Mitchell JC (1984) Phytophotodermatitis from mokihana fruits (*Pelea anisata* H. Mann, fam. Rutaceae) in Hawaiian lei. Contact Dermatitis 10: 224–226

227. Marchant YY, Turjman M, Flynn T, Balza F, Mitchell JC, Towers GNH (1985) Identification of psoralen, 8-methoxypsoralen, isopimpinellin, and 5, 7-dimethoxy-coumarin in *Pelea anisata* H. Mann. Contact Dermatitis 12: 196–199

228. Jarvis WM (1968) The photosensitizing furanocoumarins of *Phebalium argenteum* (blister bush). Aust J Chem 21: 537–538

229. Brener S, Friedman J (1985) Phytophotodermatitis induced by *Ruta chalepensis* L. Contact Dermatitis 12: 230–232

230. Gawkrodger DJ, Savin JA (1983) Phytophotodermatitis due to common rue (*Ruta graveolens*). Contact Dermatitis 9: 224

231. Zobel AM, Brown SA (1990) Dermatitis-inducing furanocoumarins on leaf surfaces of eight species of rutaceous and umbelliferous plants. J Chem Ecology 16: 693–700

232. Sidi E, Bourgeois-Gavardin J (1955) Accidents provoqués par les applications locales d' "Ammi majus". In: Accidents therapeutiques en dermatologie. Masson, Paris, pp 337–338

233. Coste F, Marceron L, Boyer J (1943) Dermite à l'angèlique. Bull Soc Fr Dermatol Syphiligr 50: 316–317

234. Benezra C, Ducombs G, Sell Y, Foussereau J (1985) Plant contact dermatitis Decker, Toronto, pp 90–91

235. Birmingham DJ, Key MM, Tubich GE, Perone VB (1961) Phototoxic bullae among celery harvesters. Arch Dermatol 83: 73–87

236. Seligman PJ, Mathias CGT, O'Malley MA, Beier RC, Fehrs LJ, Serrill WS, Halperin WE (1987) Phytophotodermatitis from celery among grocery store workers. Arch Dermatol 123: 1478–1482

237. Austad J, Kavli G (1983) Phototoxic dermatitis caused by celery infected by *Sclerotinia sclerotiorum*. Contact Dermatitis 9: 448–451

238. Kavli G, Midelfart K, Raa J, Volden G (1983) Phototoxicity from furocoumarins (psoralens) of *Heracleum laciniatum* in a patient with vitiligo. Action spectrum studies on bergapten, pimpinellin, angelicin and sphondin. Contact Dermatitis 9: 364–366

239. Weimarck G, Nilsson E (1980) Phototoxicity in *Heracleum sphondylium*. Planta Med 38: 97–100

240. Picardo M, Cristaudo A, de Luca C, Santucci B (1986) Contact dermatitis to *Pastinaca sativa*. Contact Dermatitis 15: 98–99

241. Schwartz L (1938) Cutaneous hazards in the citrus fruit industry. Arch Dermatol Syphilol 37: 631–649

242. Vickers HR (1941) The carrot as a cause of dermatitis. Br J Dermatol 53: 52–57

243. Peck SM, Spolyar LW, Mason HS (1944) Dermatitis from carrots. Arch Derm Syphilol 49: 266–269

244. Kaluder JV, Kimmich JM (1956) Sensitization dermatitis to carrots. Report of cross-sensitization phenomenon and remarks on phytophotodermatitis. Arch Dermatol 74: 149–158

245. van Dijk E, Berrens L (1964) Plants as an etiological factor in phytophotodermatitis. Dermatologica 129: 321–328

246. Hausen BM (1981) Woods injurious to human health. A manual. De Gruyter, Berlin

247. Willis JH (1982) Nasal carcinoma in woodworkers: a review. J Occup Med 24: 526–530

248. Woods B, Calnan CD (1976) Toxic woods. Br J Dermatol 95 [Suppl 13]: 1–97

249. Benezra C, Ducombs G, Sell Y, Foussereau J (1985) Plant contact dermatitis. Decker, Toronto, pp 269–299

250. Hausen BM (1986) Contact allergy to woods. Clin Dermatol 4: 65–76

251. Hausen BM, Adams RM (1990) Woods. In: Adams RM (ed) Occupational skin disease, 2nd edn. Saunders, Philadelphia, pp 524–536

252. Fernández de Corres L, Leanizbarrutia I, Muñoz D (1988) Cross-reactivity between some naturally occurring quinones. Contact Dermatitis 18: 186–187

253. Weber LF (1953) Dermatitis venenata due to native woods. Arch Derm Syphilol 67: 388–394
254. Karlberg A-T (1988) Contact allergy to colophony. Chemical identifications of the allergens, sensitization experiments and clinical experiences. Acta Derm Venereol Suppl (Stockh) 139: 1–43
255. Karlberg A-T, Bohlinder K, Boman A, Hacksell U, Hermansson J, Jacobsson S, Nilsson JLG (1988) Identification of 15-hydroperoxyabietic acid as a contact allergen in Portuguese colophony. J Pharm Pharmacol 40: 42–47
256. Hellerström S, Thyresson N, Widmark G (1957) Chemical aspects of turpentine eczema. Dermatologica 115: 277–286
257. Pirilä V, Kilpiö O, Olkkonen A, Pirilä L, Siltanen E (1969) On the chemical nature of the eczematogens in oil of turpentine. V. Pattern of sensitivity to different terpenes. Dermatologica 139: 183–194
258. Dooms-Goossens A, Degreef H, Coopman S (1989) Corticosteroid contact allergy: a reality. In: Frosch PJ, Dooms-Goossens A, Lachapelle J-M, Rycroft RJG, Scheper RJ (eds) Current topics in contact dermatitis. Springer, Berlin Heidelberg New York, pp 233–237
259. Watson ES (1986) *Toxicodendron* hyposensitization programs. Clin Dermatol 4: 160–170
260. Resnick SD (1986) Poison-ivy and poison-oak dermatitis. Clin Dermatol 4: 208–212

Chapter 15
Pigmented Contact Dermatitis and Chemical Depigmentation

Pigmented Contact Dermatitis and Chemical Depigmentation

HIDEO NAKAYAMA

Contents

15.1 Hyperpigmentation Associated with Contact Dermatitis

15.1.1 Classification

Hyperpigmentation associated with contact dermatitis is classified into three categories: (1) hyperpigmentation due to incontinentia pigmenti histologica; (2) hyperpigmentation due to increase in melanin in the basal layer cells of the epidermis, i.e. basal melanosis; and (3) hyperpigmentation due to slight haemorrhage around the vessels of the upper dermis, resulting in an accumulation of haemosiderin, such as in Majocchi-Schamberg dermatitis.

It is easy to understand that when the grade of contact dermatitis is more severe, or its duration longer, the secondary hyperpigmentation following dermatitis is more prominent. However, the first type mentioned above, incontinentia pigmenti histologica, often occurs without showing any positive manifestations of dermatitis such as marked erythema, vesiculation, swelling, papules, rough skin or scaling. Therefore, patients may complain only of a pigmentary disorder, even though the disease is entirely the result of allergic contact dermatitis. Hyperpigmentation caused by incontinentia pigmenti histologica has often been called a lichenoid reaction, since the presence of basal liquefaction degeneration, the accumulation of melanin pigment and the mononuclear cell infiltrate in the upper dermis are very similar to the histopathological manifestations of lichen planus. However, compared with typical lichen planus, usually hyperkeratosis is milder, hypergranulosis and saw-tooth shape acanthosis lacking, hyaline bodies hardly seen, and the bandlike massive infiltration with lymphocytes and histiocytes lacking.

A lichenoid reaction is considered to be a scaled-down Type IV allergic reaction of the lichen planus type, based on the positive patch test reactions in patients and the negative reactions in controls, as in ordinary allergic contact dermatitis.

An increase in melanin pigment in keratinocytes is noted after allergic contact dermatitis, presumably caused by hyperfunction of melanocytes, but the same phenomenon is also seen with irritant contact dermatitis. When sodium lauryl sulphate, a typical skin irritant, was repeatedly applied on the forearms of Caucasians, the number of epidermal melanocytes was observed to have been almost doubled, suggesting hyperplasia, hypertrophy and increased function [1].

The pathological processes involved in the third form of hyperpigmentation with contact dermatitis, purpuric dermatitis, have not yet been clarified. Shiitake mushroom, very commonly eaten in Asia, has been known to produce a transient urticarial dermatitis with severe itching, which results in a purpuric scratch effect, when insufficiently cooked. This is thought to be due to toxic substances in the mushroom unstable to heat, and the pigmentation due to purpura is not caused by hypersensitivity [2]. With other forms of dermatitis, accompanying capillary fragility results in purpura. Some cases are associated with contact hypersensitivity to rubber components or textile finishes, but in many cases the causes are not known.

15.1.2 Pigmented Contact Dermatitis

15.1.2.1 History and Causative Agents

Pigmented contact dermatitis was first reported by Osmundsen in Denmark in 1969. In 8 months he had 120 patients, seven of whom showed a pronounced and bizarre hyperpigmentation. In four of these seven cases contact dermatitis preceded the hyperpigmentation, while the other three did not notice any signs of dermatitis such as itching or erythema before the pigmentation appeared [3, 4].

Hyperpigmentation, with or without dermatitis, was located mostly in covered areas, such as the chest, back, waist, arms, neck and thighs. After a patient wanted to conceal the pigmentation by wearing long sleeves and a high-neck sweater, which she washed with a washing powder every day, the hyperpigmentation extended from the neck and axillae all over the neck, chest and arms. The hyperpigmentation was brown, slate-coloured, greyish-brown, reddish-brown, bluish-brown, etc., according to the case, and often had a reticulate pattern. The histopathology of the pigmentation showed incontinentia pigmenti histologica.

Patch tests with the standard series current at that time gave no information as to the causative allergens. However, Osmundsen noticed that the patients had used washing powders which contained a new optical whitener, Tinopal or CH3566 (Table 15.1). This was one of numerous optical whiteners which became available at that time to make textiles 'whiter than white'. Patch tests with CH3566 1% pet. finally explained the pigmentary disorder, as they showed strong positive reactions in the patients and negative results in the controls. The pigmentation was persistent, but the dermatitis which often preceded hyperpigmentation was observed to disappear following the elimination of washing powders which contained CH3566. Fortunately, the identification of the causative chemical was made rapidly, and the widespread usage of CH3566 was avoided in time.

Pigmented contact dermatitis is rare in Caucasians but not uncommon in Mongoloids. The next pigmented contact dermatitis was reported by Ancona-Alayón et al. in Mexico [5]. Among 53 workers handling azo dyes in a textile factory, 12 developed a spotted hyperpigmentation without pruritus, and 18 suffered from hyperpigmentation to a lesser extent. This new occupational

Table 15.1. The main contact sensitizers producing secondary hyperpigmentation

Name	Chemical structure	Purpose	Patch test concentration and base
Tinopal CH3566		Optical whitener in washing powder	1% pet.
Naphthol AS		Dye for textile	5% aq. 2%–0.2% acet.
Benzyl salicylate		Fragrance	5%–1% pet.
Hydroxycitronellal		Fragrance	5%–1% pet.
D&C Red 31 and		Pigment for cosmetics	1% pet.

Table 15.1. Continued

Name	Chemical structure	Purpose	Patch test concentration and base
Phenyl-azo-2-naphthol (PAN)		Impurity	0.1% pet.
D & C Yellow 11		Pigment for cosmetics	0.1% pet.
Ylang-ylang oil	(main sensitizer, dehydrodiisoeugenol)	Fragrance, incense	5% pet.
Jasmin absolute	Main sensitizers not yet identified	Fragrance	10%–5% pet.
Synthetic sandalwood	Main sensitizers not yet identified	Fragrance	10% pet.
Cinnamic alcohol		Fragrance	1% pet.
Musk ambrette		Fragrance, incense	5% pet.
Biocheck 60®		Pesticide for textiles	0.2% aq.
PPP-HB		Textile finish	5% eth.
Impurity of commercial CI, Blue 19 (Brilliant Blue®)	Main sensitizers not yet identified	Dye	5% eth.
Mercury compounds	Hg^{2+}	Bactericides	0.05% aq. or pet. (not with AL chambers)
Nickel (sulphate)	Ni^{2+}	Metal products	5%–2% aq. or pet.
Chromate (K dichromate)	Cr^{6+}	Leather, soap	0.5%–0.4% aq. or pet.

skin disorder appeared 4 months after the introduction of a new dyeing process of azo-coupling on textiles, and most of the patients had contact with azo dyes on weaving machines. Hyperpigmentation varied from a bizarre dark pigmentation to a streaky milder pigmentation of the neck, arms, face and, in exceptional cases, covered areas.

Histopathological examination of the pigmentary disorder showed spongiosis, irregular acanthosis, oedema of the dermis, pericapillary lymphocytic infiltration, basal liquefaction degeneration and incontinentia pigmenti histogica. Melanocyte proliferation at the affected sites was also noted.

Patch tests showed that 24 of the 53 workers were positive to 5% Naphthol AS in water, while the other 29, as well as 10 controls, were negative to Naphthol AS. The dermatoses disappeared after the dyeing process was changed so that the workers did not directly touch Naphthol AS.

In the early 1980s, pigmented contact dermatitis due to Naphthol AS appeared in central Japan, but this time it was not occupational. A textile factory manufacturing flannel nightwear, a traditional Japanese garment called a *yukata,* economized on water for washing the products after the process of azo-coupling using Naphthol AS. This modification of production resulted in the appearance of pigmented contact dermatitis of the covered areas of skin in people living in the districts where the products were distributed and worn. Kawachi et al. [6] and Hayakawa et al. [7] reported such cases, and the hyperpigmentation was mainly located on the back and neck. The factory was said to have improved the washing process and the materials quickly, but the presence of such cases indicates that whenever the textile industry uses Naphthol AS, and at the same time economizes on water for washing the products, there must be a risk of producing pigmented contact dermatitis of the covered areas. According to Hayakawa et al. [7] the amount of Naphthol AS detected in the patients' nightwear was 4900–8700 ppm, a considerable amount.

In 1984, the city of Tokyo decided to investigate new textile finishes which seemed to have produced contact dermatitis of the covered skin areas, including pigmented contact dermatitis (Fig. 15.1). Based on information about the textile finishes which actually came into contact with the patients' skin or were very commonly used, 115 chemicals were finally chosen and patch tested. The test materials included 50 dyes of all colours, 13 whiteners, 5 fungicides, 32 resin components, 13 softening agents, and 15 other miscellaneous textile finishes which were widely used at that time by the textile industry in Japan. They were chosen from approximately 1200 textile finishes, either imported or produced in Japan. They were checked as to solubility in water, ethanol, acetone, etc., diluted to 5% (except bactericides, fungicides and other pesticides for textiles which were diluted to 1%), and then applied to dry paper discs 8 mm in diameter, to make dry allergen-containing discs named 'instant patch test allergens'. They were peeled off silicon-treated covering paper before use.

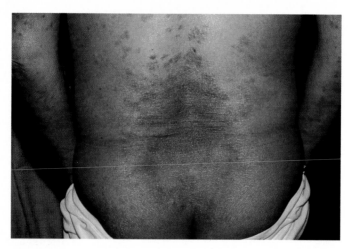

Fig. 15.1. Pigmented contact dermatitis in a 67-year-old man who was sensitized by several textile finishes, including commercial grade red and brown dyes and fungicides

The results obtained from five hospitals in and around Tokyo revealed that several new contact sensitizers were responsible for producing textile dermatitis and secondary hyperpigmentation. These textile finishes included Biochek 60, a very toxic fungicide which seemed also to have acted as a sensitizer, a phosphite polymer of pentaerythritol and hydrogenated bisphenol A (PPP-HB), impurities in a dye CI Blue 19 (or Brilliant Blue R) and mercury compounds [8].

The research on these 115 chemicals was performed in the five hospitals on 80 to 101 subjects, among whom 51 to 62 were patients suffering from textile contact dermatitis, and the rest, 29 to 39, were controls with atopic dermatitis and dermatitis due to causes other than textiles. Among those with textile contact dermatitis, 27 to 33 had pigmented contact dermatitis. Such cases had been deliberately chosen for patch testing because the investigators hoped to find out the causative contact sensitizers producing such hyperpigmentation. Of these pigmented contact dermatitis patients, nine showed positive reactions suggestive of an allergy to Biochek 60, and one to several textile finishes. The results were rather disappointing, but they did show that it is not easy to discover the contact sensitizers producing pigmented contact dermatitis from contact with textile finishes. The discoveries of CH3566 and Naphthol AS can be regarded as having been important and valuable.

Besides the above-mentioned textile finishes, rubber components can also produce dermatitis resulting in hyperpigmentation, mainly around the waist. Sometimes in such cases the pigmentation is not due to incontinentia pigmenti histologica but to purpura (see Sect. 15.1.3). Thus far, only cases of pigmented contact dermatitis in which causative allergens were found have been reported. Causes other than contact sensitivity have not yet been well investigated, except for friction melanosis which is described in Sect. 15.1.2.2.

15.1.2.2 Differential Diagnosis

Differential diagnosis of pigmented contact dermatitis due to washing powder or textile components includes Addison's disease, friction melanosis, amyloidosis cutis, drug eruption, atopic dermatitis with pigmentation and dermatitis and secondary hyperpigmentation due to dental metal sensitivity (dental metal eruption).

Friction melanosis was frequently seen in Japan in the 1970s and 1980s, the disease consisting of dark brown or black hyperpigmentation unaccompanied by dermatitis or itching [9]. Friction melanosis occurred predominantly on the skin over or along bones, such as the clavicles, ribs, scapulae, spine, knees and elbows. The colour and distribution of friction melanosis sometimes leads to confusion with pigmented contact dermatitis. The disease, however, is produced by patients vigorously rubbing the skin with a hard nylon towel or nylon brush every day when bathing. Patch testing with various contact allergens failed to demonstrate allergens which seemed to be correlated with the disease. It was Tanigaki et al. [10] in 1983 who pointed out the causative association of rubbing with a nylon towel or brush, and the disease has gradually decreased since this hazard has become known to the public.

The use of nylon towels or brushes in washing the skin should therefore be checked before the diagnosis of pigmented contact dermatitis due to textiles is made. If the dark hyperpigmentation of the skin over bones gradually fades and disappears after use of nylon towels or brushes is discontinued and patients change their mode of washing to a milder technique, the diagnosis of friction melanosis should be considered. Curiously, the histopathology of friction melanosis shows incontinentia pigmenti histologica, which is a characteristic feature of pigmented contact dermatitis. However, liquefaction degeneration of basal layer cells of the epidermis is not present [9].

Another skin disorder to be distinguished is skin amyloidosis, especially lichen amyloidosus or papular amyloidosis. It is possible that a small amount of amyloid, which can be demonstrated by Dylon staining, is found in lichenoid tissue reactions, probably because amyloid in the upper dermis is considered to be derived from degenerate epidermal cells produced by epidermal inflammation. Special staining with Congo red or thioflavine T and electron-microscopical study of the skin specimen are also helpful in the differential diagnosis.

15.1.2.3 Prevention and Treatment

It is essential that the use of textiles and washing powders containing strong contact sensitizers be avoided, in order to prevent contact dermatitis and pigmented contact dermatitis of the areas of skin which come into contact with the fabric and washing powders or softening agents that remain on them even after rinsing. There are, however, so many textile finishes available today, with more than 1200 commercial finishes being sold to the textile industry, and unfortunately their components are mainly secret. The purity of dyes is, in general, very low and some of the many impurities are allergenic. For example, the very commonly used CI Blue 19 (or Brilliant Blue R) turned out to be allergenic and caused some patch-test-positive cases of pigmented contact dermatitis in 1985 [8]. Purified CI Blue 19, in contrast, never produced positive patch test reactions at the same 5% concentration.

The experiences accumulated in the past show that, when entirely new textile finishes are introduced to textile industry, the minimum safety evaluation tests such as LD 50, Ames test and skin irritation test should be performed, and their sensitization potential should be investigated by a research team including dermatologists. Strong contact sensitizers can be detected by several experimental procedures using animals (see Chap. 18). Although animal experiments are now the subject of ethical scrutiny in connection with such investigations, they remain indicated if the irritability and allergenicity of textile finishes are to be adequately investigated.

The textile industry should cooperate with dermatologists when pigmented contact dermatitis has once occurred by immediately informing them of the components of the chemical finishes of the textile suspected to have caused the disease, and a precise study of impurities and quality control in the factory should also be performed. Shortening of the washing process should be strictly refrained from, otherwise surplus dyes, their impurities and other chemical finishes may remain and produce a problem.

When a causative allergen is discovered, the solution of pigmented contact dermatitis is not difficult [4, 5, 7]. However, when causative allergens are not identified, the solution of the pigmentary disorder is usually very difficult. In 1985, in Japan, a new strategy for the treatment of both recurrent textile dermatitis and pigmented contact dermatitis was introduced. Based on the research project for finding out contact sensitizers and irritants in textiles [8], underwear with only four or five kinds of textile finishes which showed no evidence of positive reactions in patients with contact dermatitis, pigmented contact dermatitis, atopic dermatitis and healthy controls was put into mass production and became available. This is a measure to prevent the patients coming into contact with the responsible allergen in ordinary underwear again, and keeps the patients out of range of the responsible allergens.

Such allergen-free underwear for patients is called allergen-controlled wearing apparel (ACW) and has successfully counteracted pigmented contact dermatitis. The idea was inspired by the success of allergen-controlled cosmetics in 1970, which is discussed later (Sect. 15.1.3.3). It is not surprising that persistent secondary hyperpigmentation only disappears very slowly when the causative contact allergens are completely eliminated from the patient's environment for a long period, as the hyperpigmentation is considered to be brought about by frequent and repeated contact with a very small amount of contact sensitizer in the textile or washing material. Patients were requested to use allergen-free soaps and allergen-eliminated washing materials for their clothing at the same time, so that their skin was not contaminated by the responsible allergens in ordinary soaps and washing materials. Matsuo et al. reported several cases in which this treatment was successful [11, 12].

Even though cases are very rare, pigmented contact dermatitis can also occur following systemic contact dermatitis. In a 50-year-old man, for example, recurrent and persistent dermatitis accompanied diffuse secondary hyperpigmentation. The use of corticosteroid ointments, oral antihistamines and allergen-free soaps did not improve the condition at all. A patch test with nickel sulphate 5% aq. showed a strong positive reaction, with a focal flare of most of the original skin lesion. This implied not only that the patient was sensitive to nickel but also that only a few hundred parts per million of nickel ions absorbed from the patch test site into the bloodstream were enough to provoke an allergic reaction over a wide area of the site of the original skin lesions. This observation led to a search for a source of nickel ions in the patient, and five nickel alloys were subsequently found in the patient's oral cavity. He agreed to eliminate these nickel crowns, as they turned out to have been acting as cathodes, attracting an electric current of 1–3 mA at 100–200 mV. According to Faraday's law of electrolysis, cations elute from the cathode in proportion to the amount of electric current passing into the cathode.

The complete elimination of nickel-containing alloys from his oral cavity and their substitution with gold alloys, which did not contain any nickel at all, resulted in complete cure of the dermatitis and secondary hyperpigmentation in 3 months, and there has never been any recrudescence of the disease. The patient's pigmented contact dermatitis had been kept going for a long period by metal allergens continuously supplied from his own oral cavity [13].

15.1.3 Pigmented Cosmetic Dermatitis

15.1.3.1 Signs

The most commonly seen hyperpigmentation due to contact dermatitis in the history of dermatology must have been the pigmented cosmetic dermatitis which affected the faces of oriental women [14]. Innumerable patients with this pigmentary disorder presented in the 1960s and 1970s in Japan, and similar patients were also seen in Korea, India, Taiwan and China.

The signs of pigmented cosmetic dermatitis are diffuse or reticular, black or dark brown, hyperpigmentation of the face, which cannot be cured by the use of corticosteroid ointments or the continuous ingestion of vitamin C. The border of pigmented cosmetic dermatitis is not sharp, as in lichen planus or melasma, and it is not spot-like as in naevus of Ota tardus bilateralis.

Slight dermatitis is occasionally seen with hyperpigmentation, or dermatitis may precede hyperpigmentation. In contrast to Addison's disease, pigmented cosmetic dermatitis does not show any systemic symptoms such as weakness, fatigue and emaciation. Laboratory findings such as full blood count, liver function tests, daily urinary excretion of 17-ketosteroid and 17-hydroxy corticosteroid, and serum immunoglobulins and electrolytes are normal in the majority of patients with pigmented cosmetic dermatitis [14].

Histopathological examination of pigmented cosmetic dermatitis shows basal liquefaction degeneration of the epidermis and incontinentia pigmenti histologica. The epidermis is often atrophic, presumably the effect of frequently applied corticosteroid ointments for the treatment of itchy dermatitis of the face, and cellular infiltrates of lymphocytes and histiocytes are seen perivascularly, as is often seen in ordinary allergic contact dermatitis (Fig. 15.2).

In some cases, the dark brown or black hyperpigmentation is also seen on the skin other than on the face. The neck, chest and back can be involved and in a few exceptional cases, hyperpigmentation may extend to the whole body. In these cases, the allergens, cinnamic alcohol and its derivatives, sensitize the patients first from cosmetics and then provoke allergic reactions from soaps, domestic fabric softeners and food, all of which sometimes contain cinnamic derivatives. The ingestion of 1 gram cinnamon sugar from a supermarket in

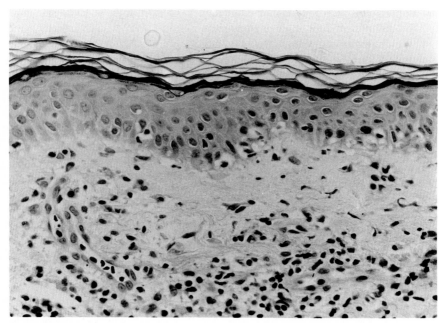

Fig. 15.2. Histopathology of a typical lichenoid reaction, with incontinentia pigmenti histologica of pigmented cosmetic dermatitis. The epidermis is atrophic, and liquefaction degeneration can be seen in the basal layer of the epidermis, which drops melanin into the upper dermis. Note that the cellular infiltration in the upper dermis is not as dense as in lichen planus

a cup of tea was enough to provoke a mild focal flare of dermatitis at the sites of diffuse reticular black hyperpigmentation of the whole body in one reported case [15]. When one of the common potent sensitizers producing pigmented cosmetic dermatitis, D & C Red 31 (Japanese name R-219), was discovered, a focal flare of dermatitis at the site of facial hyperpigmentation was occasionally noted. These findings show that the allergen could provoke the dermatitis not only by contact with the skin surface but also from within the skin, by allergens transported via blood vessels, just as allergic contact dermatitis can be provoked by the administration of small amounts of nickel or drugs.

15.1.3.2 Causative Allergens

The term 'pigmented cosmetic dermatitis' was introduced in 1973 for what had previously been known as melanosis faciei feminae when the mechanism (Type IV allergy), most of the causative allergens and successful treatment with allergen control for this miserable pigmentary disorder were clarified for the first time [16, 17]. The name was adopted by modifying Osmundsen's designation, pigmented contact dermatitis, for the disease caused by CH3566 on the trunk.

Historically, the first description of the disease goes back to 1948, when Japanese dermatologists encountered this peculiar pigmentary disorder for the first time, and were greatly embarrassed as to the diagnosis. Bibliographical surveys showed that Riehl's melanosis, described in 1917 [18], seemed probable, because World War II had ended just three years before the investigation. Subsequently, the disease was erroneously called Riehl's melanosis for almost 30 years in Asian countries. Riehl's melanosis, however, was a dark brown hyperpigmentation observed during World War I in Caucasian men, women and children, when food was extremely scanty and the patients had to eat decayed corn and weed crops instead of the normal food of peacetime. Besides hyperpigmentation of the face, ears and scalp, there were nodules and, histopathologically, dense cellular infiltration was present in the dermis. Cosmetics could be excluded as a cause, because it was during World War I, and it was not possible for all these people, especially the men and children, to have used cosmetics before they had the disease. Riehl could not discover the true cause of this pigmentary disorder, but suspected the role of the abnormal wartime diet [18]. Riehl's melanosis disappeared when World War I ended, when the people obtained normal food again, to reappear for a short period in France during the German occupation in World War II, when food again became scarce.

Consequently, Riehl's melanosis, a wartime melanosis having no relationship to cosmetic allergy, should not be confused with pigmented cosmetic dermatitis, which involved many Asian women in peacetime for many years. In 1950, Minami and Noma [19] designated the disease melanosis faciei feminae, and recognized the disease as a new entity. The causation was not known for many years. However, Japanese dermatologists gradually became aware of the role of cosmetics in this hyperpigmentation. Firstly, it occurred only on those women, and very exceptionally men, who used cosmetics and, secondly, even though the bizarre brown hyperpigmentation was so conspicuous, the presence of slight, recurrent, or preceding dermatitis was observed. The problem for the dermatologists at that time was that the components of cosmetics were completely secret, and the kinds of cosmetic ingredients were too many (more than 1,000) for their allergenicity to be evaluated.

Finally, in 1969, a research project was set up to identify the causative allergens from 477 cosmetic ingredients by patch and photopatch testing. It was a new idea, because melanosis faciei feminae had been regarded as a metabolic disorder rather than a type of contact dermatitis. This was 7 years before Finn Chambers became available: therefore, small patch test plasters of 10 × 2 cm with six discs 7 mm in diameter (Miniplaster) were put into production to enable 48–96 samples to be patch tested at one time on the backs of volunteer control subjects and patients. Many cosmetic ingredients, adjusted to nonirritant concentrations with the cooperation of 30–40 volunteers, were subsequently patch and photopatch tested in the patients. Results for each ingredient were obtained from 172 to 348 patients, including 79 to 121 with melanosis faciei feminae. Statistical evaluation brought to light a number of newly discovered contact sensitizers amongst the cosmetic ingredients, mainly fragrance materials and pigments, including jasmine absolute, ylang-ylang oil, cananga oil, benzyl salicylate, hydroxyc-itronellal, sandalwood oil, artificial sandalwood, geraniol, geranium oil, D & C Red 31 and Yellow No. 11 [14, 16, 17, 20].

15.1.3.3 Treatment

The above-mentioned research project at the same time included a plan to produce soaps (acylglutamate) and cosmetics for the patients from which the causative allergens were completely eliminated, as even those who suffered from severe and bizarre hyperpigmentation usually could not accept abandoning their use of cosmetics to remove this pigmentary disorder. Patch testing with a series of 30 standard cosmetic ingredients to find the allergens causing the disease, followed by the exclusive use of soaps and cosmetics that were completely allergen-free for such patients, designated the allergen control system, produced dramatic effects. Around 1970, most textbooks of dermatology in Japan said that melanosis faciei feminae was very difficult to cure and that the causation was unknown. However, after allergen control was introduced, the disease became completely curable. Table 15.2 shows the effect of allergen control in 165 cases reported to the American Academy of Dermatology in 1977, and also the long-term follow-up results of allergen control obtained by Watanabe after 3–11 years (mean, 5 years). In 50 cases of pigmented cosmetic dermatitis cured by allergen control (i.e.patch tests with

Table 15.2. Effect of allergen-controlled cosmetics on pigmented cosmetic dermatitis patients

	Nakayama 1977	Watanabe 1989 [43]
Total	165	53
Complete cure	52	40
Almost complete cure	21	0
Remarkable improvement	51	13
Improvement	22	0
Not Effective	19	0
Follow-up	3 months to 5 years	3–11 years (mean 5 years)

30 cosmetic series patch test allergens [22] followed by the exclusive use of allergen-free soaps and cosmetics), there were, on average, 2.5 allergens for each patient. It usually required 1–2 years for a patient to regain normal nonhyperpigmented facial skin (Fig. 15.3). Contamination with ordinary soaps and cosmetics was the most influential and decisive factor inhibiting therapy, because it was such ordinary daily necessities that contained the allergens producing the disease. The patients were therefore requested to visit the dermatologist once a month to be checked for improvement, and were persuaded every time to avoid such contamination, including products used in beauty parlours [14, 43].

In 1979, Kozuka [21] discovered a new contact sensitizer, phenylazo-2-naphthol (PAN), as an impurity in commercial supplies of D & C Red 31. Its sensitizing and ability and ability to produce secondary hyperpigmentation was as great as Yellow No. 11, so many industries began to eliminate or considerably decrease the amount of PAN and Yellow No. 11 in their products. The legal partial restriction of Red No. 31 and Yellow No. 11 by the Japanese government and the voluntary restriction by cosmetic companies of the use of allergenic fragrances, bactericides and pigments resulted in a remarkable decrease in pigmented cosmetic dermatitis after 1980. One of the reasons for the proposal to change the name from 'melanosis faciei feminae' to 'pigmented cosmetic dermatitis' [16] was that the latter name makes it easier for the patients to understand the causation of the disease and, at the same time, for industry to recognize the danger cosmetics represent in producing such disastrous pigmentary disorders through contact sensitization.

15.1.4 Purpuric Dermatitis

In 1896 Majocchi described purpura annularis telangiectodes and, 4 years later, Schamberg described a progressive pigmentary dermatitis which is now well-known as Schamberg's disease. The pigmentation in this dermatitis is due to the intradermal accumulation of haemosiderin, the predominant sites

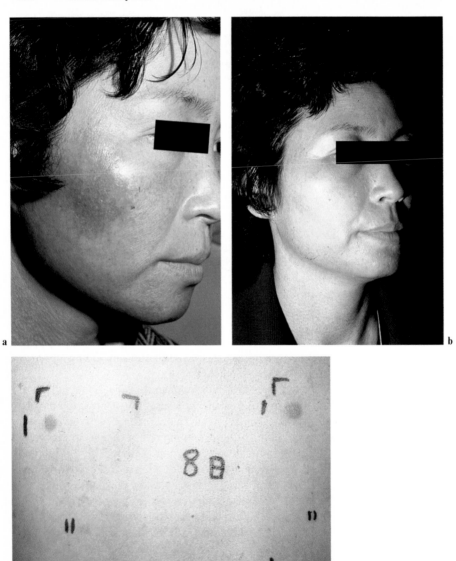

Fig. 15.3. a Pigmented cosmetic dermatitis in a 43-year-old woman, caused by cotact hypersensitivity to jasmin absolute. **b** Jasmin absolute 10% in petrolatum-produced (#) reactions (site 1) which were still positive even on the eighth day of the patch test. **c** The exclusive use of soaps and cosmetics that did not contain common and rare cosmetic sensitizers cleared the persistent dermatitis with pigmentation completely after year and 8 months of use

being the legs and thighs. Later, Gougerot and Blum described a similar dermatosis as pigmented purpuric lichenoid dermatitis.

The disease was rare but most often occurred in middle-aged or old men. However, when a similar disease occurred in many British soldiers during World War II, especially in those who sweated freely or experienced friction when wearing khaki shirts or woollen socks, or who suffered from severe pruritus, dermatitis and pigmentation due to purpura, dermatologists became aware that some textile finishes must have been responsible for the disease [23, 24]. Patch tests and use tests revealed that a blend of vegetable oils and oleic acid seemed to have been responsible.

In 1968, Batschvarov and Minkov [25] reported that rubber components such as 'N-phenyl-N'-isopropyl-p-phenylendiamine (IPPD), N-phenyl-β-naphthylamine (PNA), 2-mercaptobenzothiazole (MBT) and dibenzothiazole disulphide (DBS), i.e. derivatives of p-phenylenediamine, naphthylamine and benzothiazoles, were the allergens responsible for a purpuric dermatitis around the waist underneath the elastic of underwear. A similar pigmented dermatitis was recognized on the shoulders, breasts, groins and thighs. The capillary resistance (Rumpel-Leede) test was positive in all 23 cases studied. Similar test results were obtained in a smaller proportion of patients with the khaki dermatitis mentioned above. In Bulgaria, over 600 patients were recorded, and the necessity for dermatologists to investigate contact allergens in textiles to solve the problem of purpuric dermatitis of covered areas of skin was stressed [25].

15.2 Depigmentation from Contact with Chemicals

15.2.1 Mechanism of Leucoderma Due to Chemicals

There are at least three kinds of mechanism producing leucoderma from contact with chemicals:
1. Leucoderma due to selective destruction of melanocytes.
2. Leucomelanoderma or photoleucomelanoderma due to pigment blockade
3. Hypopigmentation due to reduction of melanin synthesis

Either allergic contact dermatitis or irritant contact dermatitis can produce a secondary leucoderma which is almost impossible to differentiate from idiopathic vitiligo. The incidence is low, except for certain phenol derivatives and catechols which produce a much higher incidence in workers who frequently come into contact with them.

Monobenzyl ether of hydroquinone (MBEH) has been known as a cause of occupational vitiligo since the 1930s [26], the main source of contact having been rubber, in which it is used as an antioxidant to prevent degeneration. The use of MBEH in the rubber industry today is rare, as it had a long history of causing occupational leucoderma by destroying melanocytes.

Instead, MBEH came to be used as a bleaching agent for melanotic skin, being used to treat diseases such as melasma and senile lentigo and by dark-skinned people for cosmetic purposes. However, as its toxic effect on melanocytes was too strong, the treatment often resulted in a mottled pattern of leucoderma (confetti-like depigmentation), which was worse than simple hyperpigmentation, and produced problems [42].

Historically, the next chemical to produce leucoderma by contact was 4-tert-butylcatechol (PTBC), known since the 1970s [28, 29]. Approximately half of the 75 workers in a tappet assembly plant in the United States were reported to have various grades of leucoderma from daily occupational contact with PTBC. Four severe cases reported in 1970 by Gellin et al. [28] initially had itchy erythematous reactions at the sites of contact, then developed sharply outlined or confluent leucoderma on the face, scalp, hands, fingers, forearms, etc. The patients were all Caucasians.

Patch tests revealed that 0.1% PTBC in acetone produced positive reactions in three of these four cases, one of whom later developed leucoderma at the site of the patch test. However, an exposure test with 1% PTBC in the assembly oil, carried out with occlusion of the forearms in six volunteers, failed to produce leucoderma artifically. Animal tests revealed that PTBC was an irritant, producing erythema and necrosis in albino rabbits, and a bleaching test with 10% PTBC in black guinea pigs resulted in depigmentation of the black skin, both macroscopically and histologically, by the loss of pigment in the epidermis and follicles.

Almost at the same time, at the begining of the 1970s, occupational contact leucoderma due to p-tert-butylphenol (PTBP) began to be recognized. The incidence of vitiligo vulgaris in the general population was considered to be less than 1%. Therefore, the presence of several cases of vitiligo, mainly located on exposed areas of skin, in the same factory of 20–30 workers alerted dermatologists to the fact that the depigmentation was an occupational dermatosis [30]. PTBP is contained in cobblers' glues, shoes cemented with rubber glues, resins, industrial oils, paints, adhesives, bactericides, plasticizers for cellulose acetate, printing inks, etc. [30–33].

The changes produced by PTBP are similar to those caused by p-tert-butylcatechol, and can occur with or without sensitization. Kahn [31] and Romaguera et al. [34] reported cases who were apparently sensitized to PTBP with positive reactions on a closed patch test with 1% PTBP.

Hydroquinone is an excellent depigmenting agent for clinical treatment of various pigmentations [35]. However, it may rarely produce leucoderma which is similar to vitiligo vulgaris [36–38]. The mechanism of the hypopigmentation caused by hydroquinone is thought to be decreased formation of melanosomes and destruction of the membranous organelles in the melanocytes, thus causing degeneration of melanocytes [39].

These historically accumulated cases of contact leucoderma caused by phenol derivatives indicate that selective toxicity of these chemicals to melanocytes is the main cause of leucoderma, judging from the degeneration

Table 15.3. Chemicals producing leucoderma or hypopigmentation on contact

Hydroquinone	
Monobenzyl ether of hydroquinone	
p-*tert*-butylcatechol (PTBC)	
p-*tert*-butylphenol (PTBP)	
Kojic acid (hypopigmentation only)	
Catechol	
MOnomethyl ether of hydroquinone (MMEH)	
Alstroemeria components (tulipalin A)	
Squaric acid dibutylester	
Cerium oxide CeO₂	

of melanocytes, the irritation often noted, and the fact that sensitization is not always demonstrated.

Another hazard of using hydroquinone as a bleaching agent is ochronosis, especially when it is used at high concentrations (eg. 3.5–7.5%) [46]. Ochronosis means 'yellow disease', and black Africans suffer from hyperpigmentation of the face due to the degeneration of elastic fibres caused by this topical agent [47]. Therefore, the use of hydroquinone as a bleaching agent by blacks should be advised carefully, and high concentrations are not recommended.

15.2.2 Contact Leucoderma Caused Mainly by Contact Sensitization

Very rarely, allergic contact dermatitis produces a secondary depigmentation like vitiligo. A gardner was reported to have developed secondary leucoderma after allergic contact dermatitis due to alstroemeria [40] and, when squaric acid dibutylester was used for immunotherapy in a 26-year-old male with alopecia areata, depigmentation over the whole scalp was reported after repeated contact dermatitis produced by nine courses of treatment. Regrowth of hair was also noted [41]. A herbicide, Carbyne R, and musk ambrette have also been reported to produce contact hypersensitivity and secondary leucoderma [44, 45].

15.3 References

1. Papa CM, Kligman AM (1965) The behavior of melanocytes in inflammation. J Invest Dermatol 45: 465–474
2. Nakamura T (1977) Toxicoderma caused by "Shiitake", lentinus edodos. Rinsho-Hifuka 31: 65–68 (in Japanese)
3. Osmundsen PE (1969) Contact dermatitis due to an optical whitener in washing powders. Br J Dermatol 81: 799–803
4. Osmundsen PE (1970) Pigmented contact dermatitis Br J Dermatol 83: 296–301
5. Ancona-Alayón A, Escobar-Márques R, González-Mendoza A et al. (1976) Occupational pigmented contact dermatitis from Naphthol AS. Contact Dermatitis 2: 129–134
6. Kawachi S, Kawashima T, Akiyama J et al. (1985) Pigmented contact dermatitis due to dyes from nightgown. Hifuka no Rinsho 27: 91–92, 181–187 (in Japanese)
7. Hayakawa R, Matsunaga K, Kojima S, et al. (1985) Naphthol AS as a cause of pigmented contact dermatitis. Contact Dermatitis 13: 20–25
8. Nakayama H, Suzuki A (1985) Investigation of skin disturbances caused by the chemicals contained in daily necessities, Part 1. On the ability to produce dermatitis of textile finishes. Tokyo - To Living Division Report: 1–27 (in Japanese)
9. Takayama N, Suzuki T, Sakurai Y, et al. (1984) Friction Melanosis. Nishinihon Hifuka (West Japan Dermatol) 46: 1340–1345 (in Japanese)
10. Tanigaki T, Hata S, Kitano M, et al. (1983) On peculiar melanosis occuring on the trunk and extremities. Rinsho-Hifuka 37: 347–351 (in Japanese)
11. Matsuo S, Nakayama H & Suzuki A (1989) Successful treatment with allergen controlled wearing apparel of textile dermatitis patients. Hifu 31, Suppl. 6: 178–185 (in Japanese)
12. Nakayama H (1989) Allergen control, an indispensable treatment for allergic contact dermatitis. Dermat Clinics 8: 197–204
13. Nakayama H (1987) Dental metal and allergy. Jpn J Dent Ass 40: 893–903 (in Japanese)
14. Nakayama H, Matsuo S, Hayakawa K et al. (1984) Pigmented cosmetic dermatitis. Int J Dermatol 23: 299–305
15. Matsuo S & Nakayama H (1984) A case of pigmented dermatitis induced by cinnamic derivatives. Hifu 26: 573–579 (in Japanese)
16. Nakayama H (1974) Perfume allergy and cosmetic dermatitis. Jpn J Dermatol 84: 659–667 (in Japanese)
17. Nakayama H, Hanaoka H, Ohshiro A (1974) Allergen controlled system. Kanehara Shuppen, Tokyo, pp 1–42

18. Riehl von G (1917) Ueber eine eigenartige Melanose. Wien Klin Wochenschr 30: 780–781
19. Minami S, Noma Y (1950) Melanosis faciei feminae. Dermatol Urol 12: 73–77 (in Japanese)
20. Nakayama H, Harada R, Toda M (1976) Pigmented cosmetic dermatitis. Int J Dermatol 15: 673–675
21. Nakayama H (1983) Cosmetic series patch test allergens, types 19 and 20. Fragrance Journal Publications, Tokyo, pp 1–121 (in Japanese, with English abstract)
22. Kozuka T, Tashiro M, Sano S et al. (1979) Brilliant Lake Red R as a cause of pigmented contact dermatitis. Contact Dermatitis 5: 297–304
23. Greenwood K (1960) Dermatitis with capillary fragility. Arch Dermatol 81: 947–952
24. Twiston Davies JH, Neish Barker A (1944) Testile dermatitis. Br J Dermatol 56: 33–43
25. Batschvarov B, Minkov DM (1968) Dermatitis and purpura from rubber in clothing. Trans St John's Hosp Dermatol Soc 54: 178–182
26. Oliver EA, Schwartz L, Warren LH (1939) Occupational leukoderma: preliminary report. JAMA 113: 927–928
27. Van der Veen, JPW, Neering H, DeHaan P et al. (1988) Pigmented purpuric clothing dermatitis due to Disperse Blue 85. Contact Dermatitis 19: 222–223
28. Gellin GA, Possik PA, Davis I H (1970) Occupational depigmentation due to 4-tertiarybutyl catechol (TBC). J Occup Med 12: 386–389
29. Gellin GA, Maibach HI, Mislaszek MH, Ring M (1979) Detection of environmental depigmenting substances. Contact Dermatitis 5: 201–213
30. Malten KE, Sutter E, Hara I, Nakajima T (1971) Occupational vitiligo due to parateriary butylphenol and homologues. Trans St John's Hosp Dermatol Soc 57: 115–134
31. Kahn G (1970) Depigmentation caused by phenolic detergent germicides. Arch Dermatol 102: 177–187
32. Malten KE (1967) Contact sensitization caused by *p-tert*-butylphenol and certain phenolformaldehyde-containing glues. Dermatologica 135: 54–59
33. Malten KE (1975) Paratertiary butylphenol depigmentation in a consumer. Contact Dermatitis 1: 180–192
34. Romaguera C, Grimalt F (1981) Occupational leukoderma and contact dermatitis from paratertiary-butylphenol. Contact Dermatitis 7: 159–160
35. Arndt KA, Fitzpatrick TB (1965) Topical use of hydroquinone as a depigmenting agent. JAMA 194: 965–967
36. Frenk E, Loi-Zedda P (1980) Occupational depigmentation due to a hydroquinone-containing photographic developer. Contact Dermatitis 6: 238–239
37. Kersey P, Stevenson CJ (1981) Vitiligo and occupational exposure to hydroquinone from servicing self-photographing machines. Contact Dermatitis 7: 285–287
38. Whittington CV (1981) Hypopigmentation from UV resin additive. Contact Dermatitis 7: 289–292
39. Jimbow K, Obata H, Pathak M, Fitzpatrick TB (1974) Mechanism of depigmentation by hydroquinone. J Invest Dermatol 62: 436–449
40. Björkner BE (1982) Contact allergy and depigmentation from alstromeria. Contact Dermatitis 8: 178–184
41. Valsecchi R, Cainelli T (1984) Depigmentation from squaric acid dibutyl ester. Contact Dermatitis 10: 108
42. Yoshida Y, Usuba M (1958) Monobenzyl ether of hydroquinone leukomelanodermia. Rinsho Hifuka Hinyokika 12: 333–338 (in Japanese)
43. Watanabe N (1989) Long term follow-up of allergen control system on patients with cosmetic dermatitis. Nishinihon Hifuka 51: 113–130 (in Japanese)
44. Brancaccio RR, Chamales MH (1977) Contact dermatitis and depigmentation produced by the herbicide carbyne. Contact Dermatitis 3: 108–109

45. Rapaport MJ (1982) Depigmentation with cerium oxide. Contact Dermatitis 8: 282–283

46. Findlay GH (1982) Ochronosis following skin bleaching with hydroquinone. J Am Acad Dermatol 6: 1092–1093

47. Hoshaw RA, Zimmerman KG, Menter A (1985) Ochronosis - like pigmentation from hydroquinone bleaching creams in American Blacks. Arch Dermatol 121: 105–108

Chapter 16
The Management
of Contact Dermatitis

The Management of Contact Dermatitis

John D. Wilkinson

Contents

Contact dermatitis can be properly treated only if it is first recognized. Management of contact dermatitis therefore involves the following stages: (a) suspicion and recognition [1] (see also Chap. 7), (b) identification of the factors involved, (c) interpretation of patch test results (see also Sect. 10.1).

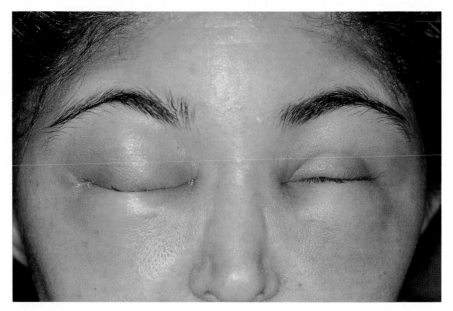

Fig. 16.1. Acute contact dermatitis in a patient allergic to *p*-phenylenediamine in a hair dye, mimicking angio-oedema

16.1 Suspicion and Recognition of Contact Dermatitis

At times the diagnosis of contact dermatitis is straightforward. At other times, it may mimic constitutional eczema [2] and even angio-oedema (Fig. 16.1). Certain occupational groups are more susceptible to irritant contact dermatitis (Table 16.1), as are those with atopic eczema. For allergic contact dermatitis, there are particular at-risk sites, such as the lower legs in patients with stasis eczema/ulceration, and certain allergen-related occupational groups [3] (Sect. 11.17).

When considering the possibility of contact dermatitis, it is helpful to divide a patient's life into separate environmental areas (Table 16.2). At

Table 16.1. Occupations with a high risk of cumulative irritant contact dermatitis

Housework
Catering
Cleaning
Nursing
Building and construction
Hairdressing
Motor mechanics
Engineering (cutting oils)
Gardening and horticulture
Dairy farming

Table 16.2. Environmental areas

Personal space:	clothes, cosmetics
Near space:	house, garden flowers
Occasional space:	holidays, neighbours, relatives
Play space:	hobbies, cars
Work space:	factory, office

the centre is the patient's personal environment, with potential exposure to cosmetics, toiletries, clothing and connubial [4] contact allergens. The next most immediate environment can be divided into work and home (including the garden). Beyond this is the general environment.

When assessing contamination of a working environment (Sect. 11.12.13), allergens are more critical than irritants. Airborne patterns of dermatitis may, however, be due to both irritants and allergens. Low ambient humidity may also be a factor in some cases of dermatitis [5].

Sites of frequent medicament use (especially damaged or occluded skin, e.g. perianal dermatitis, otitis externa, etc. [6–9]) and chronic or recurrent hand eczema are always worth patch testing since allergy may be occult. Allergy also frequently exists in patients with hand and face dermatitis. The hands are a common site as well for irritant contact dermatitis. Patch testing sometimes reveals a hidden allergen which was not known to be present in a product [10].

16.2 Identification of the Factors Involved in Contact Dermatitis

Contact dermatitis may be simultaneously irritant and allergic. Constitutional factors (especially atopy) may coexist [11].

Whether a patient is atopic is best determined on the basis of history, examination and prick testing. These individuals are at greater risk of irritant contact dermatitis, particularly if they have had atopic eczema or eczema involving the hands [12, 13]. They are not, however, at increased risk of allergic contact dermatitis (except, debatably, from nickel) [14–16]. The principal irritants are listed in Table 16.3. It is important not to forget the role of frictional and

Table 16.3. Principle irritants in contact dermatitis

Water
Skin cleansers
Detergents and solvents
Acids and alkalis
Cutting oils
Chemicals, e.g. peroxides, reducing agents
Physical and mechanical factors
Biological agents

climatic factors. Repeated trauma from swarf (metal fragments) in cutting oils, for example, may be contributory. Wet work increases the risk of hand dermatitis [14, 17, 18]. A history of metal sensitivity also increases the risk of developing hand eczema [19].

Allergens can be identified only by patch testing. At least 50% of relevant allergens are missed unless patch testing is undertaken both to standard allergens and to allergens relevant to the patient's home, personal and work environments [20]. In cases in which occupational dermatitis is suspected, a visit to the factory or place of employment is often extremely helpful [21] (Sect. 11.12.4).

16.3 Interpretation of Patch Test Results

As a general rule, patch tests tend to be 'over-read'. Only definite (+) positive reactions should be regarded as significant. Weak (?+) and follicular reactions are less reproducible and may represent nonspecific irritant responses, especially in atopics [22] or in those with an 'angry back' [23]. Doubtful reactions should therefore be retested singly or tested in a range of dilutions. The problems of false-positive and false-negative patch test reactions and the phenomena of compound allergy [24–26] and compound irritancy are discussed in more detail elsewhere (Sect. 10.1).

Clearly, establishing whether someone is truly allergic to a substance is crucial to the management of all patients with contact dermatitis. Too often, those with atopic or seborrhoeic eczema who have mild, follicular responses to metals and other patients with marginally irritant responses to various standard allergens such as potassium dichromate, carba mix, formaldehyde or lanolin are told that they are allergic to these allergens and then given misleading medical or medicolegal advice [27]. It is therefore particularly important to repeat tests showing dubious and weaker reactions and to test individually any component of a mix or proprietary product, especially in individuals susceptible to irritant reactions and in those with multiple positive reactions. Controls are necessary for all nonstandard allergens.

Not all errors, however, occur as a result of over-reading. Sometimes an ingredient may be present in a product at too low a concentration for sensitivity to be elicited on just one exposure, Properly, in addition to the actual product, the ingredients of each cosmetic or medicament need to be tested individually at appropriate concentrations and in appropriate vehicles. Sometimes repeat testing may be necessary. A repeat open application test is often helpful in establishing allergy [28], as is a use test on previously affected skin (Sect. 10.1). Most strong allergies persist – particularly those to metals – but weaker allergies may be lost with time, probably because of downregulation [29] and/or successful avoidance of the allergen. New allergies also occur with time. Some consider that a history of metal sensitivity with negative patch tests suggests atopy [30], but others disagree [31].

16.4 Advice and Counselling

Patients require precise counselling both on the primary cause of their dermatitis and as regards any cofactors that may exist, such as constitutional factors, reduced barrier function, complicating secondary allergies, type I sensitivities (contact urticaria) and irritant factors at work and at home. They need information as to the main sources of any allergen to which they are sensitive and details of cross-reacting chemicals [32], and they also need advice on the complicating role of secondary infection. Sometimes simple changes in handling routines or the avoidance of solvent-based cleansers may be sufficient to cure a case of contact dermatitis. Dermatitis induced by either irritants or allergens not only damages the skin barrier but may also stimulate inflammation and lead to an excited-skin syndrome [33], thus reducing the threshold for development of further dermatitis. Chronic exposure to low concentrations of marginal irritants may, conversely, in some individuals, lead to hardening and hyporeactivity [34].

16.5 Creation of a Low-Risk Environment

Helping a patient to create a low-risk environment may well necessitate a visit to the factory and liaison with management, factory hygienists/engineers and specialists in occupational health [35] (Sect. 11.12.4). For those with a specific allergy, the possibility of allergen avoidance or allergen substitution needs to be discussed [36]. Sometimes this can be achieved by a change in the chemicals used at work; other times it is possible to achieve the same result by mechanization or automation. For both irritants and allergens, one must consider the appropriateness and choice of protective gloves and the possible use of 'barrier' creams, after-work emollients and the provision of mild cleansing agents [37] (Sect. 11.14.4). Back-up knowledge of the 'break-through' times of various chemicals as regards different types of glove is also required [38–40]. Polyvinyl chloride gloves, for instance, give good protection against methyl methacrylate [41]. Gloves are, however, sometimes impractical and in certain situations may actually be dangerous. Rubber gloves may themselves be a cause of contact dermatitis [42] or contact urticaria [43], and plastic gloves may generally be preferred.

In situations in which the allergen cannot be avoided, and when exposure to this allergen causes persistent or recurrent dermatitis, a change of employment should be considered (Sect. 11.13.2). Often it should be possible for an individual to be relocated within the same company. Adequate retraining and protection of income are two important factors for such relocation to be a success.

In patients with chronic irritant contact dermatitis, efforts should be made to reduce both the severity and frequency of the irritant load both at work and at home. A period off work to allow the skin to heal may be necessary to allow time for the skin barrier to recover. This may take much longer than overt clinical cure. Resuming work should proceed slowly to allow for hardening, and as many of the adverse factors as possible must be corrected before the patient returns to work, or the dermatitis will recur. In those working with 'soluble' cutting oils, dermatitis is practically endemic but can usually be minimized by appropriate care and training. Prevention of such dermatitis is important, since, once established, soluble oil dermatitis may fail to resolve even after specialist treatment and change of job [44]. Preemployment screening, hand care advice, good machine care and attention to the correct dilution of soluble oil help to minimize the risk of dermatitis (Sect. 11.16.1).

16.6 Treatment of Acute Contact Dermatitis

Acute irritant reactions range from a mild transient irritant reaction through eczematous reactions indistinguishable from allergic contact dermatitis to chemical burns such as are sometimes seen with cement. Avoidance of the primary cause, with suitable protection and reconditioning of the skin with emollients, and treatment of ulcerated areas as for burns, lead to healing. Caustic burns may lead to scarring and, when severe, may best be treated by immediate excision and grafting.

It should be remembered that, even in milder cases of dermatitis, the skin barrier is damaged, and the skin remains vulnerable for several weeks after apparent clinical resolution. For eczematous reactions, a topical corticosteroid cream can be prescribed to reduce inflammation. For more severe reactions, wet compresses or wet soaks – saline, aluminium subacetate (Burow's solution) and/or dilute (1 in 10000) potassium permanganate solution – may be useful initially. Where there is skin loss, antiseptic creams and occlusive nonadherent dressings may be required.

Acute allergic contact reactions may require systemic corticosteroids if widespread or severe. Poison ivy/oak dermatitis [45] and erythema-multiforme-like reactions [46, 47] sometimes require treatment with systemic corticosteroids. Otherwise, topical corticosteroid creams with wet soaks (if indicated) and symptomatic measures such as sedative antihistamines usually suffice. Occlusive polythene gloves can be applied on top of corticosteroid for short periods in those with early acute vesicular eczema, as long as there is no secondary infection.

16.7 Treatment of Subacute Contact Dermatitis

Treatment is mainly with topical corticosteroids. These can be divided into four groups according to potency (Table 16.4) [48]. Usually, mild topical corticosteroids such as 1% hydrocortisone suffice for facial contact eczema. Potent topical corticosteroids such as betamethasone valerate 0.1% are,

Table 16.4. Topical corticosteroids [48]

Mild
Hydrocortisone base or acetate 0.1%–2.5%
Alclometasone dipropionate 0.05%
Fluocinolone acetonide 0.0025%[a]
Hydrocortisone 0.5% with sodium chloride and urea[a]
Methylprednisolone 0.25%

Moderately Potent
Clobetasone butyrate 0.05%
Desoxymethasone 0.05%
Fluocinolone acetonide 0.00625%[a]
Flucortolone hexanoate 0.1%
Fluocortolone privalate 0.1%
Flucocortolone 0.25%
Fluocortolone hexanoate 0.25%
Fluandrenolone 0.0125%
Fluandrenolone 0.05%
Hydrocortisone 1% with urea[a]

Potent
Beclomethasone dipropionate 0.025%
Betamethasone dipropionate 0.05%
Betamethasone valerate 0.025%[a]
Betamethasone valerate 0.1%
Budesonide 0.025%
Desoxymethasone 0.25%
Diflucortolone valerate 0.1%
Fluclorolone acetonide 0.025%
Fluocinolone acetonide 0.025%
Fluocinonide 0.05%
Hydrocortisone 17-butyrate 0.1%
Triamcinolone acetonide 0.1%

Very Potent
Clobetasol propionate 0.05%
Diflucortolone valerate 0.3%
Halcinonide 0.1%

---

[a]therapeutic potency is dependent on the inherent potency of the steroid as well as percutaneous absorption and other factors.

however, often necessary to treat eczema of the hands or feet. Sometimes a very potent corticosteroid such as clobetasol proprinate 0.05% may be required for a short time in cases of vesicular or hyperkeratotic eczema of the palms and soles.

These potent corticosteroids should not be used for long, however, or otherwise steroid atrophy results (especially on the backs of the hands or when used elsewhere than on the hands). A potent corticosteroid can also be used to treat localized areas of contact eczema elsewhere (avoiding the face or flexures), but for more widespread eczema a moderately potent cortico-steroid such as clobetasone butyrate 0.05% is preferred. Weak or moderately potent corticosteroids are also advised for flexures and for children.

When there is coexistent secondary infection, a corticosteroid-antimicrobial combination is often helpful. Some such combinations, however, contain well-known sensitizers such as neomycin and ethylenediamine, and combinations with less sensitizing antimicrobials such as fusidic acid, tetracyclines, hydrox-yquinolines and imidazoles are therefore to be preferred. Systemic antibiotics may be used when there is significant secondary bacterial infection.

When prescribing a topical corticosteroid, it is important to choose not only an appropriate strength but also an appropriate vehicle. Gels, lotions and creams are suitable for hairy areas. Greams are normally best for flexures, for more acute eczemas and for eczema of the hands. Ointments can be used for chronic, dry and hyperkeratotic eczema. Customarily they are applied twice daily, but a very nearly equal therapeutic effect can often be obtained by once daily or even alternate day application.

With a weak topical corticosteroid few restrictions need to be applied to its use. Continued use, however, should suggest the possibility that the cause of the dermatitis has not been adequately identified or avoided. For potent topical corticosteroids such as betamethasone valerate 0.1%, short-term use should not exceed 100 g/week, and for very potent corticosteroids such as clobetasol proprionate 0.05% short-term use should not exceed 30–50 g/week.

Soap substitutes such as aqueous cream (ung. emulsif. aquos.) and Unguentum Merck (E. Merck) can be used to avoid the detergency and irritant effects of soaps and detergents. Some soaps and detergents are probably milder than others. Each country has its favourites. In the United States Dove soap has a reputation for mildness and in the United Kingdom Neutrogena. Few comparative studies have been published, and the results of closed patch testing or scratch-patch tests may not adequately reflect the situation in real life. Emollients may be helpful to counter dryness.

Patients with hand eczema and those merely with dry skin usually prefer oil-in-water (aqueous) emollient creams. Those with atopic eczema and those with very dry skins require a high fat oil-in-water cream, a water-in-oil (oily) cream or ointments. Again, preferences and options vary from country to country and from patient to patient. During the winter, especially in situations of low ambient humidity, a more occlusive emollient may be preferred.

Topical corticosteroids are often used for all types of contact dermatitis, but at least experimentally they have not been shown to have much effect in restoring the skin barrier or reducing chronic irritant contact dermatitis [49]. One would expect them, however, to exert an antiinflammatory and healing effect, whatever the cause of an eczema. Systemic antibiotics may be used when there is significant secondary infection.

16.8 Treatment of Chronic and Chronic-Relapsing Dermatitis

In some situations, dermatitis may continue in spite of all advice. For some with atopic eczema the total environmental irritant load (at work and at home) is simply too much for their vulnerable skin, and their skin barrier never completely heals. Others unable to change their employment accept a degree of chronic dermatitis. This situation is common among atopics exposed to irritants, i.e. housewives, nurses, hairdressers, caterers, cleaners, etc.

Some individuals are unable to avoid further contact with the allergen to which they are sensitized. This is particularly so with certain allergens such as nickel (hairdressers, cleaners, nurses) [50, 51], chromate (builders, construction workers, etc.) [15] and sesquiterpene lactones (e.g. foresters exposed to *Furllania* horticulturalists exposed to Compositae; on the latter, see Sect. 10.5.3.1). I have also seen similar chronic dermatitis in those sensitive to wood dust. Appropriate advice to minimize exposure, coupled with longterm use of medium-potency topical corticosteroids may allow some of these patients to continue at work, albeit with some degree of dermatitis. For others, more potent treatments may be necessary, such as low-dose oral corticosteroids (combined with azathioprine in those with chronic actinic dermatitis due to Compositae). In others, psoralen + ultraviolet A (PUVA) therapy may be considered. Occlusive mild tar bandages can be effective in patients with chronic fissured dermatitis of the fingers and may be applied over corticosteroid at night.

16.9 Information Sheets and Test Kits

Most patients benefit from being given information sheets. These are normally one of two types: general sheets giving advice about hand care both at home (Appendix A) and at work (Appendix B [52]) and allergen-related advice sheets giving information as to the main sources of allergen, cross-reacting chemicals, synonyms, etc. These are well-known and an example only is given in Appendix C.

The dimethylglyoxime spot test is very useful for patients who are nickel allergic (Sect. 10.3). Not only can they then identify any nickel-releasing items of jewellery or clothing accessories, but they can also use the test kit at home and at work to identify other sources of nickel contact [53]. Some very sensitive individuals may, however, react to jewellery below the threshold of detection of the nickel test kit [54]. Other spot tests such as the test for formaldehyde [55] can be undertaken only in the clinic but, again, are useful for identifying the allergen, particularly when ingredients are not declared by the manufacturer.

Knowledge of occupational allergens and the risks inherent in each type of employment is necessary for the successful therapy of contact dermatitis (Sect. 11.17). In general, even relatively modest exposure to the allergen is sufficient to induce a flare-up of allergic contact dermatitis. Irritants – apart from certain strong irritants (mainly acids or alkalis) – usually cause dermatitis only by repetitive exposure. The actual irritant is not always the same, and frictional [56] and chemical factors may combine to cause a cumulative irritant contact dermatitis [57, 58].

There remain two widespread misconceptions about irritants: the first is that all irritants act in the same way and induce a similar pattern of response [59]; the second is that irritant and allergic contact dermatitis can usually be easily differentiated both clinicaly and histologically. Although some patterns of irritant and allergic contact dermatitis are characteristic, the clinical appearance, and often the histology and even the immunocytochemistry, may be indistinguishable. It is also becoming apparent that irritants are diverse in their pattern of damage to the skin and not nearly as stereotyped as was once thought (see Sect. 2.2).

16.10 Causes of Persistence

Dermatitis, once initiated, may persist even if the primary insult is removed and even following change of employment [60]. This may in part be due to a damaged skin barrier allowing penetration of secondary irritants at work and at home. Exposure at home, in second jobs or in the course of leisure pursuits is often significant but overlooked [13]. It may also be due to persistence of low levels of the primary allergen or cross-reacting allergens, or it may be due to underlying constitutional factors. A hand eczema that begins as an allergic or irritant contact dermatitis may continue as a hand eczema even when the original cause has been removed, the initial dermatitis perhaps acting simply as a 'trigger'. These post-insult eczemas, which frequently mimic constitutional-type eczemas, are often poorly served by both the legal and the medical professions.

Dermatitis may also persist due to secondary allergens (often the result of treatment), such as medicaments, topical corticosteroids [61–64] and chemicals in rubber gloves [42]. There are probably other, as unknown, factors causing persistence of an eczema. Eczema may certainly induce eczema elsewhere [65], and an eczema, once initiated, may persist even when all primary and secondary factors have been dealt with (Sect. 11.11). Chromate dermatitis is notorious for its persistence. This has, in the past, been ascribed to the ubiquitousness of this allergen, but a recent study showed no excess of chromate in air samples, and more evidence for this hypothesis is still required [66].

Secondary infection is a frequent cause of some eczemas not responding to conventional treatment. Environmental factors such as cold, heat, low or high humidity may also be important, as may coexistent physical trauma from swarf, abrasives and dust.

It is important to discuss with the patient the fact that skin barrier function remains impaired for some weeks after an episode of dermatitis [57] and to adjust his or her work accordingly. A too-early return to work increases the risk of recurrence, which may worsen the long-term prognosis. Recurrent occupational dermatitis has a worse prognosis.

Other potential causes of persistence such as hidden allergens, occult atopy and/or persisting anxiety should be sought. Occasionally, financial and medicolegal considerations have an adverse effect on the healing of the dermatitis.

Some cases of persistence are due to incorrect diagnosis, for instance, psoriasis and fungal infection. Also, the longer the delay until the patient receives specialist care, the worse may be the prognosis for the eczema.

In reality, however, we simply do not know why some eczemas persist.

16.11 Theoretical Aspects and Mechanisms of Action in Respect of Treatment of Contact Dermatitis [67]

Topical corticosteroids have been shown to inhibit nickel-positive patch test reactions and to reduce the number of Langerhans' cells and T cells in the skin [67, 68]. They do not, experimentally at least, appear to have any effect on chronic irritant dermatitis, nor do they improve barrier function [49].

Application of a strongly sensitizing chemical such 2, 4-dinitrofluoroben-zene to irradiated skin or skin treated with arachidonic acid leads to antigen-specific tolerance [69]. Both UVB and higher concentrations of topical arachidonic acid reduce Langerhans' cell counts in the skin and alter immune response [70]. Several mechanisms have been proposed for the immunosuppressive and tolerogenic effects of UVL (UVB). UVL stimulates the development of suppressor T lymphocytes [71] and causes the release of UVL-mediated cytokines (prostaglandin E_2 and nonprostaglandin substances) which inhibit cellular hypersensitivity [69, 72, 73]. Langerhans' cell depletion is greatest with PUVA and UVB but also occurs with UVL and tape stripping [74]. UVA alone does not have the same effect [75]. Recent work suggests that UVL has both hapten-specific and nonspecific effects [76], and that DNA pyrimidine dimers may also be involved in suppression of contact sensitivity following UVB [77]. Interleukin 1 also depresses the cellular response, probably through the generation and action of prostaglandins [78].

Local and systemic desensitization has also been induced – albeit on only a temporary basis – by repeat epicutaneous application of hapten [79]. Induction of specific tolerance can also be achieved by prior application of another strongly sensitizing chemical. This technique has been used experimentally to induce tolerance to urushiol (poison oak/ivy) [80]. Thlerance to urushiol-type haptens has also been achieved by blocking C5 position on the catechol ring [81].

Animal experiments have shown that interleukin 2 is necessary to convert a tolerogenic stimulus induced by intravenous injections of hapten-modified cells [82]. Cyclosporin A has also been shown to prevent induction and expression of cellular hypersensitivity, with inhibition of interleukin 2, which leads to a reduction in patch test response [83], a reduction in lymphocytes and inhibition of allergic reactions to 2, 4-dinitrofluorobenzene.

Irritants may also cause a decrease in the number of Langerhans' cells within the epidermis. At present, it is not always possible to separate irritant and allergic responses by means of their cellular responses.

Sensitization has been shown to vary with concentration of allergen applied per square centimetre [84]; density of allergen and activity of Langerhans' cells may therefore both be important.

One other observation which may help to unravel the mechanisms of allergic contact dermatitis is the reduction in reactivity that is often seen in vitiliginous skin [85, 86].

Whereas at present it does not seem possible to induce tolerance in patients already sensitized to an allergen, there do now appear to be ways in which one could, in theory at least, induce tolerance to specific allergens before accidental exposure and sensitization. This is possible either by epicutaneous application of allergen following UVL, by application of arachidonic acid, or possibly by prior oral induction of tolerance [87, 88], as appears to occur in some patients who received dental prosthetic work prior to any sensitizing contact from nickel-containing earrings [89] (see Sect. 2.1).

16.12 Other Specific Forms of Treatment

Apart from topical and systemic corticosteroids and the occasional use of cytotoxic/immunosuppressive drugs, little has been written on the treatment of contact dermatitis [90].

Phototherapy. PUVA therapy has been used to treat nickel contact dermatitis and has also been shown to be superior to UVB in the treatment of chronic palmar eczema [91]. Both cause a reduction in the number of epidermal Langerhans' cells [92]. UVB has both a local and a systemic effect on allergic contact dermatitis. UVB alone has no such effect [93]. Patch testing should not therefore be performed during a course of UVB therapy or when there is excessive sun exposure. PUVA has also been used to suppress nonimmunological immediate contact reactions [94].

Grenz Rays. The use of grenz ('borderline') rays [95] has been shown to be of benefit in treating chronic hand eczema. These reduce the OKT6+ Langerhans' cell population within the epidermis and inhibit nickel-positive patch test reactions [96]. However they have little effect on the infiltrate of irritant contact dermatitis [97]. From this it has been postulated that Langerhans' cells may be necessary for the effector phase of allergic contact dermatitis as well as for the induction of allergic contact dermatitis [98].

Chelation. Both disulfiram (Antabuse) [99–101] and triethylenetetramine (Trientine) [102] have been used as chelators of metals in patients with contact sensitivity, and topical ethylenediaminetetraacetate has been proposed as a barrier cream for those with nickel sensitivity [103]. Antabuse appears to be effective but requires abstinence from alcohol, and often there is an initial flare-up of contact dermatitis due to release of metal from stores within the body. Subsequently, dermatitis is often improved. The hazards, however, of using either Trientine or Antabuse have tended to limit this form of treatment.

Immunosuppressives. Corticosteroids are well established in the treatment of contact dermatitis (particularly allergic contact dermatitis), and azathioprine is used both as a steroid-sparing drug and, more particularly, in patients with actinic dermatitis/actinic reticuloid, especially in those patients sensitive to Compositae. Cyclosporin A has also been shown specifically to inhibit the cellular hypersensitivity response but seems to have no nonspecific effect on irritant-type reactions [104].

Induction of Tolerance. Attempts to induce tolerance [105, 106] have occasionally been successful for urushiol (poison oak/ivy) [107] and for *Parthenium* [108–110]. Other researchers, however, have found the technique unsuccessful [111].

Other treatments. Dapsone has been used to treat cement dermatitis. It was thought that this perhaps acts by reducing oxygen intermediates in the skin [112]. Post-insult emollients failed to reduce the severity of irritant contact dermatitis [113]. It has also not been possible to confirm inhibition of positive patch test reactions by the use of topically applied disodium cromoglycate [114].

16.13 Management of Specific Types of Contact Dermatitis

Hydrofluoric Acid Burns. Calcium gluconate gel can be used to treat burns from hydrofluoric acid [115].

Chromate Sensitivity. Cement can be made less sensitizing by the addition of ferrous sulphate. This seems to have led to a reduction in the incidence of chromate sensitivity in Scandinavia [116]. The addition of ferrous sulphate does not, however, make the cement any less irritant. A barrier cream containing 10% ascorbic acid has also been used [117]. In addition, PUVA therapy has been used with some success in patients with chronic chromate dermatitis.

Cosmetic Intolerance. Some patients complain that they are 'allergic to everything'. In such situations, they may often be found to be suffering from cosmetic intolerance [118]. Atopics, patients with underlying rosacea or seborrhoeic eczema and those with fair or Celtic skins often have reduced tolerance to cosmetics. Some patients also seem to develop 'cosmetic exhaustion' due to the marginal irritant effects of frequent and cumulative cosmetic exposure. Other patients may be 'stingers', reacting with immediate-type sensations to lactic acid and other chemicals [119] (see Sect. 2.2.10). Cosmetic intolerance is best managed by the avoidance of all but the most essential cosmetics, by the use of bland/nonirritant preparations and perhaps a little hydrocortisone cream. Preparations which include chemicals with a propensity to sting or smart should be avoided. Even though there is often little to see, noninvasive measurement of water loss or other parameters confirms damage to the skin.

Contact Urticaria. Two types of contact urticaria can be distinguished: immune and nonimmune types [120] (see Chap. 2.3). Immune-type contact urticaria normally occurs in atopics and is a specific IgE-type response, mostly to protein allergens. Treatment is by avoiding the responsible allergen and by measures which help to restore the skin barrier. Oral antihistamines also help. Nonimmune contact urticaria is an inflammatory response that is nonallergic in origin, and which may occur in atopics and in nonatopics. Some chemicals such as cinnamic aldehyde, cinnamic acid, methyl nicotinate, diethyl fumarate, benzoic acid and dimethyl sulphoxide may trigger this response in susceptible individuals. Nonimmune contact urticaria is mostly blocked by corticosteroids and nonsteroidal antiinflammatories [121, 122] (although some chemicals seem to have other mechanisms). The contact urticaria and anaphylaxis that may sometimes occur following contact with rubber gloves has been shown to be an IgE-mediated response to rubber latex [43, 123]. Mild cases of contact urticaria may present simply as discomfort when gloves are worn [124]. Individuals allergic to latex may use plastic undergloves, vinyl gloves [125] or nonlatex (Elastyren) gloves [126].

Atopic Dermatis. Individuals with a history of atopic dermatitis are more susceptible to irritant contact dermatitis [127–129] and also to type I skin reactions. These may be contact urticarial in type, but airborne type I allergens (such as house dust mite, grass and animal dander) may lead to exacerbation of eczema on exposed sites. Whether this is simply the result of local urticaria leading to itching, scratching and secondary eczematization, or whether this is the result of cutaneous basophil hypersensitivity which, itself, leads to a clinical eczematous response remains uncertain. Persistent contact with type I allergen can, however, undoubtedly lead to eczema.

Career advice for atopics – particularly in respect of irritants – is important. Atopics form a large proportion of those compensated for work-related skin disease [130]. Where there is a coexistent history of metal allergy, the prognosis seems to be worse [13]. Secondary staphylococcal skin infection is also often a significant factor in the persistence and lack of response to conventional treatment of some cases of irritant/atopic hand dermatitis. It is also a risk as regard cross-infection and food handling (Sect. 11.14.1). Avoidance of type I allergens may also be important in some patients. Oral antihistamines can be tried, but the response is usually disappointing. Measures to redcuce house dust mite should be tried in those with the 'volatile' pattern of atopic eczema. Treatment is otherwise as for other eczemas. Occasionally, atopics also become light sensitive and may require treatment with systemic corticosteroids and/or azathioprine. PUVA therapy can also be tried. Finding suitable sunscreens can be difficult due to the atopic's increased susceptibility to even marginal irritants.

Topical Corticosteroids. The use of topical corticosteroids can be an important cause of persistence of contact eczema [131, 132]. Cross-sensitivity among certain groups of cortico steroids is common [133]. This subject is covered in more detail in Sect. 14.2.

Hairdressers. Persons employed as hairdressers are particularly susceptible to contact dermatitis [134] (Sect. 11.16.2). Not only are they regularly and frequently exposed to water and detergent and to irritant hairdressing chemicals, but they are also exposed to several potent allergens, including glyceryl monothioglycolate (acid perms), hair dyes containing p-phenylene-diamine, biocides in shampoos, and nickel (metal) [135–138], Glyceryl monothioglycolate may persist on hair for some months and may be the cause of persistent or recurrent dermatitis [139]. Atopics should be advised against hairdressing as a career [140]. Some, particularly those who have only had asthma or hay fever, may tolerate the work. When there is also coexisting allergy, the prognosis is very poor, and many must then give up their work [135, 137], but even then, their dermatitis may persist [134]. Hairdressers should be advised always to wear appropriate gloves when handling these chemicals and to follow manufacturers' use instructions closely.

Dental. In patients allergic to mercury with lichen planus of the mouth, (particularly if adjacent to teeth containing amalgam), it may be necessary to remove amalgam fillings, and in such patients the oral lichen planus may then fade away [141] (see Sect. 9.4). In most patients with oral lichen planus, however, mercury sensitivity is not a significant factor. Mucosal soreness may also relate to metals, resins or other substances in dental prostheses [142, 143].

Prostheses. In patients receiving prostheses [144–146] it is not usually necessary to do prospective patch testing, except in patients who are to receive a metal-on-metal prosthesis [147, 148]. Patients with metal-on-plastic prostheses rarely appear to have any such problems [148, 149]. Sensitivity is now thought to be more likely a consequence of joint loosening than its cause [150, 151]. In patients known to be highly nickel sensitive, it is nevertheless wise to avoid implanting a nickel-releasing plate or other device, since both local and more generalized reactions have occurred [152]. For those in whom vitallium (cobalt-chromium-nickel) or stainless steel (nickel-chromium) prostheses would be inappropriate, a titanium prosthesis can be used.

Formaldehyde Sensitivity. Formaldehyde is widely used in shampoos and as a biocide, and even quite low levels may sensitize or elicit dermatitis. A spot test helps to detect those products containing formaldehyde [55] (see Chap. 10.3.4). It is important to remember that other biocides, such as quaternium 15 (Dowicil 200), imidazolidinyl urea (Germall 115), 2-bromo-2-nitropropane-1,3-diol (Bronopol) etc., are formaldehyde releasers. Many clothing finishes also contain formaldehyde resins.

Nickel Allergy. The incidence of nickel allergy has reached epidemic proportions in Europe and North America [153]. Most women are sensitized either by ear piercing or by inexpensive metal jewellery and clothing accessories [54, 154, 155]. Nickel sensitivity, once established, tends to persist and may be an important factor in housewives' hand dermatitis and in certain occupations. It is helpful to advise young women about nickel-free earrings [156], and manufacturers should be encouraged to use some of the safer nickel-containing alloys in jewellery and clothing accessories [157, 158]. Legislation in this regard has recently been passed in Scandinavia and will, hopefully, soon become universal throughout Europe.

Chronic Actinic Dermatitis. Secondary development of chronic actinic dermatitis following photosensitivity to perfume ingredients such as musk ambrette has been reported [159]. Even very small amounts of musk ambrette may then be enough to maintain such dermatitis [160], some such patients become persistent light reactors. A similar situation occurs in patients sensitive to sesquiterpene lactones (Compositae) [161, 162], and to other fragrance ingredients and lichens [163]. Although primarily a volatile type of allergic contact dermatitis, the dermatitis often seems to be exacerbated by light, and patients may develop chronic actinic dermatitis or actinic reticuloid (see Sect. 2.4.6). Such patients need to avoid contact with their allergen, so far as is possible, and also to avoid light. Prior to the advent of azathioprine therapy and more complete sunblocks, these patients often had to spend much of the year indoors. Nowadays, they can be managed on a combination of systemic corticosteroid and azathioprine. Sometimes treatment can be reduced during the winter months. Opaque-type sunscreens and topical corticosteroids (moderate potency) are also helpful. Many patients with Compositae sensitivity also have chronic vesicular hand eczema. In India, *Parthenium* dermatitis is normally treated with systemic corticosteroids, is often severe enough to cause generalized exfoliative dermatitis and may be associated with significant mortality [164]. Chloroquine and oral hyposensitization have been reported to have been successful in some patients [109].

Diaper dermatitis. The role of faecal proteases, lipases and increased pH from bacterial breakdown of urea is now well-recognized in causing diaper dermatitis (napkin rash; see also Sect. 12.2.1) [165–167]. Cellulose core/absorbent gel diapers have been shown to be superior to conventional cloth diapers in preventing the development of dermatitis [168]. Regular mild cleansing, use of emollient/silicone barrier creams and frequent changing of diapers have all been shown to be helpful. Hydrocortisone and imidazole combinations can be used to treat any eczema. Microbiological studies should be carried out to exclude significant secondary infection.

Frictional Contact Dermatitis. Typically frictional contact dermatitis occurs with juvenile plantar dermatosis. A similar condition is sometimes seen on the hands. Occlusion and sweating may be facilitating factors. Nonocclusive and absorbent footwear is helpful. Tar and greasy emollients are normally more successful than topical corticosteroids in the management of such patients.

Carbonless Copy Paper. Contact urticaria has been reported, which may be prostaglandin induced [169]. More general effects are controversial and have recently been reviewed by Murray [170]. Frictional dermatitis may occur, as with other paper [56].

Eyelid Dermatitis. Although some allergens such as nickel, fragrance, resins (toluenesulphonamide-formaldehyde; Santolite) and occasional cosmetic biocides may be implicated in eyelid dermatitis, and sometimes also primula and wood dusts, the majority of cases of eyelid dermatitis are negative on patch testing. Many such patients have atopic eczema [171] in which volatile irritants or volatile type I allergens may possibly be to blame. Prick testing may often be as helpful as patch testing in the investigation of such patients.

Dietary Factors. Some patients with nickel sensitivity experience chronic relapsing, vesicular hand eczema [172, 173]. Some of these patients may react to oral challenge with nickel (2,5 or 5 mg) or cobalt (1 mg) [174]. In these patients, if flares of eczema can be confirmed by double-blind challenge [175], it may be worth trying a low-nickel diet. It remains somewhat controversial as to whether this is really helpful [176–179]. Nickel may also be released from cooking utensils [180].

A similar situation obtains with balsams and spices [181]. In patients who are allergic to balsam of Peru, when their eczema does not readily respond to conventional treatment, it may be worth trying a balsam challenge [182] and a low-balsam diet [183, 184]. Otherwise, foods have a low incidence of causing eczematous-type reactions. The normal response is urticarial. Ingestion of allergens to which a patient is sensitive may lead not only to flares of vesicular hand eczema but also to urticaria [185], toxic erythemas, erythemamultiforme-like reactions, the baboon syndrome [186] and to other patterns of dermatitis [47, 187–190] (see Sect. 7.4.1.14).

16.14 Prognosis

The prognosis of contact dermatitis is worse for atopics and also for those allergic to certain allergens, particularly chromate and nickel. Experimental sensitivity does not seem to persist, or at least seems to have a low incidence of patch test recall when patients are tested after 1 year. Some other allergies also seem to be transient, although patients may be left with an altered capacity to react with accelerated response at subsequent challenge.

16.15 Prevention of Allergic Contact Dermatitis: Theoretical Considerations

There is now the possibility of inducing immune tolerance by oral ingestion, exposure to UVL, or application of arachidonic acid with subsequent application of antigen, leading to induction of a specific suppressor cell population. Once allergy has developed, however, the induction of tolerance seems to be much more difficult and recent studies on oral desensitization in patients sensitive to poison oak/ivy were unsuccessful [111].

16.16 Prevention of Contact Dermatitis: Practical Aspects

Prevention of contact dermatitis can be achieved by the following measures (Sect. 11.14).

1. The wearing of appropriate gloves [38, 40, 191–193] and specific advice as regards protection of the hands [194] is important. Damaged, contaminated or inappropriate gloves may be as harmful as wearing no gloves at all [195]. A damaged glove may allow penetration of allergen or irritant, retaining this in occlusive contact with the skin for sufficient time to result in severe dermatitis. Nitrile and nitrile-butatoluene-rubber gloves may give some protection against the bisphenol A type of epoxy resins [196]. For more general guidance see Sect. 11.14.4.1 and 17.3.1.

2. Use of appropriate barrier creams, for example, polyamine salt of linoleic acid as protection against poison ivy dermatitis [197]. In general, however, the performance of barrier creams has been disappointing [198–202] (Sects. 11.14.4.2 and 17.3.2). Both gloves and barrier creams may allow penetration of chemicals and solvents [193, 203], and care needs to be exercised to ensure that recommendations are both effective and appropriate.

3. Although after-work emollients are often recommended and may protect against dryness and chapping, they do not, experimentally at least, appear to speed healing of irritant contact dermatitis [113].

4. Specific measures include the addition of ferrous sulphate to cement, which has led to a reduction in chromate allergy in Scandinavia [116].

5. Surveillance of allergens can be monitored by population studies, studies of occupational groups, labour or compensation analyses, analysis of interval occupational or patch test material, monitoring trends in sensitivity on patch test clinic computers and predictive testing of chemicals prior to their use (Chaps. 6, 14, 18, 20). Prediction of allergy by theoretical models is still in its infancy but may be a possibility in the future.

6. Contact dermatitis can also be reduced by education both of industry/government and of the community. It may also be possible to screen at-risk groups in the community, such as patients with stasis eczema and ulceration [7]. Work-related skin disorders are the result of predisposing factors in the environment and in the host and awareness of these factors, combined with appropriate counselling and advice, should improve their prognosis. If a substance has the potential to irritate or sensitize, it is essential that this be made clear, not only on the containers but also in the workplace, and appropriate safeguards and precautions must then be taken [205]. Training should also be provided in the safe handling of that substance. Suitable washing facilities and protective clothing should be provided. This is largely the responsibility of the company. Expert advice should be sought if necessary. Good housekeeping and cleanliness at the work place is critical. Good ventilation may also be important.

7. Worker screening and preemployment medical examinations may also help to prevent patients with atopic eczema and/or nickel sensitivity from taking on unsuitable employment [51, 206, 207].

Physicians and nurses can also help by giving appropriate advice [208] on cross-reacting chemicals [209] and by avoiding the use of sensitizing medicaments, especially on areas of damaged skin. Injury to the skin is an important predisposing factor as regards the development of allergic contact dermatitis [210].

The use of only mild cleansing products and avoidance of their overuse [140] is also important.

The risk of irritant contact dermatitis can be diminished by reducing exposure to strong acids and alkalis and by reducing the frequency of exposure to other milder irritants. Gloves and barrier creams may be of assistance. Patients with a previous history of hand dermatitis or a previous history of severe eczema are at particular risk and should be advised against further wet work. The irritancy of many cleansers, soaps and detergents should also be explained.

16.17 General Preventive Measures

In Europe and North America, the prevalence of allergic contact dermatitis from nickel is such that appropriate legislation as regards the nickel content of jewellery and clothing accessories is now indicated. Safer nickel alloys already exist, and earrings, jewellery and clothing accessories should now all be nickel free [154]. In Europe, many recurrences of contact dermatitis would also be avoided if we were to follow the example of North America and institute a system of full cosmetic ingredient labelling [211]. All medicaments should also have full ingredient labelling.

It is not only the allergenicity of the individual substances that is important but also the total allergen load. There is rarely such a thing as a 'safe' or 'unsafe' chemical as far as allergic contact dermatitis is concerned. A chemical is 'safe' for a certain use at a certain concentration, and the prevalence of sensitivity also reflects the total environmental load. Prevention needs to be pursued not only in our work environment but also in our home and general environment.

16.18 Appendices

16.18.1 Appendix A: Hand Dermatitis – Advice to Housewives

To speed healing and prevent relapse of your dermatitis you should:
1. *Handwashing* – use lukewarm water and, if possible, a mild soap or detergent (nonmedicated and preferably without any perfume). The soap

should be used sparingly and the hands thoroughly rinsed. Dry carefully between the fingers. Often no soap is necessary and a 'soap substitute' cleansing cream can be used instead.

2. As far as possible *avoid direct contact with detergents and other strong cleansing agents.* Wear gloves when using any irritant household product. Keep containers clean and free of contamination and always use according to manufacturers' instructions.

3. *Avoid direct contact with shampoo.* Let somebody else shampoo your hair, or use plastic gloves.

4. Avoid direct contact with *metal polish, wax polish, shoe, floor, car, furniture* and *window polishes.*

5. Be careful not to get *solvents* and *stain-removers* such as white spirit, petrol, trichlorethylene, turpentine and thinners on the skin. Never use solvent or industrial cleansers to wash your hands.

6. Don't peel or squeeze *oranges, lemons* or *grapefruit* with bare hands. Wear gloves for all food preparations.

7. Don't apply hair dye or alcohol-based hair lotions with bare hands.

8. Wear gloves in cold weather.

9. *Rings* should not be worn during housework or other work, even when the dermatitis has healed. Rings should be cleaned on the inside frequently with a brush and left in ammonia water (1 tablespoon to 500 ml water) overnight, then rinsed thoroughly. Never wash your hands with soap when wearing a ring.

10. Regularly use a *hand cream* to prevent the skin from becoming dry.

11. *Gloves* should always be used for washing dishes, for hand-washing clothes and for all wet or irritant work. Gloves should also be worn for gardening (cloth or leather). Household gloves – plastic or rubber – should be cotton lined, or cotton gloves can be worn under rubber or plastic. They should not be worn for more than 15 – 20 minutes at a time. If water happens to enter a glove, it must be immediately taken off. Turn the gloves inside out, and leave to dry. Some people become allergic to rubber (with a sensation of discomfort or with the dermatitis becoming worse), and in these individuals plastic or PVC gloves should be used instead.

12. *Remember that the resistance of the skin is lowered for many months after the dermatitis appears to be completely healed: so continue to follow the instructions.*

13. Washing machines and dishwashers are the ideal way of preventing further attacks.

16.18.2 Appendix B: Eczema at Work – Patient Advice/Information Pack [52]

Dermatitis most commonly affects the hands, as these bear the brunt of all contact in any job. Therefore the comments in this leaflet are mostly about hand eczema/dermatitis – these two words are synonymous, neither being more serious than the other.

The two main factors involved in the development of hand eczema are *the effects of irritants* and *the development of allergy*. The two problems are quite distinct.

Irritant Dermatitis
The problem of irritants is by far the commoner and this is influenced by two factors:
(a) the nature of the skin and
(b) the nature of the work.

1. The Nature of the Skin
The skin acts as a *barrier* which both keeps *irritants out* and *moisture in*. The integrity of this barrier is the key to irritant dermatitis.

If you are *'atopic'* (had 'childhood' eczema or asthma/hay fever) then you have a constitutional or 'inborn' weakness of the skin, in that the skin is 'leaky' and therefore lets water out and irritants in more easily. This increases your chances of developing occupational hand eczema.

Atopic eczema has many forms. You may not remember having had eczema at all. It may only have been presented for a short while as a baby, or as a toddler/teenager, or it may have been present lifelong to some degree. This inborn weakness of the skin persists and is still present even when the eczema has cleared. The chances of developing occupational dermatitis is increased in those who have had atopic eczema at any site, but is particularly high in those who have had atopic eczema of the hands.

Other groups of people with vulnerable skin include:
– Fair-skinned people
– Women after childbirth
– Older people as their skin gets drier
– Those with eczema (of any sort) elsewhere
– Anyone with a delicate or fragile skin

2. The Nature of the Work
Substances encountered at work vary in their irritancy from strong acids or alkalis (which give an immediate burn) down to very minimal irritants which need prolonged exposure day after day, week after week, e.g. water/detergents. This is called cumulative irritancy or 'wear and tear' dermatitis, and is the commonest cause of eczema at work. Jobs with an increased risk of developing occupational dermatitis from cumulative irritants include the following:
– Jobs that involve repeated contact with water/detergents
– Jobs that involve repeated contact with solvents/thinners
– Jobs that involve repeated contact with cement/plaster
– Jobs that involve repeated contact with cutting oils or soluble oils
– Jobs that involve handling food and/or food preparation

Apart from chemical substances, other irritants include friction, extremes of humidity/temperature and irritant dusts/fumes. In 'low-humidity dermatosis' the commonly affected sites are face, hands and lower legs. The skin at these sites is especially prone to drying out. Fumes in the air often give a facial dermatitis. Dusts often give dermatitis around the neck and wrists due to the combined effects of sweating and friction of collars and cuffs. High temperature/high humidity causes 'sweat rash' in the axillae/groins and other sites of friction from clothing.

Allergic Dermatitis

Allergy is *less common* but *extremely important.* Once an allergy has developed, even minute quantities of an apparently innocuous substance may cause severe dermatitis. It is therefore very important that allergic factors are not missed. To be able to diagnose allergy, the most reliable way is to be patch tested. This involves having small amounts of known allergens and suspected allergens placed on your back in correct form and in correct concentration. The patches have to stay on for 2 days and are normally looked at again 2 days later. If you are allergic to something, then this will show up as a small patch of eczema at the test site. Once your have an allergy, this will tend to remain with you for life. Allergy may cause eczema at work.

1. Pre-existing Allergy

Many people become allergic to substances encountered at home or from hobbies, or from personal belongings/toiletries, e.g. to nickel in costume jewellery or from earnings. Even though you may subsequently avoid such jewellery and no longer get eczema, when you subsequently handle metal-containing implements in your job, such as taps, hair pins or scissors in hairdressing, or knives/pans in catering, you will again develop eczema but this time at your new site of contact, e.g. hands.

2. The Development of a new Allergy

Sometimes an allergy develops following contact with a substance first encountered at work, e.g. epoxy glue or chromate in cement. It may take years for such an allergy to develop or it may develop in a matter of weeks. Once established, however, eczema will develop *every time* you have contact with the allergen, even in the *smallest amounts.* Eczema will occur on subsequent exposure to the compound wherever it is found, and this could be at home or even following a change of job. Obviously eczema is extremely disruptive to the skin barrier and this in itself tends to lead to the development of further eczema – the skin becomes increasingly vulnerable and is adversely affected by even mild irritants (including those previously well tolerated such as shampoos, soaps, etc.).

Whether occupational dermatitis occurs or not is dependent on: (a) the presence or absence of a specific allergy and (b) the ability of an individual's skin barrier to remain intact in spite of the cumulative irritants to which his hands are exposed at work, at home and during leisure activities. To prevent occupational dermatitis, one has to minimize contact with potential irritants and all sensitisers and do what one can to improve the resistance of the skin. If allergy is suspected or proven, then one should avoid all further contact with the allergen. This is often difficult with some widely distributed allergens such as nickel and chromate, but easier with specific industrial allergens, e.g. industrial resins, glues, rubber chemicals, etc., when a move to another part of the factory, or the replacement of the allergen by a different substance, may lead to complete recovery.

Treatment
Eczema should be treated promptly. This normally involves:
- Supportive measures, e.g. mild cleansers, emollient hand creams, etc.
- Fairly potent topical steroids (the skin of the hands is relatively thick, so steroids have to be quite strong and applied frequently to do any good).
- Topical steroids/antibacterial combinations or oral antibiotics are necessary when the eczema is infected (this is a common cause of the eczema failing to respond to treatment).

Simply treating the eczema is, however, not enough. The root cause – whether allergic or irritant – must be identified and dealt with.

How to Reduce the Risk of Occupational Dermatitis
1. Career advice
This is necessary for 'high-risk people' and 'high-risk jobs'. It is very important that those with vulnerable skins, especially those with a past history of atopic eczema, be advised – *whilst they are still at school* – against entering high-risk jobs, otherwise it is very likely that they will suffer from occupational hand eczema. An inappropriate choice of job will only lead to unnecessary time off work, a bad work record and subsequent difficulties with employment.

2. Health Education
- Hands are tough, but if the thinner you spill takes the paint off your workbench, consider what it is doing to your skin!
- Damage to the skin is not always immediately apparent, and mild irritants such as detergents, solvents or cutting oils may simply lead to progressive weakening of the skin. Only when all your reserves are exhausted will dermatitis develop.
- Even the mildest of irritants will keep the dermatitis going, and it may take many weeks/months before the skin returns to normal again. Sometimes it is necessary to have time off work to allow the eczema to heal.
- Prevention is always easier than cure. Once dermatitis has developed, the risk of subsequent episodes of dermatitis is high.

3. Workplace Education
Awareness of potential allergens and irritants at work is important, as is the provision of adequate protection.

- There should be adequate washing facilities and a good/clean working environment.
- Health and safety data sheets should be held on all substances used in the place of work and suitable safety precautions instituted for all potentially noxious chemicals.

4. Hand care
- *Washing* – avoid solvent or abrasive hand cleansers. If your hands are irritated, your doctor can prescribe, or you can buy, soap substitutes such as aqueous cream or emulsifying ointment to use instead of soap.
- *Dry hands well* – especially between fingers and wrists. A barrier cream should *not* be relied on for protection, but may help with subsequent removal of dirt.
- The use of an emollient 'after-work' *hand cream* is important and may be used regularly throughout the day, especially in those suffering from dry, eczematous or chapped skin.
- *Protective gloves and garments* – must be appropriate to the job, e.g. solvents will pass straight through some gloves, affording no protection. The degree of protection varies both according to the composition of the glove, the nature of the chemicals with which one is in contact and the duration of contact. Rubber gloves generally afford good protection against water-based compounds and restrict movement only marginally, but offer little protection against solvents. Gloves also, of course, have some drawbacks – they get sweaty inside, for some jobs they may be dangerous/impracticable and, if pierced, subsequent irritant dermatitis may be worse than if the worker had not worn gloves at all. Some individuals become allergic to rubber. PVC gloves with cotton linings are often preferable but are somewhat stiff and unmanageable.
- *Follow instructions* – use things for the correct purpose. Dilute liquids to the correct dilution and dispose of waste safely.
- Try not be a *messy worker.* Keep your environment clean from contamination.

16.18.3 Appendix C: You are Allergic to Nickel

This allergy may persist all your life. Nickel is used in white metal for hardness and because it is cheap.

Contact with nickel-containing objects will tend to bring you out in eczema – red, itchy areas perhaps with some scaling or small water-blisters.

This may occur not only at sites of contact but also at sites where you have had trouble with metal (nickel) previously, e.g. earlobes, wrists, etc.

To help yourself recover from this present episode and to help prevent relapse, total avoidance of nickel contact is necessary. This may not be very easy but is something you must aim for.

Nickel is commonly found in the following items:

1. *Personal Objects*

    Earrings – only 18 ct. gold, platinum, British sterling silver, good quality stainless steel or plastic should be worn. Plated jewellery should be avoided as the plating quickly wears off, exposing the underlying nickel.

    Watches – it is usually the strap buckle that causes trouble, but other parts, such as the winder, back of the watch, bracelet, may also cause trouble.

    Other jewellery – brooches, necklaces, bracelets, etc.

    Jeans studs or metal studs on denim and canvas clothing are a common source of trouble. The surface electroplating or plastic film/paint is very thin and quickly wears away to expose the underlying nickel. Covering these with fabric or wearing a blouse/T-shirt tucked in is not enough. Sweating will cause the nickel to leach through.

    Other sources of nickel in clothing and one's personal possessions include:

    Bra fasteners and adjusters, zips, 'poppers', metal bits on handbags, umbrellas, etc., keys, silver coins, hair styling brushes, clips and pins.

2. *At Home*

    Drawer handles, fridge and cooker handles, lavatory handles and taps, metal wool scouring pads, sewing machines, pins, needles, thimbles, scissors, tools, pram frames.

3. *At the Office*

    Shiny metal edging on desks, trolleys, drawers, filing cabinets, paper clips.

    It is best, wherever possible, to remove or replace any nickel-containing objects with which you are in close, regular contact.

    If alternatives cannot be found, you should try covering the object with masking tape or clear nail varnish, always remember that the covering will wear off, especially if only varnish. Keep money and keys in bags or coat pockets (not trouser pockets).

    We are happy to test objects for nickel or, alternatively, can supply you with a kit for you to test for yourself at home.

16.19 References

1. Sadhra S (1987) Dermatitis: identifying the culprit. Occup Health 3: 222–224
2. de Boer EM, Bruynzeel DP, van Ketel WG (1988) Dyshidrotic eczema as an occupational dermatitis, in metal workers. Contact Dermatitis 19: 184–188
3. Rycroft RJG (1986) Occupational dermatoses. In: Rook A, Wilkinson DS, Ebling FJG, Champion RH, Burton JL (eds) Textbook of dermatology, 4th edn. Blackwells Oxford, pp 581–586
4. Dooms-Goossens A, Swinnen E, Vandermaesen J, Marien K, Dooms M (1987) Connubial dermatitis from a hair lotion. Contact Dermatitis 16: 41–47

5. Rycroft RJG (1986) Environmental aspects of occupational dermatology. Derm Beruf Umwelt 34: 157–159

6. Fraki JE, Kalimo K, Tuohimaa P, Aantaa E (1985) Contact allergy to various components of topical preparations for treatment of external otitis. Acta Otolaryngol 100: 414–418

7. Kulozik M, Powell SM, Cherry G, Ryan TJ (1988) Contact sensitivity in community-based leg ulcer patients. Clin Exp Dermatol 13: 82–84

8. Paramsothy Y, Collins M, Smith AG (1988) Contact dermatitis in patients with leg ulcers. Contact Dermatitis 18: 30–36

9. Hatinen A, Terasvirta M, Fraki JE (1985) Contact allergy to components in topical ophthalmologic preparations. Acta Ophthalmol 63: 424–426

10. Beck MH, Burrows D, Fregert S, Mendelsohn S (1985) Allergic contact dermatitis to expoy resin in ostomy bags. Br J Surg. 72: 202–203

11. Nilsson E (1985). Contact sensitivity and urticaria in 'wet' work. Contact Dermatitis 13: 321–329

12. Rystedt I (1985) Atopic background in patients with occupational hand eczema. Contact Dermatitis 12: 247–254

13. Nilsson E, Mikaelson B, Andersson S (1985) Atopy, occupation and domestic work as risk factors for hand eczema in hospital workers. Contact Dermatitis 13: 216–223.

14. Lammintausta K, Kalimo K, Aantaa S (1982) Course of hand dermatitis in hospital workers. Contact Dermatitis 8: 327–332

15. Fregert S (1975) Occupational dermatitis in a 10-year material. Contact Dermatitis 1: 96–107

16. Clemmensen OJ, Menné T, Kaaber K, Solgasard P (1981) Exposure to nickel and the relevance of nickel sensitivity among hospital cleaners. Contact Dermatitis 7: 14–18

17. Singgih SIR, Pantinga H, Nater JP, Woest TE, Kruyt-Gaspersz JA (1986) Occupational hand dermatoses in hospital cleaning personal. Contact Dermatitis 14: 14–19

18. Hansen KS (1983) Occupational dermatoses in hospital cleaning women. Contact Dermatitis 7: 14–18

19. Nilsson E, Back D (1986) The importance of amnestic information of atopy, metal dermatitis and earlier hand eczema for the development of hand dermatitis in women in wet hospital work. Acta Derm Venereol (Stockh) 66: 45–50

20. Eiermann HJ, Larsen W, Maibach HI, Taylor JS (1982) Prospective study of cosmetic reactions: 1977–80. J Am Acad Dermatol 6: 909–917

21. Rycroft R (1988) Looking at work dermatologically. Dermatol Clin 6: 1–5

22. Fischer T, Rystedt I (1985) False positive, follicular and irritant patch test reactions to metal salts. Contact Dermatitis 12: 93–98

23. Bruynzeel DP, van Ketel WG, von Blomberg, van der Flier M, Schreper RJ (1983) Angry back or the excited skin syndrome. J Am Acad Dermatol 8: 392–397

24. Fisher AA (1986) Compound ('synergistic') allergy to contactants. Cutis 38: 101–102

25. Smeenk G, Kerchoffs HP, Scheurs PH (1987) Contact allergy to a reaction product in Hirudoid cream: an example of compound allergy. Br J Dermatol 116: 223–231

26. Kellett JK, King CM, Beck MH (1986) Compound allergy to medicaments. Contact Dermatitis 14: 45–48

27. Burrows D, Andersen KE, Camarasa JG, Dooms-Goossens A, Ducombs G, LaChappelle JM, Menné T, Rycroft RJG, Wahlberg JE, White IR, Wilkinson JD (1989) Trial of 0.5% versus 0.375% potassium dichromate. Contact Dermatitis 21: 351–352

28. Hannuksela M, Salo H (1986) The repeated open application test (RDAT). Contact Dermatitis 14: 221–227

29. Andersen KE (1985) Sensitivity and subsequent 'down regulation' of sensitivity induced by chlorocresol in guinea pigs. Arch Dermatol Res 277: 84–87

30. Möller H & Svensson A (1986) Metal sensitivity: positive history but negative test indicates atopy. Contact Dermatitis 14: 57–60

31. Todd DJ, Burrows D, Stanford CF (1989) Atopy in subjects with a history of nickel allergy but negative patch tests. Contact Dermatitis 21: 129–133
32. Goh CL, Kwok SF, Rajan VS (1984) Cross sensitivity to colour developers. Contact Dermatitis 10: 280–285
33. Bruynzeel DP, Maibach HI (1986) Excited skin syndrome. Arch Dermatol 122: 323–328
34. Lammintausta K, Maibach HI, Wilson D (1987) Human cutaneous irritation: induced hyporeactivity. Contact Dermatitis 17: 193–198
35. Ross D (1987) Tackling dermatitis. Occup Health 39: 220–221
36. Calnan CD (1970) Studies in contact dermatitis. XXIII. Allergen replacement. Trans St John's Hosp Derm Soc 55: 131–138
37. Strube DD, Nicholl G (1987) The irritancy of soaps and syndets. Cutis 39: 544–545
38. Moursiden HT, Faber O (1973) Penetration of protective gloves by allergens and irritants. Trans St John's Hosp Derm Soc 59: 230–234
39. Wall LM (1980) Nickel penetration through rubber gloves. Contact Dermatitis 6: 461–463
40. Adams RM (1990) Prevention, rehabilitation, treatment. In: Adams RM (ed) Occupational skin disease, 2nd edn. Saunders, Philadelphia, pp 261–279
41. Darre E, Vedel P, Jensen JS (1987) Skin protection against methylmethacrylate. Acta Orthop Scand 58: 236–238
42. Estlander T, Jolanski R, Kanerva L (1986) Dermatitis and urticaria from rubber and plastic gloves. Contact Dermatitis 14: 20–25
43. Meding B, Fregert S (1984) Contact urticaria from natural latex gloves. Contact Dermatitis 10: 52–53
44. Pryce DW, White I, English JS, Rycroft RJ (1989) Soluble oil dermatitis: a review. J Soc Occup Med 39: 93–98
45. Baer RL (1986) Poison ivy dermatitis. Cutis 37: 434–436
46. Irvine C, Reynolds A, Finlay AY (1988) Erythema multiforme-like reactions to rosewood. Contact Dermatitis 19: 224–225
47. Menné T, Hjorth N (1982) Reactions from exposure to contact allergens. Semin Dermatol 1: 15–24
48. Monthly Index of Medical Specialities (1990) MIMS, London
49. Van der Valk PG, Maibach HI (1989) Do topical corticosteroids modulate skin irritation in human beings? Assessment by transepidermal water loss and scoring. J Am Acad Dermatol 21: 519–527
50. Menné T, Bachmann E (1979) Permanent disability from hand dermatitis in females sensitive to nickel, chromium and cobalt. Dermatosen 5: 129–135
51. Lindemayr H (1989) Das Friseurekzem. Dermatosen 32: 5–13
52. Shaw S (1989) Eczema at work. National Eczema Society (UK) Adult Information Pack
53. Rudzki E, Rebandel P, Napiórowska T, Dynowska D, Legiéc C (1985) Nickel objects causing sensitization and relapses. Contact Dermatitis 13: 335–336
54. Fischer T, Fregert S, Gruvberger B, Rystedt I (1984) Nickel release from ear piercing kits and earrings. Contact Dermatitis 10: 39–41
55. Fregert S, Dahlquist I, Gruvberger B (1984) A simple method for the detection of formaldehyde. Contact Dermatitis 10: 132–134
56. Menné T, Hjorth N (1985) Frictional contact dermatitis. Am J Ind Med 8: 401–402
57. Malten KE (1981) Thoughts on irritant contact dermatitis. Contact Dermatitis 7: 238–247
58. Malten KE, den Arend JA (1985) Irritant contact dermatitis. Traumiterative and cumulative impairment by cosmetics, climate and other daily loads. Derm Beruf Umwelt 33: 125–132
59. Willis CM, Stephens CJ, Wilkinson JD (1989) Epidermal damage induced by irritants in man: a light and electron microscopic study J Invest Dermatol 93: 695–699

60. Wilkinson DS (1985) Causes of unexpected persistence of an occupational dermatitis. In: Griffiths WAD, Wilkinson DS (eds) Essentials of Industrial Dermatitis. Blackwells, Oxford, pp 111–129

61. Förström L, Lassus A, Salde L, Niem K-M (1982) Allergic contact eczema to topical corticosteroids. Contact Dermatitis 8: 128–133

62. Guin JD (1984) Contact sensitivity to topical corticosteroids. J Am Acad Dermatol 10: 773–782

63. Spiro J-G, Lawrence CM (1986) Contact sensitivity to clobetasol proprionate. Contact Dermatitis 14: 116–117

64. Boyle J, Peachey RDG (1984) Allergic contact dermatitis to Dermovate and Eumovate. Contact Dermatitis 11: 50–51

65. Mitchell JC (1975) The angry back syndrome: eczema creates eczema. Contact Dermatitis 1: 193–194

66. Goh CL, Wong PH, Kwok SF, Gau SL (1986) Chromate allergy: total chromium and hexavalent chromate in the air. Derm Beruf Umwelt 34: 132–134

67. Belsito DV (1989) The immunologic basis of patch testing. J Am Acad Dermatol 21: 822–829

68. Prens EP, Benne K, Geursen-Reitsun AM, van Dijk G, Benner R, van Joost T (1989) Effects of topically applied glucocorticosteroids on patch test responses and recruitment of inflammatory cells in allergic contact dermatitis. Agents Actions 26: 125–127

69. Rheins LA, Barnes L, Amorusiroanitch S, Collins CE, Nordland JJ (1987) Suppression of the cutaneous immune response following topical application of the prostaglandin PGE 2. Cell Immunol 106: 33–42

70. Rheins CA, Nordlund JJ (1986) Modulation of the population density of epidermal Langerhans cells associated with enhancement or suppression of cutaneous reactivity. J Immunol 136: 867–876

71. Morison WJ, Kripke ML (1984) Systemic suppression of contact hypersensitivity by ultraviolet B radiation or methoxysalen/ultraviolet A radiation in the guinea pig. Cell Immunol 85: 270–277

72. Chung HT, Burnham DK, Robertson B, Roberts LK, Daynes RA (1986) Involvement of prostaglandins in the immune alterations caused by the exposure of mice to ultraviolet light. J Immunol 137: 2478–2484

73. Schwarz T, Urbanska A, Hschnait F, Luger TA (1986) Inhibition of the induction of contact hypersensitivity by a UV-mediated epidermal cytokine. J Invest Dermatol 87: 289–291

74. Baker D, Parker DD, Turk JL (1985) Effect of depletion of epidermal dendritic cells on the induction of contact sensitivity in the guinea pig. Br J Dermatol 113: 285–294

75. Morison WL, Pike RA, Kripke ML (1985) Effect of sunlight and its component wavebands on contact hypersensitivity in mice and guinea pigs. Photodermatol 2: 195–204

76. Yee GK, Ullrich SE, Kripke MC (1989) The role of suppressor factors in the regulation of immune suppressor cell culture sonicates. Cell Imunol 121: 88–89

77. Applegate CA, Ley RD, Alcalay J, Kripke MC (1989) Identification of the molecular target for the suppression of contact hypersensitivity by ultraviolet light. J Exp Med 170: 1117–1131

78. Robertson B, Gahring L, Newton R, Daynes R (1987) In vivo administration of interleukin 1 to normal mice depresses their capacity to elicit contact hypersensitivity responses: prostaglandins are involved in this modification of immune function. J Invest Dermatol 88: 384–387

79. Boerrigter GH, Scheper RJ (1987) Local systemic desensitization induced by repeated epicutaneous hapten applications. J Invest Dermatol 88: 384–387

80. Hanan D, Stampf JL, Fabre M, Grosshaus E, Benezra C (1985) Induction of tolerance to urushiol by epicutaneous application of this hapten on dinitrofluorobenzene-treated skin. J Invest Dermatol 85: 9–11
81. Dunn IS, Liberato DJ, Castagnoli N Jr, Byers NS (1986) Influence of chemical reactivity of urushiol-type haptens on sensitization and the induction of tolerance. Cell Imunol 97: 189–196
82. Collizzi V, Malkovsky M, Lang G, Asherson GL (1985) In vivo activity of interleukin 2: conversion of a stimulus causing unresponsiveness to a stimulus causing contact hypersensitivity by the injection of interleukin 2. Immunology 56: 653–658
83. Xue B, Dersarkissian RM, Baer RL, Thorbecke GJ, Belsito DV (1986) Reversal by lymphokines of the effect of cyclosporin A on contact sensitivity and antibody production in mice. J Immunol 136: 4128–4133
84. Friedman PS, Moss C, Shuster S, Simpson JM (1983) Quantitative relationships between dose of DNCB and reactivity in normal subjects. Clin Exp Immunol 53: 709–715
85. Singh KK, Srinivas CR, Balachandran C, Menon S (1987) *Parthenium* dermatitis sparing vitiliginous skin. Contact Dermatitis 16: 1974
86. Vehara M, Miyanchi H, Tanak S (1984) Diminished contact sensitivity response in vitiliginous skin. Arch Dermatol 120: 195–198
87. Tomasi TB (1980) Oral tolerance. Transplantation 29: 353–356
88. Vreeburg KJJ, de Groot K, von Blomberg M, Scheper RJ (1984). Induction of immunological tolerance by oral administration of nickel and chromium. J Dent Res 63: 112–128
89. van der Burg CKH, Bruynzeel DP, Vreeburg KJJ, von Blomberg BME, Scheper RJ (1986) Hand eczema in hairdressers and nurses: a prospective study. Contact Dermatitis 14: 275–279
90. Cronin E (1982) The management of allergic contact dermatitis. Clin Exp Dermatol 7: 281–284
91. Rosen K, Mobacken H, Swanbeck G (1987) Chronic eczematous dermatitis of the hands: a comparison of PUVA and UVB treatment. Acta Derm Venereol (Stockh) 67: 48–54
92. Rosen K, Jontell M, Mobacken H, Rosdahl I (1989) Epidermal Langerhans cells in chronic eczematous dermatitis of the palms treated with PUVA and UVB. Acta Derm Venereol (Stockh) 69: 200–205
93. Sjövall P, Christensen OB (1986) Local and systemic effect of ultraviolet irradiation (UVB and UVA) on human allergic contact contact dermatitis. Acta Derm Venereol (Stockh) 66: 290–294
94. Larmi E (1989) PUVA treatment inhibits non-immunologic immediate contact reactions to benzoic acid and methyl nicotinate. Int J Dermatol 28: 609–611
95. Lindelof B, Wrangsfo K, Liden S (1987) A double-blind study of grenz ray therapy in chronic eczema of the hands. Br J Dermatol 117: 77–80
96. Lindelof B, Liden S, Lagerholm B (1985) The effect of grenz rays on the expression of allergic contact dermatitis in man. Scand J Immunol 21: 463–469
97. Lindelof B, Lindberg M (1987) The effects of grenz rays on irritant skin reactions in man. Acta Derm Venereol (Stockh) 67: 128–132
98. Ek L, Lindelof B, Lidens S (1989) The duration of grenz ray-induced suppression of allergic contact dermatitis and its correlation with the density of Langerhans cells in human epidermis. Clin Exp Dermatol 14: 206–209
99. Kaaber K, Menné T, Tfell JC, Veien N (1979) Antabuse treatment of nickel dermatitis. Chelation – a new principle of nickel dermatitis. Contact Dermatitis 5: 221–228
100. Christensen OB, Kristensen M (1982) Treatment with disulphuram in chronic nickel hand dermatitis. Contact Dermatitis 8: 59–63

101. Kaaber K, Menné T, Hougard P (1983) Treatment of nickel dermatitis with Antabuse: a double-blind study. Contact Dermatitis 9: 297–300
102. Burrows D, Rogers S, Beck M, Kellett J, McMaster D, Merrett D, Eedy DJ (1986) Treatment of nickel dermatitis with Trientine. Contact Dermatitis 15: 55–57
103. van Ketel WG, Bruynzeel DP (1984) Chelating effect of EDTA on nickel. Contact Dermatitis 11: 311–314
104. Anderson C (1985) The effect of selected immunomodulating agents on experimental contact reactions. Acta Derm Venereol (Stockh) 116: 1–48
105. Turk JL, Parker D, Long PV, Bull JE (1985) Induction of immunologic tolerance: desensitization to occupational allergens. J Allergy Clin Immunol 78: 1082–1085
106. Mekori YA, Claman HN (1986) Desensitization of experimental contact sensitivity. J Allergy Clin Immunol 78: 1073–1081
107. Kligman AM (1958) Poison ivy (Rhus). Arch Dermatol 77: 149–180
108. Epstein WK, Baer H, Dawson CR et al. (1974) Poison oak hyposensitization: evaluation of purified urushiol. Arch Dermatol 109: 356–360
109. Epstein WK, Byers VS, Bazer H (1981) Induction of persistent tolerance to urushiol in humans. J Allergy Clin Immunol 68: 20–25
110. Srinivas CR, Krupashanker DS, Singh KK, Balachandran C, Shenoi SD (1988) Oral hyposensitization in Parthenium dermatitis. Contact Dermatitis 18: 242–243
111. Marks JG, Trantlein JJ, Epstein WL, Laws DM, Sicard GR (1987) Oral hyposensitization to poison ivy and poison oak. Arch Dermatol 123: 476–478
112. Miyachi Y, Uchida K, Komura J, Asada Y, Niwa Y (1985) Auto-oxidative damage in cement dermatitis. Arch Dermatol Res 277: 288–292
112. Blanken R, van der Valk PG, Water JP, Dijkstra H (1987) After-work emollient creams: effects on irritant skin reactions. Derm Beruf Umwelt 35: 95–98
114. Christensen OB, Christensen MB, Wall LM (1986) Does sodium cromoglycate have an effect on contact dermatitis? Contact Dermatitis 15: 183–185
115. Upfal M, Doyle C (1990) Medical management of hydrofluoric acid exposure. J Occup Med 32: 726–731
116. Avnstorp C (1989) Prevalence of cement eczema in Denmark before and since the addition of ferrous sulphate to Danish cement. Acta Derm Venereol (Stockh) 69: 151–155
117. Valsecchi R, Cainelli T (1984) Chromium dermatitis and ascorbic acid. Contact Dermatitis 10: 252–253
118. Maibach HI, Engasser P (1988) Management of cosmetic intolerance syndrome. Clin Dermatol 6: 102–1–7
119. Lammintausta K, Maibach HI, Wilson D (1988) Mechanisms of subjective (sensory) irritation. Propensity to non-immunologic contact urticaria and objective irritation in stingers. Derm Beruf Umwelt 36: 45–49
120. Krogh von G, Maibach HI (1981) The contact urticaria syndrome – an updated review. Contact Dermatitis 5: 328–341
121. Lahti A, McDonald DM, Tammi R, Maibach HI (1986) Pharmacological studies on non-immunological contact urticaria in guinea pigs. Arch Dermatol Res 279: 44–49
122. Lahti A, Väänänen A, Kokkonen E-L, Hannuksela M (1987) Acetylsalicylic acid inhibits non-immunologic contact urticaria. Contact Dermatitis 16: 133–135
123. Frosch RJ, Wahl R, Bahmer FA (1986) Contact urticaria to rubber gloves is IgE mediated. Contact Dermatitis 14: 241–245
124. Wrangsjö K, Mellström G, Axelsson G (1985) Discomfort from rubber gloves indicating contact urticaria. Contact Dermatitis 15: 79–89
125. Turjanmaa K, Reunala T (1988) Contact urticaria from rubber gloves. Dermatol Clin 6: 47–51
126. Turjanmaa K, Laurila K, Mäkinen-Kiljunen S, Reunala T (1988) Rubber contact urticaria. Contact Dermatitis 19: 362–367
127. Rystedt I (1985) Work-related hand eczema in atopics. Contact Dermatitis 12: 64–171

128. Lammintausta K, Kalimo KK (1981) Atopy and hand dermatitis in hospital wet work. Contact Dermatitis 7: 301–308
129. Glickman FS, Silvers SH (1967) Hand eczema and atopy in housewives. Arch Dermatol 95: 407–409
130. Shmunes E, Keil J (1984) The role of atopy in occupational dermatoses. Contact Dermatitis 11: 174–178
131. Cox NH (1988) Contact allergy to clobetasol proprionate. Arch Dermatol 124: 911–913
132. Feldman SB, Sexton FM, Buzas J, Marks JG Jr (1988) Allergic contact dermatitis from topical steroids. Contact Dermatitis 19: 226–228
133. Coopman S, Degreef H, Dooms-Goossens A (1989) Identification of cross-reaction patterns in allergic contact dermatitis from topical corticosteroids. Br J Dermatol 121: 27–34
134. Cronin E, Kullivanijaya P (1979) Hand dermatitis in hairdressers. Acta Derm Venereol [Suppl 85] 59: 47–50
135. Nethercott JR, MacPherson M, Choi BCK, Nixon P (1986) Contact dermatitis in hairdressers. Contact Dermatitis 14: 73–79
136. Matsunaga K, Hosokawa K, Suzuki M, Arimi Y, Hayakawa R (1988) Occupational allergic contact dermatitis in beauticians. Contact Dermatitis 18: 30–36
137. Wahlberg J (1975) Nickel allergy and atopy in hairdressers. Contact Dermatitis 1: 161–165
138. Schubert H, Prater E (1982) Nickel allergy in hairdressers. Contact Dermatitis 8: 414–415 (letter)
139. Morison M, Storrs FJ (1988) Persistence of an allergen in hair after glycerol monothioglycolate containing permanent wave solutions. J Am Acad Dermatol 19: 52–59
140. Wilkinson DS, Hambly EM (1978) Prognosis of hand eczema in hairdressing appretices. Contact Dermatitis 4: 63
141. Lind PO, Hurlen B, Lybergg T, Aas E (1986) Amalgam-related oral lichenoid reaction. Scand J Dent Res 94: 448–451
142. Fernandez JP, Veron C, Hildebrand HF, Martin P (1988) Nickel allergy to dental prostheses. Contact Dermatitis 14: 312
143. van Joost TH, van Ulsen J, van Loon LAJ (1988) Contact allergy to dental materials in the burning mouth syndrome. Contact Dermatitis 18: 97–99
144. Rostoker G, Rolbin J, Binet O, Paupe T (1986) Dermatoses d'intolerance aux metaux des matériaux d'osteosynthèse et des prosthèses. Ann Dermatol Venereol 113: 1097–1108
145. Waterman AH, Schrik JJ (1985) Allergy in hip arthroplasty. Contact Dermatitis 13: 294–301
146. Wilkinson JD (1989) Nickel allergy and orthopaedic prostheses. In Eds. Maibach HI, Menné T (eds) Nickel and the skin: immunology and toxicology. CRC Press, Boca Raton, pp 187–193
147. Kubba R, Taylor JS, Marks KE (1981) Cutaneous complications of orthopaedic implants. Arch Dermatol 117: 554
148. Rooker G, Wilkinson JD (1980) Metal sensitivity in patients undergoing hip replacement. J Bone Joint Surg [Br] 62: 502–505
149. Burrows D, Creswell S, Merrett JD (1981) Nickel hands and hip prostheses. Br J Dermatol 105: 437–444
150. Dentmann R, Mulder J, Brian R, Nater JP (1977) Metal sensitivity before and after hip arthroplasty. J Bone Joint Surg [Am] 59: 862
151. Langlais F, Postel M, Berry JP et al. (1980) L'intolerance and débris d'usure des prosthèses, bilan immunologiques et anatomopathologie de 30 cas. Int Orthop 4: 145
152. Nurse DS (1980) Nickel sensitivity induced by skin clips. Contact Dermatitis 6: 497

153. Schubert H et al. (1987) Epidemiology of nickel allergy. Contact Dermatitis 16: 122–128
154. Fischer T, Fregert S, Gruvberger B, Rystedt (1984) Nickel release ear piercing kits and earrings. Contact Dermatitis 10: 39–41
155. Larsson-Stymne B, Widstrom L (1985) Ear piercing – a cause of nickel allergy in schoolgirls. Contact Dermatitis 13: 289–293
156. Emmett EA, Risby TH, Jian L, Ng Sk, Feinman S (1988) Allergic contact dermatitis to nickel: bioavailability from consumer products and provocation threshold. J Am Acad Dermatol 19: 314–322
157. Romaguera C, Grimalt F, Vilaplana J (1988) Contact dermatitis from nickel: an investigation of its sources. Contact Dermatitis 19: 52–57
158. Menné T, Brandrup F, Thiestrup-Pedersen K, Veien NK, Andersen JR, Yding F, Valleur G (1987) Patch test reactivity to nickel alloys. Contact Dermatitis 16: 255–259
159. Cirne de Castro JL, Pereira MA, Prates Nunes F, Pereira dos Santos A (1985) Musk ambrette and chronic actinic dermatitis. Contact Dermatitis 13: 302–306
160. Shall L, Reynolds AJ, Holt PJA (1986) Photosensitivity to musk ambrette in toilet soap and hair gel. Contact Dermatitis 14: 324
161. Pecegueiro M, Brandão FM (1985) Airborne contact dermatitis to plants. Contact Dermatitis 13: 277–278
162. Hjorth N, Roed-Petersen J, Thomsen K (1976) Airborne contact dermatitis from Compositae oleoresins simulating photodermatitis. Br J Dermatol 95: 613–620
163. Thune P, Eeg-Larsen T (1984) Contact and photocontact allergy in persistent light reactivity. Contact Dermatitis 11: 98–107
164. Picman J, Picman AK (1985) Treatment of dermatitis from *Parthenium*. Contact Dermatitis 13: 9–13
165. Austin AP, Milligan MC, Pennington K, Tweito DH (1988) A survey of factors associated with diaper dermatitis in thirty-six pediatric practices. J Pediatr Health Care 2: 295–299
166. Campbell RC, Bartlett AV, Sarbaugh FC, Pickering LK (1988) Effects of diaper types on diaper dermatitis associated with diarrhoea and antibiotic use in children in day-care centres. Pediatr Dermatol 5: 83–87
167. Buckingham KW, Berg RW (1986) Etiologic factors in diaper dermatitis – the role of faeces. Pediatr Dermatol 3: 107–112
168. Seymour JC, Keswick BH, Milligan MC, Jordan WP, Hanifin JM (1987) Clinical and microbial effects of cloth, cellulose core and cellulose core/absorbent gel diapers in atopic dermatitis. Pediatrician 14 [Suppl 1]: 39–43
169. Marks JG, Tranklein JJ, Zwillich CW, Demers LM (1984) Contact urticaria and airway obstruction from carbonless copy paper. JAMA 252: 1038–1040
170. Murray R (1991) Health aspects of carbonless copy paper. Contact Dermatitis 24: 321–333
171. Svennson A, Möller H (1986) Eyelid dermatitis: the role of atopy and contact allergy. Contact Dermatitis 15: 178–182
172. Christensen OB, Möller H (1975) External and internal exposure to the antigen in hand eczema of nickel allergy. Contact Dermatitis 1: 136–141
173. Brun R (1979) Nickel dans les aliments et eczémade contact. Dermatologica 159: 365–370
174. Veien NK, Hattel T, Justesen O, Norholm A (1987) Oral challenge with nickel and cobalt in patient with positive patch tests to nickel and/or cobalt. Acta Derm Venereol (Stockh) 67: 321–325
175. Veien NK, Hattel T, Justesen O, Norholm A (1985) Dietary treatment of nickel dermatitis. Acta Derm Venereol (Stockh) 65: 138–142
176. Burrows D, Creswell S, Merrett JD (1981) Nickel, hands and hip prostheses. Br J Dermatol 105: 437–444

177. Jordan WP, King SE (1979) Nickel feeding in nickel sensitive patients with hand eczema. J Am Acad Dermatol 1: 506–508
178. Gawkrodger DJ, Fell GS, Hunter JAA (1985) Nickel dermatitis: the reaction to oral nickel challenge. Br J Dermatol 113: 222–223
179. Gawkrodger DJ, Shuttler IL, Delves HTR (1988) Nickel dermatitis and diet: clinical improvement and a reduction in blood urine nickel levels with a low-nickel diet. Acta Derm Venereol (Stockh) 68: 453–455
180. Christenson OB, Möller H (1978) Release of nickel from cooking utensils. Contact Dermatitis 4: 343–348
181. Niinimaki A (1984) Delayed type allergy to spices. Contact Dermatitis 11: 34–40
182. Veien NK, Hattel T, Justesen O, Norholm A (1985) Oral challenge with balsam of Peru. Contact Dermatitis 12: 104–107
183. Veien NK, Hattel T, Justesen O, Norholm A (1985) Reduction of intake of balsams in patients sensitive to balsam of Peru. Contact Dermatitis 12: 270–273
184. Fisher AA (1979) The clinical significance of positive patch test reactions to balsam of Peru. Cutis 13: 909–913
185. De Groot AC, Conemans J (1986) Allergic urticarial rash from oral codeine. Contact Dermatitis 14: 209–214
186. Andersen KE, Hjorth N, Menné T (1984) The baboon syndrome – systemically induced allergic contact dermatitis. Contact Dermatitis 10: 97–100
187. Nater JP, De Groot AC (1985) Unwanted effects of cosmetics and drugs used in dermatology, 2nd edn. Elsevier, Amsterdam, pp 215–220
188. Menné T (1987) Reactions to systemic exposure to contact allergens. In: Marzulli FN, Maibach HI (eds) Dermatotoxicology, 3nd edn. Hemisphere, Washington, pp 535–552
189. Holti G (1974) Immediate and Arthus-like hypersensitivity to nickel. Clin Allergy 4: 37
190. Andersen KE (1988) Systemic contact dermatitis. Acta Derm Venereol (Stockh) 135: 62–63
191. Mellstrom G (1985) Protective effect of gloves – compiled in a data base. Contact Dermatitis 13: 162–165
192. Rietschel RL, Huyggins R, Levy N, Pruitt PM (1984) In vivo and in vitro testing of gloves for protection against UV-curable acrylate resin systems. Contact Dermatitis 11: 279–282
193. Sansone EB, Tewari YB (1978) The permeability of laboratory gloves to selected solvents. Am Ind Hyg Assoc J 39: 169–173
194. Estlander J, Jolanki R (1980) How to protect the hands. Dermatol Clin 6: 105–114
195. Pegum JS (1979) Penetration of protective gloves by epoxy resin. Contact Dermatitis 5: 281–283
196. Blanken R, Nater JP, Veenhoff E (1987) Protection agains epoxy resins with glove materials. Contact Dermatitis 16: 46–47
197. Orchard S, Feldman JH, Storrs FJ (1986) Poison oak dermatitis. Use of polyamide salts of a linoleic acid dimer for topical prophylaxis. Arch Dermatol 122: 783–789
198. Loden M (1986) The effect of 4 barrier creams on the absorption of water, benzene and formaldehyde into excised human skin. Contact Dermatitis 14: 292–296
199. Reiner R, Rossman K, van Hooikdonk C, Centen B, Bock J (1982) Ointments for the protection against organophosphate poisoning. J Drug Res 32: 630
200. Fischer T, Rystedt I (1983) Skin protection against ionised cobalt and sodium lauryl sulphate with barrier creams. Contact Dermatitis 9: 125–130
201. Wahlberg JE (1972) Antichromium barrier creams. Dermatologica 145: 175–181
202. Boman A, Wahlberg JE, Johansson E (1982) A method for the study of the effect of barrier creams and protective gloves on the percutaneous absorption of solvents. Dermatologica 164: 157–160

203. Lauwerys RR, Dath T, LaChapelle J-M, Buchet JP, Roels H (1978) The influence of two barrier creams on the percutaneous absorption of m-xylene in man. J Occup Med 20: 17–20
204. Lammintausta K, Maibach HI (1988) Dermatologic considerations in worker fitness evaluation. State Art Rev Occup Med 3: 341–350
205. Burrows D (1985) Industrial dermatitis today and its prevention. In: Griffiths WAD, Wilkinson DS (eds) Essentials of industrial dermatology. Mosby St Louis, pp 12–23
206. Shmunes E, Keil JE (1983) Occupational dermatoses in South Carolina: a descriptive analysis of cost variables, J Am Acad Dermatol 9: 861–866
207. Lammintausta K, Kalimo K, Havn VK (1982) Occurrence of contact allergy and hand eczema in hospital wet work. Contact Dermatitis 8: 84–90
208. Edman B (1988) The usefulness of detailed information to patients with contact allergy. Contact Dermatitis 19: 43–47
209. Rudzki E (1975) Pattern of hypersensitivity to aromatic amines. Contact Dermatitis 1: 248–249
210. Meneghini CL (1985) Sensitization in traumatised skin. Am J Ind Med 8: 401–402
211. de Groot AC (1990) Labelling cosmetics with their ingredients Br Med J 300: 1636–1638

Chapter 17
Principles of Prevention and Protection in Contact Dermatitis

Principles of Prevention and Protection in Contact Dermatitis (with Special Reference to Occupational Dermatology)

JEAN-MARIE LACHAPELLE

Contents

17.1 Introduction

Preventing occupational (and nonoccupational) contact dermatitis is the cornerstone of all our projects. It is crucial that over the next few years the number of cases be reduced. This is particularly true for certain occupations: bakers, hairdressers, the staff of hospitals, nursing homes and restaurants, and many others (see Chap. 11). Two types of considerations must be borne in mind: individual aspects (some workers are disabled by many interruptions to their activities in the course of a year) and socio-economical aspects. Prevention is a difficult task, with many different facets, including both general and individual measures of protection [1]; unavoidably, it also implies a wide range of treatment procedures. There is a general principle: general measures of prevention and protection are more effective than individual measures, since the latter depend upon the personal will and constant application of each individual worker; it is clear that preventive dermatology is not yet accepted as a routine procedure [2]. In most industrialized countries, a relatively safe working environment is provided by most of the largest plants [3]. Nevertheless, at other workplaces contacts with irritants and/or allergens could be avoided more effectively.

Occupational dermatologists are all agreed on a multidimensional approach to the prevention of occupational skin disease. Such a system has been described and recommended by Mathias and Morrison [4]. It includes: identification of potential irritants and allergens, engineering controls or chemical substitution to prevent exposure, personal protection with appropriate clothing or barrier creams, personal and environmental hygiene, regulation of potential allergens and irritants within the workplace, educational efforts to promote awareness of potential allergens and irritants, motivational techniques to establish safe work conditions and practices, and pre-employment and periodic health screening.

17.2 General Measures of Prevention

The various measures are intended to reduce contact with irritants and/or allergens.

17.2.1 Use of Potent Allergens in Closed Systems

It is absolutely essential that very potent allergens be kept in closed systems; any contact with the intact or damaged skin of workers must be avoided. For instance 2,4-dinitro-1-chlorobenzene has been used extensively as an algicide in air-conditioning cooling systems [1]. It is clearly kept in a closed system; nevertheless, maintenance or repair activities involve insidious occasional contact between some categories of workers and the allergen; this can provoke epidemics of contact dermatitis involving such workers. A similar situation can occur with various amines used in the plastics industry [3].

17.2.2 Automation

Automation is the only practical means of avoiding some epidemics of contact dermatitis in industry. There are many examples of industrial airborne irritant contact dermatitis that could not be solved by individual measures of protection. Automation of the industrial procedure has been advised in several such cases. This is especially true when dust particles are responsible for skin irritation [5]. I have reported an epidemic of slag dermatitis [6] in a metallurgical plant where permanent-mould casting techniques had been introduced. At one stage of production, workers poured slag (mixture of silicon oxide and calcium oxide powders) into ingot moulds. Dust, penetrating through protective clothes or between sleeves and gloves, accumulated in the flexures and on the extensor aspects of the thighs and arms. Subjective and objective skin symptoms were similar to those of fibreglass dermatitis.

Scratch marks, papules and pustules were sometimes present. Microscopic examination of powder particles revealed that some were oblong and sharpedged (length $10 - 80$ mμ). Dermatitis was considered to be related to mechanical irritation of the skin by sharp-edged particles. Recently, we have reviewed the problem and dispersed several samples of different slag particles in distilled water. The pH of the supernatant measured between 8 and 12. Slag dermatitis could therefore be due not only to the roughness of particles, but also to irritation by alkali. This occupational problem, the large scale of which needed effective measures, has been solved by complete automation.

Among photographers, the problem of allergic contact dermatitis from colour developers has been solved almost completely in Scandinavian countries by the widespread use of automatic procedures [7, 8]. The drawback of automation is also related to maintenance and repair procedures, during the course of which workers may be off their guard.

17.2.3 Allergen Replacement or Removal

Allergen replacement (or removal) is a possible solution to many problems of allergic contact dermatitis. Some of the following examples are difficult to apply, whereas other are easy:

- Replacement of epoxy resins by other types of resins [3]. Theoretical; not easy in practice.
- Use of epoxy resins with a molecular weight greater than 1 kDa [9]. Theoretical; not easy in practice.
- Substitution of a catalyst or curing agent in an epoxy resin system [3]. Can be discussed and realized in practice.
- Replacement of accelerators and antioxidants in rubber factories. Conceivable in practice.
- Addition of ferrous sulphate to cement. Cement causes dermatitis not only in areas directly exposed to the dust but also in areas covered with dust-impregnated clothing. Premixed cement delivered wet to the work place eliminates the dust hazard to some extent. The addition of ferrous sulphate to cement immediately before mixing reduces the hexavalent chromium to the trivalent state and may thus prevent dermatitis [3]. In some countries, ferrous sulphate is available (in sacks), to be added to cement (Mesalt); its use is not always possible in practice for various reasons.
- Removal of chromate from household and/or industrial products is essential [10]. Calnan has emphasized that "chromate sensitization produces such a chronic and recalcitrant dermatitis that dermatologists should always try to limit its use in materials or fluids which may contaminate the skin, even in low concentrations." The presence of sodium dichromate in eau de Javel is no longer justified, either as a colouring agent or a stabilizer. The decision to remove sodium dichromate from eau de Javel by the French Trade Society of producers in Paris was a notable example of such an effort in

preventive dermatology. In this case, one of the arguments in favour of removal was the fear raised by the medical authorities of provoking and/or perpetuating allergic contact dermatitis from chromate among users. It is interesting to note that this measure is of importance not only in preventing housewives' dermatitis but also in occupational dermatology, since eau de Javel is used on a large scale for cleaning or antisepti purposes [11].

– Replacement of a biocide, as an additive in many industrial products, such as soluble oils. This is a fairly common problem, relatively easy to solve in practice.

The removal of irritants or allergens can also at least partly be achieved by general local exhaust ventilation.

17.2.4 Measures for More Appropriate Use of Industrial Irritants or Allergens

One very important measure to be applied in factories is the proper use of many chemicals. It is noteworthy that some products are not used as advised on notices. Two examples serve to illustrate this situation. (a) Biocides are very often used at excessively high concentrations in industrial fluids. Workers attempt to 'rejuvenate' solutions by reducing bacterial contamination with unacceptable amounts of biocides. Increased concentrations of biocides can be responsible for outbreaks of irritant or allergic contact dermatitis. (b) Glutaraldehyde solutions are used nowadays in hospitals to disinfect rooms. Cases of allergic contact dermatitis can be observed among members of staff when glutaraldehyde solutions are sprayed, for instance, over radiators, vapours being responsible for airborne contact dermatitis.

17.2.5 Measures for Better Knowledge of the Chemical Composition of End-Products

A better knowledge of the chemical nature of the various products used at work is of prime importance. Needless to say, such information is difficult to acquire in many instances. More than one paper has been devoted to this question [3, 12]. It is also very important that dermatologists have accurate knowledge of working conditions. Visiting factories or other work facilities is therefore very rewarding [13, 14]; it can provide useful information regarding many aspects of occupational life (see Chap. 11).

17.3 Individual Measures of Prevention

Individual measures of prevention (and/or protection) involve a three-step strategy [2]: (a) the use of protective clothing and/or creams adapted to each workplace, (b) correct skin cleansing, and (c) the use of skin care products after work.

17.3.1 Protective Clothing (with Special Attention to Gloves)

Protective clothing that meets a variety of requirements is nowadays available. Gloves adapted for each type of work are required. Specialist manufacturers of protective clothing provide information about the technical properties of various items. This is true particularly for different types of gloves [15]. General recommendations for the use of appropriate gloves have been made by Estlander and Jolanki [16]. These recommendations are summarized in Table 17.1 (see also Table 11.14, Chap. 11). A new glove material protective against epoxy and acrylate monomer has been produced recently [17]; this glove, termed 4-H Glove, has several layers (two outer layers of polyethylene and one inner layer of a copolymer of ethylene and vinylalcohol, separated by adhesive). The problem of contact urticaria due to latex gloves has become very important in some hospitals. Many cases have been reported from all over the world. Many efforts have been made to obtain hypoallergenic latex gloves. A possible alternative is the use of a thin polyethylene glove (such as Ethiparat, Johnson and Johnson) under the latex glove.

Table 17.1. Glove materials recommended for protection against various chemicals. (From [15])

Group of chemicals	Recommended materials
Aliphatic hydrocarbons	Nitrile rubber, viton, polyvinyl alcohol (cyclohexane excluded)
Aromatic hydrocarbons	Polyvinyl alcohol (ethylbenzene excluded), viton, nitrile rubber
Halogenated hydrocarbons	Polyvinyl alcohol, viton (FPM) (methyl chloride and halothane excluded)
Aldehydes, amines, amides	Butyl rubber (butylamine and triethylamine excluded)
Esters	Butyl rubber (butylacrylate excluded) Polyvinylalcohol (di-n-octylphthalate excluded)
Alkalis	Neoprene rubber, nitrile rubber, polyvinylalcohol
Organic acids	Neoprene rubber (acrylic acid and methacrylic acid excluded), butyl rubber, nitrile rubber (acrylic acid, methacrylic acid, and acetic acid excluded)
Inorganic acids	Neoprene rubber (chromic acid excluded), polyvinylchloride (30%–70% nitric acid, >70% sulphuric acid excluded), nitrile rubber (30%–70% hydrofluoric acid, 30%–70% nitric acid, 30%–70% sulphuric acid excluded)

17.3.2 'Barrier' Creams

Adams [3] has written an excellent summary of what we may expect from the use of barrier creams or gels:

Barrier creams, also known as protective ointments or invisible gloves, are employed as substitutes for protective clothing in situations in which gloves, sleeves, and face guards cannot be safely or conveniently used or when workers refuse to wear them. At best, barrier creams are an inferior substitute for protective clothing; however, because they must be washed off before coffee breaks and meals and before going home, they encourage cleanliness, at the same time removing industrial soil from the skin.

A most important requirement for a barrier cream is that it does not interfere with work performance. Many workers like them because they are easy to apply and in most situations are comfortable during use. They are rarely a satisfactory replacement for gloves, but on the face (especially around the eyes) they are fairly effective against some airborne substances.

'Active' barrier creams, i.e. creams containing active ingredients that are supposed to work by trapping or transforming allergens (ascorbic acid, glutathione, cysteine, ion exchangers, etc.) can be considered as ineffective. Therefore, barrier creams cannot be considered as protective against allergens.

Barrier creams or gels are recommended only against irritants. Most products on the market have not been submitted to laboratory experiments to prove their usefulness. Various methods have been proposed to evaluate the potential efficacy of barrier creams or gels. At Louvain University we have developed an animal (guinea pig) model involving the application of various irritants on the skin with and without protection. The methodology is invasive in nature, since it is based mainly on the analysis of histopathological lesions of the various compartments of the skin and therefore requires several skin biopsies on the same animal [18]. However, animal studies are to be avoided as far as possible and are tending to be replaced by noninvasive methods in man (laser Doppler flowmetry, evaporimetry, skin capacitance, etc.: see Sect. 10.7). This requires work on human volunteers. We have conducted several studies using such noninvasive methodology. From these studies, we conclude that protection against organic solvents (within certain limits of time and excluding trichloroethylene) can be achieved by antisolvent gels such as Antixol (Laphi) or Phyprol 12 (Sorefa), which are mixtures of proteins and lipoprpoteins, cellulose esters, triethanolamine, ethanol and water. Oil-in-water creams are of no value against solvents. Water-in-oil creams can be efficacious against irritants present in water (such as acids, alkalis, detergents, antiseptics, soluble oils, etc.), though for a limited period of time. Silicone creams (5%) are somewhat more effective than the same creams without silicone [19]; in some experiments the difference is substantial, whereas in others it is less so [20]. More studies are needed, including those on various schedules of application of irritants and also of barrier creams, in order to duplicate working conditions more accurately.

There is a current flood of protective foams (or 'foam gels') in many European countries. Some are marketed as 'invisible gloves' – a term previously adopted 40 years ago for barrier creams. Some contain 1% silicone (Marly Skin, Dermofilm, Epiguard, etc.) but not all (Ecoderm). At present we are conducting experimental studies on various of these foam gels. Preliminary studies indicate a protective effect, within certain time limitations and constraints of type and concentration of irritants.

An extensive programme of evaluation of the protective effect of barrier creams has been conducted recently by Frosch et al., including use of their repetitive irritation test (RIT) in humans [21–23]

17.3.3 Skin Cleansers with Low Irritant Potential

It is advisable to use skin cleansers with low irritant potential [2]. There are different options available to the clinical researcher studying irritancy. For example, a test schedule appropriate for the testing of liquid soaps used in a hospital might involve three types of test: repeated application under occlusion (Frosch-Kligman); single application under occlusion, the equivalent of acute toxicity testing (as practised at Louvain); and repeated open applications mimicking use conditions. The general methodology used in most laboratories at the present time is limited by a serious drawback: the fact that most experiments are conducted as 'acute toxicity' experiments. Applying a cleanser once (under occlusion) for 24 h is to some extent misleading since this does not reflect the real-life situation. This clearly raises questions about the usefulness of such tests.

A more useful approach would be to reproduce, as far as possible, experimentally the use applications. Use tests are therefore favoured by researchers. In the particular case of cleansing agents, repeated open applications on the forearms of volunteers, according to various schedules, have been started in our research unit. This type of investigation aims to achieve two things: better understanding of the mode of action of irritants in general and empirical knowledge about the comparative irritant potential of various chemicals and, in particular, of cleansing agents.

17.4 References

1. Lachapelle JM (1984) Abrégé de dermatologie professionnelle. Masson, Paris
2. Lachapelle JM (1990) A European overview of occupational dermatology. Occup Health Rev 27: 21–24
3. Adams RH (1990) Prevention, rehabilitation, treatment. Adams RM (ed) Saunders, Philadelphia, Occupational skin diseases 2nd Edn, pp 261–279
4. Mathias CGT, Morrison JH (1988) Occupational skin disease, United States. Arch Dermatol 124: 1519–1524
5. Lachapelle JM (1987) Industrial airborne irritant contact dermatitis due to dust particles. Boll Dermatol Allerg Prof 2: 83–89

6. Lachapelle JM (1984) Occupational airborne irritant contact dermatitis to slag. Contact Dermatitis 10: 315–316
7. Liden C, Brehmer-Andersson E (1988) Occupational dermatoses from colour developing agents. Clinical and histopathological observations. Acta Derm Venereol (Stockh) 68: 514–522
8. Liden C, Sollenberg J, Hansen L, Arvidson A (1989) Contact allergy to colour developing agents. Analysis of test preparations, bulk chemicals and tank solutions by high-performance liquid chromatography. Derm Beruf Umwelt 37: 47–52
9. Thorgeirsson A, Fregert S, Fammas O (1978) Sensitization capacity of epoxy resin oligomers in the guinea pig. Acta Derm Venereol (Stockh) 58: 17–21
10. Calnan CD (1978) Chromate in coolant water of gramophone record presses. Contact Dermatitis 4: 246–247
11. Lachapelle JM, Lauwerys R, Tennstedt D, Andanson J, Benezra C, Chabeau G, Ducombs G, Foussereau J, Lacroix M, Martin P (1980) Eau de Javel and prevention of chromate allergy in France. Contact Dermatitis 6: 107–110
12. Cohen SR (1988) Sources of information for occupational dermatology. Dermatol Clin 6: 15–19
13. Rycroft RJG (1988) Looking at work dermatologically. Dermatol Clin 6: 1–5
14. Rycroft RJG (1986) Occupational site survey: principles and significance. In: Maibach HI (ed) Occupational and industrial dermatology, 2nd edn. Year Book Medical Publishers, Chicago, pp 3–5
15. Berardinelli SP (1988) Prevention of occupational skin disease through use of chemical protective gloves. Dermatol Clin 6: 115–119
16. Estlander T, Jolanki R (1988) How to protect the hands. Dermatol Clin 6: 105–114
17. Roed-Petersen J (1989) A new glove material protective against epoxy and acrylate monomer. In: Frosch PJ, Dooms-Goossens A, Lachapelle JM, Rycroft RJ, Scheper RJ (eds) Current topics in contact dermatitis. Springer Berlin Heidelberg New York, pp 603–606
18. Mahmoud G, Lachapelle JM (1987) Uses of a guinea pig model to evaluate the protective value of barrier creams and/or gels. In: Maibach HI, Lowe NJ (eds) Models in dermatology, vol 3. Karger, Basel, pp 112–120
19. Nouaigui H, Antoine JL, Lachapelle JM (1988) Evaluation expérimentale du pouvoir protecteur d'une crème siliconée versus son excipient vis-à-vis de l'irritation cutanée par soude caustique. Arch Mal Prof 49: 383–387
20. Nouaigui H, Antoine JL, Masmoudi ML, van Neste D, Lachapelle JM (1989) Etudes invasive et non invasive du pouvoir protecteur d'une crème siliconée et de son excipient vis-à-vis de l'irritation cutanée induite par le laurylsulfate de sodium. Ann Dermatol Venereol 116: 389–398
21. Frosch PJ, Schulze-Dirks A, Hoffmann M, Axthelm I, Kurte A (1993) Efficacy of skin barrier creams, I. The repetitive irritation test (RIT) in the guinea pig. Contact Dermatitis 28: 94–100
22. Frosch PJ, Schulze-Dirks A, Hoffmann M, Axthelm I (1993) Evaluation of skin barrier creams, II. Ineffectiveness of a popular "skin protector" against various irritants in the repetitive irritation test in the guinea pig. Contact Dermatitis 29: 74–77
23. Frosch PJ, Kurte A, Pilz B (1993) Efficacy of skin barrier creams, III. The repetitive irritation test (RIT) in humans. Contact Dermatitis 29: 113–118

Chapter 18
Predictive Assays:
Animal and Man,
and In Vitro and In Vivo

Predictive Assays:
Animal and Man, and In Vitro and In Vivo[*]

Esther Patrick and Howard I. Maibach

Contents

---

[*] Adapted from E. Patrick and H. Maibach (1989) Dermatotoxicology: In: A. Wallace Hayes (ed.) Principles and Methods of Toxicology, 2nd edn. Raven Press, New York, Chap. 13.

18.1 Introduction

Assuming that data from predictive tests are interpreted prudently by dermato-toxicologists with extensive training in quantitative structure-activity relationships, animal and human predictive assays combined with broad clinical experience should aid rational risk-benefit decision making.

The policies of agencies such as the Occupational Health and Safety Administration, Department of Transportation, Consumer Product Safety Commission, and Food and Drug Administration in the United States and the Organization for Economic Cooperation and Development and European Economic Community, internationally, indicate that the identification of chemicals hazardous to the skin and the protection of society from exposure to those chemicals should be given high priority. These agencies mandate specific assays to evaluate the effects of skin exposure before registration, transport, or marketing of chemicals or formulated products.

The adverse skin responses associated with repetitive, low-dose exposure to industrial chemicals and consumer products all too often are not accurately predicted by the required assays. The need to market products with low risk of producing dermal and systemic injury to increase consumer satisfaction has led to the development of numerous assays to rank chemicals for their ability to injure the skin. Although these assays are often not mandated by regulatory agencies, the frequency with which they are conducted and their utility warrant attention.

The field of dermatoxicology includes measurement of absorption of materials as well as assays that evaluate the ability of topically applied chemicals to induce or promote the development of neoplasia, trigger an immune response in the skin, directly destroy the skin (corrosion), irritate the skin, provoke urticaria, and produce noninflammatory painful sensations. The inflammatory responses of skin are the most common chemically induced dermatoses in humans.

18.2 Dermatopharmacokinetics: Relation to Predictive Assays

Until the beginning of the twentieth century, skin was considered a relatively inert barrier to chemicals that might enter the body [148]. We now know that this view is incorrect. Although the skin's barrier properties are impressive, many chemicals penetrate the skin, and the skin can metabolize exogenous compounds. Because of its large surface area, the skin may be a major route of entry into the body for some exposure situations. Delivery of drugs through the skin to treat systemic conditions has become almost commonplace. Interest in cutaneous pharmacokinetics has increased as the skin has been reconsidered to be a route for systemic administration of drugs and chemicals, as well as a route of entry for toxins. A variety of assays, both *in vivo* and *in vitro*, for measuring absorption through the skin have been developed [4, 5, 139, 178], and many factors that govern absorption through the skin have been determined. A major diffusion barrier of the skin is considered to be the stratum corneum. Removal of the stratum corneum by tape stripping increases the rate of absorption of some chemicals [10]. Absorption of chemicals through shunts, openings of skin appendages, and gaps in the stratum corneum associated with these structures have been considered [157, 164]. Absorption can be described as passive diffusion across this membrane by the equation, $J = (K_m C_v D_m)\pi d$, or, rate of absorption = (vehicle/stratum corneum partition coefficient = concentration = diffusion constant of penetrant in stratum corneum) divided by thickness of stratum corneum [31]. It is clear that skin from different animals or sites of different thickness from the same animal vary in barrier properties to absorption. The concentration term refers to that at the skin surface. Application of suspensions of penetrant with slow dissolution rates, of emulsions, or of penetrants in vehicles in which diffusion rate is slow alters surface concentration and may control the rate of penetration [15, 19, 23, 66]. Other factors that affect thermodynamic activity of the solution at the skin surface, such as pH and temperature, may vary the absorption rate [149, 149]. Vehicle influence cannot be overstated; for a specific concentration of chemical, thermodynamic activity may vary by 1000-fold from one vehicle to another [30]. Some vehicles may promote penetration by altering the characteristics of the stratum corneum [87]. Other factors that affect percutaneous absorption include condition of the skin [42], age, surface area to which the material is applied [178], penetrant volatility, temperature and humidity [48], substantivity, and wash-and-rub resistance to removal from the skin and binding to the skin [137]. Skin may become saturated by a penetrant and thus resist penetration from subsequent applications.

Once a chemical has gained access to the viable epidermal layers, it may initiate a local effect, be absorbed into the circulation and produce an effect or produce no local or systemic effects. The viable epidermis contains many enzymes capable of metabolizing exogenous chemicals [132], including a cytochrome P-450 system, mixed function oxidases, and gluconyltransferases. Early studies indicated that enzymatic activity is skin was only a fraction of the activity of the liver. These studies were conducted *in vitro* using whole skin; the enzymatic activity is in the epidermis, which makes up under 5% of the whole skin. When enzymatic activities of the epidermis were calculated, activities ranged from 80% to 240% of those in liver. Comparison of metabolites formed after dermal and oral administration of [3H]cortisol demonstrated that different metabolites were formed. The skin does not have the capacity to metabolize all chemicals. For example, topically applied hexachlorophene does not appear to be metabolized. At present, it is not possible to predict metabolic pathways or rates following topical application; these must be determined experimentally.

Percutaneous absorption can be determined by applying a known amount of chemical to a specified surface area and then measuring levels of the chemical in the urine and/or feces. To correct for excretion of the material through the lungs, sweat, or retention in the body, levels measured following topical administration are usually expressed as a percentage of levels following parenteral administration of the chemical [179]. Because the analytical techniques to measure the chemical are not always available and because some chemicals may be metabolized, radioactively labelled chemicals, usually carbon-14 or tritium, are customarily used in these assays. Although studies with radiolabelled compounds accurately reflect absorption, they may not provide accurate estimates of bioavailability. For example, comparision of bioavailability from nitroglycerin (unmetabolized drug) levels and levels of radioactive tracer indicates that use of the tracer overestimates available drug by as much as 20%. This corresponds to the metabolism of the drug to an inactive form.

In vivo studies have been conducted in humans and in a number of species [5]. Comparison of absorption rates of a number of compounds showed that absorption rates in the rat and rabbit tend to be higher than in humans, and that the skin permeability of monkeys and swine more closely resembles that of humans. No significant mouse – human skin flux comparisons exist. Currently available, but limited, guinea pig – human comparisons offer some promise for refinement of guinea pig – human irritation and sensitization extrapolations. Although these differences are not predicted by any single factor, for example epidermal thickness, they are not unexpected in the light of differences in routes of excretion of some chemicals as well. This may be due in part to metabolism of the chemical, and the metabolic capabilities of the species should be considered when selecting an animal model and designing the experiment. Ingestion of the test material by the animal must be prevented, and this may require restraint of the animal or designing specialized protective apparatus for the site of application. Because urine and feces are collected for analysis, specialized cages are also required. The difficulty of conducting these types of pharmacokinetic assays is obvious: collection of excrement requires a relatively long period of time (>24 h), the use of specialized cages and specialized protective apparatus, and the increased space requirements for housing animals individually. Although there is no question that pharmacokinetic studies of this type in humans or animals provide the best estimate of percutaneous absorption, the cost and difficulty in conducting well-controlled studies has led to the use of other *in vivo* assays that are poorer predictive tools and to the development of *in vitro* models.

18.2.1 In Vitro Percutaneous Penetration Assays

The excised skins of humans or animals can be used to measure penetration of chemicals. *In vitro* assays using excised skin utilize specially designed diffusion cells [4, 46]. The skin is stretched over the opening of a collecting receptacle, epidermal side up. The chemical to be studied is applied to the epidermis, and fluid from the receptacle is assayed to measure the penetration of the chemical. Chemicals are usually radioactively labelled. Although some investigators have used diffusion cells in which the epidermis was covered with fluid containing the chemical, the preferred method for toxicological relevance is often a one-chambered cell in which the stratum corneum is exposed to the air, and the underside of the skin is bathed in saline or other receptacle fluid. Because diffusion through a membrane depends on relative concentrations on each side, some chambers have been designed to allow periodic replacement of the receptacle fluid. Fluid in the receptacle base is usually constantly stirred and maintained at a physiological temperature. Either full-thickness skin or epidermis alone may be used in *in vitro* assays. With relatively hairless skin, epidermis can be separated from the dermis by heat treatment.

This type of *in vitro* assay offers some advantages over *in vivo* assays: highly toxic compounds can be studied in human skin; large numbers of cells can be run simultaneously; diffusion through the membrane, eliminating other pharmacokinetic factors, can be studied; and these assays may be cheaper and easier to conduct.

These assays do not mimic human exposure in some important areas. Because excised skin must often be stored before use, it cannot be assumed that the skin will retain full enzymatic activity. This may alter the metabolic profile of compounds entering the receptacle. In intact skin, chemicals penetrating the epidermis enter the circulation through vessels and lymphatics located just below the epidermis. In excised full-thickness skin, the dermis is also involved in the absorptive process. The influence of the dermis can be minimized by using heat-separated epidermis or by removal of the skin with a dermatome at the level of the upper dermis. In the intact animal, the chemical enters the peripheral circulation in plasma; the collecting fluid of diffusion chambers is usually saline or water. The relative solubilities of hydrophobic and hydrophilic chemicals in these collecting fluids may alter the rate at which they leave the skin. Surface conditions of excised skin may vary from normal skin; changes in the surface emulsion occurring during storage have not been studied. Storage conditions and procedures for preparing the tissue may affect skin absorption and metabolism. When possible, the suitability of each specimen of excised skin should be verified by measurement of penetration of a standard, tritiated water, through the tissue before its use to study penetration of other chemicals.

Comparison of penetration rates obtained from *in vitro* and *in vivo* assays have been made [4]. Often a good correlation between the two methods was obtained. However, with some compounds the correlation between methods was poor. Differences in the methods for some compounds could be explained on the basis of solubilities in the receptacle fluid and blood; others could not be explained. *In vitro* penetration rates through skin of various species have also been compared. Skin of the weanling pig and miniature swine appears to be a good *in vitro* model for most compounds [5]. Although a limited number of studies have been reported, the skin of monkeys also appears to be a good model [178]. For most compounds, mouse and hairless mouse skin appears more permeable than skin of other species. Rat skin appears to be a good model for some compounds; however, when differences have been noted, they have been large.

A few investigators have estimated percutaneous absorption using 'model' membranes, and physicochemical data have been used to predict absorption. Lipid:water partition coefficients have been correlated with skin permeability. Smaller molecules (molecular weight <400) are more readily absorbed than large. Molecules with polar groups generally do not penetrate as well as nonpolar molecules [147]. The addition of hydroxyl groups also lowers the permeability. Substitutions that increase lipid solubility may increase penetration, depending on the vehicle in which the chemicals are applied [148]. Electrolytes do not penetrate the skin well [149].

18.2.2 Specific Examples in Predictive Testing

Predictive assays generally require data on the dose-response relationship for prudent and optimal interpretation. Until recently such experiments listed the applied dose but offered no possibiity of interpretation as to the acutal dose reaching the tissue of interest, i.e., penetrated dose in epidermis and dermis. Now that more investigators are trained in designing, performing and interpreting such assays, we are beginning to understand the complexity of the relationship of absorbed dose and biologic effect.

For instance, the effect of patch test chamber design on the penetration of an allergen in the guinea pig revealed a several-fold difference in absorption from the least to most efficient system. These differences permit one to describe relative delivered rather than just applied dose and offer easier interpretations when attempting to extrapolate from an experimental system to the others.

Other critical variables which, when data are available, can facilitate more robust and sound information include:
- Effect of species as related to man (some guinea pig – human correlative studies exist)
- Vehicle effects (may be 100-fold)
- Dose-response relationships ($\mu g/cm^2$; linear, flat, or inverse)
- Anatomic site (more completely studies in man than in animals)
- Duration of occlusion (more completely studied in man than in animals)
- Experimentally damaged skin (may not increase bioavailability)

18.3 Allergic Contact Dermatitis

Jadassohn [73, 74] demonstrated that in some patients dermatitis is due to increased sensitivity following repeated contact with a substance and not to the toxic (irritant) properties of the material. By 1930 a procedure for producing this hypersensitivity to chemicals in guinea pigs had been developed [12]. The pioneering work of Landsteiner and associates [100–102] demonstrated that low molecular weight chemicals conjugate with proteins to form an antigen that stimulates the immune system to form a hyperreactive state [102]; that immunogenicity is related to chemical structure [101]; and that two types of immunological response exist, one transferable by serum and another transferred by suspensions of white blood cells [100]. Most cases of allergic contact dermatitis are of the cell-mediated type, transferable by lymphocytes.

Some understanding of the processes by which this hypersensitivity develops is helpful in selecting and interpreting results of predictive sensitization tests (see also Sect. 2.1). During ontogenesis, stem cells from the yolk sac, fetal liver, and bone marrow migrate to the central lymphoid organs, i.e. the thymus and bone marrow in mammals. After birth, stem cells derive from bone marrow. In the central lymphoid organs, stem cells differentiate into immunocompetent lymphocytes. This results in two classes of lymphocytes: thymus-processed T lymphocytes, and B lymphocytes processed in bone marrow. B lymphocytes are precursors of antibody-producing cells responsible for immune responses transferable by serum; T lymphocytes are responsible for producing delayed-type hypersensitivity (DTH) and for regulation of the immune system. This regulation is accomplished by subsets of T cells, i.e., T-helper and T-suppressor cells. Lymphocytes leaving the lymphoid organs are 'programmed' to recognize a specific chemical structure via a receptor molecule(s). If, during circulation through body tissues, a cell encounters the structure that it is programmed to recognize, an immune response may be induced. The ability to develop and express a hypersensitivity response is determined by the relative activities of the T-helper and T-suppressor cell types [141].

To stimulate an immune response, a chemical must be presented to lymphocytes in an appropriate form [101, 102]. Chemicals are usually haptens, which must conjugate with proteins in the skin or in other tissues in order to be recognized by the immune system. Haptens conjugate with multiple proteins to form a number of different antigens that may stimulate an allergic response by stimulating T lymphocytes with different recognition capabilities [142]. Hapten-protein conjugates are processed by macrophages or other cells expressing I a proteins on their surface. Although the exact nature of this processing is not completely understood, it is known that physical contact between macrophage and T cells is required [166], suggesting that receptor interactions are necessary. Physical interaction is accompanied by the release of interleukins, a family of soluble regulatory proteins that stimulate cell division, act as growth factors, and increase expression of immune proteins on the surface of some cells [41, 70, 124].

Following stimulation by antigen in the skin, lymphocytes enter the lymphatic system and migrate to the draining lymph nodes. Disruption of lymphatic drainage prevents sensitization of an animal [47]. Stimulated T lymphocytes settle in the paracortial regions of the lymph nodes and differentiate into immunoblasts. This differentiation involves interaction with other cell types. Immunoblasts eventually give rise to T-effector cells that enter the systemic circulation and, on encountering the antigen that they are programmed to recognized, release lymphokines that initiate a local inflammatory response. Immunoblasts also give rise to memory cells, which enter the systemic circulation. These memory cells are capable of similar activities to the T-processed lymphocytes; they recognize antigen and can be stimulated to divide. Memory cell production is essentially an expansion of the number of cells capable of recognizing a given antigen.

The lymphokines released by primed effector cells that encounter their stimulating antigen directly, and indirectly by stimulation of other white blood cells, produce a local inflammatory response. Actions of lymphokines include direct tissue damage, chemotactic factors, stimulation of mitosis, increased phagocytic activity of macrophages, and factors that inhibit migration of some cell types from the area [25]. Only a small percentage of lymphocytes in an area of skin exhibiting a DTH response is specifically stimulated by antigen [128]. Most cells in the lesion are 'recruited' by lymphokines. Histologically, the response has been described as a hyperproliferative epidermis with intracellular edema, spongiosis, intraepidermal vesiculation, and mononuclear cell inflitrate by 24 h. The dermis shows perivenous accumulation of lymphocytes, monocytes, and edema. No reaction occurs if the local vascular supply is interrupted, and the appearance of epidermal changes follows the invasion of monocytes. Vascular changes, for example, increased blood flow, occur early – at 5–6 h into the response. The histology of the response varies somewhat by species. For example, a higher proportion of polymorphonuclear cells in the cellular infiltrate has been observed in DTH reaction sites of mice than in guinea pigs or humans [75]. These differences may be due in part to mixed immune responses. Mice develop both antibody and DTH responses to haptens applied to the skin [3]. Exposure via the skin is thought to lead preferentially to DTH in guinea pigs and humans.

Many factors modulate development of DTH in experimental animals and in humans. Keratinocytes produce interleukin [25], an important regulatory protein for induction of DTH. Langerhans cells express I a antigen and may act as antigen-presenting cells [104, 161]. Intradermal injection in animals bypasses these processes but assures entry of the chemical into the skin. Factors that govern rate of penetration also influence rate of sensitization. The effects of vehicle and occlusion are well documented [110]. Application of haptens to damaged skin (e.g., irritated or tape stripped) usually increases the sensitization rate. Increasing the dose per unit area increases the sensitization rate. Repeated applications to the same site are more effective in inducing sensitization than application to new sites each time [37, 110]. The incidence of sensitization increases with increased numbers of exposures (this applies through 10–15 exposures) [110]. An interval between exposures of 2–7 days increased the sensitization rate [110]. This may be due to the 'booster' effect of memory cells. Materials such as Freund's complete adjuvant (FCA) nonspecifically enhance development of immune responses. Treatment of animals with adjuvant, either simultaneously or shortly after hapten exposure, increases sensitization rates [112, 113]. The development of DTH is under genetic control; all individuals do not have the capability to respond to a given hapten [110]. The status of the immune system determines whether an immune response can be induced. For example, young animals may become tolerant to a hapten, and pregnancy may suppress expression of allergy [110]. The intrinsic biological variables controlling sensitization can be influenced only by selection of animals likely to be capable of mounting an immune response to the hapten. The extrinsic variables of dose, vehicle, route of exposure, adjuvant, etc., can be manipulated to develop sensitive predictive assays.

Appropriate planning and execution of predictive sensitization assays is critical. All too often techniques are discredited when, in fact, the performance of the tests was inferior, or the study design (e.g., choice of dose) was inappropriate. The first priority is to choose an appropriate experimental design. Often the assay to be used is chosen on a *pro forma* basis, without realizing the inherent weakness and strengths of the method. A common error in choosing an animal assay is using FCA when setting dose response relationships. The adjuvant provides such sensitivity that dose-effect relationships are muted.

Choice of dose and vehicle appropriate to the assay and the study question is the second priority. Although dose must be high enough to ensure penetration, it must be below the threshold at challenge to avoid misinterpretation of irritant inflammation as allergic. For instance, the quaternary ammonium compounds, such as benzalkonium chloride, rarely sensitize but have been identified as allergens in some guinea pig assays. Knowing the irritation potential of compounds allows the investigator to design and execute these studies appropriately. Vehicle choice determines in part the absorption of the test material and can influence sensitization rate, ability to elicit response at challenge, and the irritation threshold. Inappropriate selections effectively invalidate studies.

18.3.1 Quantitative Structure-Activity Relationships

Quantitative structure-activity relationship studies examine the relationship of chemical structure to biologic activity – in this case allergic contact dermatitis. A computer-assisted database describing the chemical structure and biological parameters of several thousand entries provides a convenient approach to designing appropriate *in vitro* animal and human sensitization studies. Chap. 4 summarizes the current status of this database.

In essence, searching the prior experimental data permits not only determination of relationship between structures and allergenicity but provides insight into planning a given experiment. For example, if a closely related structure to the chemical of interest has been shown to be a potent allergen, a new chemical may be examined with a more quantitative assay, such as open epicutaneous test, rather than the less quantitative maximization test.

18.3.2 Guinea Pig Sensitization Tests

Predictive animal tests to determine the potential of substances to induce DTH reactions in humans are conducted most often in guinea pigs. Several tests have been described. Each offers its own advantages and disadvantages; most have many features in common. All utilize young, randomly bred albino guinea pigs (1–3 months old, 250–550 g). To reduce the possibility of seasonal variability in reactivity, animals are maintained in facilities with temperature approximately $20° \pm 1°C$, 40%–50% relative humidity, 12-h automatic light cycle, a standard vitamin C-supplemented chow, and water available at all times. Test sites are clipped free of hair; some assays specify chemical depilation as well. Most evaluate the responses visually, using descriptive scales for erythema and edema. There is some disagreement about which sex, if either, is more susceptible to sensitization. Males are more aggressive and may damage the skin of cage mates. Some assays specify use exclusively of one sex or one-half of each sex. The tests differ significantly in route of exposure, use of adjuvants, induction interval, and number of exposures. The principal features of the most commonly used assays and assays acceptable to regulatory agencies [24, 36, 129, 136] to predict sensitization are summarized in Table 18.1.

Even if proper assay, dose, and vehicles are chosen, improper conduct of the study may result in incorrect conclusions. Sensitization assays are often assigned to the novitiate, when they should be performed and read by the experienced. Experienced investigators often recognize that marginal reactions should be investigated further or that positives may be irritant in nature. Working with laboratories and personnel with extensive experience greatly decreases errors and increases the reliability and relevance of all standard assays described below [69, 80, 83, 146].

18.3.3 Draize Test

The Draize sensitization test [29, 81, 82] was the first predictive sensitization test accepted by regulatory agencies, and it is still widely used. One flank of 20 guinea pig is shaved and 0.05 ml of a 0.1% solution of test material in saline, paraffin oil, or polyethylene glycol is injected into the anterior flank on day 0. The next day and every other day through day 20, 0.1 ml of the test solution is injected into a new site on the same flank. Challenge follows a 2-week rest period. The opposite untreated flank is shaved, and 0.05 ml of test solution is injected into each animal. Twenty previously untreated controls are injected at the same time. The test site is visually evaluated 24 and 48 h

Table 18.1. Principal features of guinea pig sensitization assays

Feature	Draize test epicutaneous test	Open test	Buehler complete adjuvant test	Freund's test	Optimization test	Split adjuvant maximization	Guinea pig
Number in test group	20	6–8	10–20	8–10	20	10–20	20–25
Number in control group	20	6–8	10–20	8–10	20	10–20	20–25
Induction exposure route	i.d.	Open	Patch	i.d.	i.d.	–	i.d. and patch
Number of exposures	10	20 or 21	3	3	9	4	1 i.d., 1 dermal
Duration patches	–	Continuous open	6 h each	–	–	48 h each	48 h
Concentration (%)	0.1	Nonirritating	Nonirritating	5–50	0.1	–	Max. tolerated
Test group(s)	TS	TS	TS	TS in FCA	TS in FCA	TS, FCA	TS, TS+FCA, FCA
Control group	–	V only	–	FCA only	–	–	FCA, FCA+V, V
Site	L flank	R flank	L flank	Shoulder	Back	Midback	Shoulder
Frequency of exposure	Every 2nd day	Daily	Every 7 days	Every 4 days	Every 2nd day	0, 2, 4, 7 days (patch)	0 (i.d.)
Duration (days)	1–18	0–20	0–14	0–9	0–21	0–9	0–7
Miscellaneous	–	–	–	–	–	Dry ice pre-treatment	SLS pretreatment
Rest period (days)	19–23	21–34	15–27	9–21, 22–34	22–34	10–21	9–20
Challenge exposure route	i.d.	Open	Patch	i.d., patch	i.d.	–	Patch
Number of exposures	1	2	1	2	2	1	1
Day(s)	35	21 and 35	28	22 and 35	14–28	22	21

FCA, Freund's complete adjuvant; SLS, sodium lauryl sulphate; V, vehicle; TS, test substance.

after injection. The intensity of the responses of test animals is compared with that of controls; a larger or more intensely erythematous response than that of controls is considered a positive response. Results are expressed as the percentage of animals positive or as the ratio of positive animals to the number tested (actual numbers listed).

18.3.4 Open Epicutaneous Test

The open epicutaneous test [80–82] simulates the conditions of human use by topical application of the test material. The procedure determines the doses required to induce sensitization and to elicit a response in sensitized animals. The irritancy profile is determined by applying 0.025 ml of varying concentrations, typically undiluted, 30%, 10%, 3%, and 1% in ethanol, acetone, water, polyethylene glycol, or petrolatum, to a 2-cm^2 area of the shaved flanks of six to eight guinea pigs. Vehicle solubility and use conditions (e.g., direct application to skin or dilution during normal use) is considered in selecting the concentration. Test sites are visually evaluated 24 h after application of test solutions for the presence or absence of erythema. The dose not causing a reaction in any animal (maximal nonirritant concentration) and the dose causing a reaction in 25% of the animals (minimal irritant concentration) are determined. During induction, 0.10 ml of test solution is applied to an 8-cm^2 area of flank skin of six to eight guinea pigs for 3 weeks, or five times a week for 4 weeks. Up to six groups of animals are treated with different doses; a control group is treated with vehicle only. The highest dose tested is usually the minimal irritant concentration; lower doses are based on usage concentration or a stepwise reduction, for example, 30–10–3–1. Solutions are applied to the same site each day unless a moderate inflammatory response develops. A new site on the same flank is treated when inflammation develops.

Each animal is challenged on the previously untreated flank 24–72 h after the last induction treatment. The minimal irritant concentration, the maximum nonirritant concentration (from irritancy screen), and five solutions of lower concentrations are applied, 0.025 ml to a 2-cm^2 area. Skin reactions are read on an all-or-none basis at 24, 48, and 72 h after application of the solutions. The maximum nonirritating concentration in the vehicle-treated group is calculated. Animals in test groups that develop inflammatory responses to lower concentrations are considered sensitized. The dose required to sensitize is determined by comparing the number of positive animals in the test groups. The minimal concentration necessary to elicit a positive response in a sensitized animal is apparent from the challenge responses.

18.3.5 Buehler Test

The Buehler test [17, 18, 58, 81, 82] also employs topical application of the test material. An absorbent patch 20 × 20 mm Webril, backed by Blenderm tape and saturated with 0.4 ml of the test material, is placed on the shaved flanks of 10–20 guinea pigs. Test concentration varies from undiluted to usage levels. A concentration that produces slight erythema is optimum and is selected based on an irritancy screen conducted in other animals. The patch is held in place by wrapping the animal with an occlusive wrapping, then placing the animal in a special restrainer fitted with a rubber dam to maintain even pressure over the patch for a 6-h exposure period. This procedure is repeated 7 and 14 days after the initial exposure. A control group of 10–20 animals is patched with vehicle only. Two weeks after the last induction patch, animals are challenged with patches saturated with a nonirritating concentration of test material applied to both flanks and with the vehicle (if other than water or acetone). Wrapping and restraint are as during induction. After 6 h, the patch is removed and the area depilated. Test sites are visually evaluated 24 and 48 h after patch removal. Animals developing erythematous responses are considered sensitized (if irritant control animals do not respond). The incidence of positive reactions and the average intensity of the response are calculated.

18.3.6 Freund's Complete Adjuvant Test

The FCA test is an intradermal technique incorporating test material in a 50/50 mixture of FCA and distilled water. The test has been significantly modified since originally described [81]. The latest published description [82] is summarized here. A 6 × 1 cm area across the shoulders of two groups of 10–20 guinea pigs is shaved and used as the injection site. Animals of one group are injected with 0.1 ml of a 5% solution of the test material in FCA/water. Control animals are injected with FCA/water. Injections are repeated every 4 days until three injections are given. The minimal irritating and maximum nonirritating concentration following topical application of 0.025 ml solutions to a 2-cm^2 area of skin is determined on a minimum of four naive guinea pigs (see Sect. 18.3.4). Twenty one days after the first induction injection, 0.025 ml of the minimal irritant concentration, the maximum nonirritant concentration, and two lower concentrations are applied to 2-cm^2 areas of the shaved flank. Test sites are not covered and are evaluated for the presence of erythema at 24, 48, and 72 h after application. The minimum nonirritating concentration in FCA/water-treated controls is determined. Animals injected with the test material during induction that respond to lower doses are considered sensitized. The incidence of sensitization and the threshold concentration for elicitation of the response in these animals are calculated.

18.3.7 Optimization Test

The optimization test resembles the Draize test but incorporates the use of adjuvant for some induction injections and both intradermal and topical challenges [81, 82, 121]. Injections during induction are 0.1 ml of 0.1% concentration of test material in 0.9% saline or in 50/50 FCA/saline. A total of ten injections are given. On day 1 of the 1st week, one injection into the shaved flank and one into a shaved area of dorsal skin are given. After 2 and 4 days, one injection into a new dorsal site is given. The test material is administered in saline during the 1st week. During the 2nd and 3rd weeks, test material is administered in FCA/saline every other day to a shaved area over the shoulders. Twenty test animals are treated; 20 controls are injected with saline during week 1 and FCA/saline during weeks 2 and 3. The intensity of the 24-h responses during week 1 is calculated as reaction volume. Thickness of a skin fold over the injection site is measured with a caliper (millimeters), and the two largest diameters of the erythematous reaction are recorded (millimeters). The reaction volume is calculated by multiplying fold thickness times by both diameters and is expressed as micro-liters. The mean reaction volume of each animal to the intradermal injections using saline as a vehicle (week 1) is calculated.

Thirty-five days after the first injection, animals are challenged with 0.1 ml of 0.1% test material in saline. The challenge reaction volume for each animal is calculated and compared to the mean reaction volume for that animal. Any animal developing a reaction volume at challenge greater than the mean plus one standard deviation during induction is considered sensitized. Vehicle control animals are injected with saline at challenge. A second challenge is conducted 45 days after the first injection. A nonirritating concentration of the test material in a suitable vehicle is applied to the flank skin, away from injection sites; 0.05 ml is applied to approximately 1 cm^2. The area is covered with a 2×2 cm #2 filter paper backed by an occlusive dressing, which remains in place for 24 h. Reactions are visually evaluated using the four-point erythema scale of the Draize primary irritancy scale (see Sect. 18.4.3). The control animals are patched with vehicle alone. The number of positive animals in the test group is statistically compared with the number of 'pseudo-positive' animals in the control groups, using the exact Fisher's test. Separate comparisons of intradermal and epicutaneous challenges are made; a p value of <0.01 is considered significant. To classify materials as strong/moderate/weak/not sensitizer, a classification scheme has been devised using results of the exact Fisher's test and number of positives detected (Table 18.2).

18.3.8 Split Adjuvant Test

The split adjuvant test [82, 112, 113] utilizes skin damage and FCA as adjuvants; application of the test material is topical. An area of back skin just

Table 18.2. Classification scheme based on results of the optimization test

Intradermal positive animals	Epidermal positive animals	Classification
77S, >75%	And/or S, >50%	Strong sensitizer
S, 50%–75%	And/or S, 30%–50%	Moderate sensitizer
S, 30%–50%	NS, 0%–30%	Weak sensitizer
NS, 0%–30%	NS, 0%	Not sensitizer

S, significant; NS, not significant (using exact Fisher test).

behind the scapulas of 10–20 guinea pigs is clipped, shaved to glistening, then treated with dry ice for 5–10s. A dressing of a layer of loose mesh gauze and stretch adhesive with a 2×2 cm^2 opening over the shaved area is placed around the animal and secured with adhesive tape. This dressing remains in place throughout induction. Approximately 0.2 ml of creams or solid test material, 0.1 ml if liquid, is spread over the test site and covered with two layers of #2 filter paper backed by occlusive tape and attached to the dressing by adhesive tape. The concentration tested varies by irritancy potential, use conditions, etc. Two days later, the filter paper is lifted from the test site, the test material reapplied, and the filter paper covering replaced. On day 4, the filter paper cover is removed, two injections of 0.075 cm^3 FCA are given into the edges of the test site, the test material is reapplied, and the site is resealed. On day 7 the test material is reapplied, and on day 9 the dressing is removed. Twenty-two days after the initial treatment, animals are challenged by topical application of 0.5 ml of test material to a 2×2 cm area of the shaved midback. The test site is covered by filter paper backed with adhesive tape, held in place by wrapping the animal with an elastic adhesive bandage secured with adhesive tape. A group of naive controls, 10–20 animals, is treated by the same procedure at challenge. Twenty-four hours after application, the dressing is removed, and the test site is visually evaluated at 24, 48, and 72 h using a seven-point descriptive visual scale. Sensitization of individual animals is indicated by significantly stronger reactions than those of controls.

18.3.9 Guinea Pig Maximization Test

The guinea pig maximization test [81, 82, 110] combines FCA, irritancy, intradermal injection, and occlusive topical application during the induction period. The shoulder region of two groups of 20–25 guinea pigs is shaved. Two identical sets of 0.1 ml intradermal injections of 50/50 FCA/water, test material in water, paraffin oil, or propylene glycol, and the same dose of test material in FCA/vehicle are placed on a 2×4 cm filter paper, placed over the injection site, covered with approximately 4×8 cm occlusive surgical tape, and secured in place with an elastic bandage wrapped around the animal. If the test material is nonirritating, the test site is pretreated with 10% sodium lauryl sulfate in petrolatum on day 6 to provoke an irritant reaction. If a vehicle

Table 18.3. Classification of materials by maximization test

Sensitization rate	Grade	Class
0%–8%	I	Weak
9%–28%	II	Mild
29%–64%	III	Moderate
65%–80%	IV	Strong
81%–100%	V	Extreme

other than petrolatum is used for topical application of the test material, the filter is saturated with the solution. Control animals are patched with the vehicle alone. The dressing is removed from the animals 48 h after application. Test and control animals are challenged on the shaved flank with the highest nonirritating concentration, approximately one-half of the highest nonirritating concentration, and with the vehicle. Solutions are applied to 1×1 cm pieces of filter paper secured in place as during induction. Patches are removed 24 h later. The challenge area is shaved, if needed, 21 h after patch removal. Reactions are visually evaluated 24 and 48 h after patch removal. The intensity of responses to test material and vehicle in the test group is compared to the responses in controls. Reactions are considered positive when they are more intense than the response to vehicle and the responses to the test materials in controls. The test material is rated as a weak-to-extreme sensitizer, based on the incidence of positives in the test group (Table 18.3).

18.3.10 Mouse Sensitization Tests

Over the last few years increasing use has been made of the mouse as an alternative animal model to the guinea pig [80a, 115a] (see Sect. 2.1.3).

18.3.11 Human Sensitization Assays

Chemicals can be tested for their ability to induce contact hypersensitivity in panels of human volunteers from whom informed consent is obtained. Generally, materials shown to be sensitizers in animals are not tested on humans. However, if the potential benefit of the material warrants it, a small group of human subjects may be tested with materials inducing sensitization in animals. Such situations should be reviewed by an Institutional Review Board, test subjects should be informed of the risks, and the number of subjects exposed should be limited (additional subjects can be exposed if members of a small group do not respond).

Subjects should be randomly selected; however, some precautions are indicated. Recurrence of skin conditions in remission (e.g., psoriasis or eczema) has been associated with patch testing, as well as other minor physical traumas. Subjects at risk should be informed of this possibility and encouraged to consult their dermatologists before testing. Allergic contact dermatitis from materials already commercially available is sometimes detected by early induction patches. This does not reflect the particular test material's ability to induce sensitization: it indicates merely that, under patch conditions, the material may elicit a response in presensitized individuals. The incidence of preexisting sensitization is not helpful in evaluating a material's ability to induce sensitization. Subjects should not be tested with materials to which they are known to be allergic, i.e., as demonstrated by diagnostic patch test or in previous predictive assays. It is wise to question potential subjects routinely concerning their history of dermatological disease and allergies. Records of positive responses of individuals participating in multiple predictive assays should be reviewed before testing, to eliminate presensitized subjects.

Although numerous variations have been reported, there are four basic predictive human sensitization tests in current use: (a) single-induction/single-challenge patch test, (b) repeated insult patch test (RIPT), (c) RIPT with continuous exposure (modified Draize test), and (d) the maximization test. Principal features of human sensitization assays are summarized in Table 18.4. As originally described, all used customized patches. Patch selection was governed by available adhesive systems. Description of customized patches would be of historical interest only; as currently conducted, all human assays use similar patches. Occlusive patches, consisting of a nonwoven pad, usually Webril, or four-ply gauze sponges, backed by a good occlusive surgical tape (e.g., Blenderm) are commercially available or may be custom-made in strips of four or five pads. Acceptable alternatives include the Hilltop Chamber [79], which contains a Webril pad inside an occlusive plastic disc backed by a porous tape; the Duhring chamber [54], a stainless steel disc that contains a Webril pad; and the large Finn Chamber. Duhring and Finn Chambers are usually secured in place by porous surgical tape. Occassionally, semiocclusive patches made of Webril backed by porous tape may be used; these are decidedly inferior to occlusive patches in inducing sensitization.

For assays other than maximization, 150 to 200 subjects are usually tested. Henderson and Riley [65] showed statistically that if no positive reactions are observed in 200 randomly selected subjects, as many as 15/1000 of the general population *may* react (95% confidence interval). As sample size is reduced, the likelihood of unpredicted adverse reactions in the general population increases.

18.3.12 Schwartz-Peck Test (and Modification)

A single application induction patch followed by a single application patch test was described by Schwartz [150, 151] and Schwartz and Peck [152], with a use test 1 month after challenge to verify patch results. The test has been modified by some to eliminate the use test [16], to eliminate patching

Table 18.4. Principal features of human sensitization tests

	Complete Schwartz/Peck	Shelanski/Shelanski	Draize	Griffith/Voss/Stotts	Modified Draize	Human maximization
Number of subjects	200	200	200	200	200	25
Induction site	Upper arm	Upper arm; same site	Upper back; upper arm; new sites	Upper arm; same site	Lower back; upper back; same site	upper arm; same site
777Number of exposures	1	15	10	9	10	5
Duration of exposures (h)	24–72	24	24	24	48–72	48
Frequency of exposure	–	3/week	3/week	3/week	Continuous	24 h rest periods
Evaluations at	Removal 24, 48 h	Patch removal	Patch removal	48–72 h	30 min	
Miscellaneous	4-week usage period	Fatiguing index		Pilot group		Irritant does or SLS used
Rest period (days)		14–21	10–14	14	14	14
Challenge site	Upper arm	Upper arm; upper arm; new site	Upper back; (2 patches)	Upper arms upper back; new site	Upper arm; upper arm; new site	Lower back;
Duration of challenge	24–72 h	48 h	24 h	24 h	72 h	48 h
Evaluations at	Removal, 24, 48 h	Removal	Removal	48, 96 h	Removal, 24 h	Removal, 24, 48 h
Miscellaneous				Challenge induct. and fresh site	May do two 48-h challenge patches	SLS provocative patch, sensitization index

SLS, Sodium lauryl sulphate

altogether, and to place a period of use between induction and challenge patches [163]. The term 'complete Schwartz-Peck' refers to a single induction patch, period of use, single challenge patch test. This may also be referred to as the Traub-Tusing-Spoon method. Incomplete Schwartz-Peck test do not incorporate a period of use.

A patch saturated with the test material, diluted if necessary, is applied to the outer upper arm of 200 test subjects and remains in place for 24–72 h. The dose tested and duration of patch contact vary with intended use. Cosmetics may be tested without a covering (open application) or with semiocclusive patches. The test site is visually evaluated at patch removal and at 24 and 48 h after removal for erythema and edema. A 4-week period of normal use follows the induction patch in the complete Schwartz-Peck test. A challenge patch is applied to the same site on the upper arm at the conclusion of the period of use or 10–14 days after the induction patch of the incomplete Schwartz-Peck test. Duration of contact and evaluation of site are performed as during induction. The development of dermatitis at challenge, not present or much stronger than during induction, signifies sensitization. Schwartz originally described the incomplete Schwartz-Peck test. A use test was to be conducted after the challenge patch, using 1000 different subjects.

Although Schwartz and Peck [152] referred to their assay as a 'prophetic patch' test, experience has shown that only potent haptens induce sensitization in this assay. The test was originally designed to evaluate the effect of nylon garments on the skin. It was intended to detect adverse effects, irritation, and 'secondary irritation' (sensitization). The mechanism of DTH was not understood by most scientists when the test was designed. Although the test was useful for its original purposes, its use was unfortunately expanded by its designers without considering new information generated by immunologists. Clearly, the assay is inferior to all other predictive human sensitization assays.

18.3.13 Repeat Insult Patch Tests

Three major variations on the RIPT are in common use: (a) the Draize human sensitization test [27, 28], (b) the Shelanski-Shelanski test [153–155], and (c) the Voss-Griffith test [18, 57, 58, 171]. Although the Shelanskis first published a description of a RIPT, they based its development on a verbal description of a method that Draize was devising [154]. Voss modified the Shelanski-Shelanski test [171], and his assay was later modified by Griffith [57]. As one would expect, the three assays have much in common. There are, however, some significant differences in the assays as originally described.

In the Draize human sensitization test, an occlusive patch containing the test material is applied to the upper arm or upper back of 200 volunteers. The patch remains in place for 24 h and is then removed. The test site is evaluated at patch removal for erythema and edema. A second patch test is applied to a new site 24 h after the first patch is removed. This process is repeated until a total of ten patches are applied. For convenience, the test may be run on a Monday-to-Friday schedule, with subjects removing their own patches on Saturday (72 h between Friday and Monday applications). Ten to 14 days after application of the last induction patches, subjects are challenged via a patch applied to a new site. Duration of contact is 24 h; sites are evaluated visually at removal of the patch. The response at challenge is compared to the response to patches applied early in induction. The incidence of sensitization is reported.

Like the Draize RIPT, the Shelanski-Shelanski test employs occlusive patches that remain in contact with the skin of the upper arm for 24 h. The patching cycle is the same; however, patches are placed on the same test site each time, and a total of 15 patches is applied during induction. The test site is evaluated before application of a new patch to the site; if inflammation has developed, the patch is placed on an adjacent uninflamed site. Two or 3 weeks after the induction period, subjects are challenged by application of a patch that remains in place for 48 h. Test sites are evaluated at patch removal for erythema and edema. The incidence of positive response is reported. Patch responses during induction were considered by Shelanski-Shelanski to be evidence of 'skin fatigue' (cumulative irritation); the time to development, i.e., number of patches, was reported as a fatiguing index.

Voss [171] reduced the number of 24-h patch exposures to nine over a 3-week period. At challenge 2 weeks after the last induction patch, duplicate patches applied to the original test site are worn for 24 h. Patch sites are evaluated 48 and 96 h after patch application. A pilot group of 10–12 subjects was tested before exposing the full panel of 60–70 subjects. Griffith later published more detailed accounts of the method [57, 58]. Up to four dissimilar materials were simultaneously tested, and duplicate challenges were applied to the sites of induction and to the opposite arm, thus testing on areas drained by different regional lymphatics. Griffith also described characteristics of allergic reactions at challenge, stronger reactions than during induction, persistence of the response through 96 h, and reactions in a few subjects with no reactions in the test of the panel. The concept of a rechallenge of subjects with reactions difficult to interpret was also introduced. The number of subjects was increased to 200 by conducting tests on multiple panels.

As currently conducted, the differences in Draize and Voss-Griffith RIPT are minimal. Many investigators apply patches to the same site during induction and refer to the procedure as a Draize RIPT. The value of multiple grades at challenges is widely recognized and utilized. Multiple test materials are simultaneously tested in all RIPT for reasons of efficiency and economy. Although the distinctions between Draize and Voss-Griffith procedures have blurred with common usage, the Shelanski-Shelanski test with five to six more induction applications remains distinct.

18.3.14 Human Maximization Test

Kilgman [84] reviewed the common human predictive sensitization test methods in use in 1966 and found them to be unsatisfactory in inducing sensitization to nine clinical allergens. In panels of 200 subjects, the Shelanski-Shelanski method induced sensitization to four materials; the original Draize test and the complete Schwartz-Peck test induced sensitization to two allergens each; and the incomplete Schwartz-Peck test failed to induce sensitization to any allergen. He concluded that 'emphasis must shift from prophecy to the more practical objective of identifying potential allergens ... Once the allergenic potential is known with reasonable certainty, a judgement of risk might be ventured after examining all the pertinent variables' [86]. This represented a profound change in the intent of predictive sensitization assays. Based on his studies of factors affecting rates of sensitization in predictive assays [85, 88], Kligman designed the human maximization test [86]. He later modified the procedure somewhat to reduce difficulties in performing and interpreting the test [89].

The maximization test utilizes irritancy as an adjuvant. During induction, compounds that are irritating are tested at a concentration that produces a moderate erythema within 48 h. For materials that are nonirritating, the test site is pretested with a 24-h patch of 5% sodium lauryl sulfate (SLS); a second pretreatment of SLS patch may be applied to produce a brisk erythema, and induction concentrations are at least five times higher than use levels. Petrolatum is the preferred vehicle. Often custom-made Webril/Blenderm patches of Duhring chambers are used. Patches are applied to either the outer aspect of the arm or lower back, and up to four dissimilar materials may be tested at one time. Wrapping with extra tape is often necessary to ensure occlusion. Bandage sprays may be used to ensure sealing of the test site. Five sets of patches are worn on the same site for 48 h each, with a 24-h rest period between removal and reapplication. Following a 2-week rest period after the last induction patch, an SLS provocative patch procedure is performed to prepare the skin for challenge. A patch saturated with a 2.5%–5% solution of SLS is applied to previously untreated sites on the lower back. SLS concentration is based on the season and on individual subject response. The SLS patch is removed after 1 h and a patch containing the test material applied. A control site is patched with SLS (1 h) and petrolatum (48 h) to aid in interpretation of the results. Forty-eight hours after application, the patch is removed and test sites are evaluated. Test sites are reexamined 24 and 48 h after patch removal. The number of subjects developing a positive response is reported, and a sensitization index based on percent of subjects responding is assigned to the test material. Although it is clear that the maximization test is a sensitive tool for detection of allergenicity, the skin damage produced is dramatic and unacceptable to many subjects.

18.3.15 Modified Draize Human Sensitization Test

The RIPT procedure was modified to provide for continuous patch exposure to the test material during the 3-week induction period [117, 118]. Patches containing test material are applied to the outer upper arm each Monday, Wednesday, and Friday until a total of ten patches have been applied. Patches remain in place until about 30 min before application of a fresh patch. (This allows some clearing of responses to tape and facilities grading). Fresh patches are applied to the same site unless moderate inflammation has developed; the patches are placed on adjacent noninflamed skin if inflammation becomes pronounced. This produces a continuous exposure of 504–552 h (some investigators apply only nine patches), compared to a total exposure period of 216–240 h for RIPT of comparable induction periods. In addition, induction concentration was increased to levels above usage exposure. Two weeks after induction, subjects are challenged by exposure of a new site to a patch of 72-h duration at a nonirritating concentration. Test suites are evaluated at patch removal and 24 h after removal. Jordan and King [77] modified the challenge procedure to two consecutive 48-h patch periods.

18.3.16 General Comment

It is emphasized that, as in animal testing, the greater the experience in designing and executing the test, the more useful will be the result. Numerous artifacts may lead to either false-positive or false-negative results. These assays are best run by scientists with specific training in their planning and execution.

18.4 Irritant Contact Dermatitis

Historically, skin irritation has been described by exclusion as localized inflammation not mediated by either sensitized lymphocytes or by antibodies, for example, that which develops by a process not involving the immune system. Application of some chemicals directly destroys tissue, producing skin necrosis at the site of application. Chemicals producing necrosis that results in formation of scar tissue are described as corrosive. Chemicals may disrupt cell functions and/or trigger the release, formation, or activation of autocoids that produce local increases in blood flow, increase vascular permeability, attract white blood cells in the area, or directly damage cells. The additive effects of the mediators result in local skin inflammation. A number of as yet poorly defined pathways involving different processes or mediator generation appear to exist. Although no agent has yet met all the criteria to establish it as a mediator of skin irritation, histamine, 5-hydrotryptamine, prostaglandins, leukotrienes, kinins, complement, reactive oxygen species, and products of white blood cells have been strongly implicated as mediators of some irritant reactions [144]. Chemicals that produce inflammation as a result of a single exposure are termed acute irritants.

Some chemicals do not produce acute irritation from a single exposure but may produce inflammation following repeated application to the same area of skin. The cumulative irritation from repeated exposures has also been called skin fatigue [153]. Because of the possibility of skin contact during transport and use of many chemicals, regulatory agencies have mandated screening chemicals for the ability to produce skin corrosion and acute irritation. These studies are conducted in animals, using standardized protocols. However, the protocols specified by some agencies vary somewhat. It is not appropriate to conduct screening studies for corrosion in humans, but acute irritation is sometimes evaluated in humans after animals studies have been completed. Tests for cumulative irritation in both animals and humans have been reported.

Recently, knowledge of the biology of irritation has progressed sufficiently to provide insights into the extraordinary complexity of the process. Lammintausta et al. have succinctly summarized some of the data [99a].

18.4.1 Quantitative Structure-Activity Relationships

Computerized databases providing assistance in predicting irritancy potential and designing efficient experiments do not yet exist. However, experienced investigators with extensive knowledge of irritancy in animal and man can utilize their knowledge of specialized situations with certain classes of chemicals to execute more appropriate assays.

18.4.2 In Vitro Assays

Numerous in vitro assays for irritation exist. Basom summarizes these assays and offers guidelines as to their potential validation [5a]. An indepth summary of the recent advances in this field is provided in the Rougier et al. textbook listed under "Additional References."

18.4.3 Irritation Tests in Animals

18.4.3.1 Draize-Type Tests

Primary irritation and corrosion are most often evaluated by modifications of the method described by John Draize and colleagues in 1944 [29]. The Federal Hazardous Substance Act (FHSA) adopted one modification as a standard procedure [24]. The backs of six albino rabbits are clipped free of hair. Each material is tested on two 1 × 1 in. sites on the same animal; one site is intact, and one is abraded in such a way that the stratum corneum is opened but no bleeding produced. Abrasion can be performed using the tip of a hypodermic needle repeatedly drawn across the skin or commercial instruments such as the Berkely Scarifier [64] or the Maryland Plastics skin abrader. Materials

Table 18.5. Draize-FHSA scoring system

Skin reaction	Score
Erythema and eschar formation	
No erythema	0
Very slight erythema (barely perceptible)	1
Well-defined erythema	2
Moderate to severe erythema	3
Severe erythema (beet redness)	4
to slight eschar formations	
(injuries in depth)	
Edema formation	
No erythema	0
Very slight erythema (barely perceptible)	1
Slight edema (edges of area well defined	2
by definite raising)	
Moderate edema (raised $\sim$ 1 mm)	3
Severe edema (raised > 1 mm and	4
extending beyond the area of exposure)	

are tested undiluted; 0.5 ml liquid or 0.5 g solid or semisolid material is applied. In some cases the skin may be moistened to help solids adhere to the site, or an equal volume of solvent may be used to moisten the material. Each test site is covered with two layers of 1 × 1 in. surgical gauze secured in place with tape. The entire trunk of the animal is then wrapped with rubberized cloth or other occlusive impervious material to retard evaporation of the substances and to hold the patches in one position. Twenty-four hours after application, the wrappings are removed, and the test sites are evaluated for erythema and edema, using a prescribed scale (Table 18.5). Evaluations of abraded and intact sites are separately recorded. Test sites are evaluated again 48 h later (72 h after application) by the same procedure. The reproducibility of the FHSA procedure [168, 176] and the relevance of test results to human experience [26, 69, 105, 119, 131, 143, 159] have been questioned. NUmerous modifications to the Draize procedure have been proposed to improve its prediction of human experience. Modifications that have been proposed include changing the species tested [127], reduction of exposure period, use of fewer animals, and testing on intact skin only [60]. Several governmental bodies utilized their own modification of the Draize procedure for regulatory decisions. The FHSA, Department of Transportation, Environmental Protection Agency, Federal Insecticide, Fungicide, and Rodenticide Act, and the guidelines of the Organization for Economic Cooperation and Development are contrasted to the original Draize methods in Table 18.6.

Summaries and evaluations of the scores vary somewhat. Draize reported values for individual animals at each time point, combined the erythema and edema values at each time point, and then averaged the 24- and 72-h evaluations for intact and abraded sites separately. He also calculated

Table 18.6. Comparison of skin irritation tests based on the Draize method

	Draize	FHSA	DOT	FIFRA	OECD[a]
No. of animals	3[b]	6	6	6	6
Abrasion	Abraded & intact	Abraded & intact	Intact	2 abraded & 2 intact	Intact
Dose liquids	0.5 ml undiluted	0.5 ml undiluted	0.5 ml	0.5 ml undiluted	0.5 ml
Dose solids	0.5 g	0.5 g in solvent	0.5 g	0.5 g moistened	0.5 g moistenend
Wrapping materials	Gauze and rubberized cloth	Impervious material			Semiocclusive
Exposure period (h)	24	24	4	4	4
Examination (h)	24, 72	24, 72	4, 48	0.5, 1, 24, 48, 72[c]	0.5, 1, 24, 48, 72[c]
Removal of test materials	Not specified	Not specified	Skin washed	Skin wiped -not washed	Skin washed
Excluded from testing	–	–	–	Toxic materials pH $\leq$ 2 or $\geq$ 11.5	Toxic materials pH $\leq$ 2 or $\geq$ 11.5

DOT, Department of Transportation; FHSA, Federal Hazardous Substance Act; FIFRA, Federal Insecticide, Fungicide, and Rodenticide Act; OECD, Organization for Economic Cooperation and Development.

[a] Although other species are acceptable, the albino rabbit is the preferred species.

[b] Draize tested four materials on six rabbits. Three abraded and three intact sites were tested with each material.

[c] Times listed are after patch removal for FIFRA and OECD. Times listed for Draize, FHSA, and DOT are after each material.

a primary irritation index (PII), which was the average of the intact and abraded sites. Agents producing PII under 2 were considered only mildly irritating. The primary irritation calculated for the FHSA is essentially the PII of Draize. A minimum PII of 5 defines an irritant by Consumer Product Safety Commission (CPSC) standards. The National Institute of Occupational Safety and Health (NIOSH) does not combine responses of abraded sites and includes probable effects on normal and damaged skin in their evaluation.

Although vesiculation, ulceration, and severe eschar formations are not included in the Draize scoring scales, all Draize-type tests are used to evaluate corrosion as well as irritation. When severe reactions that may not be reversible are noted, test sites are observed for a longer period. Delayed evaluations are usually made on days 7 and 14. However, evaluations have been made as late as 35 days after application. EPA bases its interpretation on 7-day observations.

The basic exposure procedures for skin irritation/corrosion in the guidelines of the Organization for Economic Cooperation and Development have been further modified to test for corrosion during shorter periods [136]. Under a directive of the European Economic Community, a 3-min exposure was added (with no wrapping procedure) and the United Nations recommendations for the Transport of Dangerous Goods are based on exposure times of 4 h, 1 h, and 3 min, with the recommendation that the 1-h exposure be conducted first. Evaluations are made 1, 24, 48, 72 h, and 7 days after dosing.

18.4.3.2 Non-Draize Animal Studies

Animal assays to evaluate the ability of chemicals to produce cumulative irritation have been developed [140]. The impetus for their use is largely the development of products that are better tolerated by consumers. Although many such tests have been described, only a few are used extensively enough to summarize. Even those used more often are not as well standardized as Draize-type tests, and many variables have been introduced by multiple investigators.

Repeat application patch tests in which diluted materials are applied to the same site each day for 15–21 days have been reported, using several species [140]. The guinea pig or rabbit is most commonly used. Patches used vary considerably, with gauze Draize-type dressings and metal chambers being the extremes. Some authors recommend testing the materials with no covering, presumably with a restraining collar to prevent grooming of the area and ingestion of the material. Because the degree of occlusion is an important determinant of percutaneous penetration, the choice of covering materials may determine the sensitivity of a given test [107]. A reference material of similar use or one that produces a known effect in humans is included in almost all repeat application procedures. The degrees of inflammation produced by the materials in a single assay are compared. Test sites are evaluated for erythema and edema, using either the scales of the Draize-type tests or more descriptive scales developed by the investigator. Although interpretation ratings such as 'slight', 'moderate', or 'severe' irritation are not usually made, the data from cumulative irritancy assays in rabbits have been used to predict reactions in humans. Other investigators used multiple application with shorter periods of time to evaluate materials [78].

The guinea pig immersion assay has been used to evaluate the irritancy of aqueous detergent solutions [21, 85, 124, 135]. Ten guinea pigs are placed in restraining devices that are immersed in a 40°C test solution for 4 h. The apparatus is designed to maintain the guinea pig's head above the solution. Immersion is repeated daily for three treatments. Twenty-four hours after the final immersion, the flank is shaved and skin is evaluated for erythema, edema, and fissures. Concentration of test materials varies somewhat, but is usually under 10% to limit systemic toxicity of the agents. Some materials are unsuitable for this assay because death may result from systemic absorption of toxic materials. A second group of animals is usually tested with a reference material for comparison to the material of interest.

Uttley and van Abbé [167] developed a mouse ear test in which undiluted shampoos were applied to one ear daily for 4 days. The degree of inflammation was quantified visually as vessel dilation, erythema, and edema, using a visual scale. The degree of inflammation produced by materials of interest was compared to that produced by a reference material tested on another group of mice. Others have used ear thickness to quantify degree of inflammation and have either pretreated the ear with a strong irritant to simulate damaged skin or increased the frequency of application to increase the sensitivity of the assay.

18.4.4 Human Irritation Tests

Because only a small area of skin need be tested, it is possible to conduct predictive irritation assays in humans, provided systemic toxicity (from absorption) is low and informed consent is obtained. Although regulatory agencies do not routinely require testing in humans, human tests are preferred to animal tests in some cases because of the uncertainties of interspecies extrapolation. New materials, i.e., those of unknown or unfamiliar composition, should be tested on animal skin first to determine if application to humans is warranted [129].

Many forms of a single application patch test have been published. Duration of patch exposure has varied between 1 and 72 h. Custom-made apparatus to hold the test material has been designed [79, 107, 154, 156]. A variety of adhesives no longer commercially available have been used [109]. Although the individual assays provided important information to the investigators of the period, they were never standardized or gained wide acceptance.

The single application patch procedure outlined by the National Academy of Sciences [129] incorporates important aspects of assays used by many investigators. The procedure is similar to FHSA tests in rabbits. Commercial patches, chambers, gauze squares, or cotton bandage material (e.g., Webril) may be applied either to the intrascapular region of the back or to the dorsal surface of the upper arms [108]. Patches are secured in place with surgical tape without wrapping the trunk or arm. For new materials or volatiles, a relatively nonocclusive tape (e.g., Micropore, Dermicel, or Scanpor) should be used. Increasing the degree of occlusion with occlusive tapes (e.g., Blenderm) or chamber devices (e.g., the Duhring chamber or Hilltop chamber) generally increases the severity of responses.

A 4-h exposure period was suggested by the National Academy of Sciences panel. However, it is desirable to test new materials and volatiles for shorter periods – 20 min – 1 h – and many investigators apply materials intended for skin contact for 24- to 48-h periods. Subjects should routinely be instructed to remove patches immediately if any unusual discomfort develops. After the period of exposure, the patches should be removed, the area cleaned with water to remove any residue, and the test site marked by study personnel. Responses are evaluated 30 min – 1 h after patch removal (to allow hydration and pressure effects to subside) and again 24 h after the patch is removed. Persistent reactions may be evaluated for 3–4 days. The Draize scales for erythema and edema (Table 18.5) have been used for grading human skin responses. However, they have no provision for scoring papular, vesicular, or bullous responses. Integrated scales ranging from 4 to 16 points have been published and are generally preferred to the Draize scales (for example, Table 18.7). Up to ten materials can be tested simultaneously on each subject. The position where the materials are placed on the skin, for example, upper right back or lower left back, should be systematically varied, because skin reactivity differs by body region, and some locations may receive more pressure from chairs, clothing, etc., than others. Each battery of patches should include at least one reference material. Scores from all subjects are averaged for each material, and comparisons between standards and other test materials are made. Some investigators have accepted an average difference of 1 unit on the grading scale as meaningful. Other investigators analyze the data by

Table 18.7. Simple integrated scale for irritant patch test

0	No sign of inflammation; normal skin
±(1/2)	Glazed appearance of the sites, or barely perceptible erythema
1	Slight erythema
2	Moderate erythema, possibly with barely perceptible edema at the margin; papules may be present
3	Moderate erythema, with generalized edema
4	Severe erythema with severe edema, with or without vesicles
5	Severe reaction spread beyond the area of the patch

standard statistical tests. It is also possible to test multiple doses and calculate median irritant dose (ID_{50}) responses.

The development of inflammation after repeated application of patches contain a test material to the same are of skin was referred to as 'skin fatigue' by Shelanski [153], to explain the development of inflammation late in the induction phase of sensitization tests without positive responses at challenge. The phenomenon was also referred to as secondary irritation and later as cumulative irritation. As with single application patch tests, many investigators developed their own version of a repeat application patch test. Most were patterned after human sensitization studies with 24-h exposures, with or without a rest period between patches. Kligman and Wooding [90] applied the Litchfield and Wilcoxon probe analysis to cumulative irritation testing, with calculation of ID_{50} values (irritant dose 50) and statistical comparison of those values for different materials. Their early work forms the basis for the 21-day cumulative irritation assay that currently is widely used.

The cumulative irritation assay as described by Lanman and coworkers [103] was used to compare antiperspirants, deodorants, and bath oils to provide guidance for product development. A 1×1 in. area Webril was saturated with liquid or up to 0.5 g of viscous substances and applied to the surface of the pad to be applied to the skin. The patch was applied to the upper back and sealed in place with occlusive tape. After 24 h the patch was removed, the area evaluated, and a fresh patch applied. The procedure was repeated daily for up to 21 days. The sensitivity of the assay was increased by increasing the number of test subjects from 10 to 24. The IT_{50} as described by Kligman and Wooding [90] was used to evaluate and compare test materials.

Modifications of the cumulative irritation assay have been reported. Data generated have been compared using other evaluation schemes [119], and the interval between application of fresh patches [145] has been varied. The newer chamber devices have replaced Webril with occlusive tape in some laboratories. Some investigators currently use cumulative scores to compare test materials and do not calculate an IT_{50}. The necessity of 21 applications has recently been questioned [7]. Although the procedure came to be known as the 21-day cumulative irritation assay, the number of applications used was varied by Lanman et al. [103], depending on the types of material to be tested. Twenty-one days was the *maximum* period of testing Kligman and Wooding applied to damaged skin. Light-skinned Caucasians who developed severe erythema with edema and vesicles following a 24-hr exposure to 5% SLS in Duhring chambers applied to the inner forearm are preselected as subjects. Six to eight 10-mm-square areas on the midvolar forearm are scarified with eight criss-cross scratches made with a 30-gauge needle. Four scratches are parallel, with another four at right angles. In scarifying the tissue, the bevel of the needle is to the side and is drawn across the tissue at a 45° angle with enough pressure to scratch the epidermis without drawing blood. Duhring chambers containing the test material, 0.1 g for ointments, creams, and powders or Webril saturated with 0.1 ml for liquids, are placed over the scarified areas and are secured in place with nonocclusive tape wrapped around the forearm. Fresh chambers containing the same materials are applied serially for 3 days. Thirty minutes after removal of the last set of chambers, the test sites are evaluated on a 0-to-4 scale. The responses are averaged and materials are classified as low (0–0.4), slight (0.5–1.4), moderate (1.5–2.4), or severe iritants. In some cases, a scarification index is calculated by comparing responses on intact or scarified skin (scores from scarified sites divided by scores from intact skin). The scarification index is used to estimate the relative risk for damaged and normal tissue. It is not used to rank test materials.

Many variables of the chosen test procedure (e.g., vehicle, type of patch, concentration tested) may modify the intensity of the response [34, 121]. Selection of subjects tested may also influence the outcome. Differences in intensity of responses has been linked to differences in age [87], sex [87], and race [174, 175]. Some investigators select the test population based on proposed use of the test materials.

In addition to patch test procedures, exaggerated exposure tests simulating extreme uses and use tests have been used to compare the irritation potential of a variety of consumer products. These tests include skin washing procedures [43], arm or hand immersion studies [44, 59, 78], and clinical use tests in which subjects use exaggerated concentrations of test materials [22, 76, 92] or materials treated with the agent under investigation [173]. The study designs vary significantly, and it is not possible to describe generally accepted procedures because of variabilities in design. Special emphasis should be placed on design in terms of statistical validity [1]. Although some toxicologists specializing in the skin as a target organ are involved in tests of this type, they are more often conducted by groups specializing in clinical testing and claim support.

18.5 Contact Urticaria

Contact urticaria has been defined as a wheal-and-flare response that develops within 30–60 min after exposure of the skin to certain agents [170] (see Sect. 2.3). Symptoms of immediate contact reactions can be classified according to their morphology and severity:
- Itching, tingling, and burning with erythema is the weakest type of immediate contact reaction.
- Local wheal-and-flare with tingling and itching represents the prototpye reaction of contact urticaria.
- Generalized urticaria after local contact is rare but may occur from strong urticaria.
- Symptoms in other organs may appear with the skin symptoms in cases of immunological contact urticaria syndrome.

The strength of the reactions can vary greatly, and often the whole range of local symptoms – from slight erythema to strong edema and erythema – can be seen from the same substance if different concentrations are used in skin tests [95]. Not only the concentration but also the site of the skin contact affects the reaction. A certain concentration of contact urticant may produce strong edema and erythema reactions on the skin of the upper back and face but only erythema on the volar surfaces of the lower arms or legs. In some cases, contact urticaria can be demonstrated only on damaged or previously eczematous skin, and it may be part of the mechanism responsible for maintenance of chronic eczemas [2, 114, 135]. Some agents, such as formaldehyde, produce urticaria on healthy skin following repeated but not single applications to the skin. Diagnosis of immediate contact urticaria is based on a thorough history and skin testing with suspected substances. Skin tests for human diagnostic testing are summarized in a recent review [170]. Because of the risk of systemic reactions, such as anaphylaxis, human diagnostic tests should be performed only by experienced personnel with facilities for resuscitation on hand. Contact urticaria has been divided into two main types on the basis of proposed pathophysiological mechanisms, nonimmunological and immunological [115]. Recent reviews list agents suspected of causing each type of urticarial response [97].

Nonimmunological contact urticaria is the most common form and occurs without previous exposure in most individuals. The reaction remains localized and does not cause systemic symptoms or spread to become generalized urticaria. Typically, the strength of this type of contact urticaria reaction varies from erythema to a generalized urticarial response, depending on the concentration, skin site, and substance. The mechanism of nonimmunological contact urticaria has not been delineated, but a direct influence on dermal vessel walls or a non-antibody-mediated release of histamine, prostaglandins, leukotrienes, substance P, or other inflammatory mediators represent possible mechanisms. Recent reports suggest that nonimmunologcal urticaria produced by different agents may involve different combinations of mediators [97].

The most potent and best studied substances producing nonimmunological contact urticaria are benzoic acid, cinnamic acid, cinnamic aldehyde, and nicotinic esters. Under optimal conditions, more than half of a random sample of individuals show local edema and erythema reactions within 45 min of application of these substances if the concentration is high enough. Benzoic acid and sodium benzoate are used as preservatives for cosmetics and other topical preparations at concentrations of 0.1%–0.2% and are capable of producing immediate contact reactions at the same concentrations [118]. Cinnamic aldehyde at a concentration of 0.01% may elicit an erythematous response associated with a burning or stinging feeling in the skin. Mouthwashes and chewing gums contain cinnamic aldehyde at concentrations high enough to produce a pleasant tingling or 'lively' sensation in the mouth and enhance the sale of the product. Higher concentrations produce lip swelling or typical contact urticaria in normal skin. Eugenol in the mixture inhibits contact sensitization to cinnamic aldehyde and inhibits nonimmunological contact urticaria from this same substance. The mechanism of the quenching effect is not certain, but a competitive inhibition at the receptor level may be the explanation [61].

Immunological contact urticaria is an immediate type 1 allergic reaction in people previously sensitized to the causative agent [170]. The molecules of a contact urticant react with specific IgE molecules attached to mast cell membranes. The cutaneous symptoms are elicited by vasoactive substances, mainly histamine, released from mast cells. The role of histamine is conspicuous, but other mediators of inflammation, for example, prostaglandins, leukotrienes, and kinins, may influence the degree of response. Immunological contact urticaria reactions can extend beyond the contact site, and generalized urticaria may be accompanied by other symptoms, such as rhinitis, conjunctivitis, asthma, and even anaphylactic shock. The term 'contact urticaria syndrome' was therefore suggested by Maibach and Johnson [115]. The name generally has been accepted for a symptom complex in which local urticaria occurs at the contact site with symptoms in others parts of the skin or in target organs such as the nose and throat, lung, and gastrointestinal and cardiovascular systems. Fortunately, the appearance of systemic symptoms is rare, but it may be seen in cases of strong hypersensitivity or in a widespread exposure and abundant percutaneous absorption of an allergen.

Foodstuffs are the most common causes of immunological contact urticaria. The orolaryngeal area is a site where immediate contact reactions are frequently provoked by food allergens, most often among atopic individuals. The actual antigens are proteins or protein complexes. As a proof of immediate hypersensitivity, specific IgE antibodies against the causative agent can typically be found in the patient's serum using the radioallergosorbent test technique and skin test for immediate allergy. The passive transfer test (Prausnitz-Kustner) also often gives a positive result.

18.5.1 Guinea Pig Ear Swelling Test

Predictive assays for evaluating the ability of materials to produce nonimmunological contact urticaria have been developed. No predictive assays for immunological contact urticaria have been published. Lahti and Maibach [96] developed an assay in guinea pigs using materials known to produce urticaria in humans: 0.1 ml of the material is applied to one ear of the animal and an equal volume of the solvent in which the test material is dissolved or suspended is applied to the opposite ear as a control. Ear thickness is measured before application and then every 15 min for 1–2 h after application. The swelling response is dependent on the concentration of the eliciting substance. The maximum response is about a 100% increase in ear thickness, and it appears within 50 min after application of a contact urticant. In histological sections, marked dermal edema and intra-

and perivascular infiltration of heterophilic granulocytes appear 40 min after application of test substances.

This assay is the predictive test of choice for nonimmunological contact urticaria if animals are to be tested. Guinea pig body skin reacts with quickly appearing erythema to cinnamic aldehyde, methyl nicotinate, and dimethyl sulphoxide but not to benzoic acid, sorbic acid, or cinnamic acid. Analogous reactions can be elicited in the earlobes of other animal species. Cinnamic aldehyde and dimethyl sulfoxide produce a swelling reaction in guinea pig, rat, and mouse. Benzoic acid, sorbic acid, cinnamic acid, diethyl fumarate, and methyl nicotinate produce no response in the rat or mouse, but the guinea pig ear reacts to all of them [97]. This suggests that either there are several mechanisms of nonimmunological contact urticaria, or there are differences in the activation of sensitivity to mediators of inflammation amoung guinea pig, rat, and mouse.

Materials can also be screened for nonimmunological contact urticaria in humans. A small amount of the test material is applied to a marked site on the forehead, and the vehicle is applied to a parallel site. The areas are evaluated at about 20–39 min after application for erythema and/or edema [170].

Differentiation between nonspecific irritant reactions and contact urticaria may be difficult. Strong irritants (e.g., hydrochloric acid, lactic acid, cobalt chloride, formaldehyde, and phenol) can cause clear-cut immediate whealing if the concentration is high enough, but the reactions do not usually fade away within a few hours. Instead, they are followed by sings of irritation; erythema, scaling, or crusting are seen 24 h later. Some substances have only urticant properties (e.g., benzoic acid, nicotinic acid esters), some are pure irritants (e.g., SLS) and some have both these features (e.g., formaldehyde, dimethyl sulphoxide).

Contact urticaria reactions are much less frequently encountered than either skin irritation or skin allergy [98]. However, increasing awareness of contact urticaria may expand the list of etiological agents and hopefully will lead to the development of adequate predictive assays for detecting causative agents of other forms of urticaria.

18.6 Subjective Irritation and Paraesthesia

Cutaneous application of some chemicals elicits sensory discomfort, tingling, and burning without visible inflammation (see Sect.2.2.10). This noninflammatory painful response has been termed subjective irritation [52, 55]. Materials reported to produce subjective irritation include dimethyl sulphoxide, some benzoyl preparations, and the chemicals salicylic acid, propylene glycol, amyl-dimethyl-*p*-aminobenzoic acid, and 2-ethoxyethyl-*p*-methoxy cinnamate, which are ingredients of cosmetics and over-the-counter drugs. Pyrethroids, a group of broad-spectrum insecticides, produce a similar condition that may lead to temporary numbness, which has been called paraesthesia [20, 45, 91]. As in subjective irritation, the nasolabial folds, cheeks, and periorbital areas are frequently involved. The ear is also sensitive to the pyrethroids.

Only a portion of the human populations seems to develop nonpyrethroid subjective irritation. Frosch and Kligman [52] found that they needed to prescreen subjects to identify 'stingers' for conducting predictive assays. Only 20% of subjects exposed to 5% aqueous lactic acid in a hot, humid environment developed a stinging response. All stingers in their series reported a history of adverse reactions to facial cosmetics, soaps, etc. A similar screening procedure by Lammintausta et al. [99] identified 18% of their subjects as stingers. Prior skin damage, for example, sunburn, pretreatment with surfactants, and tape stripping, increases the intensity of responses in stingers, and persons not normally experiencing a response report pain on exposure to lactic acid or other agents that produce subjective irritation [52]. Attempts to identify reactive subjects by association with other skin descriptors, such as atopy, skin type, or skin dryness, have not yet been fruitful. However, recent data show that stingers develop stronger reactions to materials causing nonimmunological contact urticaria and some increase in transepidermal water loss and blood flow following application of irritants via patches than those of 'nonstingers' [99].

The mechanisms by which materials produce subjective irritation have not been extensively investigated. Pyrethroids act directly on the axon by interfering with the channel gating mechanism and impulse firing [169]. It has been suggested that agents causing subjective irritation act via a similar mechanism because no visible inflammation is present.

An animal model was developed to rate paraesthesia to pyrethroids and may be useful for other agents [20, 123]. The test site is the flank of 300 to 450-g guinea pigs. Both flanks are shaved, and animals are individually housed in observation cages. A volume of 100 μl of the test material is spread over approximately 30 mm^2 on one flank. The same amount of the vehicle is applied to the other flank. The animal's behavior is monitored by an unmanned video camera for 5 min at 0.5, 1, 2, 4, and 6 h after application of the materials. Subsequently, the film is analyzed for the number of full turns of the head made to the control and pyrethroid-treated flank. Head turns were usually accompanied by attempted licking and biting of the application sites. Using this technique, it was possible to rank pyrethroids for their ability to produce paraesthesia. The ranking corresponded to the ranking available from human exposure.

18.6.1 Human Assay

As originally published, the human subjective irritation assay required the use of a 110° F environmental chamber with 80% relative humidity [52]. Volunteers were seated in the chamber until a profuse facial sweating was observed. Sweat was removed from the nasolabial fold and cheek; then a 5% aqueous solution of lactic acid was briskly rubbed over the area. Those who reported stinging for 3–5 min within the first 15 min were designated as stingers and were used for subsequent tests. Subjects were asked to evaluate the degree of stinging as nil (0), slight (1), moderate (2), or severe (3): stinging was evaluated 10 s, 2.5, 5 and 8 min after application of the test material. Other investigators [99] used a 15-min treatment with a commercial facial sauna to produce facial sweating, had subjects turn away from the sauna for application of the test materials, and then turn back to face the sauna for the observation period. The facial sauna technique is less stressful to both subjects and investigators and produces similar results.

Additional References

General:
   Dermatotoxicology 4th ed. by Marzulli and Maibach; Hemisphere, 1991.

Clinical Aspects:
   Contact Dermatitis 3rd ed. by Fisher; Lea & Febiger, 1986.
   Contact Dermatitis by Cronin; Churchill Livingstone, 1980.
   Patch Testing Guidelines by Malten, Nater & Van Ketel; Nijmegen; Dekker & Van de Vogt, 1976.
   Manual of Contact Dermatitis 2nd ed. by Fregert; Muskgaard, 1981.

Percutaneous Penetration:
   In Vitro Percutaneous Absorption by Bronaugh and Maibach; CRC Press 1991.
   Dermatological Formulations by Barry; Marcel Dekker, 1983.
   Percutaneous Absorption 2nd ed. by Bronaugh & Malibach; Marcel Dekker, 1990.

Occupational Dermatology:
   Occupational Contact Dermatitis by Foussereau, Benezra & Maibach; Munksgaard, 1982.
   Occupational and Industrial Dermatology 2nd ed. by Maibach; Year Book Publishers, 1987.
   Occupational Skin Diseases 2nd ed. by Adams; Grune & Stratton, 1990.

Predictive Testing:
   Contact and Photocontact Allergens by Maurer; Marcel Dekker, 1983.
   Contact Allergy Predictive Tests in Guinea Pigs by Anderson & Maibach; Karger, 1985.
   In Vitro Skin Irritation by Rougier, Goldberg & Maibach; Mary Ann Liebert, 1994.
   Health Risk Assessment: Dermal and Inhalation Exposure by Wang, Knaak & Maibach; CRC Press, 1992.

18.7 *References*

1. Allen AM (1978) Clinical trial design in dermatology: experimental design. I. Int J Dermatol 17: 42–51
2. Andersen KE, Maibach HI (1983) Multiple-application delayed-onset contact urticaria: possible relation to certain unusual formalin and textile reactions. Contact Dermatitis 10: 227–234
3. Asherson CL, Ptak W (1968) Contact and delayed hypersensitivity in the mouse. I. Active sensitization and passive transfer. Immunology 15: 405–416
4. Bartek MJ, LaBudde JA (1975) Percutaneous absorption *in vitro*. In: Maibach HI (ed) Animal models in dermatology. Churchill Linvingstone, New York, pp 103–120
5. Bartek MJ, LaBudde JA, Maibach HI (1972) Skin permeability *in vivo*: comparision in rat, rabbit, pig and man. J Invest Dermatol 58: 114–123
5a. Bason MM, Gordon V, Maibach HI (1991) Skin irritation in vitro assays. Int J Dermatol 30: 623–626
6. Battista CW, Rieger MM (1971) Some problems of predictive testing. J Soc Cosmet Chem 22: 349–359
7. Berger RS, Bowman JP (1982) A reappraisal of the 21-day cumulative irritation test in man. J Toxicol Cutan Ocular Toxicol 1: 109–115
8. Bergstressor PR, Paniser RJ, Taylor JR (1978) Counting and sizing of epidermal cells in human skin. J Invest Dermatol 70: 280–284
9. Bjornberg A (1975) Skin reactions to primary irritants in men and women. Acta Derm Venereol (Stockh) 55: 191–194
10. Blank HI (1953) Further observations on factors which influence the water content of the stratum corneum. J Invest Dermatol 21: 259–269
11. Blank I (1952) Water content of stratum corneum. J Invest Dermatol 18: 433–440
12. Bloch B, Steiner-Wourlisch A (1930) Die Sensibilisierung des Meerschweinchens gegen Primeln. Arch Dermatol Syph 162: 349–378
13. Boutwell RK (1981) Chemical carcinogenesis. A. Biochemical role. In: Laerum DD, Iverson OH (eds) Biology of skin cancer (excluding melanomas). International Union against Cancer, Geneva, pp 134–150
14. Boutwell RK, Urbach F, Carpenter G (1981) Chemical carcinogenesis. B. Experimental models. In: Laerum DD, Iverson OH (eds) Biology of skin cancer (excluding melanomas). International Union against Cancer, Geneva, pp 109–123
15. Bronaugh RL, Congolon ER, Scheuplein RJ (1981) The effect of cosmetic vehicles on the penetration of *N*-nitro-diethanolamine through excised skin. J Invest Dermatol 76: 94–96
16. Brunner MJ, Smiljanic A (1952) Procedure for evaluation of skin sensitizing power of new materials. Arch Dermatol 66: 703–705
17. Buehler EV (1964) A new method for detecting potential sensitizers using the guinea pig. Toxicol Appl Pharmacol 6: 341
18. Buehler EV (1965) Experimental skin sensitization in the guinea pig and man. Arch Dermatol 91: 171
19. Busse MJ, Hunt P, Lees KA, Maggs PND, McCarthy TM (1969) Release of betamethasone derivatives from ointments – *in vivo* and *in vitro* studies. Br J Dermatol 81: 103
20. Cagen SZ, Malloy LA, Parker CM, Gardiner TH, van Gelder CA, Jud VA (1984) Pyrethroid mediated skin sensory stimulation characterized by a new behavioral paradigm. Toxicol Appl Pharmacol 76: 270–279
21. Calandra J (1971) Comments on the guinea pig immersion test. CTFA Cosmet J 3(3): 47
22. Carter RO, Griffith JF (1965) Experimental basis for the realistic assessment of safety of topical agents. Toxicol Appl Pharmacol 7: 60–73

23. Christie GA, Moore-Robinson M (1970) Vehicle assessment – methodology and results. Br J Dermatol 82: 93
24. Code of Federal Regulations (1985) Office of the Federal Registrar, National Archives of Records Service. General Services Administration, title 16, parts 1500.50–1500.41
25. Cunningham-Rundles S (1981) Cell-mediated immunity. In: Safai B, Good RA (eds) Immunodermatology. Plenum, New York, pp 1–33
26. Davies RE, Harper KH, Kynoch SR (1972) Interspecies variation in dermal reactivity. J Soc Cosmet Chem 23: 371–381
27. Draize JH (1955) Procedures for the appraisal of the toxicity of chemicals in foods, drugs, and cosmetics. VIII. Dermal toxicity. Food Drug Cosmet Law J 10: 722–731
28. Draize JH (1959) Dermal toxicity. US appraisal of the safety of chemicals in food, drugs and cosmetics. Association of Food and Drug Officials, Texas State Department of Health, Austin, pp 46–59
29. Draize JH, Woodard G, Calvery HO (1944) Methods for the study of irritation and toxicity of substances applied topically to the skin and mucous membrane. J Pharmacol Exp Ther 82: 377–390
30. Drill VA, Lazar P (1983) Cutaneous toxicity. Raven, New York
31. Dugard PJ (1983) Skin permeability theory in relation to measurements of percutaneous absorption. In: Marzulli FN, Maibach HI (eds) Dermatotoxicology, 2nd edn. Hemisphere, New York
32. Elias PM (1987) Lipids and the epidermal permeability barriers. Arch Dermatol Res 270: 95–117
33. Elias PM, Cooper ER, Korc A, Brown BE (1981) Percutaneous transport in relation to stratum corneum structure and lipid composition. J Invest Dermatol 76: 297–301
34. Emergy BE, Edwards LD (1940) The pharmacology of soaps. II. The irritant action of soaps on human skin. J Am Pharm Assoc 29: 251–254
35. Emmett EA (1975) Occupational skin cancer: a review. J Occup Med 17: 44–49
36. Environmental Protection Agency (1982) Pesticides registrations: proposed data requirements, sect 158.135: toxicology data requirements. Fed Reg 47: 53192
37. Epstein WL, Kligman AM, Senecal IP (1963) Role of regional lymph nodes in contact sensitization. Arch Dermatol 88: 789
38. Everall JD (1981) Chemical carcinogenesis. A. Environmental carcinogens. In: Laerum DD, Iverson OH (eds) Biology of skin cancer (excluding melanomas). International Union against Cancer, Geneva, pp 105–108
39. Everall JD, Dowd PM (1978) Influence of environmental factors excluding ultraviolet radiation on the incidence of skin cancer. Bull Cancer 65: 241–24840
40. Fare G (1966) Rat skin carcinogenesis by topical applications of some azo dyes. Cancer Res 26: 2466–2468
41. Farrar JJ, Benjamin WR, Hilficker ML, Howard M, Farrar WL, Fuller-Farrar JF (1982) The biochemistry, biology, and role of interleukin in the induction of cytotoxic T-cell and antibody-forming B-cell responses. Immunol Rev 63: 129–166
42. Feldman RJ, Maibach HI (1967) Regional variation in percutaneous penetration of [^{14}C]cortisone in man. J Invest Dermatol 48: 181–183
43. Finkelstein P, Laden K, Meichowski W (1963) New methods for evaluating cosmetic irritancy. J Invest Dermatol 40: 11–14
44. Finkelstein P, Laden K, Meichowski W (1965) Laboratory methods for evaluating skin irritancy. Toxicol Appl Pharmacol 7: 74–78
45. Flannigan SA, Tucker SB (1986) Variation in cutaneous sensation between synthetic pyrethroic insecticides. Contact Dermatitis 13: 140–147
46. Franz TJ (1975) Percutaneous absorption. On the relevance of in vitro data. J Invest Dermatol 64: 190–195
47. Frey JR, Wenk P (1957) Experimental studies on the pathogenesis of contact eczema in the guinea pig. Int Arch Allergy Appl Immunol 11: 81–100

48. Fritsch WC, Stoughton RB (1963) The effect of temperature and humidity on the penetration of [^{14}C]acetyl-salicylic acid in excised human skin. J Invest Dermatol 41: 307

49. Frosch PJ (1982) Irritancy of soap and detrgent bars. In: Frost P, Horwitz SN (eds) Principles of cosmetics for the dermatologist. Mosby, St Louis, pp 5–12

50. Frosch PJ, Kligman AM (1976) The chamber scarification test for irritancy. Contact Dermatitis 2: 314–324

51. Frosch PJ, Kligman AM (1977) The chamber scarification test for assessing irritancy of topically applied substances. In: Drill VA, Lazar P (eds) Cutaneous toxicity. Academic, New York, pp 127–144

52. Frosch PJ, Kligman AM (1977) A method for appraising the stinging capacity of topically applied substances. J Soc Cosmet Chem 28: 197–207

53. Frosch PJ, Kligman AM (1979) The soap chamber test. A new method for assessing the irritancy of soaps. J Am Acad Dermatol 1: 35–41

54. Frosch PJ, Kligman AM (1979) The Duhring chamber: an improved technique for epicutaneous testing for irritant and allergic reactions. Contact Dermatitis 5: 73

55. Frosch PJ, Kligman AM (1982) Recognition of chemically vulnerable and delicate skin. In: Frost P, Horwitz SN (eds) Principles of cosmetics for the dermatologist. Mosby, St Louis, p 287

56. Gilman MR, Evans RA, DeSalva SJ (1978) The influence of concentration, exposure duration, and patch occlusivity upon rabbit primary dermal irritation indices. Drug Chem Toxicol 1(4): 391–400

57. Griffith JF (1969) Predictive and diagnostic test for contact sensitization. Toxicol Appl Pharmacol [Suppl] 3: 90–102

58. Griffith JF, Buehler E (1976) Prediction of skin irritancy and sensitization potential by testing with animals and man. In: Drill V, Lazar P (eds) Cutaneous toxicity. Academic, New York

59. Griffith JF, Weaver JE, Whitehouse HS, Poole RL, Newman EA, Nixon CA (1969) Safety evaluation of enzyme detergents. Oral and cutaneous toxicity, irritancyi and skin sensitization studies. Food Cosmet Toxicol 7: 581–593

60. Guillot JP, Gopnnet JF, Clement C, Caillard L, Truhauf R (1982) Evaluation of the cutaneous-irritation potential of compounds. Food Chem Toxicol 20: 563–572

61. Guin JD, Meyer BN, Drake RD, Haffley P (1984) The effect of quenching agents on contact urticaria caused by cinnamic aldehyde. J Am Acad Dermatol 10: 45–51

62. Guy RH, Wester RC, Tur E, Maibach HI (1983) Noninvasive assessments of the percutaneous absorption of methyl nicotinate in humans. J Pharm Sci 72: 1077–1079

63. Guy RH, Tur E, Bugatto B, Gaebel C, Sheiner L, Maibach HI (1984) Pharmacodynamic measurements of methyl nicotinate percutaneous absorption. Pharmacol Res 1: 76–81

64. Haley T, Hunziger J (1974) Instrument for producing standardized skin abrasions. J Pharm Sci 63: 106

65. Henderson CR, Riley EC (1945) Certain statistical considerations in patch testing. Invest Dermatol 6: 227–230

66. Higuchi T (1960) Physical chemical analysis of percutaneous absorption process from creams and ointments. J Soc Cosmet Chem 11: 85–97

67. Holbrook KA, Odland GF (1974) Regional differences in the thickness (cell layers) of the human stratum corneum: an ultrastructural analysis. J Invest Dermatol 62: 415–422

68. Holbrook KA, Smith LT (1981) Ultrastructural aspects of human skin during the embryonic, fetal, premature, neonatal, and adult periods of life. In: Blandau RJ (ed) Morphogenesis and malforming of the skin. Liss, New York, pp 9–38

69. Hood DB, Neher RJ, Reinke RE, Zapp JA (1965) Experience with the guinea pig in screening primary irritants and sensitizers. Toxicol Appl Pharmacol 7: 485–486

70. Ihle JN, Rebar K, Keller J, Lee JC, Hapel AJ (1982) Interleukin 3: possible roles in the regulation of lymphocyte differentiation and visual assessment. Br J Dermatol 92: 131–142

71. Iverson OH (1981) Chemical carcinogenesis. E. Short term tests for carcinogens. In: Laerum DD, Iverson OH (eds) Biology of skin cancer (excluding melanomas). International Union Against Cancer, Geneva, pp 151–163

72. Jackson R, Grainge JW (1975) Arsenic and cancer. Can Med Assoc J 113: 396–401

73. Jadassohn J (1896) Zur Kenntniss der medicamentösen Dermatosen. Verh Dtsch Dermatol Ges 5: 103–129

74. Jadassohn J (1896) A contribution to the study of dermatoses produced by drugs. Verh Dtsch Dermatol Ges 207–229

75. Jaffee BD, Maguire HC Jr (1981) Delayed-type hypersensitivity and immunological tolerance to contact allergens in the rat (Abstr). Fed Proc 40: 991

76. Johnson SAM, Kile RL, Kooyman DJ, Whitehouse HS, Brod JS (1953) Comparison of effects of soaps and detergents on the hands of housewives. Arch Dermatol Syph 68: 643–650

77. Jordan WP, King SE (1977) Delayed hypersensitivity in females during the comparison of two predictive patch tests. Contact Dermatitis 3: 19–26

78. Justice JD, Travers JJ, Vinson LJ (1961) The correlation between animals tests and human tests in assessing product mildness. Proc Sci Sect Toilet Goods Assoc 35: 12–17

79. Kaminsky M, Szivos MM, Brown KR (1986) Application of the Hill Top patch test chamber to dermal irritancy testing in the albino rabbit. J Toxicol Cutan Ocular Toxicol 5(2): 81–87

80. Kero M, Hannuksela M (1980) Guinea pig maximization test, open epicutaneous test and chamber test in induction of delayed contact hypersensitivity. Contact Dermatitis 6: 341–344

80a. Kimber I, Mitchell JA, Griffin AC (1986) Development of a murine local lymph node assay for the determination of sensitizing potential. Food Chem Toxicol 24: 585–586

81. Klecak G (1982) Identification of contact allergens: predictive tests in animals. In: Marzulli FN, Maibach HI (eds) Dermatotoxicology, 2nd edn. Hemisphere, New York, pp 200–219

82. Klecak G (1985) The Freund's complete adjuvant test and the open epicutaneous test. In: Maibach HI, Anderson KE (eds) Contact allergy, predictive tests in guinea pigs. Karger, Basel, pp 152–171

83. Kligman A (1964) Quantitative testing of chemical irritants. In: Steinberg M (ed) Evaluation of therapeutic agents and cosmetics. McGraw-Hill, New York, pp 186–192

84. Kligman AM (1966) The identification of contact allergens by human assay. I. A critique of standard methods. J Invest Dermatol 47: 369–374

85. Kligman AM (1966) The identification of contact allergens by human assay. II. Factors influencing the induction and measurement of allergic contact dermatitis. J Invest Dermatol 47: 375–392

86. Kligman AM (1966) The identification of contact allergens by human assay. III. The maximization test. A procedure for screening and rating contact sensitizers. J Invest Dermatol 47: 393–409

87. Kligman AM (1983) A biological brief on percutaneous absorption. Drug Dev Ind Pharm 521–560

88. Kligman AM, Epstein W (1959) Some factors affecting contact sensitization in man. In: Shaffer JH, Lo Grippo GA, Chase WM (eds) Mechanism of hypersensitivity. Little, Brown, Boston, pp 713–722

89. Kligman AM, Epstein W (1975) Updating the maximization test for identifying contact allergens. Contact Dermatitis 1: 231–239

90. Kligman AM, Wooding WM (1967) A method for the measurement and evaluation of irritants on human skin. J Invest Dermatol 49: 78–94

91. Knox JM, Tucker SB, Flannigan SA (1984) Paresthesia from cutaneous exposure to synthetic pyrethroid insecticide. Arch Dermatol 120: 744–746

92. Kooyman DJ, Snyder FH (1942) Tests for the mildness of soaps. Arch Dermatol Syph 46: 846–855

93. Kral F, Schwartzman RM (1964) Veterinary and comparative dermatology. Lippincott, Philadelphia

94. Kuroki T, Nemoto N, Kitano Y (1980) Use of human epidermal keratinocytes in studies on chemical carcinogenesis. In: Pullman B, Ts'o POP, Gelboin H (eds) Carcinogenesis: fundamental mechanism and environmental effects. Redel, Boston, pp 417–426

95. Lahti A (1980) Nonimmunologic contact urticaria. Acta Derm Venereol [Suppl] (Stockh) 60: 1–49

96. Lahti A, Maibach HI (1984) An animal model for nonimmunologic contact urticaria. Toxicol Appl Pharmacol 76: 219–224

97. Lahti A, Maibach HI (1985) Species specificity of nonimmunologic contact urticaria: guinea pig, rat and mouse. J Am Acad Dermatol 13: 66–69

98. Lahti A, von Krogh G, Maibach HI (1985) Contact urticaria syndrome. An expanding phenomenon. In: Stone J (ed) Dermatologic immunology and allergy. Mosby, St Louis, pp 379–390

99. Lammintausta K, Maibach HI, Wilson D (1988) Mechanisms of subjective (sensory) irritation: propensity of nonimmunologic contact urticaria and objective irritation in stingers. Derm Beruf Umwelt 36: 45–49

99a. Lammintausta K, Maibach H (1990) Irritation insights: epidemiology of experimented status. In: Menné T, Maibach H (eds) Exogenous dermatoses: environmentet dermatitis. CRC, Boca Raton, pp 179–186

100. Landsteiner K, Chase MW (1937) Studies on the sensitization of animals with simple chemical compounds. IV. Anaphylaxis induced by pictyl chloride and 2:4 dinitrochlorbenzene. J Exp Med 66: 337–351

101. Landsteiner K, Jacobs J (1935) Studies on the sensitization of animals with simple chemical compounds. J Exp Med 61: 643–648

102. Landsteiner K, Jacobs J (1936) Studies on the sensitization of animals with simple chemical compounds. II. J Exp Med 64: 625–629

103. Lanman BM, Elvers WB, Howard CS (1968) The role of human patch testing in a product development program. In Proceedings of the Joint Conference on Cosmetic Sciences. The Toilet Association, Washington, pp 135–145

104. Lever WF, Schaumburg-Hevor's (1983) Histopathology of the skin, 6th edn. Lippincott, Philadelphia

105. MacMillan FSK, Rafft RR, Elevers WB (1975) A comparison of the skin irritation produced by cosmetic ingredients and formulations in the rabbit, guinea pig, beagle dog to that observed in the human. In: Maibach HI (ed) Animal models in dermatology. Churchill Livingstone, Edinburgh, pp 12–22

106. Magee PN (1970) Tests for carcinogenic potential. In: Paget GE (ed) Methods in toxicology. Davis, Philadelphia, pp 158–196

107. Magnusson B, Hersle K (1965) Patch test methods. I. A comparative study of six different types of patch tests. Acta Dermatol 45: 123–128

108. Magnusson B, Hersle K (1965) Patch test methods. II. Regional variations of patch test responses. Acta Dermatol 45: 257–261

109. Magnusson B, Hersle K (1966) Patch test methods. III. Influence of adhesive tape on test response. Acta Dermatol 46: 275–278

110. Magnusson B, Kligman AM (1969) The identification of contact allergens by animals assay. The guinea pig maximization test. J Invest Dermatol 52: 268–276

111. Magnusson B, Kligman AM (1970) Allergic contact dermatitis in the guinea pig. Thomas, Springfield
112. Maguire HC (1973) Mechanism of intensification by Freund's complete adjuvant of the acquisition of delayed hypersensitivity in the guinea pig. Immunol Commun 1: 239–246
113. Maguire HC (1974) Alteration in the acquisition of delayed hypersensitivity with adjuvant in the guinea pig. Monogr Allergy 8: 13–26
114. Maibach HI (1976) Immediate hypersensitivity in hand dermatitis: role of food contact dermatitis. Arch Dermatol 112: 1289–1291
115. Maibach HI, Johnson HL (1975) Contact urticaria syndrome. Contact urticaria to diethyltoluamide (immediate-type hypersensitivity). Arch Dermatol 111: 726–730
115a. Maisey J, Miller K (1986) Assessment of the ability of mice fed on vitamin A supplemented diet to respond to a variety of potential contact sensitizers. Contact Dermatitis 15: 17–23
116. Malkinson FD (1958) Studies on the percutaneous absorption of ^{14}C labeled steroids by use of the gas-flow cell. J Invest Dermatol 31: 19
117. Marzulli FN, Maibach HI (1973) Antimicrobials: experimental contact sensitization in man. J Soc Cosmet Chem 24: 399–421
118. Marzulli FN, Maibach HI (1974) The use of graded concentration in studying skin sensitizers: experimental contact sensitization in man. Food Cosmet Toxicol 12: 219–227
119. Mathias CGT, Maibach HI (1978) Dermatoxicology monogaphs. I. Cutaneous irritation: factors influencing the response to irritants. Clin Toxicol 13: 333–346
120. Mathias CGT, Chappler RR, Maibach HI (1980) Contact urticaria from cinnamic aldehyde. Arch Dermatol 116: 74–76
121. Maurer T, Thomann P, Weirich EG, Hess R (1975) The optimization test in the guinea pig. A method for the predictive evaluation of the contact allergenicity of chemicals. Agents Actions 5: 174–179
122. McKenzie AW, Stoughton RM (1962) Method for comparing percutaneous absorption of steroids. Arch Dermatol 86: 608–610
123. McKillop CM, Brock JAC, Oliver CJA, Rhodes C (1987) A quantitative assessment of pyrethroid-induced paresthesia in the guinea pig flank model. Toxicol Lett 36: 1–7
124. Mizel SB (1982) Interleukin 1 and T cell activation. Imunol Rev 63: 51–72
125. Montagna W (1962) The structure and function of skin. Academic, New York
126. Montagna W (1962) The epidermis. Academic, New York
127. Motoyoshi K, Toyoshima Y, Sato M, Yoshimura M (1979) Comparative studies on the irritancy of oils and synthetic perfumes to the skin of rabbit, guinea pig, rat, miniature swine, and man. Cosmet Toilet 94: 41–42
128. Najarian JS, Feldman JD (1963) Specificity of passive transfer or delayed hypersensitivity. J Exp Med 118: 341–352
129. National Academy of Sciences, Committee for the Revision of NAS Publication 1138 (1977) Principles and procedures for evaluating the toxicity of household substances. National Academy of Sciences, Washington, pp 23–59
130. Nicolaides N (1963) Human skin surface lipids – origins, composition and possible function. In: Montagna W, Ellis RA, Silver AF (eds) The sebaceous glands. Pergamon, Oxford, pp 167–187 (Advances in biology of skin, vol 4)
131. Nixon GA, Tyson CA, Wertz WC (1975) Interspecies comparisons of skin irritancy. Toxicol Appl Pharmacol 31: 481–490
132. Noonan PK, Wester RC (1983) Cutaneous biotransformations and some pharmacological and toxicological implications. In: Marzulli FN, Maibach HI (eds) Dermatotoxicology. Hemisphere, New York, pp 71–90
133. Odom RB, Maibach HI (1976) Contact urticaria: a different contact dermatitis. Cutis 18: 672–676

134. Opdyke D (1971) The guinea pig immersion test – a 20 year appraisal. CTFA Cosmet J 3(3): 46–47
135. Opdyke DL, Burnett CM (1965) Practical problems in the evaluation of the safety of cosmetics. Proc Sci Sect Toilet Goods Assoc 44: 3–4
136. Organization for Economic Cooperation and Development (1981) OECD guidelines for testing of chemicals, 4. OECD, Paris
137. Ostrenga J, Steinmetz C, Poulsen B, Yett S (1971) Significance of vehicle composition. II. Prediction of optimal vehicle composition. J Pharm Sci 60: 1180–1183
138. Page NP (1977) Concepts of a bioassay program in environmental carcinogenesis. In: Kraybill HF, Mehlmann MA (eds) Advances in modern toxicology. Hemisphere, New York, pp 87–171 (Environmental cancer, vol 3)
139. Palotay JL, Adachi K, Dobson RL, Pinto JS (1986) Carcinogen-induced cutaneous neoplasms in non-human primate. JNCI 57: 1269–1272
140. Phillips L, Steinberg M, Maibach HI, Akers WA (1972) A comparison of rabbit and human skin response to certain irritants. Toxicol Appol Pharmacol 21: 369–382
141. Polak L (1977) Immunological aspects of contact sensitivity. In: Marzulli FN, Maibach HI (eds) Dermatotoxicology and pharmacology. Hemisphere, New York, pp 225–288
142. Polak L, Polak A, Frey JR (1974) The development of contact sensitivity to DNFB in guinea pigs genetically differing in their response to DNP-skin protein conjugate. Int Arch Allergy Appl Immunol 46: 417–426
143. Potokar M (1985) Studies on the design of animal tests for the corrosiveness of industrial chemicals. Food Chem Toxicol 2: 615–617
144. Prottey C (1978) The molecular basis of skin irritation. In: Breuer MM (ed) Cosmetic science, vol 1. Academic, London, pp 275–349
145. Rapaport M, Anderson D, Pierce U (1978) Performance of the 21 day patch test in civilian populations. J Toxicol Cutan Ocular Toxicol 1: 109–115
146. Ritz HL, Buehler EV (1980) Planning conduct and interpretation of guinea pig sensitization patch tests. In: Drill VA, Lazar P (eds) Current concepts in cutaneous toxicity. Academic, New York, p 25
147. Rothman S (1954) Physiology and biochemistry of the skin. University of Chicago Press, Chicago
148. Scheuplein RJ (1978) Permeability of skin: a review of major concepts. Curr Probl Dermatol 7: 58–68
149. Scheuplein RJ, Bronough RL (1983) Percutaneous absorption. In: Goldsmith LA (ed) Biochemistry and physiology of the skin. Oxford University Press, New York, pp 1255–1295
150. Schwartz L (1951) The skin testing of new cosmetics. J Soc Cosmet Chem 2: 321–324
151. Schwartz L (1969) Twenty-two years' experience in the performanced of 200,000 prophetic patch tests. South Med J 53: 478–484
152. Schwartz L, Peck SM (1944) The patch test in contact dermatitis. Public Health Rep 59: 546–557
153. Shelanski HA (1951) Experience with and considerations of the human patch test method. J Soc Cosmet Chem 2: 324–331
154. Shelanski HA, Shelanski MV (1953) New technique of patch tests. Drug Cosmet Ind 73: 186
155. Shelanski HA, Shelanski MV (1953) A new technique of human patch tests. Proc Sci Sect Toilet Goods Assoc 19: 46–49
156. Shellow WVR, Rapaport MJ (1981) Comparison testing of soap irritancy using aluminum chamber and standard patch methods. Contact Dermatitis 7: 77–49
157. Simpson WL, Cramer W (1943) Fluorescnece studies: carcinogens in skin. Cancer Res 3: 362–369

158. Sokolov UE (1982) Mammal skin. University of California Press, Berkeley
159. Steinberg M, Akers WA, Weeks M, McCreesh AH, Maibach HI (1975) I. A comparison of test techniques based on rabbit and human skin responses to irritants with recommendations regarding the evaluation of mildly or moderately irritating compounds. In: Maibach HI (ed) Animal models in dermatology. Livingstone, Edinburgh, pp 1–11
160. Stingl G, Abever W (1983) The Langerhans' cell. In: Goldsmith LA (ed) Biochemistry and physiology of the skin. Oxford University Press, New York, pp 907–921
161. Stingl G, Katz SI, Clement L, Green I, Shevach E (1978) Immunologic functions of la-bearing epidermal Langerhans' cells. J Immunol 121: 2005–2013
162. Sweeney TM, Downing DT (1970) The role of lipids in the epidermal barrier to water diffusion. J Invest Dermatol 55: 135–140
163. Traub EF, Tusing TW, Spoor HJ (1954) Evaluation of dermal sensitivity; animal and human tests compared. Arch Dermatol 69: 399–409
164. Tregear RT (1964) Relative penetrability of hair follicles and epidermis. J Physiol (Lond) 156: 303–313
165. Tregear RT (1966) Physical function of skin. Academic, New York
166. Unanue ER (1984) Antigen-presenting function of the macrophage. Annu Rev Immunol 2: 395–428
167. Uttley M, van Abbé NJ (1973) Primary irritation of the skin; mouse ear test and human patch test procedures. J Soc Cosmet Chem 24: 217–227
168. Vinegar MB (1979) Regional variation in primary skin irritation and corrosivity potentials in rabbits. Toxicol Appl Pharmacol 49: 63–69
169. Vivjeberg HP, VandenBercken J (1979) Frequency dependent effects of the pyrethroid insecticide decamethrin in frog myelinated nerve fibers. Eur J Pharmacol 58: 501–504
170. Von Krogh C, Maibach HI (1982) The contact urticaria syndrome. Semin Dermatol 1: 59–66
171. Voss JG (1958) Skin sensitization by mercaptans of low molecular weight. J Invest Dermatol 31: 273–279
172. Wasserman SJ (1983) The mast cell and its mediators. In: Goldsmith LA (ed) Biochemistry and physiology of the skin. Oxford University Press, New York, pp 878–898
173. Weaver JE (1976) Dermatologic testing of household laundry products: a novel fabric softener. Int J Dermatol 15: 297–300
174. Weigand DA, Gaylor JR (1976) Irritant reaction in Negro and Caucasian skin. South Med J 67: 548–551
175. Weigand DA, Haygood C, Gaylor JR (1974) Cell layer and density of Negro and Causcasian stratum corneum. J Invest Dermatol 62: 563–568
176. Weil CS, Scala RA (1971) Study of intra- and interlaboratory variability in the results of rabbit eye and skin irritation tests. Toxicol Appl Pharmacol 19: 276–360
177. Wester RC, Maibach HI (1975) Rhesus monkey as an animal model for percutaneous absorption. In: Maibach HI (ed) Animal models in dermatology. Livingstone, New York, pp 133–137
178. Wester RC, Maibach HI (1983) Cutaneous pharmacokinetics: 10 steps to percutaneous absorption. Drug Metab Rev 14: 169–205
179. Whitton JT, Ewell JD (1973) The thickness of epidermis. Br J Dermatol 89: 467–478
180. Wooding WH, Opdyke DL (1967) A statistical approach to the evaluation of cutaneous responses to irritants. J Soc Cosmet Chem 18: 809–829

Chapter 19
International Legal Aspects
of Contact Dermatitis

International Legal Aspects of Contact Dermatitis

PETER J. FROSCH and RICHARD J. G. RYCROFT

Contents

19.1 Introduction

In a European textbook on contact dermatitis a chapter on legal aspects is entirely appropriate. In many cases an occupational cause is suspected and proven after careful diagnostic procedures. There then arise a number of questions that are handled in different ways in the different European countries. Facing the Europe of 1992, with its expected migrations of labour, the occupational physician needs to know the essential differences between legislation in the major countries.

As a basis for this chapter, a questionnaire was sent to members of the European Environmental and Contact Dermatitis Research Group (EECDRG) and other colleagues experienced in this field. The underlying concept of handling an occupational contact dermatitis in (West) Germany, and three typical examples, were described. Fifteen questions were asked about various aspects (institutions involved, report forms, requirements for recognition, retraining, pension, etc.). Due to the nomenclature and country-specific legal rules it often proved difficult for respondents to answer these questions and to make clear statements. Nevertheless, some major differences became apparent.

In the following, the authors have tried to characterize the principle legal characteristics in the various countries. The frequent comparisons with the German system are made only for ease of understanding and definitely not made with any intention of suggesting that this should be regarded as a 'standard'. In the years to come it will probably be necessary to create more uniform joint legislation in this area, so as to avoid socially injust decisions.

19.2 Occupational Dermatitis in Germany

In Germany, the legal basis for dealing with occupational diseases is fixed in the 3rd book of the state insurance code *Reichsversicherungsordnung* (RVO) and the 7th decree on the extension of accident insurance to occupational diseases (*7. Verordnung über die Ausdehnung der Unfallversicherung auf Berufskrankheiten*). Occupational skin diseases are defined in paragraphs 551.1 and 551.2 RVO and are classified in the list in the 7th decree under:
- No. 5101: Severe or repeatedly relapsing dermatoses which have clearly necessitated the cessation of all occupational activities which were or could be responsible for causing the disease or its relapse or aggravation, and
- No. 5102: Cancers or precanceroses caused by soot, unpurified paraffins, tar, anthracene, pitch or similar substances.

The list is updated from time to time. The responsibility for dealing with occupational incidents and diseases is held by nonprofit-making insurance institutions, the *Berufsgenossenschaften* (BG). There are 36 BGs, each responsible for a different field of work, such as administrative work and trade, construction, health care, mechanical engineering and the iron and steel industry, mining, transport, food production, forestry and the wood industry, and so on.

Every employee must by law be insured against occupational accidents, injuries and diseases. Employers have to pay for the insurance. The system for the settlement of claims about occupational incidents and diseases is quite elaborate and has a very 'social' touch.

Even when there is only a slight suspicion that a dermatosis is work related, a dermatologist's report (*Hautarztbericht*) is filed with the competent insurance institution (BG). This report needs the consent of the person concerned. It is based on a detailed examination including patch tests and atopy screening. It also includes recommendations concerning therapy, protection, skin care, or even changing of the workplace. This attempt to handle occupational dermatoses as quickly and unbureaucratically as possible is in the forefront of change in legal regulations. If the dermatosis continues, and the suspicion that the disease has an occupational origin, is confirmed, any doctor in contact with the person concerned is obliged *by law* to fill in a special initial report form (the medical report of an occupational disease, (*Ärztliche Anzeige über eine Berufskrankheit*). This form is then sent to the competent BG or to an official government physician dealing with occupational diseases (*Staatlicher Gewerbearzt*). This does not need the consent of the person concerned.

The BG, after obtaining the report, investigates the case further, quite often by sending a specially trained adviser to inspect the workplace. The adviser gives detailed advice to the worker regarding avoidance of irritants and potential allergens, and can recommend the use of barrier creams, gloves and appropriate cleansing agents. These must be provided by the employer. If the patient continues to have skin symptoms he is referred to a dermatologist. A detailed work-up, including patch testing and atopy screening, is carried out and a dermatologist's report (*Hautarztbericht*) is sent to the BG. The BG makes a moderate payment for both the initial report and the *Hautarztbericht*. The dermatologist must make a clear statement as to the origin of the disease, including occupational and nonoccupational factors, and provides detailed suggestions for avoidance of occupational risks and recommendations for preventive measures. If all such measures fail (as in the case of the bricklayer given below), the patient must stop working in his or her occupation and an expert opinion from a dermatologist (usually a different one) is ordered by the BG. This opinion provides the basis for rejecting or recognizing the condition as an occupational skin disease, and for payment of compensation or for retraining.

A copy of the initial report (*Ärztliche Anzeige*) is also sent to an official government physician (*Staatlicher Gewerbearzt*), who can then investigate the case further, order an expert opinion or decide independently whether the disease is to be classified as occupational or nonoccupational. If the *Gewerbearzt* and the BG disagree on a case, particularly if a monthly pension is at stake, a second or third expert's opinion is obtained. A commission (see below) then makes a decision. If the patient is dissatisfied with the decision, he or she may take the matter to court (*Sozialgericht*). The judge, after reviewing the case, often orders another expert opinion from a recognized specialist in occupational dermatology.

According to German law (7th decree on occupational diseases, (*7. Berufskrankheitenverordnung*), to be regarded as an occupational contact dermatitis an eczema must be either 'severe' or 'repeatedly relapsing' and must have given the accomplished cause to cease all activities which are or could be causing the disease or aggravation or relapse of the disease (No. 5101: "schwere oder wiederholt rückfällige Hauterkrankungen, die zur Unterlassung aller Tätigkeiten gezwungen haben, die für die Entstehung, die Verschlimmerung oder das Wiederaufleben der Krankheit ursächlich waren oder sein können"). There is no clear definition of 'severe', although most physicians consider a disease as severe if practically continuous medical treatment is necessary for at least 6 months and if the patient is seriously handicapped. 'Repeatedly relapsing' (*'wiederholt rückfällig'*) is defined, and means that at least three bouts of the disease must have occurred. By definition it is also necessary that the disease has healed or at least considerably improved between two bouts.

A further specific term in the German legislation is *'Minderung der Erwerbsfähigkeit'* (MdE), meaning 'diminution of working ability'. The physician must estimate in an abstract manner how many occupations available in the overall labour market the patient is unable to work in because of the occupational disease. For instance, a bricklayer who has acquired a chromate allergy and is suffering from severe hand eczema will receive an MdE of 20%–30%, which means that he cannot enter about 20%–30% of the occupations available in the labour market because chromate is such a ubiquitous allergen. If the estimate is below 20% (e.g., 10%–15% in the case of a nickel allergy with *slight* hand eczema), the case is still recognized as an occupational disease (*'Anerkennung dem Grunde nach'*, 'basic recognition' or 'admission in law'). However, 20% is a critical figure because a patient with an MdE of 20% or more receives compensation: he or she is paid a pension equivalent to the appropriate percentage of the pension that would have been awarded if he or she were totally disabled, i.e. two-thirds of the annual earnings in the year before stopping work. This pension is paid by the insurance institution (BG) for as long as the disability lasts, sometimes for life. Withdrawing the compensation is difficult and depends on the percentage MdE, which can change for medical and/or occupational reasons. In every case, though, once an occupational disease has been legally acknowledged to exist, this acknowledgement can never be withdrawn.

The *Arbeitsgemeinschaft für Berufsdermatologie* (Task Force on Occupational Dermatoses of the German Dermatological Society) has published recommendations regarding the degree of MdE based on the presence and severity of skin lesions, intensity of allergic contact sensitization(s) and spread (occurrence) of the allergen(s) in daily life. Each item scores on a scale from 0 to 20. If the total score reaches 20 points the MdE is considered to be 20%, and a score of 50 points or more implies an MdE of 30% [4].

19.2.1 Examples

In the following, three typical examples of occupational 'legal cases' are given, as they were handled by the German authorities.

Example A. A bricklayer, aged 35 years, has to stop all occupational activities because of severe hand eczema which has resulted in at least three sick leaves of several weeks' duration. A patch test is positive for dichromate. He cannot avoid contact with cement and the suggestion of the dermatologist in the expert opinion is to retrain him, to recognize his disease as occupational (*Berufskrankheit* 5101) and to grant him a pension of 20%.

The retraining is paid for by the insurance company (BG for construction workers). The retraining programme takes 2 years and costs about DM 120 000. This procedure is performed according to paragraph 3 of the *Berufskrankheitenverordnung,* which states that the insurer has to do everything possible to prevent the development, the aggravation or the recurrence of an occupational disease. In general, retraining procedures are not implemented on persons older than 40 to 45 years.

Example B. A nurse suffers from atopic eczema, which began in childhood. She suffers from hay fever and, when she started her training as a nurse, she had slight eczema on the flexures, but not on the hands. After 2 years she develops a hand eczema, which is considered to be irritant because patch tests with occupational allergens are negative. She has had three sick leaves and has occasionally seen a dermatologist. She has voluntarily given up her occupation and wants to be retrained for a clean, dry office job. In the expert opinion the physician denies the existence of an occupational skin disease because the patient is suffering from a mild atopic eczema which has been precipitated on the hands by her occupational activities. After stopping nursing she is not free from skin symptoms on the hands. This is interpreted as the expression of a primarily endogenous skin disease, and not an occupational dermatitis. The physician also recommends retraining but the costs are not covered by the insurer. In most cases like this the ministry of labour will cover part of the cost of retraining.

Comment. Cases like this one are often difficult to assess. some dermatologists would recognize this case as occupational because the patient had never had symptoms on the hands before her occupational activity triggered off the eczema at this site. Other dermatologists would recognize the occupational cause of the hand eczema but argue that, due to the mildness of the disease, there was no objective need to cease all occupational activities. They might, however, recommend measures according to paragraph 3 (i.e. therapy, protective measures) in order to prevent relapses of a severe hand dermatitis if the patient returned to working as a nurse. This could, in fact, mean that the nurse would be retrained for a new job at the cost of the insurer.

If a patient appeals, the case is frequently taken to a commission (*Widerspruchsausschuß*) which includes a representative of the employers and a union representative. Every detail of the individual case is scrutinized and the opinion of a dermatologist may be heard once more.

If the commission's decision is not accepted by the patient, he or she can appeal and take the insurer to court (*Sozialgericht*). There are no court costs here, and the costs for a lawyer are covered by the patient's union, if he or she is a member.

Example C. A surgeon, 40 years of age, develops a contact allergy to rubber gloves. Patch testing confirms that he is allergic to thiurams and must use more expensive thiuram-free latex gloves. He is free from symptoms when he uses this type of gloves. In the expert opinion the disease is recognized as occupational but the surgeon can continue his work with special precautions.

He does not receive any compensation because he is not obliged to stop working. The cost of the more expensive gloves has to be covered by the insurance institution (BG). This is a procedure according to paragraph 3 to keep the surgeon in his occupation.

19.3 Occupational Contact Dermatitis in Other European Countries and the USA

Table 19.1 lists the institutions primarily involved in dealing with a case of occupational dermatitis. In nearly all countries except the United Kingdom, where two separate systems exist (see below), such cases are initially handled

Table 19.1. Institutions primarily involved in the settlement of an occupational dermatitis

Country	Institution	Institution collecting data on occupational dermatitis
Austria	1. AUVA (Allgemeine Unfallversiche-rung), Unfallverhütungsdienst, Webergasse 4, A-1203 Vienna, Austria 2. Insurance companies	AUVA
Belgium	Belgian Fund for Occupational Diseases, Ave. de l'Astronomie 1, B-1030 Brussels, Belgium	
Denmark	Arbeijdsskadestyrelsen, AEbelO-gade 1, DK-2100 Copenhagen O, Denmark	
Finland	1. Private insurance companies 2. Institute of Occupational Health 3. Työsuojeluhallitus (Government Board for Occupational Safety)	same same
France	Caisse Nationale d'Assurance Mala-die des Travailleurs Salariés, 66, av-enue du Maine, F-75694 Paris Cedex 14, France	Ministère du Travail, de l'Emploi et de la Formation Professionnelle, Inspection Médicale du Travail, 1, place Fontenoy, F-75007 Paris, France
Germany	1. Hauptverband der Gewerblichen Be-rufsgenossenschaften, Lindenstrasse 78, W-5202 St. Augustin 2, FRG 2. Ministerium für Arbeit und Soziales, Gewerbeärztilcher Dienst, W-5300 Bonn, FRG 3. Bundessozialgericht	same

Table 19.1. (Continued)

Country	Institution	Institution collecting data on occupational dermatitis
Spain	1. Instituto Nacional de la Salud 2. Private insurance companies	Instituto Nacional Medicina y Seguridad del Trabajo, Com Evaluac. de Incapacidad, Alcala 56, E-28071 Madrid, Spain
Sweden	1. National Board of Occupational Safety and Health	Occupational Injury Information System (ISA), S-17184 Solna, Sweden Labour Market No-Fault Liability Insurance (TFA), S-11388 Stockholm, Sweden
United Kingdom	1. National Insurance (state compensation), Department of Social Security, Newcastle Central Office, Newcastle-upon-Tyne, NE98 1YX, UK 2. Courts and lawyers (common law action) 3. Private insurance companies	
United States of America	1. State authorities (each state's Division of Occupational Medicine) 2. Private insurance companies	NIOSH, Taft Highway Cincinnati, Ohio, USA

outside the system of common law. Insurance institutions – private, semiprivate or governmental – deal with the first stage after the case has been reported to them. In most countries this report is filed by the family physician, by a dermatologist or by a company physician and the suspicion, not the proof, of an occupational cause is sufficient. Further details are discussed below. Most of the institutions listed in Table 19.1 regularly compile data on occupational skin diseases: the reader may obtain these directly from them.

19.3.1 Austria

In Austria, the equivalent to the German BGs is the *Allgemeine Unfallversicherungsanstalt* (AUVA), a state-owned insurance institution that is independent of other health insurers or employers. Every employer must pay a small fee for each of his employees (1.4% of the total income) to be insured by the AUVA. Every physician must report a case of suspected occupational skin disease to the AUVA; the patient's consent is not necessary. The AUVA can then inspect the workplace and will order an expert opinion. The expert will review the case and will make detailed suggestions, in the same way as described in the three German examples. He will also make an estimate of the degree of disability and suggest a pension (e.g. 20% for the bricklayer, example A). In general, the main cause of the disease must be occupational in order for it to be judged as a 'legal case'. A primarily endogenous disease (e.g. atopic eczema) does not qualify for compensation. A cumulative insult dermatitis may be recognized, if severe, disabling and associated with frequent sick leaves.

Negligence on the part of the employer does not have to be proven. Retraining is available to patients even if they are older than 40 years and costs are met mostly by the AUVA, partly by other state authorities.

The three examples of occupational contact dermatitis given would be handled in a very similar way in Austria to that in Germany.

19.3.2 Belgium

In Belgium, occupational dermatoses are handled primarily by the Belgium Fund for Occupational Diseases. The family physician, dermatologist, company physician or the physician of the Labour Ministry can initiate the case, suspicion being sufficient rather than proof, using a special report from *(Déclaration de Maladie Professionelle)*. The patient's consent is not necessary in order to make such a report, but it is required before demanding compensation.

The Belgian Fund for Occupational Diseases investigates the case. A consulting engineer may inspect the workplace. The occupational physician also reports the case to the Ministry of Employment and Labour, from where the expert opinion of a dermatologist is requested, and a pension granted if the disease is severe and continuous (including cumulative irritant contact dermatitis). If a sensitization is proven, compensation may be paid. The dermatitis does not have to be wholly occupational to qualify, negligence does not have to be proved, and the patient need not leave his or her job. Retraining is restricted to those below 55 years. Social workers and specialists in the job market may be involved in this decision as well as doctors, the cost of such retraining being borne by the state fund.

In example A, the system would be quite different: the pension and retraining procedure would be paid by the state fund. In example B, the previous condition would not exclude the nurse from compensation. In example C, the gloves would not be paid for by the state fund, but possibly by the hospital; only medications are paid by the State Fund.

19.3.3 Denmark

In Denmark the system is very similar to the German one. The patient's consent is not necessary for the report to the state authority. In the expert opinion the doctor makes an estimate of the patient's disability and the size of pension awarded is in accordance with the severity and course of the disease. Compensation is paid if the *degree of permanent injury* exceeds 5%. A lump sum, not a monthly payment, is given. If the patient cannot work at all because of the skin disease, he or she can apply for a permanent disability pension through the county authorities.

The disease may still be recognized as an occupational disease even if it is only partially due to the occupation. Therefore, the nurse's case (example B) would be accepted as being an occupational dermatosis.

Retraining is also carried out even after the age of 40 years, costs being met by the state.

19.3.4 Finland

In Finland the whole matter of occupational diseases is primarily in the hands of private insurance companies. There is one exception: financial compensation for civil servants comes from government funds but the principles for the compensation are the same as in the private systems. Not only the physicians involved but also the patient can initiate an investigation by filling out a special report form. This special report is forwarded to the provincial administrative board and to the local department of occupational safety and health, which usually do not take any actions of their own. The insurance company can order an expert opinion, but apparently this is not obligatory in every case.

The reviewing doctor recommends recognition or refusal. The estimate of disability seems, in general, to be higher than in Germany: the bricklayer in example A would receive 20%–40%, depending on the severity of the disease. Under Finnish legislation the 'inconvenience' and suffering resulting from the occupational disease clearly carry more weight in determining the financial compensation.

Retraining is recommended for patients up to 50 years of age, costs being met by the insurance companies. The lawyer of the insurance company is also involved in the decision as to the new occupation that the patient is to be retrained for.

A cumulative insult dermatitis may be recognized as an occupational dermatitis under special circumstances if severe and disabling. It is not accepted as such if endogenous factors clearly predominate. Worsening of nonoccupational diseases for occupational reasons will also be compensated by the insurance companies.

Otherwise, the three examples of occupational contact dermatitis given above would be handled in a very similar fashion according to Finnish legislation. The costs for dealing with all suspected and not-proven cases of occupational dermatitis are also covered by the private insurance companies.

19.3.5 France

In France, the legal basis for handling occupational diseases is fixed in the *Code de la Sécurité Sociale* (social security code) and in the *Code Rural* (for agriculture). The existence of 'tables of occupational diseases' is the main characteristic of the French legislation. These tables are brought up to date regularly. Each table consists of a heading and three columns entitled, respectively: 'designation of the disease', 'term of notice', 'list of work likely to provoke the disease'. More than 40 tables deal with skin diseases, and some are very specific for particular contact sensitizing compounds. The French law is rigid but very clear: a disease may be recognized as occupational only if it is mentioned in the tables. Thus, every dermatitis fulfilling medical, administrative, and occupational conditions mentioned in the tables is considered as occupational: no proof is required ('presumption of imputability'). Depending on the tables, patch tests are rarely necessary. Generally, the recurrence of the dermatitis is a sufficient argument. For instance, Table 8 dealing with cements and bricklaying does not require patch testing.

The French legislation clearly distinguishes between an occupational dermatitis officially recognized because it is mentioned in a table and a 'dermatitis with occupational features' allowing no recognition and no compensation because it is not mentioned in any table. The latter should nevertheless be reported on a special form sent to the Ministry of Labour: it could actually contribute to complete, extend and bring the tables up to date, and therefore improve the legislation.

Every employee must by law be insured against occupational accidents, injuries and diseases, but the social contributions are paid by the employer alone.

When an occupational dermatitis is suspected, notification of the Social Security service not only requires the patient's consent but it is up to the employee him- or herself to fill in an application form and send it to the *Caisse de Sécurité Sociale* along with a certificate made out by the physician. The Social Security physician then reviews the case. This physician holds the power of decision; the dermatologist can only give specialist advice. The Social Security service has the right to send a consulting engineer to inspect the workplace. When the dermatitis is recognized as an occupational disease, the physician can make an estimate of the patient's disability: compensation is paid if the degree of permanent injury exceeds 10%. A lump sum would be paid, rather than a monthly pension. However, it is very rare to be considered 10% disabled for a skin complaint.

Usually, the company physician tries to provide a new working area or a new job in the same company. In the case of repeatedly relapsing dermatitis, retraining may be carried out, but even if they are retrained many people will find it extremely difficult to get a job.

The three examples of occupational dermatitis would be handled in a different way in France.

Example A (Bricklayer). Table 8 ('diseases due to cements') applies perfectly in this case: the occupational disease is officially recognized only if the bricklayer himself makes the notification. The employer must, by law, provide another job in the same company, or is obliged to double the redundancy compensation. The situation of the bricklayer is hard to manage. Retraining procedures are slow and difficult.

Example B (Nurse). If the nurse works in a state hospital, she is considered a civil servant and the tables do not apply to her. An administrative procedure would be carried out within the hospital. Unlike the tables system, there is no presumption of imputability. On the other hand, the dermatitis may be recognized as occupational even if it is not mentioned in any table. In practice, the nurse would be appointed to another post in the same hospital (public or private).

Example C (Surgeon). The surgeon is unlikely to apply for any form of compensation. The problem would be dealt with within the hospital, and the more expensive gloves would be paid for by the employer.

19.3.6 Spain

In Spain occupational dermatoses are handled by the Instituto Nacional Salud and private insurance companies. A dermatologist, company physician or 'state doctor' can file a report on a special form. In contrast to most other countries, the suspicion of an occupational dermatitis is not sufficient, but the case has to be proved beforehand. The patient must give his consent for this report. The case is then pursued further by a commission of the Health Department (*Comision Tecnica Calcificadora Seguridad Social*). The Union Medica Valoracion Incapacidad takes further action, inspects the workplace, and orders an expert opinion. The reviewing doctor does not make any estimates of disability or size of compensation.

Another important difference in comparison to other European countries is that more responsibility is placed on the employer after a worker has contracted an occupational dermatosis. The company, together with the company physician, has to provide a new working area based on the recommendations of the expert opinion. If the patient continues to have skin symptoms and suffers from frequent sick leaves in a 2-year period, then he must be given a new job in the same company, or can claim for permanent and total disability. For skin diseases, total disability is a rare decision of the courts that is only arrived at after a long struggle with lawyers. In line with this, an irritant contact dermatitis is never accepted as occupational and no financial compensation is granted.

Examples B and C would be dealt with within the hospital without the further intervention of government institutions.

19.3.7 Sweden

In Sweden a state authority (National Board of Occupational Safety and Health) is primarily involved in dealing with occupational skin diseases. An injury at work is understood to be an injury incurred in connection with an accident at work, an injury sustained on the way to or from work or an *occupational disease* contracted as a result of *environmental* conditions at work. A person suffering from an injury at work receives compensation for loss of earnings and reimbursements of expenses, partly through statutory social insurance and partly through labour market insurance. Labour market insurance also pays the injured person for noneconomic loss, e.g. for pain and suffering as well as for disfigurement and permanent disadvantage.

The forms of social insurance primarily concerned with cases of injury at work are those provided through the National Insurance Act (AFL) and the Work Injury Insurance Act (LAF). LAF was revised in 1993, but the outcome is not yet established. The labour market insurance which gives *additional* cover to the cover provided by social insurances is the Labour Market No-fault Liability Insurance (TFA).

In contrast to most other countries mentioned in this chapter, the employer and the patient together report the suspicion of an occupational dermatosis. The special report form (Notification of a Work Injury) is also signed by the patient. The National Health Insurance and the Work Inspectorate review the case; they rarely inspect the working place, but order an expert opinion by a dermatologist. The reviewing doctor examines the case in detail with a careful work-up including patch testing. He makes no estimate regarding the degree of disability or pension.

When judging whether or not a harmful influence has existed in the work environment of an injured person, different personal factors that are characteristic of the injured person must also be taken into consideration. Examples of such personal factors, which may render a person less resistant, are previous diseases, congenital weakness or ageing. The principle that a person is insured 'in existing condition' is laid down in the legislative material as well as in established practice.

A recognized case of occupational contact dermatitis will attract retraining if the course is severe with repeated recurrences. There is no firm age limit. The decision on the new job is made in cooperation with physicians and National Health Insurance and union representatives. The costs of retraining are covered by state authorities.

A chronic irritant contact dermatitis will be recognized as an occupational disease if the course is severe.

The three examples would be handled differently. The bricklayer would also be retrained for another occupation. If he were to earn less in his new job he would receive the difference between the new income and the average income of bricklayers in Sweden. The nurse's case would be recognized as an occupational disease with full compensation, because the eczema on her *hands* started after 2 years at work due to occupational contact. The more expensive gloves for the surgeon with an allergy to thiurams would be covered by the employer and not by any insurance institution.

19.3.8 United Kingdom

There is a dual system in the United Kingdom: state compensation and suing the company in the courts under common law. Every company in the United Kingdom has to be insured for what is known as employer liability through a private insurance company for the common law action. They also pay national insurance to the government, which covers the state payment ('benefit'): in recent years this benefit has been considerably diminished.

One of the reasons that patients sue the company as well as applying for state benefit is that the state benefit is now little different from what they would receive on ordinary sickness benefit. In the state system it is left to the patient to fill in an application form. When he or she sues the firm, a lawyer would usually be consulted, either a trade union lawyer or a private lawyer. If the patient does not have sufficient means, the state will give legal aid. When a lawyer is apporached he or she will usually ask for a report from a dermatologist.

The suspicion of an occupational cause is sufficient to file a report to the state. Definite proof and positive patch tests are not essential. There is no special report form in the United Kingdom. The patient's consent is not necessary, as it is assumed that if he or she has applied or contacted a lawyer then permission is implied.

After the case has been reported to the state there is a medical appeals tribunal, which, while set up by the state, is independent of it. This tribunal assesses the person's disablement. He or she now has to be at least 14% disabled to receive any benefit. This is more difficult than it may sound, because the fact that the person cannot work at his or her own job is not considered disablement. It refers to impairment of everyday life. It must be an exceptionally bad case for a skin complaint to reach 14% disablement and, currently, only a very few such cases are recorded each year. Usually, a lump sum will be paid rather than a monthly pension. This is one of the reasons why people also sue through the courts.

In the state case, a report from a dermatologist will be the basis for a further decision. In the court case, the insurance company or union would almost invariably ask for a report from a dermatologist before proceeding.

If the worker is suing through the courts he or she must prove:
1. That the skin complaint was contracted at work
2. That it was foreseeable to a reasonable employer
3. That the employer did not take adequate precautions against it.

If the case is accepted as an occupational skin disease, compensation payments will take into account the following:
1. Loss of earnings by the person
2. Future loss of earnings
3. Pain and suffering
4. Loss of amenity (meaning that, if the patient had lost a hand, he or she might not be able to pursue a hobby, such as golf).

After recognition of an occupational skin disease the worker is not bound to leave his occupation, though very often the employer will subsequently take the opportunity to lay him off for other reasons.

Retraining in Britain for dermatological cases is not well organized and rarely done. Even if they are retrained, many people will find it extremely difficult to get a job because employers are reluctant to take on someone whose skin is vulnerable and may get skin trouble in their factory and then sue them.

A cumulative insult dermatitis will usually be accepted as occupational if severe, causing frequent sick leaves, or resulting in a job change.

Regarding institutions collecting information on occupational diseases, in Britain there is now a pilot scheme under the auspices of the British Association of Dermatology, sponsored by the Health and Safety Executive, to collect data from clinicians on occupational dermatoses. The Department of Social Security collects statistics on disability assessments (Health and Safety Commission Annual Report 1989/90. HMSO, London, 1991, pp. 79–85, 102).

In the United Kingdom, none of the three cited examples (bricklayer, nurse, surgeon) would be likely to obtain either a state disability pension or compensation through the courts. The bricklayer and the nurse would both have entered the state disability statistics, had they applied for such a pension, which they are increasingly unlikely to have done because of the growing knowledge in the community of the unlikelihood of obtaining one for skin disease. The surgeon is extremely unlikely to have applied for any form of compensation: if he were directly employed in the National Health Service, the additional expense of his gloves would be met by his or her employers; if self-employed (as, for example, are all dental surgeons), he or she would have to meet the extra cost.

No formal feedback of any kind is provided by the state or legal system as to the outcome of cases in which dermatologists have provided expert opinions. In the state system this information is also not available on request; in the legal system it will usually be granted, but the dermatologist will rarely know when to ask, since most cases are settled out of court with no further reference to him or her.

19.3.9 United States

Laws establishing worker compensation in the United States were first passed in 1911. In the first decade coverage was for accidents only. In 1920 illnesses were included, and in recent decades coverage has been extended to disorders caused by cumulative trauma and conditions arising from emotional trauma. As in the case with the laws of most other nations, the basic tenet is *liability without fault*, eliminating the requirement that the worker prove negligence on the part of the employer. The intent was to prevent an adversary climate in the workplace. The system is operated through insurance, which may be either a state-supported insurance company, private insurance company, or by self-insurance in the case of large, financially sound companies. Some states permit all methods to be used. Federal employees are covered under a special federal program. Heavy penalties exist for companies that fail to insure their workers. *Medical care* is available without restriction, and may be provided not only by MDs and DOs but also by dentists, podiatrists, optometrists, physical therapists, and chiropractors. In some states Christian Science practitioners and naturopaths are authorized to treat these patients, but only if the employer is notified of this choice prior to injury.

While some states provide a free choice of physician, certain states require treatment under a physician designated by the employer for the first 30 days or so, unless the employee makes prior arrangements.

Income protection during recovery is a basic tenet in all states, with a maximum and minimum. The employer assumes the cost through an insurance carrier or, if self-insured, through the company, usually a subsidiary.

Although unusual in dermatology, *death benefits*, when the death is due to illness related to the workplace, is provided with automatic payments to the surviving dependents. Payments usually equal the worker's temporary disability indemnity benefit. Burial expenses are included, with a maximum cost permitted.

Disputes arise in fewer than 10% of cases, but when there is disagreement and *dispute resolution* is necessary, lawyers for the opposing sides may request depositions of the various physicians. Later the case may be presented before a judicial hearing officer (often called a "referee"). The purpose of the hearing is clarification of the issues, and with intent to decide the case fairly and according to the law. If the hearing officer's decision is unacceptable to either party, an appeals board can be requested to hear the case. At that time an *independent medical examiner* is usually appointed to evaluate the case. If there are still unresolved issues, the state appeals court may be petitioned to study the problem; an appelate court is next in line, and finally the state supreme court, but the great majority of cases are settled in the lower courts.

An important difference between worker compensation law and ordinary civil law is that the court which originally decided an award may alter its decision if there is reasonable cause, or it the worker's condition changes.

Rehabilitation services are available in most states, but are unequal in extent and funding. Job training is available for workers unable to return to their previous work and is especially important for patients with allergic contact dermatitis in which a workplace allergen has been positively identified.

The following three cases present examples of the way in which compensation would be handled in the United States: (a) Rehabilitation training in most states continues indefinitely, even past the normal retirement age of 65. The rating for pension indemnity is based upon the percentage of the workplace from which the worker is precluded because of the skin condition. This determination involves a complicated process, requiring the recommendations of rehabilitation specialists, vocational disability experts, and industrial engineers, as well as the examining/reporting physicians. (b) The insurance company is required to pay for that period of time in which there was clearly work aggravation of this preexisting condition (atopic dermatitis, in this case). Furthermore, if the work appeared to have brought a previously inactive condition to clinical activity, which is not uncommon in atopics, the treatment period allowed could be longer. Even if there is no work relationship, rehabilitation services are provided. (c) In this case, the contact allergy of the surgeon would be considered work related, and the cost of the alternate gloves would be paid for the by the insurance company. However, unfortunately, the company (in this case, the hospital) might find other reasons to discharge this surgeon because of the excessive cost of the gloves and the possible increase in insurance premium, although this more commonly occurs with nonprofessional workers.

19.4 Conclusions and Comment

Profound differences in legislation on occupational skin disease become apparent by comparing the systems in the various European countries. In Germany and Scandinavian countries, recognition of a dermatosis as occupational is proposed in a relatively easy manner by initiating well-developed and frequently used governmental and insurance pathways. An irritant contact dermatitis or atopic hand eczema will be recognized in most cases if the disease is severe and causes frequent sick leaves and its relationship to occupational activities is quite clear. A patient might receive compensation or retraining for an alternative 'clean' job. In a country like Spain much more responsibility is placed on the employer to help employees after they have acquired a skin disease in the working environment. The system seems to be less institutionalized and more 'privatized'.

In most countries a bricklayer with dichromate allergy would receive financial compensation, but lump sums are preferred to monthly payments. In Germany retraining is rarely performed after the age of 40 years, while in

most other countries the patient can be older than 40. In the questionnaire, the question on the value of retraining and the course of the skin disease was answered by the overwhelming majority in the following way:
- Most patients find a job only with difficulty after retraining.
- They continue to have skin problems quite frequently.

Regarding the overall evaluation of retraining programmes, three out of seven respondents decided it was 'very valuable in some cases', two 'very valuable', one 'some value' and one 'little value'.

These judgments of experienced occupational dermatologists should stimulate further thinking and work. Should we be more restrictive with retraining, because most patients will have problems in finding new satisfying work and will continue to have major skin problems? Are we retraining patients at too late a stage, once the disease has manifested itself and taken on a more endogenous character (see Sect. 11.11)? Is more cooperation necessary between physicians, social workers and specialists in occupational safety with regard to inspecting the workplace and making far-reaching recommendations for the patient with an occupational skin disease? In every country a striking shortcoming exists: the workplace is rarely inspected by a physician! Based on many reports in the literature we know that this is an extremely important aspect of dealing with an occupational disease (see Sect. 11.12.4). The patient inevitably and unintentionally sometimes omits important details from the history that turn out to be diagnostic clues if detected by a trained observer.

In most countries the legislation seems to be rather inaccurate and unclear with regard to important aspects and the definition of terms such as 'severity of disease', 'recurrence' and 'frequency of relapses'. This also holds true for the degree of disability and estimates of the pensionable lump sum for compensation. In connection with the protection of personal data, it seems important to point out that the patient's consent for a report to be made to the insurer or governmental institution is not obligatory in every country. Considering the possibility that the patient may experience retaliation of various kinds in the workplace after the case for compensation has been initiated, consent by the patient to this procedure should be made mandatory.

In order to harmonize the various systems for dealing with occupational dermatoses, we recommend the formation of a committee under the auspices of the European Community.

Acknowledgements. The cooperation of the following colleagues in preparing this chapter is gratefully acknowledged: W. Aberer (Austria), R.M. Adams (USA), K. Andersen (Denmark), D. Burrows (UK), J. Camarasa (Spain), H. Fabry (Germany), E. Grosshans (France), M. Hannuksela (Finland), H.I. Maibach (USA), T. Menné (Denmark), J. Oleffe (Belgium), J. Roed-Petersen (Denmark), R. Tomb (France), J. Wahlberg (Sweden).

19.5 Further Reading

1. Achten G, Oleffe J (1967) Dermatoses professionelles et capacité economique. Arch Belg Dermatol Syphil 23: 280–297
2. DDG (1987) Empfehlungen für die Einschätzung der MdE bei berufsbedingten Hauterkrankungen. Stand 1.1.1987. Dermatosen 35: 102–104
3. Eck E (1989) Hauterkrankungen als Berufskrankheiten. Akt Dermatol 15: 352–356
4. Fabry H (1991) Der Dermatologe als medizinischer Sachverständiger im Bereich der Unfallversicherung. Deut Dermatol 39: 77–85
5. Kühl M, Nauroth E (1990) Gesetze und Verfahren. In: Kühl M, Klaschka F (eds) Berufsdermatosen. Urban and Schwarzenberg, Munich, pp 7–25
6. National Board of Occupational Safety and Health, the Swedish Work Environment Fund (ed) (1987) Occupational injuries in Sweden 1983. Solna
7. Nauroth E (1989) Hautarztbericht, Berufskrankheitenanzeige, Begutachtung – verwaltungsmäßig/juristische Aspekte. Akt Dermatol 15: 347–351
8. Pirilä V, Fregert S, Bandmann H-J et al (1971) Legislation on occupational dermatoses. Acta Dermatovener (Stockholm) 51: 141–145

Chapter 20
Computers and Patient Information Systems

Computers and Patient Information Systems

AN DOOMS-GOOSSENS, M. DOOMS and J. DRIEGHE

Contents

20.1 Introduction

Computer hardware and software have become part and parcel of our daily lives. Machines are available throughout the world, and there are application programs in virtually every field of human endeavour.

In the practice of medicine, a computer can assist in doing a number of things: patient administration, image processing, drug distribution, simulations, laboratory automation, word processing, and knowledge-based systems, to name a few of the common applications. In this chapter, we focus on the use of computers in the field of contact dermatitis.

The first use of electronic data processing in this field mainly concerned exposure lists and the computation of the frequency of positive patch test results [1–5]. Then, in the late 1970s, we began to compile a permanent data base on products, patients and literature [6]. Several contact dermatitis units throughout the world now have computer data bases that they use to provide information for the diagnosis and treatment of contact dermatitis patients. An overview of the existing databases was published in a special edition of *Seminars in Dermatology* [7].

The growing interest in this field led to the formation of the International Contact Dermatitis Computer Group, which holds its regular meetings around the world. The members of this group feel strongly that the diagnosis and treatment of contact dermatitis today is rapidly becoming impossible without the assistance of a computer. The patient needs the information that only a computer can provide efficiently, and the clinician will soon find that the computer, if used properly, is an indispensable diagnostic tool.

In the first part of this chapter, we present several data bases that contain information useful in the field of contact dermatitis. These data bases contain information on the composition of products used on the skin and mucous membranes or literature references to material on the subject. In the second part, we discuss the latest developments in artificial intelligence and describe the first steps we are taking to convert all the data we have been gathering over the years into knowledge that can be used to assist in the patient anamnesis.

20.2 Useful Data Bases

Before you begin to compile a data base, it would be wise to look around to see if that information does not already exist in a computer-readable form. What follows is a survey of data bases that contain data useful in the field of contact dermatitis.

20.2.1 Product Information

We list here several data bases that contain information on the complete composition of different kinds of products that come into contact with the skin and mucous membranes and that can cause a contact dermatitis reaction.

20.2.1.1 Pharmaceutical Products

In every country, there are several computer systems with compositional information on pharmaceutical products, but they concern only the active ingredients. These data bases are generally inadequate. We will list here only those databases that give the complete composition, active and nonactive ingredients alike, of pharmaceutical products.

Codex. This data base contains the complete composition of over 7000 pharmaceutical products sold on the Belgian market for application to the skin and mucous membranes [6]. Some 2400 separate ingredients are coded with the *Merck Index* [8] number and the name as it appears in *Martindale* [9]. Each patient with a contact allergy to one of these ingredients is given a computer printout of all the topical pharmaceutical products that contain it. An example of the information provided to a chlorocresol-sensitive patient and the accompanying letter is given in Table 20.1. If the patient needs to

Table 20.1. Sample letter sent to a patient who is allergic to chlorocresol

---

Kuleuven
Department of Dermatology
Prof. Dr. H. Degreef   Leuven, 16/04/90

Dear (NAME),
When you consulted our Department recently, we told you that the results of your
patch tests indicated that you are allergic to:

CHLOROCRESOL.

Should you come in contact with products containing this (these) substance(s), your
eczema may well recur.

To help you avoid it (them) in the future, the following is a list of pharmaceuticals that
contain it (them).

Brand-name pharmaceuticals you should not use:

Becalmex (cream) Vital	Emesil (cream) Essex*
Betamethasone valerate (cream) Vital	Eumovate (cream) Glaxo
Betnelan V (cream) Glaxo	Geomycine (cream) Schering
Betnelan VC (cream) Glaxo	Helipur (solution) Braun
Betnelan VN (cream) Glaxo	Hemeran (cream) Ciba-Geigy
Celestoderm V (cream) Essex	Ivisol (solution) Thissen*
Celestoderm V neomycine (cream) Essex	Lloyd adrenaline (cream) Lloyd
Creme adrenaline Lloyd's (cream) CCP	Modraderm (cream) Essex
Dermovate (cream) Glaxo	Neomedrol veriderm (ointment) Upjohn
Dettol chelate 5 N (solution) Destree	Noviderm (cream) Sopar*
Diprosone (cream) Schering	Periderm (cream) Essex

Specially prepared pharmaceuticals you should not use
Onguent emulsif aqueux FN IV
Unguentum emulsificans aquosum FN IV
Waterhoudende emulgerende zalf NF IV
Emulsifying ointment with water (National Formulary IV)

We hope we have been of service to you.

A. Dooms-Goossens, Dr. Pharm.
Contact Allergy Unit

---

* No longer on the market.

be treated with a corticosteroid, a list of the 'chlorocresol-free' corticosteroid
creams is provided (Table 20.2).

Complex natural ingredients are coded along with their main constituents,
metabolites, and impurities, which gives one the opportunity to check for co-
and cross-sensitivities. Such lists can lead to an insight into certain intolerance
reactions, as is the case with balsam of Peru, for which Table 20.3 gives the
main constituents.

Contact: A. Dooms-Goossens, Contact Dermatitis Unit, University Hospital, Kapucij-
nenover 33, B-3000 Leuven, Belgium.

Table 20.2. Corticosteroid creams without chlorocresol

Alphaderm (cream) Norwick	Locacortene Neomycine (cream)
Amicla (cream) Lederle	Ciba-Geigy
Azucort Neomycine (cream) SMB	Locacortene Vioform (cream)
Beeler base with prednisolone (cream)	Ciba-Geigy
ABL	Locoid (cream) Mycofarm
Beeler base with prednisolone and	Locoid (lipocream) Brocades
vioforme (cream) ABL	Logamel (cream) Ciba-Geigy
Cetylcream with prednisolone and	Lotriderm (cream) Essex
chloramphenicol (cream) ABL	Mecloderm (cream) Pfizer
Clotrasone (cream) Essex	Mycolog (cream) Labaz
Coderm (cream) Lederle	Neosynalar (cream) Sarva
Cremicort (cream) Chefar	Nerisona (cream) Schering
Curalon (cream) Chefar	Pevisone (cream) Cilag
Cycloderm (cream) Continental Pharma	Pimafucort (cream) Mycofarm
Daktacort (cream) Janssen	Preferid (cream) Gist Brocades
Decoderm (cream) Merck	Prosterolone (cream) Pmrobel
Decoderm composition (cream) Merck	Sential (cream) Pharmacia
Delmeson (cream) Hoechst	Sicorten (cream) Ciba-Geigy
Delphi (cream) Lederle	Sintisone (cream) Lab. Parm. D'Ohain*
Dexatopic (cream) Organon	Srilane (cream) Lipha
Diprolene (cream) Essex	Sterax (cream) Alcon-Courvreur
Dolanal (cream) Christiaens	Synalar DBO (cream) Synthex
Eoline (cream) Roerig	Synalar Forte (cream) Synthex
Florone (cream) Upjohn	Synalar Gamma (cream) Synthex
Halciderm (cream) Squibb	Tibicorten (cream) Labaz
Halog (cream) Squibb	Topicorte (cream) Roussel
Ledercort Neomycine (cream) Lederle	Topsyne (cream) Synthex
Lidex Emolliens (cream) Sarva	Travocort (cream) Schering
Lidex Gamma (cream) Sarva	Ultralan (cream) Schering
Locacortene (cream) Ciba-Geigy	Varlane (cream) Schering

Table 20.3. Main constituents of balsam of Peru

Benzyl cinnamate	Cinnamic acid
Cinnamyl cinnamate	Benzoic acid
Vanillin	Benzyl alcohol
Benzyl benzoate	

Daluk. Daluk lists more than 1 100 products and 400 associated substances on the Swedish market [10]. Substances are registered with the name and the code number of the *Merck Index* [8].

Contact: B. Edman, Dermatology, Malmö General Hospital, S-21401 Malmö, Sweden.

Infoderm. Infoderm lists 550 pharmaceuticals on the Finnish market with the complete qualitative formulas [11]. The system is used by many dermatological clinics in Finland and also by some private practitioners.

Contact: T. Rantanen, Dermatology, Savonlinna Central Hospital, SF-57120, Savonlina, Finland.

Swedis. This drug information system is supported by the Swedish National Department of Drugs and covers every registered pharmaceutical product. It contains information such as adverse reactions, the results of drugconsumption analysis and composition. Software is written to distribute information on drugs not containing specific allergens [12].

Contact: P. Manell, Uppsala University Data Center, P.O. Box 2103, S-75002 Uppsala, Sweden.

20.2.1.2 Cosmetic Products

While the number of pharmaceutical products is great, the mass of cosmetics on the market is overwhelming. The first three databases cited above also include some cosmetics, washing products, cleansers, and the like. Codex contains the complete composition of roughly 400 cosmetic products. When a patient is allergic to a listed ingredient, he or she is given a list of products that do not contain that ingredient. Table 20.4 is the list we provide to patients who should not come into contact with formaldehyde and formaldehyde releasers. In the United States, the Food and Drug Administration has compiled a large body of information on the composition of cosmetic products on the market. This data can be consulted through Derm/Allergens [13].

Contact: L. Rosenthal, American Academy of Dermatology, 1567 Maple Avenue, Evanston IL 60601, USA.

Table 20.4. Cosmetics permitted for patients allergic to formaldehyde, paraformaldehyde, imidazolidinyl urea, diazolidinyl urea, quaternium 15, bronopol, DMDM hydantoin, or hexamine

Albichtyol (soap) Couvreur	Crème au Mélilot Composée (cream)
Antipyorol (toothpaste) Qualiphar	Galenic
Aqua Coloniensis FN IV	Dentosyl (tooth paste) Debrus-Tensi
Aquatain (cream) Lederle	Dermac (soap) Stiefel
Baby Oil (oil) Diadal	Dermacide (soap) Clin
Baby Powder (powder) Diadal	Dermalotion (solution) Diadal
Baby Soap (soap) Diadal	Desquam (cream) Hermal
Balneum (bath oil) Hermal	Dylsoap (soap) Visele
Balneum Forte (oil) Merck	E.D.S. (shampoo) Schering Essex
Bebisol (bubble bath) Pharmaco	E.D.S. tar (shampoo) Schering Essex
Bebisol (shampoo) Pharmaco	E.D.S. zinc (shampoo) Schering Essex
Bergasol 1 (oil) Memo-Goupil	Eau de Cologne (solution) Diadal
Bergasol 2 (oil) Memo-Goupil	Eau de Toilette (solution) Expanscience
Bergasol 4 (oil) Memo-Goupil	Eau Précieuse (solution) Sanders
Betadermil (soap) Belgana	Edel Water (solution) Sanders
Bronze Gel Makeup (gel) Clinique	Effagel (gel) Roche Posay
Cerat Inalterable (ointment) Roche Posay	Fabrame (hair lotion) Fabram
Cetaphil (solution) Owen	Fluocaril Bifluore (toothpaste) Memo
Cold Cream (cream) Expanscience	Fluocaril Bifluore Mint (toothpaste) Memo
Cold Cream Natural (cream) Roche Posay	Galenic Honingklaver Creme (cream)
Continuous Coverage (cream) Clinique	Galenic
Cophasil (cream) Schering	Gesichtswasser (solution) Alcina
	Gingival Pâte (paste) Specia
	+ 116 further entries

Isolated efforts are also being made to compile compositional information in cooperation with the cosmetic industry (e.g. [14]).

The *Göttinger Liste* from Germany, which is available as a book or on diskette, contains compositional information on some 1 000 topical products containing UV screens. Detailed information is given on the nature of the preservative agents, and the presence of ingredients such as antioxidants and perfumes is indicated. User-friendly software is available to search the data on IBM-compatible machines running at least MS-DOS 3.2.

Contact: Dr. S. Schauder, Hautklinik, Von Sieboldstrasse 3, D-3400 Göttingen, FRG.

Most cosmetic companies also have their own formulations in a computer-readable form for their own production purposes. These files, however, are not in the public domain and cannot be consulted outside the company.

20.2.1.3 Occupational Products

The only data base with compositional information on products used at work is called EPA and can be accessed through Derm/Infonet, the network of the American Academy of Dermatology. One can obtain lists of products the allergic patient should avoid because of the allergens they contain. A list of the ingredients in a single product can also be obtained [13].

Contact: L. Rosenthal, American Academy of Dermatology, 1567 Maple Avenue, Evanston IL 60601, USA.

In order to be able to give up-to-date and relevant information to those who have to choose and recommend suitable protective gloves, a data base has been developed for the test data on protective effects against chemicals in the working environment [15].

Contact: Jan Wahlberg, Occupational Dermatology, National Institute of Occupational Health, S-17184 Solna, Sweden.

The Danish Product Register (PROBAS) is a governmental data base established in 1979 by the Danish Ministries of Environment and Labour. The data base contains data on chemical products (primarily for industrial use) reported from producers and importers, according to obligatory notification rules, surveys, and research projects. This computer data base contains some 25 000 products.

Contact: M.A. Flyvholm, Danish National Institute of Occupational Health, LersøParkallé 105, DK-2100 Copenhagen, Denmark.

20.2.2 The Literature

Medlars and Embase are two major data bases that cover the biomedical literature. Over 11 million references from 3 000 journals have been accumulated since 1966 in Medlars, and Embase has some 5 million citations on file from 3 500 journals beginning in 1973. The unit record of both of these data bases gives the author, the title, other bibliographic data, key words and an abstract in English.

Contact: Medlars, National Library of Medicine, 8600 Rockville Pike, Bethesda, Maryland 20209, USA.

Embase, Excerpta Medica, 305 Keizersgracht, NL-1016 ED Amsterdam, the Netherlands.

In addition to these two huge data bases, several institutes collect literature references in specialized areas. An overview of the data bases of interest is given elsewhere [16, 17].

On-line access is available throughout the world. Selected data from these computer-readable files can be downloaded for further use in one's own computer system. The technical problems and cost of telecommunication restrict these facilities to larger hospitals and biomedical libraries.

A CD-ROM (compact disk, read-only memory), physically identical to the well-known audio compact disc, can store and handle one full year of the entire medical literature. With a CD-ROM player and a personal computer, more users can retrive and download information cost effectively [18].

Contact: EBSCO, P.O. Box 204, NL-1430 AE Aalsmeer, the Netherlands.

20.3 Data Processing

One of the first applications of a newly acquired computer system is certainly word processing. The use of form letters that can be adapted does, indeed, save time. The software market offers an ample number of excellent packages with extras beyond the basic functions. One thing to be careful of is whether or not the printer is supported in the package. An interesting option is the ability to import 'foreign' data, such as laboratory results on diskette, into a text.

The construction of a complete and integrated medical information system belongs in the world of professional computer applications. However, this does not mean that the computer user has no resources at his disposal to set up a limited information system. While there is very little medical software available in specific areas, general packages for data storage and retrieval are, in many cases, sufficient. User-friendly input of data, rapid retrieval of specific information and the ability to exchange information with other users are necessary options. The package chosen, therefore, must be open and, if more complex functions are permitted, help screens or menus must be available.

Over the last 15 years, a great deal of experience has been accumulated in the use of software packages and hardware systems. Table 20.5 gives the hardware and software that are currently used for contact dermatitis applications. You are encouraged to contact them if you have questions about starting your own system.

Table 20.5. Some of the computer systems currently being used in contact dermatitis

Name and address	Hardware	Relevant software	Communi- cation facilities	Data stored
K.E. Andersen, MD Dept. of Dermatology University Hospital 5000 Odense Denmark	Micro 386	DSI Allergen- bank (own)	No	Patients Allergens
F. Bahmer, MD Univ. Hautklinik Homburg Germany	Micro 386/486	ALLDAT ASK SAM SPSS BTX IMAL	Yes	Patients Products
M. Beck, MD The Skin Hospital Chapel Street Salford M60 9EP United Kingdom	Mainframe CDC 7600	SPSS Kermit Fortran Janet	Yes	Patients
A. Bircher, MD Dermat. Poliklinik Petersgraben 4 Basel Switzerland	Micro Macintosh	Excel Filemaker Procite Cricket- graph	No	Patients Literature Patch test data
F. Menezes Brandão, MD Dept. of Dermatology Hospital Garcia de Orta 2800 Almada Portugal	Micro 486	Dbase 3 Open-Access SPS Own	No	Patients
D.P. Bruynzeel, MD Allergologie/Arbeidsder- matologie Vrije Univ. Acad. Zeikenh. De Boelelaan 1117 1081 HV Amsterdam The Netherlands	Micro 486	Paradox	No	Patients
T. Diepgen, MD Univ. Hautklinik Hartmannstrasse 14 91052 Erlangen Germany	Micro 386/486	Informix Kermit SPSS Own	Yes	Patients Products Literature
A. Dooms-Goossens, PhD Contact Dermatitis Unit University Hospital 3000 Leuven Belgium	Mainframe IBM-9370 Micro 486	Own expert system: Codex/E Codex/PC	Dermis	Patients Products

Table 20.5. Continued

Name and address	Hardware	Relevant software	Communi-cation facilities	Data stored
B. Edman, PhD Dept. of Dermatology General Hospital 21401 Malmo Sweden	Micro 386	Statistica Data-talk Sorto	No	Patients Products Literature
P. Elsner, MD Gloriastrasse 31 8091 Zürich Switzerland	Micro Macintosh 386/486	Informix ALLDAT SPSS	Yes	Patients
P. Fernström, BSc Nat. Inst. of Occup. Health Dept. of Occup. Dermatol. 17184 Solna Sweden	Micro Macintosh	4th Dimension	No	Question-naire Service
M.A. Flyvholm Nat. Inst. of Occupat. Health 2100 Copenhagen Denmark	Digital VAX	Adabas Natural	No	Products
P. Frosch, MD Städt. Kliniken Dortmund and University of Witten/Herdecke Beurhausstrasse 40 44123 Dortmund Germany	Micro 486	Dbase 4 Alldat Harvard-Graphics 3.0 Excel	No	Patients Literature Product list of dental materials
G. Gailhofer, MD Dept. of Dermatology University of Graz Auenbruggerplatz 8 8036 Graz Austria	Micro 386	Lotus 123 Lab Base Phamac 3.3 35 MM - (Polaroid) Harvard - Graphics Dbase 4	No	
M. Goos, MD Universitätsklinikum Hufelandstrasse 55 45147 Essen Germany	Micro AT	Own	No	Patients Products Literature
K. Kalimo, MD Dept. of Dermatology University of Turku 20520 Turku Finland	Micro 486	Paradox	No	Patients Allergens Products

Table 20.5. Continued

Name and address	Hardware	Relevant software	Communi-cation facilities	Data stored
M. Lacroix, MD Rue Général-Joubert 3 21000 Dijon France	Digital VAX	SAS	No	Patients
A. Lahti, MD Dept. of Dermatology University of Oulu 90220 Oulu Finland	Digital VAX	Own Datapak	No	Patients Products
H. MacFarlane Dept. of Dermatology Royal Infirmary Edinburgh EH3 9YW United Kingdom	Micro 386/486	Aladin Dbase 3 Modistat	No	Patients
T. Menné MD Dept. of Dermatology Gentofte Hospital 2900 Hellerup Denmark	Micro 386/486	DSI system 2.1	No	Patients Products
J. Meynadier, MD Hôpital St. Charles 300, Rue A. Broussonnet 34295 Montpellier Cedex 5 France	Micro 386	Clipper Dbase 3	No	Patients
D. Perrenoud, MD Dept. of Dermatology CHUV 1011 Lausanne Switzerland	Micro 386/486	Dbase 3 Own Access Visual basic Reference Manager	No	Products Patients Literature
T. Rantanen, MD Dept. of Dermatology Central Hospital Päijät-Häme 15850 Lahti Finland	Micro 486	Clipper 5	No	Products
L. Rosenthal, PhD Am. Acad. Dermatology 1567 Maple Avenue Evanston, IL 60601 USA	Mini IBM s36	Customized Derm/Infonet Tymnet	Yes	Patients Products Literature

Table 20.5. Continued

Name and address	Hardware	Relevant software	Communication facilities	Data stored
S. Schauder Hautklinik Von Siebold-Strasse 3 37075 Göttingen Germany	Micro 386		No	Products
A. Sertoli, MD Clinica Dermatologica Via Degli Alfani 37 50121 Florence Italy	Micro 386/486	Clipper Dbase 3	No	Patients
S. Shaw, MD J. Wilkinson, MD Dept. of Dermatology Wycombe Hospital HP11 BTT High Wycombe United Kingdom	Micro 486	Customized PC Promise	No	Patients Letters
T. Sugai, MD, PhD Dept. of Dermatology Osaka Kaisei Hospital 4-6-6 Toyosaki Kita, Osaka 531 Japan	Micro 386/486	RDB, Stax Samic-Tqc/2 Epofamily Customized	No	Patients Products Literature
K. Thestrup-Pedersen, MD Dept. of Dermatology Marselisborg Hospital 8000 Aarhus C Denmark	Micro 386/486	Rbase Symphony Customized Foxbase	No	Patients Products Literature
J.E. Wahlberg, MD C. Liden, MD Dept. of Occup. Dermatol. Karolinska Sjukhuset 10401 Stockholm Sweden	Micro 486	Focus Internet Ethernet	Yes	Patients
I.R. White, MD Dept. of Dermatology St. Thomas Hospital London SE1 7EH United Kingdom	Micro 386	Dbase 3 Own SCALC 5	No	Patients
V. Ziegler, MD Holshauser Strasse 8 32257 Bünde Germany	MediStar M 4233	Prologue Dbase 3 INPRET	No	Patients Literature

20.4 Artificial Intelligence

Artificial intelligence has several applications in medicine [19] such as speech recognition, image processing and knowledge-based systems in clinical as well as laboratory medicine [20]. A number of early reports on the use of artificial intelligence in dermatology have been published [21–25].

20.4.1 Knowledge-Based or Expert Systems

Thus far in this chapter, we have presented systems that store, transmit and manipulate data on contact dermatitis. However, medical intelligence requires more than these basic tasks. It also asks for reasoning and inference and for the combining of observations with human knowledge of the domain. At the most fundamental level, a knowledge-based system consists of a knowledge base, an inferencing system that can use the data (knowledge) in problem solving and an input-output mechanism. The knowledge base may contain facts, beliefs, rules and procedures pertinent to the problem area. The immense task of the 'knowledge engineer' is to turn all these data into knowledge.

Some of the possible legal implications of the production, marketing, and use of expert systems (professional malpractice, product liability) are discussed elsewhere [26].

20.4.2 An Example of a Knowledge-Based or Expert System: Codex-E

The knowledge base we are presently using in our system contains rules that are derived mainly from the patient data we have compiled over the last 12 years on some 12 000 patients who have passed through several contact dermatitis units [27]. By means of in-house software, the patient data is searched at night for primary rules based on sex, lesion location, exposure, occupation/hobbies and topical cosmetics and pharmaceuticals used. This procedure is conducted for the entire data set for general rules and, for the last 1000 patients, for new trends.

Here are some examples of primary rules based on sex and lesion location: female + legs = wool alcohols; female + earlobes = nickel; male + hands = chromate. For example, a primary rule based on the occupation of hairdresser gives paraphenylenediamine and related hair dyes, persulphates, as the probable eliciting allergen.

Here are some examples of primary rules based on a previous history of intolerance to specific products: an allergic reaction to adhesive tape calls attention to colophony and diphenylthiourea; a reaction to jewellery requires consideration of nickel and cobalt; and a reaction to aftershave lotion indicates a probable allergy to perfume components.

Secondary rules, which are derived from the clinical experience of the investigators and from the literature, are based on the clinical picture of the lesions. For example: a linear configuration draws attention to plant dermatitis, while erythema-multiforme-like lesions call for the consideration of mephenesin and tropical woods.

In our product file, we store ingredient information on pharmaceutical and cosmetic products. The inferencing system now lists all the ingredients of these products used by a particular patient and draws the attention of the clinician to the ingredients that have been found to be more allergenic than others.

At present, our expert system contains some 1000 rules, which are automatically adapted as a function of new patient data. The software has been developed on an IBM 9/370. It has 136 programs and procedures and includes 41 files. The system has been operational since September 1989. Since 1992 information and software have been disseminated to Belgian dermatologists on disc (Codex/PC). In 1993 on-line Communication facilities were established (DERMIS).

20.5 Conclusion

We have reported here on the first steps that we have taken in the process of converting our massive amount of data into knowledge to be used in compiling the anamnesis of our contact dermatitis patients. This process will be intensified as much as possible and also applied in other fields of contact dermatitis. For example, allergen frequency data combined with physico-chemical data on these compounds will most probably enable us to obtain primary rules for assigning risk factors to new organic compounds.

We hope that this chapter will encourage the reader to start or to continue to use computers in the diagnosis and treatment of contact dermatitis. The world of contact dermatitis is too complex to do otherwise.

Acknowledgment. We thank all the members of the International Contact Dermatitis Computer Group for their stimulating discussions and their inspiring suggestions during our meetings.

20.6 References

1. Bandmann H-J, Calnan CD, Cronin E et al. (1972) Dermatitis from applied medicaments. Arch Dermatol 106: 335–337
2. MacEachran JH, Clendenning WE, Gosselin RE (1976) Computer-derived exposure lists of common contact dermatitis antigens. Contact Dermatitis 2: 239–246
3. Panconesi E, Sertoli A, Fabbri P et al. (1975) Computer data on patch tests of 688 eczema patients. Contact Dermatitis 1: 317–318
4. Richter G (1975) Arbeitsdermatosen in Bezirk Dresden 1962 bis 1975. Dermatol Monatschr 164: 36–50

5. Fabbri P, Sertoli A (1971) Premises and preliminary programming for the use of the computer in dermato-allergological diagnosis. Folia Allergol 18: 138–144
6. Dooms-Goossens A, Degreef H, Drieghe J et al. (1980) Computer-assisted monitoring of contact-dermatitis patients. Contact Dermatitis 6: 123–127
7. Dooms-Goossens A (1989) Computers and dermatology, Saunders, Philadelphia, (Seminars in dermatology, vol 8, part 2)
8. Merck Index, 9th edn (1976) Merck, Rahway
9. Martindale. The Extra Pharmacopoeia, 29th edn (1989) Reynolds JEF (ed) Pharmaceutical Press, London
10. Edman B (1988) Computerized patch-test data in contact allergy. Dissertation, University of Lund, Malmö
11. Rantanen T (1989) Infoderm-A microcomputer database system with Finnish product files. Semin Dermatol 8(2): 94–95
12. Johannson SG, Manell P (1978) The drug information system SWEDIS and its users. International Symposium on Medical Information Systems, 2–6 Oct 1978, Osaka
13. White R (1988) Derm/Infonet. The American Academy of Dermatology's computer-based information system for the clinical dermatologist. In: Orfanos CE, Stadler R, Gollnick H (eds) Dermatology in five continents. Proceedings of the XVII World Congress of Dermatology, Berlin, 24–29 May 1987. Springer, Berlin Heidelberg New York, pp 831–832
14. Keuringsdienst van Waren voor het gebied Enschede. Jaarverslag 1987. Specialisatie Cosmetica, p 15. "Databank Cosmetische Produkten".
15. Mellström G (1985) Protective effect of gloves – compiled in a database. Contact Dermatitis 13: 162–165
16. Dooms-Goossens A, Rigel DS (1986) Computers and contact dermatitis. In: Fisher A (ed) Contact dermatitis, 3rd edn. Lea and Febiger, Philadelphia, pp 846–847
17. Dooms-Goossens A, Drieghe J, Dooms M (1990) The computer and occupational skin disease. In: Adams RM (ed) Occupational skin disease, 2nd edn. Saunders, Philadelphia, pp 254–260
18. Wertz RK (1986) CD-ROM. A new advance in medical information retrieval. JAMA 256 (24): 3376–3378
19. Miller PL (1986) The evaluation of artificial intelligence systems in medicine. Comput Methods Programs Biomed 22: 5–11
20. Spackman KA, Connelly DP (1987) Knowledge-based systems in laboratory medicine and pathology. Arch Pathol Lab Med 111: 116–119
21. Evans SJ, Norwich KH, Cobbold RSC et al. (1984) Computer diagnoses of skin disease: system desiign and preliminary results. Int J Biomed Comput 15: 271–284
22. Bell DA, Carolan M (1984) Data access techniques for diagnosis in clinical dermatology. In: Lindberg DAB, Reichertz PL (eds) Lecture notes in medical informatics. Springer, Berlin Heidelberg New York, 347–351
23. Finlay AY, Hammond P (1986) Expert systems in dermatology: the computer potential. Dermatologica 173: 79–84
24. Finlay AY, Sinclair J, Alty JL (1983) Computer-aided diagnosis in dermatology – an expert systems approach. Br J Dermatol 109 [Suppl 24]: 42 – 43
25. Cascinelli N, Ferrario M, Tonelli T et al. (1987) A possible new tool for clinical diagnosis of melanoma: the computer. J Am Acad Dermatol 16: 361–367
26. Cannataci JA (1989) Liability for medical expert systems. An introduction to the legal implications. Med Inf (Lond) 14 (3): 229–241
27. Dooms-Goossens A, Drieghe J, Degreef H, Dooms M (1990) The "Codex-E": an expert system for contact dermatitis. Contact Dermatitis 22: 180–181

Chapter 21
Contact Dermatitis
Research Groups

Contact Dermatitis Research Groups

DESMOND BURROWS

Belgium	*Belgian Contact and Environmental Contact Dermatitis Group (BCEDG)*
Chairman:	An Dooms-Goossens
	Department of Dermatology
	University Hospital
	Kapucijnenvoer 33
	3000 Leuven
	Belgium
Secretary:	Dominique Tennstedt
	Unité de Dermatologie Professionelle
	Université Catholique de Louvain
	30, Clos Chapelle-aux-Champs
	UCL 3033
	1200 Bruxelles
	Belgium
Denmark	*Danish Contact Dermatitis Group (DCDG)*
Chairman:	Klaus E. Andersen
	Department of Dermatology
	Odense Hospital
	6000 Odense C
	Denmark
Secretary:	Jytte Roed-Petersen
	Department of Dermatology
	Gentofte Hospital
	Niels Andersens Vej 65
	2900 Hellerup
	Denmark
France	*Groupe d'Etudes et de Recherches en Dermatoallergie (GERDA)*
Chairman:	Georges Ducombs
	50, avenue Thiers
	33100 Bordeaux
	France

Secretary:

Jean Marie Mougeolle
6, rue des Glacis
54000 Nancy
France

Germany
Chairman:

German Contact Dermatitis Research Group
Thomas Fuchs
Universitäts-Hautklinik
von-Siebold-Str. 3
37075 Göttingen
Germany

Secretary:

Werner Aberer
Universitäts-Hautklinik
Auenbrugger Platz 8
8036 Graz
Austria

Finland
Chairman:

Finnish Contact Dermatitis Group
Kirsti Kalimo
Departnebt of Dermatology
University of Turku
20520 Turku
Finland

Secretary:

Kaija Lammintausta
Department of Dermatology
University of Turku
20520 Turku
Finland

Hungary
President:

Hungarian Contact Dermatitis Group
Nebenfuhrer Laszlo
St Stephen's Hospital
Szt. Istvan Korhaz Borgyogyaszati Osztaly
Nagyvarad ter 1
1096 Budapest
Hungary

Scientific Secretary:

Temesvari Erzsebet
State Institute of Dermatology and Venerology
Orszagos Bor–es Nemikortani Intezet
Maria u.41
1085 Budapest,
Hungary

Organising Secretary:

Kohanka Valeria
Occupational Health Institute
Orszagos Munka–es Uzemegeszegugyi Intezet

Nagyvarad ter 2
1096 Budapest
Hungary

Italy
Chairman:

Italian Contact Dermatitis Group
Carlo Meneghini
Department of Dermatology
Policlinico
Bari
Italy

Secretary:

Achille Sertoli
Department of Dermatology
Via Degli Alfani 37
Florence
Italy

Japan
Chairman:

Japanese Society for Dermatoallergology (JSDA)
Hikotaro Yoshida
Department of Dermatology
Nagasaki University School of Medicine
1-7-1, Sakamoto-machi
Nagasaki
Japan

Japanese Society for Contact Dermatitis (JSCD)
General Secretary:

Ritsuko Hayakawa
Department of Dermatology
Nagoya University Branch Hospital
1-1-20, Daikominami, Higashiku
Nagoya 461
Japan

Netherlands
Chairman:

Dutch Contact Dermatitis Group
Jan D. Bos
Department of Dermatology
University of Amsterdam
Academisch Medisch Centrum
Meibergdreef 9
1105 AZ Amsterdam
The Netherlands

Secretary:

Pieter G.M. van der Valk
Department of Dermatology
Academic Hospital Nijmegen
Rene Descartesdreef 1
6525 GL Nijmegen
The Netherlands

Norway   *Norwegian Contact Dermatitis Group*
Chairman: Per Thune
                                 Department of Dermatology
                                 Ullevaal Hospital
                                 0407 Oslo 4
                                 Norway

Secretary: Joar Austad
                                 Department of Dermatology
                                 Rikshospitalet
                                 0027 Oslo 1
                                 Norway

Poland   *Allergology Section of the Polish*
                                 Dermatological Society
Chairman: Edward Rudzki
                                 Klinika Dermatologiczna AM
                                 ul. Koszykowa 82a
                                 02-008 Warsaw
                                 Poland

Secretary: Zdziuslawa Grzywa
                                 Klinika Dermatologiczna AM
                                 ul. Koszykowa 82a
                                 02-008 Warsaw
                                 Poland

Portugal   *Portuguese Contact Dermatitis Group (GPEDC)*
Chairman: Saudade Goncalo
                                 Dermatologic Clinic
                                 University Hospital
                                 3000 Coimbra
                                 Portugal

Secretary: Margarida Goncalo
                                 Dermatologic Clinic
                                 University Hospital
                                 3000 Coimbra
                                 Portugal

Spain   *Spanish Contact Dermatitis Group (GEIDC)*
Coordinating Secretary: Augustín Alomar
                                 Dermatology
                                 Hospital Sant Pau
                                 St. Antoni M. Claret, 167
                                 08025 Barcelona
                                 Spain

Sweden
Coordinating Secretary:

Swedish Contact Dermatitis Group
Jan E. Wahlberg
Department of Occupational Dermatology
Karolinska Hospital
104 01 Stockholm
Sweden

Switzerland
Chairman:

Swiss Contact Dermatitis Research Group
Andreas Bircher
Dermatologische Klinik
Kantonsspital Basel
4031 Basel
Switzerland

Secretary:

Peter Elsner
Dermatologische Klinik
Universitätsspital Zürich
8091 Zürich
Switzerland

United Kingdom
Chairman:

British Contact Dermatitis Group
Michael H. Beck
The Skin Hospital
Chapel Street
Salford M60 9EP
United Kingdom

Secretary:

Christopher R. Lovell
Department of Dermatology
Royal United Hospital
Combe Park
Bath BA1 3NG
United Kingdom

Meetings Secretary:

John S.C. English
Department of Dermatology
Central Outpatients Department
Hartshill
Stoke-on-Trent ST4 7PA
United Kingdom

Treasurer:

Stephanie Shaw
Department of Dermatology
Amersham General Hospital
Amersham
Bucks HP7 0JD
United Kingdom

United States
President: *American Contact Dermatitis Society*
                     Robert L. Rietschel, MD
                     1514 Jefferson Highway
                     New Orleans, LA 70121
                     USA

President-Elect: Frances J. Storrs, MD
                     Oregon Health Services University
                     Department of Dermatology L468
                     Portland, OR 97201
                     USA

Vice-President: Elizabeth F. Sheretz, MD
                     Department of Dermatology
                     Bowman Gray–WFU Medical Centre
                     Medical Centre Boulevard
                     Winston-Salem, NC 27157

Secretary-Treasurer Vincent A. Deleo, MD
                     630 West 168th Street
                     New York, NY 10032
                     USA

Europe   *European Environmental and Contact Dermatitis*
                     Research Group (EECDRG)
Chairman: I.R. White
                     St John's Institute of Dermatology
                     St Thomas Hospital
                     London SE1 7EH
                     United Kingdom

Secretary: D.P. Bruynzeel
                     Free University Hospital
                     De Boelelaan 1117
                     1081 HV Amsterdam
                     The Netherlands

                     European Society of Contact Dermatitis (ESCD)
Chairman: Ian R. White
                     St John's Institute of Dermatology
                     St Thomas Hospital
                     London SE1 7EH
                     United Kingdom

Secretary: Jan E. Wahlberg
                     Department of Occupational Dermatology
                     Karolinska Hospital
                     S-17176 Stockholm
                     Sweden

Treasurer: Derk Bruynzeel
                       Department of Occupational Dermatology
                       Free University Academic Hospital
                       De Doelelaan 1117
                       1081 HV Amsterdam
                       The Netherlands

International Contact Dermatitis Research Group (ICDRG)

Chairman: Jan E. Wahlberg
                       Department of Occupational Dermatology
                       Karolinska Hospital
                       17176 Stockholm
                       Sweden

Secretary: Matti Hannuksela
                       Kakelankatu 4 A
                       53130 Lappeenranta
                       Finland

Central American Contact Dermatitis Group

Guatemala: F. Rolando Vasquez Blanco
                       Eduardo Silva Lizama

El Salavador: Delma Lopez Lino de Salazar
Honduras: Angel Cruz Banegas
Nicaragua: Aldo Martinez
                       Francisco Gomez Urcuyo

Costa Rica: Orland Jaramillo Antillon
                       Rollanda Murillo Chavez
                       Eduardo Carbajal Rodriguez
                       Olman Riggioni Cordero

Panama: Arturo Tapia Collante
                       Homera Penangos Gonzalez
                       Marta Jaen de Oliveros

Mexican Contact Dermatitis Group

Chairman: Armando Ancona
                       Tonala 48
                       06700 Mexico
                       Mexico

                       Alfredo Arevalo
                       Roberto Blancas
                       Lourdes Alonzo
                       Atalo Alanis
                       Graciela Guzman
                       Remigio Gonzalez
                       Salvador Robles

Chapter 22
Patch Test Concentrations and Vehicles for Testing Contact Allergens

Patch Test Concentrations and Vehicles for Testing Contact Allergens

Anton C. de Groot and Peter J. Frosch

Patch testing is a sound, relatively safe and reasonably reliable method of identifying contact allergens in patients with contact dematitis. It has been clearly shown that patch testing is necessary in the majority of patients with eczema [1]. The technique of patch testing is described in Chap. 10.

All patients are tested with the European standard series, containing the most frequent contact allergens in European countries (Table 22.1). Often, standard series patch testing is not enough, and additional allergens or potential allergens are tested, based on the patient's history and clinical examination. Examples are products and chemicals to which the patient is exposed occupationally or in his home environment. Test series containing the most frequent allergens in certain products (preservatives, fragrances, dental materials, plastics and glues, medicaments) or in certain occupations (hairdressing, pesticides, oil and cooling fluid) are very helpful. Approximately 300 patch test materials are commercially available from Hermal (Reinbeck Hamburg, FRG) and Chemotechnique (Malmö, Sweden).

For other chemicals and products, the investigator must decide how to apply them as a patch test. Chemicals usually need to be diluted, and it is of the utmost importance to use an appropriate patch test concentration and vehicle to avoid both false-negative and false-positive (irritant) reactions. The most useful reference source for documented test concentrations and vehicles of chemicals, groups of chemicals and products is the book *Patch Testing* [2]. Other useful lists are provided in recent textbooks on contact dermatitis [3–5].

When chemicals or products for which insufficient information is available to decide on a test concentration and vehicle are to be patch tested, the following advice from the International Contact Dermatitis Research Group and the North American Contact Dermatitis Group may be followed [6]:

Vehicle: A test substance should be miscible with or soluble in the vehicle. The best all-purpose vehicle is pertrolatum. The materials to be tested can sometimes be dissolved in water, alcohol, methyl ethyl ketone or acetone; otherwise petrolatum is used.

Concentration: To avoid irritant reactions, an open test with different concentrations should be used first. If the result is negative, a patch test can be performed with a 10–100 times lower concentration. A suitable concentration

Table 22.1. The European standard series

Chemical	Test concentration and vehicle
Metals	
Cobalt chloride	1% pet.
Nickel sulphate	5% pet.
Potassium dichromate	0.5% pet.
Rubber chemicals	
Thiuram mix Dipentamethylenethiuram disulphide (0.25%) Tetramethylthiuram disulphide (0.25%) Tetramethylthiuram disulphide (0.25%) Tetramethylthiuram monosulphide (0.25%)	1% pet.
N-Isopropyl-N'-phenyl-p-phenylenediamine	0.1% pet.
Mercapto mix Cyclohexylbenzothiazyl sulphenamide (0.5%) Dibenzothiazyl disulphide (0.5%) Mercaptobenzothiazole (0.5%) Morpholinyl mercaptobenzothiazole (0.5%)	2% pet.
Mercaptobenzothiazole	2% pet.
Medications	
Benzocaine	5% pet.
Neomycin sulphate	20% pet.
Clioquinol	5% pet.
Cosmetic ingredients	
Balsam of Peru	25% pet.
5-Chloro-2-methyl-4-isothiazolin-3-one+2-methyl-4-isothiazolin-3-one (Me+Cl-isothiazolinone)	0.01% aq.
Colophony (rosin)	20% pet.
Formaldehyde	1% aq.
Fragrance mix α-Amylcinnamaldehyde (1%) Cinnamaldehyde (1%) Cinnamyl alcohol (1%) Eugenol (1%) Geraniol (1%) Hydroxycitronellal (1%) Isoeugenol (1%) Oak moss absolute (1%)	8% pet.
Paraben mix Butyl parahydroxybenzoate (3%) Ethyl parahydroxybenzoate (3%) Methyl Parahydroxybenzoate (3%) Propyl parahydroxybenzoate (3%)	12% pet.

Table 22.1. Continued

Chemical	Test concentration and vehicle
p-Phenylenediamine free base	1% pet.
Quaternium-15	1% aq.
Wool alcohols	30% pet.

Miscellaneous

p-tert-Butylphenol-formaldehyde resin	1% pet.
Epoxy resin	1% pet.
Primin	0.01% pet.
Sesquiterpene lactone mix	0.1% pet.
Alantolactone (0.033%)	
Dehydrocostus lactone (0.033%)	
Costunolide (0.033%)	

Table 22.2. Test concentrations and vehicles

Name of chemical	Test concentration and vehicle
Acrylated monomers	0.1% pet.
Alachlor (Lasso)	0.1% aq. or 1% pet.
Alcohol	as is
Amethocaine	5% pet.
Ametryne	0.05% aq.
Amfenac (Fenazox)	50% aq.
Aminoazobenzene	0.25% pet.
p-Aminobenzoix acid (PABA)	2% pet.
Amitrole	1% aq.
Ammoniated mercury	1% pet.
Ampholyt G®	1% aq.
Amprolium	10% aq.
Amylocaine	5% pet.
Anilazine (Dyrene)	1% pet.
Aniline	1% pet.
Arsanilic acid	10% pet.
Atrazine	0.05% aq.
Azinphos-methyl	0.25% pet.
Azodicarbonamide	0.5% pet.
Bacitracin zinc	20% pet.
Benomyl	0.1% aq. or pet.
Benzalkonium chloride	0.01%–0.1% aq.
Benzophenone-3 (oxybenzone)	2% pet.
Benzophenone-10 (mexenone)	2% pet.
2-Benzothiazyl disulphide (MBTS)	2% pet.

Table 22.2. Continued

Name of chemical	Test concentration and vehicle
1 H-Benzotriazole	1% pet.
Benzyl salicylate	1–5% pet.
Biocheck 60	0.2% aq.
2,2-Bis(4-(2-hydroxy-3-methacryloxypropoxy)phenyl)propane (BIS-GMA)	2% pet.
2,2-Bis(4-(methacryloxy)phenyl)propane (BIS-MA)	2% pet.
Bismuth neodecanoate	1% pet.
Bovine tuberculin	10% aq.
2-Bromo-2-nitropropane-1,3-diol (Bronopol)	0.5% pet.
Bromophos	0.025% pet.
Butonate	5% aq.
Butyl methoxydibenzoylmethane (Parsol 1789)	2% pet.
Butylated hydroxyanisole (BHA)	2% pet.
Captan	0.1% aq.
Carbaryl	0.5% or 1% pet.
Carbyne (barban)	10% o.o.
Cetostearyl alcohol	30% pet.
Chloral hydrate	15% aq.
Chloramine T	0.05% aq.
Chloramphenicol	1% pet.
Chlorhexidine	0.5% aq.
Chloridazon	0.1%–1% aq. or pet.
Chlormequat	0.5% aq.
Chloroacetamide	0.2% pet.
Chloromethylphenoxyacetic acid (MCPA)	5%–10% aq.
Chlorpromazine	0.5–1% pet.
Chlorpropham	0.5% pet.
Chlortetracycline hydrochloride	3% pet.
Cinchocaine	5% pet.
Cinnamon oil	2% pet.
Clove oil	2% pet.
Congo red	2% pet.
Copper 8-quinolinolate	1% pet.
Copper sulphate	0.5% or 1% aq.
Coumarone-indene resin	20% pet.
Cresol	1% pet.
Cyclomethacaine	5% pet.
2,4-D/2,4,5-T mix	0.5% o.o.
Dalapon	50% aq. or pet.
Dazomet	0.1% aq.
D & C Red 31	1% pet.
D & C Yellow 11	0.1% pet.
Demephion-O	0.25% aq.
N-N-Diallyl-2-chloroacetamide	0.01% or 0.1% pet.
4,4'-Diaminodiphenylmethane (DDM)	0.5% pet.
Diazinon	1% pet.
Diazolidinyl urea (Germall II)	2% pet.
Dibromodicyanobutane + phenoxyethanol (Euxyl K400)	1% pet.
Dibutylthiourea	1% pet.

Table 22.2. Continued

Name of chemical	Test concentration and vehicle
Dichlorodiphenyltrichloroethane (DDT techn.)	1% pet. or acet.
Dichlorophene	0.5% or 1% pet.
2,4-Dichlorophenoxyacetic acid (2,4-D techn.)	1% aq.
2,4-Dichlorophenoxybutyric acid (2,4-DB)	1% aq.
Dichlorprop	1% aq.
Dichlorvos (DDVP)	0.05% aq.
Dicyanodiamide	0.1% aq.
Diethylstilbestrol	0.1% alc.
Diethylthiourea	1% pet.
Difolatan (captafol)	0.1% pet.
Dihydrostreptomycin	0.1% pet.
Diisocyanates	0.1%–1% pet. or acet.
Dimethoate	0.5% or 1% aq.
Dimethylaminoethyl ether	1% pet.
Dimethyloldihydroxyethylene urea	5% aq.
Dimethyloldihydroxypropylene urea	10% pet.
N,N-Dimethylol-4-methoxy-5,5-dimethylpropylene urea	10% pet.
Dimethylolmethoxypropylene urea	10% pet.
Dimethylolpropylene urea	5% pet.
Dimethylol urea	10% pet.
N,N-Dimethyl-p-toluidine	5% pet.
2,4-Dinitrochlorobenzene (DNCB)	0.01% acet. or aq.
4,6-Dinitrocresol (DNOC)	50% aq.
Dinobuton	1–10% pet.
Dinocap	1% pet.
Dioctyl phthalate	5% pet.
Diorthotolyl guanidine	1% pet.
N,N'-Diphenyl paraphenylenediamine (DPPD)	1% pet.
Diquat	0.1% pet.
Disperse Black 1	1% pet.
Disperse Blue 3	1% pet.
Disperse Blue 106	1% pet.
Disperse Blue 124	1% pet.
Disperse Orange 3	1% pet.
Disperse Red 1	1% pet.
Disperse Yellow 3	1% pet.
Ditalimphos	0.01% pet.
Dithianone	1% pet.
4,4'-Dithiodimorpholine	1% pet.
N-Dodecyl mercaptan	0.1% pet.
Dowicides	1% pet.
DPPDA	1% pet.
Dyrene (anilazine)	0.1% pet.
Epoxy hardeners	0.1%–1% pet., alc. or acet.
Epoxy reactive diluents	0.1%–1% pet., alc. or acet.
Erythromycin base	1% pet.

Table 22.2. Continued

Name of chemical	Test concentration and vehicle
2-Ethoxyethyl-*p*-methoxycinnamate (cinoxate)	2% pet.
Ethoxyquin	1% pet.
Ethylbutyl thiourea	1% pet.
Ethylenediamine	1% pet.
Ethyleneglycol dimethacrylate (EGDMA)	2% pet.
Ethylene thiourea	1% pet.
Ethylene urea	10% pet.
Etophon	1% aq.
Eucalyptus oil	1% pet.
Eucerit	30% pet.
Eugenol	1% pet.
Fenazox (amfenac)	50% aq.
Fenticlor	1% pet.
Fentinhydroxide (triphenyltin hydroxide)	0.5% pet.
Folpet	0.05% or 0.1% pet.
Glutaraldehyde	1% aq.
Glyphosate	10% aq.
HCH techn. (hexachlorocyclohexane)	1% pet. or acet.
Hexachlorophene (G-11)	1% pet.
Hexahydrophthalic anhydride	1% or. 0.1% pet.
Hydrogenated lanolin	as is
Hydroxycitronellal	1%–5% pet.
2-Hydroxy-4-methoxybenzophenone	2% pet.
Imidazolidinyl urea (Germall 115)	2% pet.
4-Isopropyl dibenzoylmethane (Eusolex 8020)	2% pet.
Jasmine absolute	5%–10% pet.
Lidocaine (Xylocaine)	5% pet.
Lindane	1% pet. or acet.
Malathion	0.5% pet.
Mancozeb	1% pet.
Maneb	0.5% or 1% pet.
Medroxyprogesterone acetate	1% pet.
Melamine-formaldehyde resin	7% pet.
Menthol	1% pet.
Mercaptobenzothiazole (MBT)	2% pet.
Mercury compounds	0.05% aq. or pet.
Metaldehyde	1% pet.
Metam sodium	0.03% aq.
Methacrylated monomers	2% pet.
Methidathion	0.5% or 1% pet.
3-(4-Methylbenzylidene)-camphor (Eusolex 6300)	2% pet.
Methyl dichlorobenzene sulphonate	0.1% alc.
Methyl methacrylate	2% pet.
Methyl orange	2% pet.
Methyltetrahydrophthalic anhydride	1% or 0.1% pet.
3-Methyl thiazolidine 2-thion (Vulkacit CRV)	1% pet.
Molinate	1% pet.
Monomethylol-urea	10% pet.
Musk ambrette	5% pet.

Table 22.2. Continued

Name of chemical	Test concentration and vehicle
Naled	0.5% aq.
1-Naphthalenylthiourea (ANTU)	1% or 2% pet.
Naphthol AS	5% aq.; 0.2%–2% acet.
Nitrofen	0.5% pet. or o.o.
Nitrofurazone	1% pet.
Octyl dimethyl PABA (Escalol 507)	2% pet.
N-Octyl-4-isothiazolin-3-one (Kathon LP)	0.1% pet.
Octyl methoxycinnamate (Parsol MCX)	2% pet.
Oxydemeton methyl	0.25% pet.
Oxytetracycline	10% pet.
Paraquat	0.1% pet.
Parathion ethyl	1% pet. or aq.
Parathion methyl	1% pet.
Panethamate	1% pet.
Penicillin	10000 IU/g pet.[a]
Pentachloronitrobenzene	0.5% pet.
Pentachlorophenol (PCP)	1% aq.
Phaltan (Folpet)	0.05% or 0.1% pet.
Phenmedipham	0.2% or 0.5% aq.
Phenothiazines	2% pet.
Phenyl-azo-2-naphthol (PAN)	0.1% pet.
Phenylhydrazine	1% pet.
Phenylmercuric acetate	0.05% pet.
o-Phenylphenol	1% pet.
Phorate	1% pet.
Picric acid	1% pet.
Piperazine	1% pet.
Pirimiphos methyl	0.5% pet.
Plondrel	0.01% pet.
Potassium dicvanoaurate	0.001% aq.
PPP-HB	5% alc.
Procaine	1% pet. or 2% aq.
Propachlor (Ramrod)	0.05% or 0.1% aq.
Propanil	1% pet.
Propylene glycol	20% pet.
Propyl gallate	1% pet.
Proxymetacaine	5% aq.
Pyrethrum	2% pet.
Quindoxin	0.1% pet.
Quintozene	10% aq.
Randox	0.01% or 1% pet.
Rodannitrobenzene	1% pet.
Scarlet red (Sudan IV)	2% pet.
Simazine	5% aq.
Sodium hypochlorite	0.5% aq.
Sodium hyposulphite	1% aq.
Sodium thiosulphatoaurate	0.5% pet.
Sodium trichloroacetate (TCA)	1% aq.

[a] See warning Sect. 14.7.3.1

Table 22.2. Continued

Name of chemical	Test concentration and vehicle
Solvent Red 23 (Sudan III)	2% pet.
Spiramycin sulphate (Rovamycin)	10% pet.
Streptomycin	1% pet.
Sulphacetamide	1% pet.
Sulfiram (Tetmosol)	1% pet.
Synthetic sandalwood	10% pet.
Tego 103 G	0.1% aq.
Terpene phenolic resin	20% pet.
Tetmosol (Sulfiram)	1% pet.
Tetrachloroisophthalonitrile	0.01% or 0.001% acet.
Tetramethyl butanediamine	1% pet.
Tetramethylolacetylene urea	5% aq.
Thiabendazole	1% pet.
Thiram	1% pet.
Thymol	2% pet.
Tinopal (CH 3566)	1% pet.
Toluenesulphonamide-formaldehyde resin	10% pet.
Toluenesulphonhydrazide	0.5% alc.
p-Tolydiethanolamine	2% alc.
Tribromosalan	1% pet.
Tributyltin oxide	0.001% aq.
Trichlorfon	1% aq.
Trichlorodinitrobenzene	0.01% aq.
2,4,5-Trichlorophenoxyacetic acid (2,4,5-T)	0.5% o.o.
Triclosan (Irgasan DP-300)	2% pet.
Triethyleneglycol dimethacrylate (TREGDMA)	2% pet.
2,2,4-Trimethyl-1,2-dihydroquinoline	1% pet.
Triphenyltin hydroxide	0.5% pet.
Tuberculin	10% aq.
Tylosin tartrate	5% pet.
Urea-formaldehyde resin	10% pet.
Warfarin	0.05% pet.
Ylang-ylang oil	5% pet.
Zineb	1% pet.
Ziram	1% pet.

acet., Acetone; alc., alcohol; aq., water; comm. prep., commercial preparation; o.o., olive oil; pet., petrolatum; conc., concentration; techn., technical.

for patch testing most substances is 0.1%–1%. A positive allergic test reaction with a new substance must be validated by negative controls (minimum of six subjects). In still unclear cases a repeated open application test according to the method of Hannuksela and Salo [7] should be performed.

Table 22.2 lists alphabetically all chemicals mentioned in this book with their test concentrations and vehicles (sometimes two concentrations are suggested when insufficient data is available) as suggested by the various

Table 22.3. List of abbreviations

ANTU	1-Naphthalenylthiourea
BHA	Butylated hydroxyanisole
BIS-GMA	2,2-Bis(4-(2-hydroxy-3-methacryloxypropoxy)phenyl)propane
BIS-MA	2,2-Bis(4-(methacryloxy)phenyl)propane
2,4-D	2,4-Dichlorophenoxyacetic acid
2,4-DB	2,4-Dichlotophenoxybutyric acid
DDM	4,4'-Diaminodiphenylmethane
DDT	Dichlorodiphenyltrichloroethane
DDVP	Dichlorvos
DNCB	Dinitrochlorobenzene
DNOC	Dinitrocresol
DPPD	N,N'-Diphenyl paraphenylenediamine
EGDMA	Ethyleneglycol dimethacrylate
HCH	Hexachlorocyclohexane
MBT	Mercaptobenzothiazole
MBTS	2-Benzothiazyl disulphide
MCPA	Chloromethylphenoxyacetic acid
PABA	*p*-Aminobenzoic acid
PCP	Pentachlorophenol
PPP	Phenylpropylpyridine
2,4,5-T	2,4,5-Trichlorophenoxyacetic acid
TCA	Sodium trichloroacetate
TREGDMA	Triethyleneglycol dimethacrylate
TSCA	Tribromosalan

authors. Table 22.3 provides an alphabetical listing of commonly used abbrevations and their full chemical synonyms.

22.1 References

1. Rycroft RJG (1990) Is patch testing necessary? In: Champion RH, Pye RJ (eds) Recent advances in dermatology, vol 8. Churchill Livingstone, Edinburgh, pp 101–111
2. De Groot AC (1986) Patch testing. Test concentrations and vehicles for 2800 allergens. Elsevier, Amsterdam
3. Fisher AA (1986) Contact dermatitis, 3rd edn. Lea and Febiger, Philadelphia
4. Adams RM (1990) Occupational skin disease, 2nd edn. Saunders, Philadelphia
5. Foussereau J (1987) Les eczémas allergiques. Masson, Paris
6. Fregert S (1981) Manual of contact dermatitis, 2nd edn. Munksgaard, Copenhagen
7. Hannuksela M, Salo H (1986) The repeated open application test (ROAT). Contact Dermatitis 14: 221–227

Subject Index